Nutraceuticals in Immune Function

Nutraceuticals in Immune Function

Editors

Sok Cheon Pak
Soo Liang Ooi

MDPI • Basel • Beijing • Wuhan • Barcelona • Belgrade • Manchester • Tokyo • Cluj • Tianjin

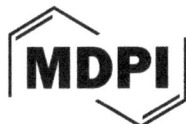

Editors
Sok Cheon Pak
School of Dentistry and
Medical Sciences
Charles Sturt University
Bathurst
Australia

Soo Liang Ooi
School of Dentistry and
Medical Sciences
Charles Sturt University
Bathurst
Australia

Editorial Office
MDPI
St. Alban-Anlage 66
4052 Basel, Switzerland

This is a reprint of articles from the Special Issue published online in the open access journal *Molecules* (ISSN 1420-3049) (available at: www.mdpi.com/journal/molecules/special_issues/Nutraceuticals_Immune_Function).

For citation purposes, cite each article independently as indicated on the article page online and as indicated below:

LastName, A.A.; LastName, B.B.; LastName, C.C. Article Title. *Journal Name* **Year**, *Volume Number*, Page Range.

ISBN 978-3-0365-2060-5 (Hbk)
ISBN 978-3-0365-2059-9 (PDF)

© 2021 by the authors. Articles in this book are Open Access and distributed under the Creative Commons Attribution (CC BY) license, which allows users to download, copy and build upon published articles, as long as the author and publisher are properly credited, which ensures maximum dissemination and a wider impact of our publications.

The book as a whole is distributed by MDPI under the terms and conditions of the Creative Commons license CC BY-NC-ND.

Contents

About the Editors vii

Preface to "Nutraceuticals in Immune Function" ix

Soo-Liang Ooi and Sok-Cheon Pak
Nutraceuticals in Immune Function
Reprinted from: *Molecules* **2021**, *26*, 5310, doi:10.3390/molecules26175310 1

Elena Genova, Maura Apollonio, Giuliana Decorti, Alessandra Tesser, Alberto Tommasini and Gabriele Stocco
In Vitro Effects of Sulforaphane on Interferon-Driven Inflammation and Exploratory Evaluation in Two Healthy Volunteers
Reprinted from: *Molecules* **2021**, *26*, 3602, doi:10.3390/molecules26123602 7

Jiyeon Choi, Joo Weon Lim and Hyeyoung Kim
Lycopene Inhibits Toll-Like Receptor 4-Mediated Expression of Inflammatory Cytokines in House Dust Mite-Stimulated Respiratory Epithelial Cells
Reprinted from: *Molecules* **2021**, *26*, 3127, doi:10.3390/molecules26113127 23

Seung-Heon Shin, Mi-Kyung Ye, Dong-Won Lee, Byung-Jun Kang and Mi-Hyun Chae
Effect of Korean Red Ginseng and Rg3 on Asian Sand Dust-Induced MUC5AC, MUC5B, and MUC8 Expression in Bronchial Epithelial Cells
Reprinted from: *Molecules* **2021**, *26*, 2002, doi:10.3390/molecules26072002 39

Suji Bae, Joo Weon Lim and Hyeyoung Kim
-Carotene Inhibits Expression of Matrix Metalloproteinase-10 and Invasion in *Helicobacter pylori*-Infected Gastric Epithelial Cells
Reprinted from: *Molecules* **2021**, *26*, 1567, doi:10.3390/molecules26061567 51

Keryn G. Woodman, Chantal A. Coles, Shireen R. Lamandé and Jason D. White
Resveratrol Promotes Hypertrophy in Wildtype Skeletal Muscle and Reduces Muscle Necrosis and Gene Expression of Inflammatory Markers in *Mdx* Mice
Reprinted from: *Molecules* **2021**, *26*, 853, doi:10.3390/molecules26040853 67

Layla Panahipour, Selma Husejnovic, Jila Nasirzade, Stephan Semelmayer and Reinhard Gruber
Micellar Casein and Whey Powder Hold a TGF- Activity and Regulate ID Genes In Vitro
Reprinted from: *Molecules* **2021**, *26*, 507, doi:10.3390/molecules26020507 81

Adil Ehmedah, Predrag Nedeljkovic, Sanja Dacic, Jelena Repac, Biljana Draskovic-Pavlovic, Dragana Vučević, Sanja Pekovic and Biljana Bozic Nedeljkovic
Effect of Vitamin B Complex Treatment on Macrophages to Schwann Cells Association during Neuroinflammation after Peripheral Nerve Injury
Reprinted from: *Molecules* **2020**, *25*, 5426, doi:10.3390/molecules25225426 93

Lien-Yu Chou, Yu-Ming Chao, Yen-Chun Peng, Hui-Ching Lin and Yuh-Lin Wu
Glucosamine Enhancement of BDNF Expression and Animal Cognitive Function
Reprinted from: *Molecules* **2020**, *25*, 3667, doi:10.3390/molecules25163667 115

Ayse Günes-Bayir, Abdurrahim Kocyigit, Eray Metin Guler and Agnes Dadak
In Vitro Hormetic Effect Investigation of Thymol on Human Fibroblast and Gastric Adenocarcinoma Cells
Reprinted from: *Molecules* **2020**, *25*, 3270, doi:10.3390/molecules25143270 . . . . **127**

Laura López-Gómez, Agata Szymaszkiewicz, Marta Zielińska and Raquel Abalo
Nutraceuticals and Enteric Glial Cells
Reprinted from: *Molecules* **2021**, *26*, 3762, doi:10.3390/molecules26123762 . . . . **139**

Mudhi AlAli, Maream Alqubaisy, Mariam Nasser Aljaafari, Asma Obaid AlAli, Laila Baqais, Aidin Molouki, Aisha Abushelaibi, Kok-Song Lai and Swee-Hua Erin Lim
Nutraceuticals: Transformation of Conventional Foods into Health Promoters/Disease Preventers and Safety Considerations
Reprinted from: *Molecules* **2021**, *26*, 2540, doi:10.3390/molecules26092540 . . . . **161**

Soo Liang Ooi, Sok Cheon Pak, Peter S. Micalos, Emily Schupfer, Catherine Lockley, Mi Houn Park and Sung-Joo Hwang
The Health-Promoting Properties and Clinical Applications of Rice Bran Arabinoxylan Modified with Shiitake Mushroom Enzyme—A Narrative Review
Reprinted from: *Molecules* **2021**, *26*, 2539, doi:10.3390/molecules26092539 . . . . **189**

Tiantian Meng, Dingfu Xiao, Arowolo Muhammed, Juying Deng, Liang Chen and Jianhua He
Anti-Inflammatory Action and Mechanisms of Resveratrol
Reprinted from: *Molecules* **2021**, *26*, 229, doi:10.3390/molecules26010229 . . . . **207**

Sahar Eshghjoo, Arul Jayaraman, Yuxiang Sun and Robert C. Alaniz
Microbiota-Mediated Immune Regulation in Atherosclerosis
Reprinted from: *Molecules* **2021**, *26*, 179, doi:10.3390/molecules26010179 . . . . **223**

Minkyung Bae and Hyeyoung Kim
The Role of Vitamin C, Vitamin D, and Selenium in Immune System against COVID-19
Reprinted from: *Molecules* **2020**, *25*, 5346, doi:10.3390/molecules25225346 . . . . **235**

Ming Xian Chang and Fan Xiong
Astaxanthin and its Effects in Inflammatory Responses and Inflammation-Associated Diseases: Recent Advances and Future Directions
Reprinted from: *Molecules* **2020**, *25*, 5342, doi:10.3390/molecules25225342 . . . . **247**

José Antonio Uranga, Vicente Martínez and Raquel Abalo
Mast Cell Regulation and Irritable Bowel Syndrome: Effects of Food Components with Potential Nutraceutical Use
Reprinted from: *Molecules* **2020**, *25*, 4314, doi:10.3390/molecules25184314 . . . . **261**

Edward J. Calabrese
Hormesis and Ginseng: Ginseng Mixtures and Individual Constituents Commonly Display Hormesis Dose Responses, Especially for Neuroprotective Effects
Reprinted from: *Molecules* **2020**, *25*, 2719, doi:10.3390/molecules25112719 . . . . **291**

Sahu Henamayee, Kishore Banik, Bethsebie Lalduhsaki Sailo, Bano Shabnam, Choudhary Harsha, Satti Srilakshmi, Naidu VGM, Seung Ho Baek, Kwang Seok Ahn and Ajaikumar B Kunnumakkara
Therapeutic Emergence of Rhein as a Potential Anticancer Drug: A Review of Its Molecular Targets and Anticancer Properties
Reprinted from: *Molecules* **2020**, *25*, 2278, doi:10.3390/molecules25102278 . . . . **341**

About the Editors

Sok Cheon Pak

Sok Cheon Pak has been teaching and researching at Charles Sturt University since 2007. His field of research is in complementary medicine and has become recognized internationally and nationally through ongoing external research collaborations in Korea, Hong Kong, and the USA. His area of expertise relates specifically to introducing evidence-based practice to complementary medicine research and practice. This has been based on laboratory experiments that incorporate modern medical technologies to identify the rationale for prescribing therapeutic substances for treatment. Over the years, his principal focus has been on the experimental/clinical application of bee venom to human diseases. He was also the Guest Editor of a Special Issue on "Bee and wasp venoms: biological characteristics and therapeutic application"for the journal *Toxins* (ISSN 2072-6651).

Soo Liang Ooi

Soo Liang Ooi is a practising nutritionist and naturopath. He holds a Bachelor of Health Science degree from Charles Sturt University, a Master of Business Administration degree from the National University of Singapore, and a Master of Mathematics degree from the University of Waterloo in Canada. He is currently pursuing his Doctor of Philosophy (PhD) at Charles Sturt University. His PhD research focuses on understanding the immunomodulating properties of rice bran arabinoxylan compound and its effects on the quality of life of cancer patients. His research interests lie in evidence-based complementary medicine, nutritional medicine, naturopathy, and herbal medicine. As an avid academic writer, Soo Liang published extensively in major peer-reviewed integrative and complementary medicine journals. He is also a co-editor of the Special Issue book on *Health Benefits of Meditation* for the journal *OBM Integrative & Complementary Medicine* (ISSN 2573-4393).

Preface to "Nutraceuticals in Immune Function"

Most diseases are preventable and are related to what we eat. Moreover, most doctor visits are for lifestyle-based diseases, which can be prevented by adopting a healthy lifestyle. Treating the causes of illness rather than symptoms of the disease is not only safer and cheaper, but it can work better. In this context, the Special Issue on "Nutraceuticals in Immune System" for the journal *Molecules* was launched in January 2020. Soon after that, the world was ravaged by the COVID-19 pandemic, causing a grave health threat. Paradoxically, the immune system can be both friend and foe of COVID-19. COVID-19 manifests only mild to moderate symptoms for most infected people who recover without hospitalization, demonstrating the proper functioning of the immune system in fighting such an infection. For some, however, the overactivation of the immune response, causing a "cytokine storm" has dire consequences, with severe respiratory distress leading to multiple organ failure, which can be fatal. In fact, most deaths from COVID-19 have come from organ inflammation due to undesirable immune system responses. As such, COVID-19 is a good case in point, demonstrating the importance of a healthy immune system.

Nutraceuticals are products derived from food sources with health benefits in addition to the basic nutritional values. Many of them can positively affect and enhance the immune system, which is particularly pertinent in the current turbulent times of COVID-19. Not surprisingly, nutraceutical sales rose dramatically during the pandemic period. However, much research is still needed to understand how natural products interact with the immune system to clarify their chemical compositions, mechanisms of action, and effects on health and illnesses.

This Special Issue provided an open forum for researchers to share their research findings in the growing interest of nutraceuticals. We received an overwhelming response with a total of 33 submissions, of which only nine original research papers and ten reviews were accepted after rigorous peer review. The articles included report research on natural substances of interest in nutraceuticals ranging from herbal medicine to vitamins to microbiota-derived metabolites. The investigated immune-related responses include cancer, neurological diseases, gastroenterological disorders, inflammatory conditions, and infections.

We thank the publisher for this excellent opportunity to serve the research community. As academic editors for this Special Issue, it has been our pleasure to review these insightful manuscripts first-hand. We thank all the authors for their contributions. The collected works represent our current understanding and latest findings on nutraceuticals in the immune system, which we hope will continue to inspire knowledge quests into the field of nutraceuticals.

Sok Cheon Pak, Soo Liang Ooi
Editors

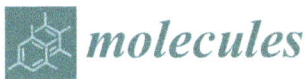

Editorial

Nutraceuticals in Immune Function

Soo-Liang Ooi and Sok-Cheon Pak *

School of Dentistry and Medical Sciences, Charles Sturt University, Bathurst, NSW 2795, Australia; sooi@csu.edu.au
* Correspondence: spak@csu.edu.au; Tel.: +61-2-6338-4952; Fax: +61-2-6338-4993

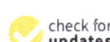

Citation: Ooi, S.-L.; Pak, S.-C. Nutraceuticals in Immune Function. *Molecules* 2021, 26, 5310. https://dx.doi.org/10.3390/molecules26175310

Received: 3 August 2021
Accepted: 24 August 2021
Published: 1 September 2021

Publisher's Note: MDPI stays neutral with regard to jurisdictional claims in published maps and institutional affiliations.

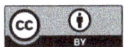

Copyright: © 2020 by the authors. Licensee MDPI, Basel, Switzerland. This article is an open access article distributed under the terms and conditions of the Creative Commons Attribution (CC BY) license (https://creativecommons.org/licenses/by/4.0/).

Nutraceutical, a term derived from 'nutrition' and 'pharmaceutical', refers to any product isolated from herbs, nutrients, specific diets, processed foods, and beverages used not only for nutritional but also for medicinal purposes. Nutraceuticals comprise many bioactive derivatives from edible sources such as anti-oxidants, phytochemicals, fatty acids, amino acids, prebiotics and probiotics. Many of them possess therapeutic properties that can affect the immune system. In this Special Issue, AlAli et al. [1] offer a comprehensive review of nutraceuticals categorized based on their source, nature and application. The authors broadly classified the mode of actions of nutraceuticals into anti-cancer, anti-inflammatory, anti-oxidant, and anti-lipid activities. Nutraceuticals can augment the immune system to prevent cancer, neurological conditions, gastroenterological disorders, inflammatory diseases, and infections.

Cancer: Henamayee et al. [2] reviewed the anti-cancer properties of rhein, a naturally derived anthraquinone found in the rhubarb (*Rheum rhabarbarum*) leaves and many *Aloe* species. Current research supports rhein to be a multitargeted cytotoxicity compound. It affects several pathways such as mitogen-activated protein kinase (MAPK), Wnt, nuclear factor-kappa B (NF-κB) and hypoxia inducible factor-1 signaling to stimulate apoptosis and inhibit cell proliferation and angiogenesis. The chemopreventive activity of rhein was demonstrated in vivo or in vitro with various cancer types, including breast, cervical, colon, glioma, leukemia, liver, lung, nasopharyngeal, ovarian, pancreatic, and oral.

Anti-cancer cytotoxicity can directly or indirectly restore the suppressed immune response within the tumor microenvironment. Ooi et al. [3] reviewed the health-promoting properties and clinical applications of rice bran arabinoxylan compound (RBAC), a hydrolyzed extract of defatted rice bran modified with the shiitake mushroom enzyme. RBAC is also an anti-cancer neutraceutical that can upregulate the cytotoxic activity of natural killer cells, enhance phagocytic cellular functions, and induce the maturation and activation of dendritic cells. Moreover, the immunomodulatory, anti-inflammatory, anti-oxidant, and anti-angiogenic properties of RBAC are also promising for a wide range of applications beyond cancer.

Thymol is a phenolic compound found in the essential oil of thyme (*Thymus spp.*). Günes-Bayir et al. [4] studied the cytotoxic, genotoxic, and anti-oxidative effects of thymol on healthy cells and gastric adenocarcinoma cells. The study demonstrated that thymol at low concentrations provides anti-oxidative protection to healthy cells in vitro while inducing toxic effects in adenocarcinoma cells. The dose-dependent hormetic impact of thymol of different cell lines makes thymol a potential anti-cancer agent.

In another in vitro experiment, Panahipour et al. [5] showed that micellar casein and whey powder maintain the transforming growth factor-β (TGF-β) activity and its capacity to regulate the inhibitor of deoxyribonucleic acid binding (ID) 1 and ID3 genes in oral fibroblasts and oral squamous carcinoma cells, respectively. While the TGF-β activity and over-expression of the ID3 gene are known to link to oral cancer, the potential application of casein and whey powder in its prevention needs further research.

Neurological conditions: Ginseng (*Panax spp.*) is a widely used immune modulator in the traditional medicine of East Asia. Ginseng is also known to protect against neurodegeneration and neuroinflammation. Calabrese [6] reviewed the available literature on the hormetic dose-response effects of ginseng and its constituents (ginsenosides Rg1, Rb1, Rc, Rd, Re, ginseng saponins, gintonin, polyacetylenes). The author found evidence supporting the generality of such effects, especially in the neuroprotective studies of Parkinson's disease, Alzheimer's disease, stroke, and neonatal brain hypoxia. Hormesis is characterized by low-dose stimulation and high-dose inhibition. Hence, due to its popularity, overconsumption of ginseng in the population can be a public health concern.

Chou et al. [7] studied the effects of glucosamine in brain cognitive performance with an in vivo model. Glucosamine is an amino sugar and a prominent precursor in the biochemical synthesis of glycosylated proteins and lipids. The study found evidence of glucosamine exerting a cognition-enhancing function in the experimental mice through upregulating the brain-derived neurotrophic factor (BDNF) levels via the dependency pathway of cyclic adenosine $3',5'$-monophosphate (cAMP), protein kinase A, and cAMP response element-binding protein. As abnormal BDNF levels might be due to the chronic inflammatory state of the brain, glucosamine may also have applications in neuroinflammatory disorders such as Alzheimer's disease, Parkinson's disease, fibromyalgia, multiple sclerosis and chronic pain.

Peripheral nerve injuries (PNI) can also induce neuroinflammation. Vitamin B complex was explored as a potential treatment by Ehmedah et al. [8] with a femoral nerve injury rat model. Treatment with B vitamins appeared to enhance the M1-to M2-macrophage polarization and accelerate the transition from the non-myelin to myelin-forming Schwann cells. Hence, B vitamins could potentially promote nerve repair through PNI-triggered processes of neuroinflammation and neurodegeneration.

Gastroenterological disorders: Uranga et al. [9] reviewed the effects of mast cells on irritable bowel syndrome (IBS), a disorder of the gut–brain axis. There is a close interaction between the immune system and the nervous system with mast cells playing a key mediation role. A variety of food components were found to affect the modulation of mast cell activity in a specific manner. These nutrient-derived bioactive compounds include fatty acids, lipid molecules, fat-soluble vitamins (D3 and E), amino acids (arginine, glutamine and glycine), carotenoids, polyphenolic compounds, and spices. They can reduce mast cell degranulation that is responsible for the de novo synthesis of mediators of the neuro-immune-endocrine alterations present in IBS.

López-Gómez et al. [10] reviewed the effects of nutraceuticals as modulators of enteric glial cells (EGC). Various compounds, particularly those with anti-oxidant activity, including L-glutamine, L-glutathione, quercetin, resveratrol, and palmitoylethanolamide, were found to exert local or systemic neuroprotective effects on the enteric nervous system. Hence, nutraceuticals targeting the EGCs can potentially prevent or reduce gastroenterological disorders.

Inflammatory diseases: Resveratrol is a natural phytoalexin polyphenol predominantly found in berries and grapes. Meng et al. [11] reviewed its anti-inflammatory actions and mechanisms. Resveratrol appeared to regulate inflammatory response through various signaling pathways, including the arachidonic acid, NF-κB, MAPK, activator protein (AP)-1 transcription factor, and anti-oxidant defense pathways. Hence, there exist multiple lines of compelling evidence that resveratrol can play a promising role in managing autoimmune and inflammatory chronic diseases. One such condition is Duchenne muscular dystrophy (DMD), a progressive and fatal neuromuscular disorder with no cure. Woodman et al. [12] treated mdx mice with a low dose of resveratrol (5 mg/kg body weight/day) for 15 weeks. The study found resveratrol to reduce exercise-induced muscle necrosis in dystrophic muscle and lower gene expression of immune cell markers cluster of differentiation (CD) 86 and CD163. Nevertheless, signaling targets associated with resveratrol's mechanism of action, including Sirtuin 1 and NF-κB, were unchanged. This study confirmed that resveratrol could be a therapeutic candidate for DMD treatment.

Astaxanthin is another nutraceutical compound with potent anti-inflammatory properties. It is a lipid-soluble, red-orange carotenoid accumulated in many marine creatures, such as lobsters, shrimp, trout, and salmon. Chang and Xiong [13] reviewed the anti-inflammatory mechanisms of astaxanthin. Astaxanthin was found to attenuate many inflammatory biomarkers through multiple signaling pathways, including phosphatidylinositol-3-kinase/protein kinase B (Akt), nuclear factor erythroid 2-like 2, NF-κB, extracellular-signal-regulated kinase, c-Jun N-terminal kinases, p38 MAPK, and the Janus kinase 2/signal transducer and activator of transcription 3. Moreover, astaxanthin was confirmed experimentally to alleviate chronic and acute inflammation in various diseases, such as neurodegenerative disorders, diabetes, gastrointestinal disease, renal inflammation, as well as skin and eye diseases.

Atherosclerosis is characterized by low-grade, chronic inflammation of the arterial wall. The review by Eshghjoo et al. [14] showed that many microbiota-derived metabolites were associated with atherosclerosis. For example, trimethylamine-N-oxide, a by-product of gut microbial metabolism of L-carnitine and choline after ingestion of eggs, meat, or fish, can elevate oxidized low-density lipoprotein and increased plaque formation. Accumulation of indoxyl sulphate, a metabolite converted from dietary tryptophan, can cause coronary calcification leading to atherosclerosis. Whereas indole, another gut microbiota-derived tryptophan catabolite, is an agonist for the aryl hydrocarbon receptor with anti-inflammatory effects that can prevent atherosclerosis. Hence, indole can be a promising nutraceutical for cardiovascular disease prevention.

Two studies investigated the role of different nutraceuticals in suppressing airway inflammation. In the first study, Shin et al. [15] studied how Korean red ginseng (KRG) could prevent airway inflammation triggered by Asian sand dust (ASD). KRG and its active compound ginsenoside Rg3 significantly suppressed ASD-induced NF-κB expression and activity. Furthermore, KRG and Rg3 inhibited ASD-induced mucin gene expression and protein production from bronchial epithelial cells in vitro. In another study, Choi et al. [16] demonstrated that the anti-oxidant lycopene could inhibit cytokine expression induced by house dust mites. Lycopene, a naturally occurring chemical that gives fruits and vegetables a red color, possibly suppressed the activation of toll-like receptor 4 and reduced the intracellular and mitochondrial oxidative stress in respiratory epithelial cells. Interferonopathies are monogenic autoinflammatory diseases characterized by disturbance of interferon-mediated immune responses. Genova et al. [17] showed that sulforaphane, a bioactive molecule in cruciferous vegetables, could modulate the stimulator of interferon genes (STING) mediated inflammation and interferon-stimulated genes expression in vitro. However, the study could only reproduce a trend towards the downregulation of STING in vivo. Further in vivo research is needed to confirm the findings.

Infectious pathogens: *Helicobacter pylori* infection can lead to gastric inflammation, ulcers, and gastric cancer progression. Bae et al. [18] confirmed β-carotene as a potential treatment to prevent *H. pylori*-induced inflammation. β-carotene is the red-orange pigment abundant in fungi, plants, and fruits. It was shown in vitro to inhibit the *H. pylori*-induced activation of MAPKs and AP-1, expression of matrix metalloproteinase-10, and cell invasion. Moreover, β-carotene promoted the expression of peroxisome proliferator-activated receptor-gamma and catalase, which reduced oxidative stress in *H. pylori*-infected cells.

Coronavirus disease 2019 (COVID-19) is currently affecting the world ferociously with multiple waves of infections and variants. Bae and Kim [19] reviewed the literature on the potentially beneficial roles of vitamin C, D, and selenium for COVID-19. Vitamin D improves the physical barrier against viruses and stimulates the production of antimicrobial peptides. Selenium enhances the function of cytotoxic effector cells, whereas vitamin C is considered an anti-viral and anti-inflammatory agent as it increases immunity. For these reasons, supplementing vitamin C, D, and selenium for COVID-19 patients may help to boost the immune system, prevent virus spread, and reduce the disease progression.

In conclusion, how natural foods and nutritional products can improve health and immunity beyond their nutritional values is a phenomenon of interest in current research. This Special Issue brings together 19 scholarly articles exploring various neutraceuticals in immune function, through reviews or experiments against cancer, neurological conditions, gastroenterological disorders, inflammatory diseases, and infections. The findings are promising. While most nutraceuticals are generally safe for consumption, many also demonstrated hormetic dose-response effects. Hence, more studies on the safety and toxicities of nutraceuticals are needed to advise on their effective utilization.

Conflicts of Interest: The authors declare no conflict of interest.

Abbreviations

The following abbreviations are used in this manuscript:

AP	activator protein
ASD	Asian sand dust
cAMP	cyclic adenosine 3′,5′-monophosphate
CD	cluster of differentiation
COVID-19	Coronavirus disease 2019
DMD	Duchenne muscular dystrophy
EGC	enteric glial cells
IBS	irritable bowel syndrome
ID	inhibitor of deoxyribonucleic acid binding
KRG	Korean red ginseng
MAPK	mitogen-activated protein kinase
NF-κB	nuclear factor-kappa B
PNI	peripheral nerve injuries
RBAC	rice bran arabinoxylan compound
STING	stimulator of interferon genes
TGF-β	transforming growth factor beta

References

1. AlAli, M.; Alqubaisy, M.; Aljaafari, M.N.; Alali, A.O.; Baqais, L.; Molouki, A.; Abushelaibi, A.; Lai, K.S.; Lim, S.H.E. Nutraceuticals: Transformation of conventional foods into health promoters/disease preventers and safety considerations. *Molecules* **2021**, *26*, 2540. [CrossRef] [PubMed]
2. Henamayee, S.; Banik, K.; Sailo, B.L.; Shabnam, B.; Harsha, C.; Srilakshmi, S.; Naidu, V.G.; Baek, S.H.; Ahn, K.S.; Kunnumakkara, A.B. Therapeutic emergence of rhein as a potential anticancer drug: A review of its molecular targets and anticancer properties. *Molecules* **2020**, *25*, 2278. [CrossRef] [PubMed]
3. Ooi, S.L.; Pak, S.C.; Micalos, P.S.; Schupfer, E.; Lockley, C.; Park, M.H.; Hwang, S.J. The health-promoting properties and clinical applications of rice bran arabinoxylan modified with shiitake mushroom enzyme—A narrative review. *Molecules* **2021**, *26*, 2539. [CrossRef] [PubMed]
4. Güneş-Bayir, A.; Kocyigit, A.; Guler, E.M.; Dadak, A. In vitro hormetic effect investigation of thymol on human fibroblast and gastric adenocarcinoma cells. *Molecules* **2020**, *25*, 3270. [CrossRef] [PubMed]
5. Panahipour, L.; Husejnovic, S.; Nasirzade, J.; Semelmayer, S.; Gruber, R. Micellar casein and whey powder hold a TGF-β activity and regulate ID genes in vitro. *Molecules* **2021**, *26*, 507. [CrossRef] [PubMed]
6. Calabrese, E.J. Hormesis and ginseng: Ginseng mixtures and individual constituents commonly display hormesis dose responses, especially for neuroprotective effects. *Molecules* **2020**, *25*, 2719. [CrossRef] [PubMed]
7. Chou, L.Y.; Chao, Y.M.; Peng, Y.C.; Lin, H.C.; Wu, Y.L. Glucosamine enhancement of BDNF expression and animal cognitive function. *Molecules* **2020**, *25*, 3667. [CrossRef] [PubMed]
8. Ehmedah, A.; Nedeljkovic, P.; Dacic, S.; Repac, J.; Draskovic-Pavlovic, B.; Vučević, D.; Pekovic, S.; Nedeljkovic, B.B. Effect of vitamin B complex treatment on macrophages to schwann cells association during neuroinflammation after peripheral nerve injury. *Molecules* **2020**, *25*, 5426. [CrossRef] [PubMed]
9. Uranga, J.A.; Martínez, V.; Abalo, R. Mast cell regulation and irritable bowel syndrome: Effects of food components with potential nutraceutical use. *Molecules* **2020**, *25*, 4314. [CrossRef] [PubMed]
10. López-Gómez, L.; Szymaszkiewicz, A.; Zielińska, M.; Abalo, R. Nutraceuticals and enteric glial cells. *Molecules* **2021**, *26*, 3762. [CrossRef] [PubMed]
11. Meng, T.; Xiao, D.; Muhammed, A.; Deng, J.; Chen, L.; He, J. Anti-inflammatory action and mechanisms of resveratrol. *Molecules* **2021**, *26*, 229. [CrossRef] [PubMed]
12. Woodman, K.G.; Coles, C.A.; Lamandé, S.R.; White, J.D. Resveratrol promotes hypertrophy in wildtype skeletal muscle and reduces muscle necrosis and gene expression of inflammatory markers in mdx mice. *Molecules* **2021**, *26*, 853. [CrossRef] [PubMed]
13. Chang, M.X.; Xiong, F. Astaxanthin and its effects in inflammatory responses and inflammation-associated diseases: Recent advances and future directions. *Molecules* **2020**, *25*, 5342. [CrossRef] [PubMed]

14. Eshghjoo, S.; Jayaraman, A.; Sun, Y.; Alaniz, R.C. Microbiota-mediated immune regulation in atherosclerosis. *Molecules* **2021**, *26*, 179. [CrossRef] [PubMed]
15. Shin, S.H.; Ye, M.K.; Lee, D.W.; Kang, B.J.; Chae, M.H. Effect of korean red ginseng and rg3 on asian sand dust-induced MUC5AC, MUC5B, and MUC8 expression in bronchial epithelial cells. *Molecules* **2021**, *26*, 2002. [CrossRef] [PubMed]
16. Choi, J.; Lim, J.W.; Kim, H. Lycopene inhibits toll-like receptor 4-mediated expression of inflammatory cytokines in house dust mite-stimulated respiratory epithelial cells. *Molecules* **2021**, *26*, 3127. [CrossRef] [PubMed]
17. Genova, E.; Apollonio, M.; Decorti, G.; Tesser, A.; Tommasini, A.; Stocco, G. In vitro effects of sulforaphane on interferon-driven inflammation and exploratory evaluation in two healthy volunteers. *Molecules* **2021**, *26*, 3602. [CrossRef] [PubMed]
18. Bae, S.; Lim, J.W.; Kim, H. β-carotene inhibits expression of matrix metalloproteinase-10 and invasion in helicobacter pylori-infected gastric epithelial cells. *Molecules* **2021**, *26*, 1567. [CrossRef] [PubMed]
19. Bae, M.; Kim, H. The roles of vitamin C, vitamin D, and selenium in the immune system against covid-19. *Molecules* **2020**, *25*, 5346. [CrossRef] [PubMed]

In Vitro Effects of Sulforaphane on Interferon-Driven Inflammation and Exploratory Evaluation in Two Healthy Volunteers

Elena Genova [1,†], Maura Apollonio [1,†], Giuliana Decorti [1,2], Alessandra Tesser [1,*], Alberto Tommasini [1,2,‡] and Gabriele Stocco [3,‡]

1. Institute for Maternal and Child Health IRCCS Burlo Garofolo, 34137 Trieste, Italy; elena.genova@burlo.trieste.it (E.G.); maura.apollonio@burlo.trieste.it (M.A.); decorti@units.it (G.D.); alberto.tommasini@burlo.trieste.it (A.T.)
2. Department of Medical, Surgical and Health Sciences, University of Trieste, 34149 Trieste, Italy
3. Department of Life Sciences, University of Trieste, 34127 Trieste, Italy; stoccog@units.it
* Correspondence: alessandra.tesser@burlo.trieste.it; Tel.: +39-040-378-5422
† These authors contributed equally to this work.
‡ These authors contributed equally to this work.

Abstract: Interferonopathies are rare genetic conditions defined by systemic inflammatory episodes caused by innate immune system activation in the absence of pathogens. Currently, no targeted drugs are authorized for clinical use in these diseases. In this work, we studied the contribution of sulforaphane (SFN), a cruciferous-derived bioactive molecule, in the modulation of interferon-driven inflammation in an immortalized human hepatocytes (IHH) line and in two healthy volunteers, focusing on *STING*, a key-component player in interferon pathway, interferon signature modulation, and *GSTM1* expression and genotype, which contributes to SFN metabolism and excretion. In vitro, SFN exposure reduced *STING* expression as well as interferon signature in the presence of the pro-inflammatory stimulus cGAMP (cGAMP 3 h vs. SFN+cGAMP 3 h p value < 0.0001; cGAMP 6 h vs. SFN+cGAMP 6 h p < 0.001, one way ANOVA), restoring STING expression to the level of unstimulated cells. In preliminary experiments on healthy volunteers, no appreciable variations in interferon signature were identified after SFN assumption, while only in one of them, presenting the *GSTM1* wild type genotype related to reduced SFN excretion, could a downregulation of *STING* be recorded. This study confirmed that SFN inhibits *STING*-mediated inflammation and interferon-stimulated genes expression in vitro. However, only a trend towards the downregulation of *STING* could be reproduced in vivo. Results obtained have to be confirmed in a larger group of healthy individuals and in patients with type I interferonopathies to define if the assumption of SFN could be useful as supportive therapy.

Keywords: sulforaphane; type I interferons; *STING*; interferon signature; *GSTM1*

1. Introduction

The mechanisms behind inflammatory diseases are complex and various, making it difficult to find targeted therapies for patients. From the second part of the last century, it was clear that glucocorticoids could represent an effective anti-inflammatory treatment for the vast majority of inflammatory diseases, although burdened by serious adverse effects [1]. However, at the end of the last century, a better knowledge of the pathogenetic mechanisms of these diseases allowed for the development of targeted therapies able to mimic the anti-inflammatory power of cortisone without its adverse effects. For example, following the discovery that some diseases are dominated by the inflammatory effect of specific cytokines, biological drugs usually based on monoclonal antibodies, soluble receptors, or receptor antagonists have been developed [2]. Indeed, anti-tumor necrosis factor-α (TNFα) antibodies have been successfully used in rheumatoid arthritis and in inflammatory bowel disease [3,4], while interleukin-1 (IL-1) inhibitors have found application in autoinflammatory diseases, such as Still's disease, recurrent pericarditis, gout arthritis, Behçet's disease, and a set of genetic conditions such as periodic fever [5]. In the last ten years, a set of genetic diseases characterized by a defective regulation of type I interferons production, the so-called interferonopathies, were identified, which often showed poor responses to conventional anti-inflammatory drugs, including biologics and glucocorticoids. Thus, their study allowed to evaluate the potential of novel targeted treatments to reduce interferon driven inflammation [6,7]. Interferonopathies are a heterogeneous group of Mendelian diseases characterized by an abnormal response to nucleic acid stimuli due to either deficiency of nucleases involved in the disposal of nucleic acids, or to defective regulation of downstream effector molecules, leading to excessive production of type I interferon, in particular α and β [6,7]. Interferons are glycoproteic cytokines classified in type I, II, and III according to their cellular origin and receptor structure. Interferons can activate several transduction pathways by different mechanisms resulting in antiviral, immunomodulatory and antiproliferative activities [8,9]. Interferonopathies include Aicardi-Goutières syndrome (AGS), monogenic forms of systemic lupus erythematosus (SLE), *STING*-associated vasculopathy with onset in infancy (SAVI), COPA syndrome and other exceptionally rare disorders [6]. Unfortunately, the measure of type I interferon in human sera is not routinely available in clinical practice, due to the short half-life and the low serum concentrations of the cytokine. Moreover, an isolated interferon dosage may not fully reflect the importance of a prolonged systemic exposure. These issues restrict the ability to diagnose and monitor treatment of these diseases [10]. So far, the assessment of interferon-mediated inflammation in these disorders relies on indirect assays, performed on peripheral blood cells, that present transcriptional changes related to their autocrine or paracrine exposition to high concentration of interferons [11]. One of these approaches consists in the relative quantification of a set of interferon-stimulated genes (ISGs), the so-called interferon signature. One of the most used set of ISGs for interferon signature assessment was proposed by Crow and his group [10], who defined the over-expression of six ISGs (*IFI27*, *IFI44L*, *IFIT1*, *ISG15*, *RSAD2*, and *SIGLEC1*) in a cohort of AGS patients compared to healthy controls. The interferon signature intensity is provided by the calculation of an "interferon score" (IFN score) as the median fold change of the six target ISGs. The validation of this score for the detection of monogenic interferonopathies made it preferred by centers involved in the screening and diagnosis of these rare conditions.

Currently, no targeted drugs for type I interferonopathies are authorized for routine clinical use and the few treatments available control principally the downstream effects of interferons [6,7]. Only a few drugs, such as antimalarial agents, Janus Kinase inhibitors, mycophenolate mofetil, and high dose glucocorticoids, have proven to demonstrate some efficacy. Moreover, anti-interferon α antibodies resulted not useful in the clinical practice while, more recently, antibodies blocking the common type I interferon receptor have been developed and are used with promising results in SLE [12]. To identify more efficient targeted drugs, and for developing drug classes already proven as partially efficient, it is important to develop or improve in vitro models already available reproducing significant disease-related pathogenic mechanisms [13,14]. During the research of new effective treatments, it is also crucial to face the possibility of the infectious risk connected to excessive suppression of cytokines and organism signaling pathways [15]. This implies that active compounds interacting with these inflammatory mechanisms should be modular in action intensity and should be selective, in order to reduce adverse effects.

Historically, medicinal chemistry finds a landmark in plants as a starting point for drug development. In the last years, the field of nutraceuticals has expanded, providing treatments that maintain the bioactive plant compound as close to its native state as possible [16,17]. In this context, sulforaphane (SFN), a bioactive molecule contained in cruciferous vegetables (e.g., broccoli), emerges as a potential phytochemical compound, able to produce positive results in conditions lacking satisfactory pharmaceutical compounds [18], by modulating an important key-component of interferon pathway production. Despite being a food-derived molecule, SFN can reach an intracellular concentration sufficient to affect gene expression, thanks to its high bioavailability [17]. In particular, based on the in vitro effect on cells from patients with SAVI syndrome, SFN may be a reasonable supplement in the treatment of patients affected by type I interferonopathies. Indeed, it is well-known that SFN is an effective activator of the transcription factor NRF2 (nuclear factor erythroid 2-related factor 2), which can modulate key components of the cellular defense processes, operating on redox- and inflammation-regulating gene expression via activation of the antioxidant responsive elements axis [19]. Cytosolic NRF2 contrasts the activity of nuclear factor NF-κB, which drives immune responses to cellular challenges such as bacterial and viral infection and inflammation [19]. As regards the interferon cascade, NRF2 activation driven by SFN leads to downregulation of *STING* (stimulator of interferon genes), an important kinase implicated in type I interferon production, through a mechanism that brings to its mRNA instability in a time and dose dependent manner [20]. In addition, SFN has been demonstrated as an important agent in the regulation of functionalizing (phase I) and conjugating (phase II) xenobiotic biotransformation enzymes [21]. Among phase II enzymes, GSTs are known to be induced by SFN through the activation of the antioxidant responsive elements axis thanks its sulphur interaction with thiol groups of the Keap1 cysteine residues [22]. In addition, GSTs, and in particular the *GSTM1* isoform, play an important role in enzymatic formation and cleavage of the GSH conjugates of isothiocyanates, contributing to SFN pharmacokinetics [23–25]. In fact, higher SFN excretion in urines after 24 h since consumption in null individuals rather than those with functional *GSTM1* was identified [25]. This evidence suggested that *GSTM1* positive individuals may have a different metabolism of SFN, with reduced SFN metabolites excretion. This may explain why *GSTM1* null individuals show less protection offered by SFN than positive subjects do [25].

In this work we studied the effect of SFN on interferon inflammation induced by cGAMP treatment, using a healthy immortalized human hepatocytes (IHH) cell line, focusing on *STING* and interferon signature modulation. The peculiar ability of SFN to induce the expression of phase II enzyme *GSTM1*, that plays an important role in its pharmacokinetics, was also evaluated in IHH cells. Moreover, as a secondary objective, we assessed the expression of *STING* and interferon signature in vivo in two healthy volunteers after the consumption of increasing doses of two commercial SFN supplements.

2. Results

2.1. Cytotoxicity of SFN on IHH Cells

To evaluate cytotoxicity of SFN on IHH cells, various concentrations were tested (1.25×10^{-6} M to 4×10^{-5} M) for 72 h by MTT assay. IHH cell line was found sensitive to SFN (EC_{50} 1.84×10^{-5} M, confidence intervals C.I. 1.37×10^{-5} M to 2.49×10^{-5} M) (Figure 1). The 10 μM concentration used for the subsequent treatment resulted in about 70% of cell viability.

2.2. STING Expression

STING expression in IHH cells was evaluated by RT-PCR. Cells were treated with 10 μM SFN in the presence or absence of the inflammatory stimulus 5.9 μM cGAMP added in the last 3 or 6 h of SFN incubation (Figure 2).

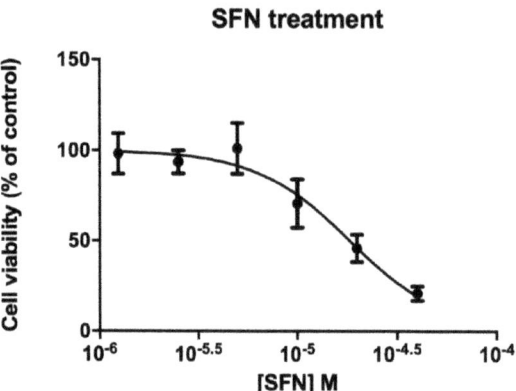

Figure 1. Cytotoxicity effects of sulforaphane (SFN) on IHH cell line. Cells were exposed for 72 h to SFN and cytotoxicity effects were analyzed by MTT assay. Data are reported as means ± SE of 3 independent experiments performed in triplicate. O.D.% observed to untreated cells.

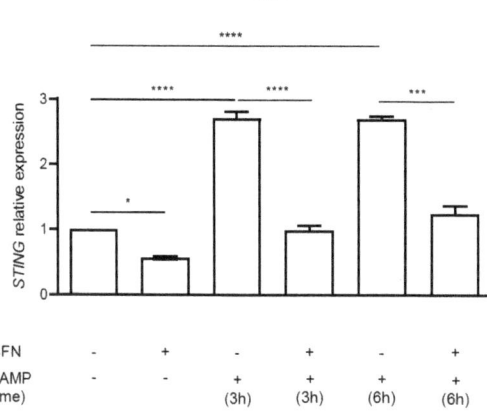

Figure 2. *STING* expression in IHH cells pretreated or not with sulforaphane (SFN, 10 μM) in presence of inflammatory stimulus cGAMP (5.9 μM). Data are shown as means and C.I. of two representative experiments and reported evaluating $2^{-\Delta\Delta Ct}$ values using untreated cells as calibrator and *HPRT1* and *G6DP* housekeeping genes as reference. *: $p < 0.05$, one way ANOVA untreated CTRL IHH cells vs. 72 h SFN 10 μM treatment. ****: $p < 0.0001$, one way ANOVA IHH exposed to 5.9 μM cGAMP for 3 h and vs. IHH pre-treated with SFN 10 μM for 72 h and 5.9 μM cGAMP for 3 h. ***: $p < 0.001$, one way ANOVA IHH exposed to 5.9 μM cGAMP for 6 h vs. IHH pre-treated with SFN 10 μM for 72 h and 5.9 μM cGAMP for 6 h. ****: $p < 0.0001$, one way ANOVA untreated CTRL IHH cells vs. IHH treated with 5.9 μM cGAMP for 3 and 6 h.

As expected, cGAMP induced a strong increase ($p < 0.0001$, one way ANOVA) in *STING* expression after 3 and 6 h of stimulation. A significant ($p < 0.05$, one way ANOVA) *STING* expression decrease was identified in cells treated with SFN for 72 h in comparison to the untreated control (CTRL) (Figure 2). The effect was even more evident when *STING* expression was induced after 3 h and 6 h of cell exposure to the inflammatory stimulus cGAMP in comparison to control. Cells pre-treated with SFN and stimulated with cGAMP showed a significant lower *STING* expression in comparison to those that were only stimulated with cGAMP (cGAMP 3 h vs. SFN+cGAMP 3 h p value < 0.0001; cGAMP 6 h vs. SFN+cGAMP 6 h $p < 0.001$, one way ANOVA) resulting in *STING* levels similar to the untreated control.

2.3. Interferon Signature Analysis of IHH Cells

Interferon signature was analyzed on IHH cells treated with SFN 10 μM in presence and absence of the inflammatory stimulus cGAMP, to evaluate whether the expression of the six ISGs decreases in the presence of SFN during an inflammatory event (Figure 3).

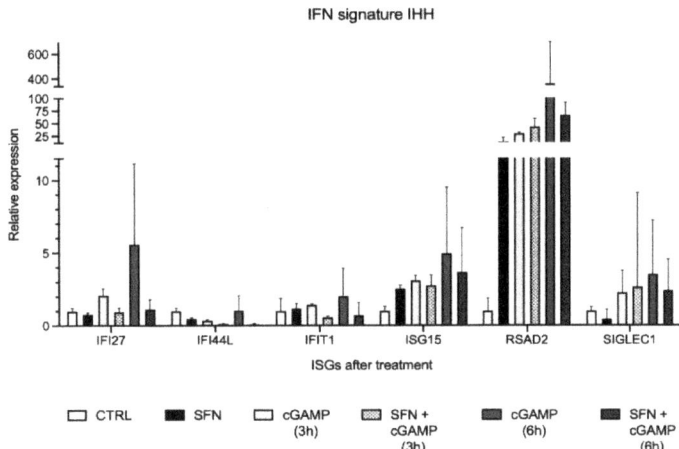

Figure 3. Interferon signature analysis of IHH cells pretreated with sulforaphane (SFN, 10 μM) for 72 h in presence of inflammatory stimulus cGAMP (5.9 μM) displayed as the expression levels of the six interferon-stimulated genes (ISGs). Data are shown as means and C.I. of one representative experiment and reported evaluating $2^{-\Delta\Delta Ct}$ values using untreated cells as calibrator (CTRL) and *HPRT1* and *G6DP* housekeeping genes as reference.

An increase of ISGs expression after cell exposure to the cGAMP inflammatory stimulus was identified (Figure 3). In particular, the increment was higher after 6 h exposure in comparison to 3 h. Most ISGs showed a lower expression level in cells pretreated with SFN and subsequently exposed to cGAMP. In particular, the effect was more evident when cells were pretreated with SFN for 72 h and stimulated with cGAMP for 6 h in comparison to the same conditions at 3 h. Above all ISGs, *RSAD2* proved the most represented and overexpressed gene during cell stimulation with cGAMP and pretreatment with SFN for 72 h significantly reduced its overexpression. However, we noticed a strong increment in *RSAD2* expression also after SFN exposure alone, in absence of the cGAMP stimulus. Also, *ISG15* expression was slightly augmented by SFN exposure. The intensity of the interferon signature analyses is reported in Table 1 as IFN scores.

Table 1. IFN scores of IHH cells treated with SFN and cGAMP.

CTRL	SFN 72 h	cGAMP 3 h	SFN 72 h + cGAMP 3 h	cGAMP 6 h	SFN 72 h + cGAMP 6 h
1.00	0.96	2.16	1.79	4.22	1.75

CTRL = untreated control; SFN = sulforaphane 10 μM; cGAMP = 5.9 μM.

IFN score (Table 1) was higher in cells stimulated with the proinflammatory stimulus cGAMP. In particular, IFN score resulted about two times higher when the stimulus was maintained for a longer time. By contrast, the IFN score was similar, considerably lower in cells pre-treated with SFN and then stimulated with cGAMP for 3 or 6 h. Cells treated only with SFN have an IFN score similar to the control.

2.4. IHH GSTM1 Analysis

GSTM1 expression was evaluated by RT-PCR after SFN exposure for 24 and 72 h at a concentration of 10 µM (Figure 4).

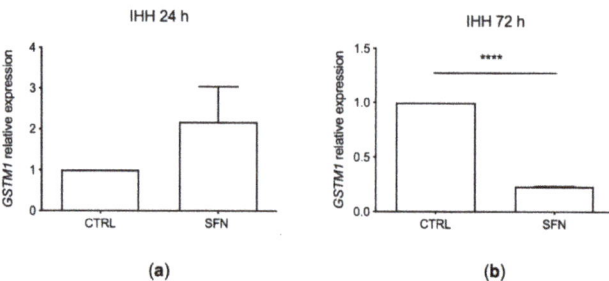

Figure 4. *GSTM1* expression in IHH cell line treated with sulforaphane (SFN, 10 µM) for 24 h (**a**) and 72 h (**b**). Data are shown as means and C.I. of three representative experiments and reported evaluating $2^{-\Delta\Delta Ct}$ values, using untreated cells as calibrator (CTRL) and beta-actin housekeeping gene as reference. ****: $p < 0.001$, one way ANOVA IHH exposed to SFN vs. untreated CTRL IHH cells.

GSTM1 expression increased after 24 h of treatment while significantly decreased after 72 h of SFN incubation ($p < 0.001$, one way ANOVA).

2.5. Basal STING Expression in Healthy Volunteers and Patients

Initially, basal *STING* expression in six patients suffering from type I interferon-related disorders (SLE, AGS, CANDLE like) and in three healthy individuals, not taking drugs or supplements, was evaluated to identify possible differences between healthy individuals and patients. The expression reported is normalized to a control (CTRL), which is represented by one of the three healthy individuals (Figure 5).

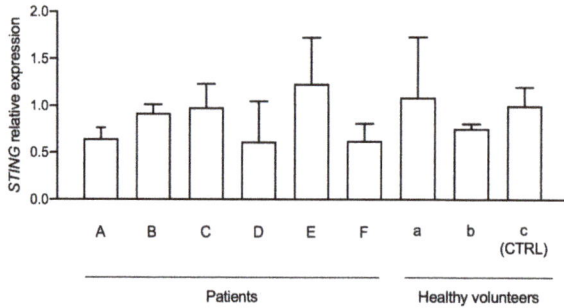

Figure 5. *STING* expression in patients (A–F) suffering from type I interferon dysregulations and healthy individuals (a–c). Data are reported evaluating $2^{-\Delta\Delta Ct}$ values, using healthy volunteer "c" as calibrator (CTRL) and *HPRT1* and *G6DP* housekeeping genes as reference.

Results indicated that STING expression in patients and healthy volunteers is heterogenous and no relevant differences between healthy individuals and patients can be observed.

2.6. STING Expression after Administration of Lower-Dose SFN Supplement in HV1

HV1 was treated with up to 25.2 mg of SFN daily for three consecutive days (T1: 24 h of treatment, T2: 72 h of treatment) and, after two weeks of interruption, for other seven days (T3) to evaluate whether oral SFN administration can decrease *STING* expression. The relative expression was evaluated considering *STING* expression measured in the last day of supplement intake as reference (T3) (Figure 6).

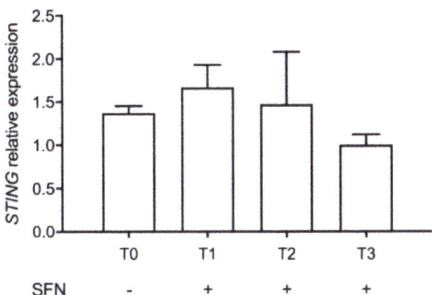

Figure 6. *STING* expression after sulforaphane (SFN) supplement consumption in the first volunteer (HV1). Data are reported evaluating $2^{-\Delta\Delta Ct}$ values considering the last day of assumption as calibrator (T3), using *HPRT1* and *G6DP* housekeeping genes as reference.

Results showed no significant changes in *STING* expression.

2.7. Interferon Signature Analysis after Administration of Lower-Dose SFN Supplement in HV1

To evaluate whether interferon signature analysis could be affected by oral SFN supplement administration, the expression levels of the six ISGs were assessed on the same samples used for *STING* analysis of the same volunteer (HV1), considering as calibrator a pool of healthy volunteers' cDNAs (CTRL) (Figure 7).

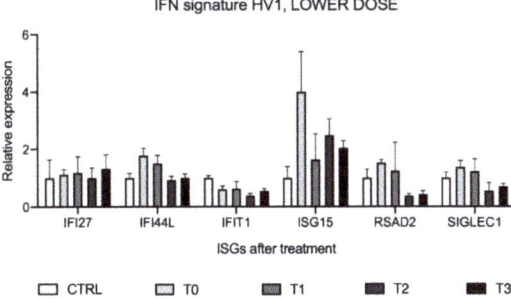

Figure 7. Interferon signature analysis after sulforaphane (SFN) supplement assumption in the first volunteer (HV1) displayed as the expression levels of the six interferon-stimulated genes (ISGs). Data are shown as means and C.I. of one representative experiment reported evaluating $2^{-\Delta\Delta Ct}$ values considering a pool of healthy volunteers' cDNAs as calibrator and using *HPRT1* and *G6DP* housekeeping genes as reference.

Relative gene expression showed a reduction of the expression levels of most of the ISGs after SFN assumption, even if not significant. The intensities of interferon signature analyses, reported as IFN scores (Table 2), did not show significant changes for different intake times.

Table 2. IFN scores calculated through the median of the relative quantifications of the six genes of the interferon signature analysis after administration of lower-dose sulforaphane (SFN) supplement in the first healthy volunteer (HV1).

CTRL	T0	T1	T2	T3
1.00	1.44	1.23	0.73	0.85

2.8. STING Expression after Higher-Dose SFN Supplement Administration in the Two Volunteers

After gene expression evaluation in HV1 taking lower supplement doses, we enrolled a second volunteer (HV2), increased the SFN dose and changed the commercial supplement (Broccoraphan®, Dieters). The dose was about four folds higher (90 mg/day) in comparison to the first one (up to 25.2 mg/day), and administration time lasted for three days (T1, T2, T3). Relative STING expression was evaluated before (T0) and after SFN assumption, considering as control the last day of supplement consumption (T3) (Figure 8).

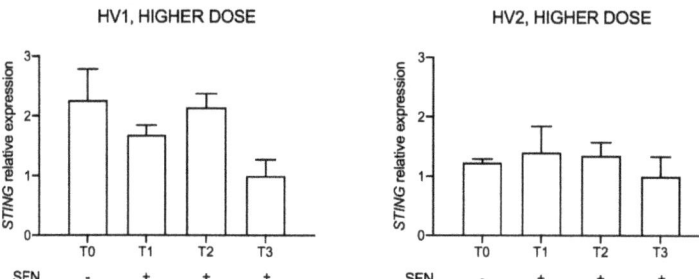

Figure 8. *STING* expression in two healthy volunteers (HV1, HV2) after sulforaphane (SFN) supplement administration at 90 mg/die for three days. Data are reported evaluating $2^{-\Delta\Delta Ct}$ values considering the last day of supplement consumption (T3) as calibrator and using *HPRT1* and *G6DP* housekeeping genes as reference.

A downward trend in *STING* expression was observed in HV1 but not in HV2.

2.9. Interferon Signature Analysis after Higher-Dose SFN Supplement Assumption in the Two Volunteers

To evaluate the ISGs expression levels after consumption of a higher dose of SFN supplement (90 mg/day), interferon signature analysis was performed before (T0) and after SFN assumption (T1, T2, T3). ISGs expression results are relative to the calibrator, which is represented by a pool of healthy volunteers' cDNAs (CTRL). Results did not highlight significant changes in ISGs after the 90 mg/day higher dose of SFN supplement in both volunteers (Figure 9).

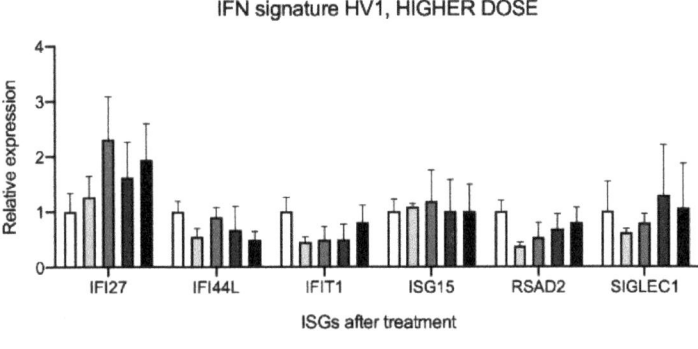

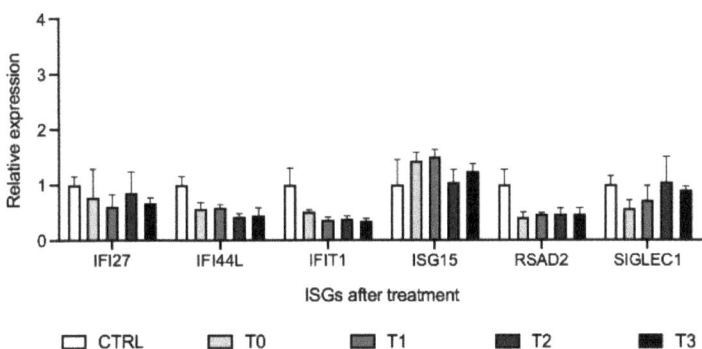

Figure 9. Interferon signature analysis in two healthy volunteers (HV1, HV2) after sulforaphane (SFN) supplement consumption at 90 mg/day for three days, displayed as the expression levels of the six interferon-stimulated genes (ISGs). Data are shown as means and C.I. of one representative experiment and reported evaluating $2^{-\Delta\Delta Ct}$ values considering a pool of healthy volunteers' cDNAs as calibrator and using *HPRT1* and *G6DP* housekeeping genes as reference.

The IFN scores did not show significant differences in both volunteers (Tables 3 and 4).

Table 3. IFN scores calculated through the median of the relative quantifications of the six interferon-stimulated genes (ISGs) of the interferon signature analysis after administration of higher-dose sulforaphane (SFN) supplement in the first healthy volunteer (HV1).

CTRL	T0	T1	T2	T3
1.00	0.58	0.85	0.84	0.91

Table 4. IFN scores calculated through the median of the relative quantifications of the six interferon-stimulated genes (ISGs) of the interferon signature analysis after administration of higher-dose sulforaphane (SFN) supplement in the second healthy volunteer (HV2).

CTRL	T0	T1	T2	T3
1.00	0.57	0.60	0.66	0.57

2.10. Healthy Volunteers' GSTM1 Genotype

To evaluate *GSTM1* genotype of the two healthy volunteers enrolled a genotype analysis was performed. Results indicated that the first volunteer (HV1) has a functional *GSTM1* gene while the second one (HV2) presents the deletion of the gene (null genotype).

2.11. GSTM1 Expression (HV1)

GSTM1 expression was evaluated by RT-PCR in HV1 with the functional *GSTM1* genotype before and after SFN assumption. Analyses were performed before (T0) and after SFN assumption (T1, T2, T3) comparing the *GSTM1* level to no assumption condition (T0) both in lower and higher dose treatments (Figure 10).

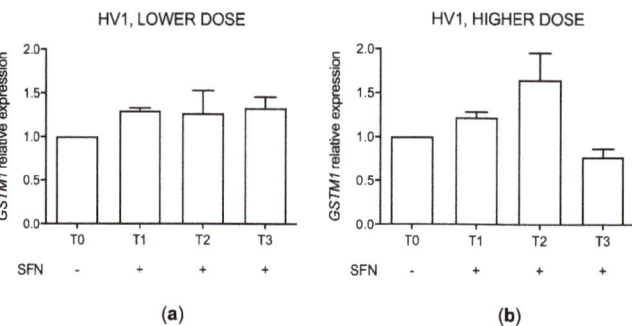

Figure 10. *GSTM1* expression in the first healthy volunteer (HV1) after sulforaphane (SFN) supplement consumption at 12.6 mg for the first day (T1), 25.2 mg for the second and third days (T2) and 25.2 mg for further seven days (T3) (**a**) and 90 mg/day for three days (**b**). Data are reported as $2^{-\Delta\Delta Ct}$ values considering the no assumption samples (T0) as calibrators and using *GAPDH* housekeeping gene as reference.

An increment trend in *GSTM1* expression after SFN assumption in both treatment conditions was identified except for the last day (T3) of 90 mg dosage.

3. Discussion

Autoinflammatory diseases are rare genetic conditions defined by systemic inflammatory episodes caused by innate immune system activation in the absence of pathogens, with early onset in childhood. For these conditions, treatment is focused on main disease manifestations and includes various classes of drugs such as glucocorticoids, immunomodulatory agents, antimalarials and biological drugs [2,15,26]. These drugs are barely effective on type I interferon generating pathway, which is constitutively active in monogenic interferonopathies like AGS, and in multifactorial interferon-related disorders like SLE, dermatomyositis, Sjögren syndrome and others [6]. In this regard, SFN, a small molecule derived from vegetables, may be useful as a possible support to dampen interferon inflammation given its ability to modulate the expression of *STING* [20], an upstream pathway component that mediates type I interferon production. Based on this evidence, we evaluated SFN effect in vitro in the hepatic IHH stable cell line and in vivo on two healthy volunteers.

After SFN exposure for 72 h, a decrease in *STING* expression in comparison to the untreated control was detected in IHH cells. This result confirmed the ability of SFN to reduce its effects in terms of *STING* expression in vitro, as described by Olagnier and colleagues work in the THP-1 human monocytic cell line after SFN treatment [20]. When the IHH cells were treated with the interferon inducer cGAMP, the treatment with SFN was able to prevent the stimulation-induced increase in *STING* expression. Similarly, we examined the so-called interferon signature, a set of characteristic overexpressed interferon-stimulated genes in patients suffering from type I interferonopathy. Interferon signature showed a similar behavior, demonstrating a considerably higher IFN score when cells were exposed to the cGAMP inflammatory stimulus with more than halved IFN score in cells pretreated with SFN and in presence of cGAMP. Therefore, our study provides additional information about *STING* expression in the presence of an inflammatory stimulus with and without pretreatment with SFN. These data provide knowledge about the role of SFN in interferon-driven inflammation suggesting a SFN preventing effect on inflammatory stimuli on IHH cell line.

Moreover, we analyzed the SFN effect on *GSTM1*, a gene encoding for a phase II xenobiotic detoxification enzyme, in IHH cells, previously confirmed wild type. In IHH cells we found an increased *GSTM1* expression after 24 h, while a decrease after 72 h using a 10 µM concentration of SFN that resulted in a 30% of cell cytotoxicity. The modulation of SNF on gene expression depends on its concentration which can cause both antioxidant and pro-oxidant effects with consequent modulation on *GSTM1* expression [27]. This result seems in line with the literature [27] where slightly toxic SFN concentrations can increase *GSTM1* levels due to the generation of ROS that interact with NRF2 pathway which can modulate key components of inflammation-promoting gene expression contrasting the action of nuclear factor NF-κB. Instead, after 48 h, when ROS was significantly reduced and could not have an effect on NRF2, *GSTM1* expression also decreased.

Interestingly, in the work of Yoon-Jin Lee and colleague [27] demonstrated that SFN increases the nuclear translocation of NRF2 via a ROS dependent mechanism in bronchial epithelial cells at a concentration of 10 µM corresponding to around 30% of cytotoxicity: the paper describes a rapid increase in intracellular ROS levels which rapidly starts within 10 min after SFN addition, peaks at 8 h and gradually declines until 48 h [27]. From this result, it is possible to assume that as the ROS peak was found 8 h after treatment, and gradually decreased until 48 h with a consequent decrement of NRF2 nuclear accumulation, also *GSTM1* induction probably could cease explaining our result of lower *GSTM1* expression after 72 h of treatment using a slight cytotoxic dose of SFN.

As a secondary objective, we performed an exploratory analysis on *STING* expression levels and IFN score after SFN assumption in two healthy volunteers, to assess the possibility of extending the study by enrolling an adequate number of subjects. After preliminary data obtained in one volunteer with low SFN doses (up to 25.2 mg/day), showing no significant effect on *STING* expression and IFN score, we increased the supplement dose (90 mg/day for three days), choosing a commercial supplement whose SFN content and indications resulted convenient to our purpose (Broccoraphan®, Dieters). At the same time, we enrolled a second volunteer (HV2) in order to evaluate potential individual differences in response. At the same time, we performed a genotype analysis of *GSTM1* since *GSTM1* genotype has an important role in SFN pharmacokinetics: in particular, *GSTM1* null or not functional individuals have a greater excretion of SFN and its metabolites in the first 24 h after SFN assumption in comparison to individuals with a functional gene [25]. Results were not consistent between the two subjects. In particular, only HV1 showed some *STING* expression decrease after treatment. In our experiment, HV1 was found to be wild type for *GSTM1*, while HV2 turned out not functional. This fact may support an interpretation of the different STING expression response to SFN in the two volunteers: the *GSTM1* functional one had a more notable decrease trend in comparison to the *GSTM1* non-functional individual. This result may suggest that, if SFN excretion is not rapid, as in *GSTM1* functional individuals, *STING* repression can be possible, in a dose and time dependent manner, according to Olagnier and colleagues [20]. In fact, the lower *STING* level was appreciable at the last day of assumption at higher doses (90 mg/day) only in the HV1 with the functional *GSTM1* gene. Regarding the SFN effect on *GSTM1*, we can appreciate an upregulation after both treatment conditions in the HV1 except for the last day of the 90 mg dose assumption. The induction of *GSTM1* by SFN is in line with the above reported results on the IHH line where, as the initial induction of *GSTM1* gradually ceases for the depletion of ROS and nuclear accumulation of NRF2, leading to the reduction of the *GSTM1* expression in the last day of SFN assumption.

The treatment with SFN did not impact the IFN score in the two volunteers. However, considering that healthy individuals did not present an inflammatory state and ISGs are downstream from *STING* and dependent on type I interferon production, results are reasonable, although this is a preliminary experiment. Thus, the real anti-interferon potential of SFN could be difficult to assess in unstimulated conditions.

The presence of other antioxidants could be a confounder in our analysis. However, beyond SFN, only the first supplement used (Broccoli Sprout, Love Life) also contained other antioxidants such as polyphenols. However, the much higher bioavailability of SFN in comparison to poorly bioavailable polyphenols [17], together with the data acquired using the second supplement devoid of other antioxidants, suggests that the effects highlighted in healthy donors are SFN-driven.

4. Materials and Methods

4.1. Cell Culture

The immortalized human hepatic IHH cell line was maintained in Dulbecco's modified Eagle's medium (DMEM) high glucose with the addition of 10% fetal bovine serum (Sigma-Aldrich, St. Louis, MO, USA), 1.25% L glutamine 0.2 M (EuroClone, Milan, Italy), 1% penicillin 0.03 M (EuroClone), streptomycin 0.02 M (EuroClone), 1% Hepes buffer 1 M (EuroClone), 0.01% human insulin 10^{-4} M (Sigma-Aldrich), and 0.04% dexamethasone 2.1×10^{-3} M (Sigma-Aldrich). Cell cultures were maintained according to standard procedures in a humidified incubator at 37 °C and with 5% CO_2, and cell passage was performed twice a week.

4.2. IHH Treatment

IHH cells (5×10^3 cells/well) were exposed for 72 h to different concentrations of sulforaphane (SFN) (1.25×10^{-6} M to 4×10^{-5} M) for cytotoxicity analysis evaluated by the MTT assay.

IHH cells were treated with SFN 10 μM for 24 h and 72 h in presence and absence of the pro-inflammatory stimulus cGAMP (Table 5) for *STING* and for interferon signature analysis. In particular, cGAMP 5.9 μM was added in the last 3 or 6 h of incubation in presence or absence of SFN 10 μM.

Table 5. Different combination treatment of SFN and cGAMP used on the IHH cell line.

SFN	cGAMP	Exposure Time
10 μM	-	24 h
10 μM	-	72 h
-	5.9 μM	3 h cGAMP
-	5.9 μM	6 h cGAMP
10 μM	5.9 μM	SFN 72 h, 3 h cGAMP
10 μM	5.9 μM	SFN 72 h, 6 h cGAMP

SFN = sulforaphane; cGAMP = cyclic guanosine monophosphate–adenosine monophosphate.

4.3. Cytotoxicity Assay

In the last 4 h of treatment, a solution of 3-(4,5-dimethylthiazol-2-yl)-2,5-diphenyltetrazolium (MTT) was added (final concentration 0.5 mg/mL) and the crystals produced by metabolically active cells were solubilized with 100 μL of DMSO. The absorbance was read by an Automated Microplate Reader EL 311s (Bio-Tek Instruments, Winooski, VT, USA) at 540/630 nm. Data are the means ± SE of at least three independent experiments performed in triplicate and are reported as % of untreated controls (absorbance treated/absorbance untreated control × 100).

4.4. Healthy Volunteers

Two individuals without clinical symptoms of diseases were selected for the study: both were of Caucasian ethnicity, one male and one female, more than 18 years old.

At first, one healthy volunteer (HV1) assumed up to 25.2 mg/day SFN (Broccoli Sprout Extract®, Love life, Cambridge, UK) for three consecutive days (T1: 24 h of assumption, T2: 72 h of assumption) and, after two weeks of stop, for other seven days (T3). Doses were decided considering the steady state concentration of SFN, which, taking 8.2 mg every 8 h resulted in the 0.3–0.6 µM range [28,29]. In particular, 4.2 mg of SFN supplement was administered every 8 h for the first 24 h (12.6 mg daily), 8.2 mg every 8 h for the next 48 h (25.2 mg daily) and, after two weeks of stop, the same dosage for 7 days. Broccoli sprout extract® Love life supplement was chosen because the amount (2.5 mg of SFN/capsule 600 mg) of SFN contained in each capsule was convenient to reach pharmacologically relevant blood concentrations of the drug. Peripheral blood samples were collected for RNA extraction before treatment (T0 no assumption), at T1, T2, and at T3 (Table 6).

Table 6. Doses and timing of sulforaphane (SFN) administrations in the first healthy volunteer enrolled (HV1).

Lower Dose	
Dose/Day	Administration Timing
-	No assumption (T0)
12.6 mg	Day 1 (T1)
25.2 mg	Day 2–3 (T2)
25.2 mg	7 days assumption (T3)

In the second treatment, both volunteers (HV1, HV2) assumed an almost four-times-higher dose (90 mg daily for 3 days). This time, the supplement chosen was *Broccoraphan®* (Dieters, Frechen, Germany) because the formulation was convenient in relation to our objectives, despite the bad taste of the supplement powder (~15 mg SFN/g supplement—90 mg corresponds to 6 g daily). Indeed, the dose should lead to an SFN steady state concentration of 1–2 µM [28,29] and was considered safe, as reported by the supplement indications. Peripheral blood samples were collected for RNA extraction before treatment (T0 no assumption), at T1, T2, and T3 for both volunteers (Table 7).

Table 7. Doses and timing of sulforaphane (SFN) administrations in both volunteers enrolled (HV1, HV2). The second-round dose treatments were considered high doses and referred as "higher dose".

Higher Dose	
Dose/Day	Administration Timing
-	No assumption (T0)
90 mg	Day 1 (T1)
90 mg	Day 2 (T2)
90 mg	Day 3 (T3)

4.5. RNA Extraction

Total RNA of the IHH cell line was extracted with TRIzol reagent (Invitrogen, Waltham, MA, USA) while healthy volunteers' total RNA was extracted using the PAXgene Blood RNA kit (PreAnalytiX, Hombrechtikon, Switzerland) according to the manufacturer's instruction. The obtained RNA was quantified using Nanodrop 2000 spectrophotometer (ThermoFisher Scientific, Waltham, MA, USA) and reversed-transcribed into cDNA using the High-Capacity RNA-to-cDNA kit (Applied Biosystem, Waltham, MA, USA).

4.6. Real-Time PCR

4.6.1. Interferon Signature and STING Analysis

Interferon signature analysis was performed by relative quantification of six interferon-stimulated genes (ISGs: *IFI27*, *IFI44L*, *IFIT1*, *ISG15*, *RSAD2*, *SIGLEC1*) by real-time PCR (RT-PCR), using UPL Probes (Roche, Basel, Switzerland), TaqMan Gene Expression Master

Mix (Applied Biosystems), and a AB 7500 Real Time PCR system (Table 8). The same analysis was also used for *STING* and the housekeeping reference genes *HPRT1* and *G6PD*.

Table 8. Universal Probe Library (UPL) probes (Roche) and primers (Eurofins Genomics) for the six interferon-stimulated genes (ISGs) of interferon signature and STING analysis by Real-Time PCR.

	Probes and Primers		
GENE	Probe (10 µM)	Primer Forward (20 µM)	Primer Reverse (20 µM)
	ISGs assessed for interferon signature analysis		
IFI27	P. n. 21	GTGGCCAAAGTGGTCAGG	CCAATCACAACTGTAGCAATCC
IFI44L	P. n. 15	TGACACTATGGGGCTAGATGG	TTGGTTTACGGGAATTAAACTGAT
IFIT1	P. n. 82	TCCACAAGACAGAGAATAGCCAGAT	GCTCCAGACTATCCTTGACCTG
ISG15	P. n. 76	GAGGCAGCGAACTCATCTTT	AGCATCTTCACCGTCAGGTC
RSAD2	P. n. 76	ACAAATGCGGCTTCTGTTTC	GAAATGGCTCTCCACCTGAA
SIGLEC1	P. n. 76	CTGCCCTGCAAGTCCTCTA	CAGCAGGTGGCTCACTGTC
	Primers and probe for measuring *STING* expression		
STING	P. n. 51	CGCCTCATTCCCTACCAG	TGCCCACAGTAACCTCCTCC
	Housekeeping genes		
HPRT1	P. n. 73	TGACCTTGATTTATTTTGCATACC	CGAGCAAGACGTTCAGTCCT
G6PD	P. n. 82	GCAAACAGAGTGAGCCCTTC	GAGTTGCGGGCAAAGAAGT

The RT-PCR protocol consists of an initial denaturation for 2 min at 50 °C and for 95 °C for 10 min, followed by 40 cycles of heating at 95 °C (15 s), and then a final extension for 1 min at 60 °C. Data were analyzed with 7500 SDS (Applied Biosystems) analysis software. Data were normalized with two housekeeping genes: *G6DP* and *HPRT1*. Relative quantification was performed using the $2^{-\Delta\Delta Ct}$ method using as reference the cDNA mix of 10 healthy controls (CTRL) for ISGs while cDNA of the last day of treatment sample (T3) for *STING*. For interferon signature analysis, the IFN score was calculated through the median of the relative quantifications of the six ISGs.

4.6.2. GSTM1 Expression

RT-PCR was performed using the TaqMan® Gene Expression Assays (Hs01683722_gH, Applied Biosystems) in a Thermal Cycler Dice Real Time System (BIO-RAD). Relative quantification is represented as $2^{-\Delta\Delta Ct}$ with respect to the housekeeping genes beta-actin (*ACTB*) and glyceraldehyde 3-phosphate dehydrogenase (*GAPDH*), setting untreated IHH and untreated donor as reference. The RT-PCR protocol for *GSTM1* analysis consists of an initial denaturation for 10 min at 95 °C, followed by 40 cycles of heating at 95 °C (15 s) and 60 °C (1 min). All experiments were carried out in duplicate and the reproducibility of the observations was confirmed in two or three independent experiments.

4.6.3. GSTM1 Genotype

GSTM1 genotype state was assessed by TaqMan® CNV genotyping Assays (Applied Biosystems) kit, containing forward and reverse specific primers for the interested amplicon, which, in that case, is *GSTM1* and a FAM conjugated probe. Additionally, TaqMan™ Copy Number Reference Assay, human RNase P was used to assess the presence of a double copy gene. In this case, too, the kit contains forward and reverse specific primers for the interested amplicon (human RNase P) and a VIC® dye–labeled TAMRA™ probe. The thermic protocol used was 95 °C for 10 min, 95 °C for 15 sec, and 60 °C for 1 min. The whole reaction was repeated for 40 cycles. Results are expressed as deleted vs. functional *GSTM1*.

4.7. Statistical Analysis

Results are presented as mean ± 95% confidence intervals (C.I.) from up to two independent experiments. Statistical analyses were performed using GraphPad Prism software (version 8.0.2). One-way ANOVA and Bonferroni's post-test were used for gene expression analysis. p values < 0.05 were considered statistically significant.

5. Conclusions

In conclusion, this study confirmed SFN inhibiting action on inflammatory stimuli response in vitro in terms of *STING* reduction and ISGs expression. We observed a *STING* reduction trend in vivo only in the HV1 after SFN administration. The higher efficacy of SFN in *STING* reduction could be related to the functional *GSTM1* genotype related to a slower elimination rate and therefore a higher SFN efficacy. Since individuals were healthy and not affected by inflammatory conditions, no effect of SFN treatment was observed on ISGs expression, as already characterized by low ISGs expression. From these premises, it will be reasonable to expand the study to a larger group of healthy individuals to further investigate the association between *STING* modulation by SFN and *GSTM1* genotype, and subsequently to evaluate these effects in patients with type I interferonopathies.

Author Contributions: Conceptualization, A.T. (Alberto Tommasini) and G.S.; data curation, E.G. and M.A.; formal analysis, E.G., M.A. and A.T. (Alessandra Tesser); funding acquisition, G.D., A.T. (Alberto Tommasini) and G.S.; investigation, E.G., M.A. and A.T. (Alessandra Tesser); methodology, E.G., M.A. and A.T. (Alessandra Tesser); project administration, E.G., M.A., A.T. (Alberto Tommasini) and G.S.; resources, G.D. and A.T. (Alberto Tommasini); software, E.G., M.A. and A.T. (Alessandra Tesser); supervision, A.T. (Alberto Tommasini) and G.S.; validation, G.D., A.T. (Alberto Tommasini) and G.S.; visualization, E.G., M.A., A.T. (Alberto Tommasini) and G.S.; writing—original draft, E.G. and M.A.; writing—review & editing, E.G., M.A., G.D., A.T. (Alessandra Tesser) and A.T. (Alberto Tommasini). All authors have read and agreed to the published version of the manuscript.

Funding: This work was supported by Institute for Maternal and Child Health—IRCCS Burlo Garofolo RC#24/2017 and RC#07/2014.

Institutional Review Board Statement: The study is part of the IRCCS Burlo Garofolo project RC#24/2017, approved by the Institutional Review Board and by the Friuli Venezia Giulia Independent Ethical Committee (2018-SPER-079-BURLO, N. 0039851, approved on 12 December 2018).

Informed Consent Statement: Written informed consent has been obtained from the participants to publish this paper.

Data Availability Statement: Raw data will be provided upon reasonable request.

Conflicts of Interest: The authors declare no conflict of interest.

References

1. Barnes, P.J. How Corticosteroids Control Inflammation: Quintiles Prize Lecture 2005. *Br. J. Pharmacol.* **2006**, *148*, 245–254. [CrossRef]
2. Diaz-Borjon, A.; Weyand, C.M.; Goronzy, J.J. Treatment of Chronic Inflammatory Diseases with Biologic Agents: Opportunities and Risks for the Elderly. *Exp. Gerontol.* **2006**, *41*, 1250–1255. [CrossRef]
3. Levin, A.D.; Wildenberg, M.E.; van den Brink, G.R. Mechanism of Action of Anti-TNF Therapy in Inflammatory Bowel Disease. *J. Crohns Colitis* **2016**, *10*, 989–997. [CrossRef]
4. Wu, C.; Wang, S.; Xian, P.; Yang, L.; Chen, Y.; Mo, X. Effect of Anti-TNF Antibodies on Clinical Response in Rheumatoid Arthritis Patients: A Meta-Analysis. *Biomed Res. Int.* **2016**, *2016*, 7185708. [CrossRef]
5. Bettiol, A.; Lopalco, G.; Emmi, G.; Cantarini, L.; Urban, M.L.; Vitale, A.; Denora, N.; Lopalco, A.; Cutrignelli, A.; Lopedota, A.; et al. Unveiling the Efficacy, Safety, and Tolerability of Anti-Interleukin-1 Treatment in Monogenic and Multifactorial Autoinflammatory Diseases. *Int. J. Mol. Sci.* **2019**, *20*, 1898. [CrossRef] [PubMed]
6. Rodero, M.P.; Crow, Y.J. Type I Interferon–Mediated Monogenic Autoinflammation: The Type I Interferonopathies, a Conceptual Overview. *J. Exp. Med.* **2016**, *213*, 2527–2538. [CrossRef]
7. Volpi, S.; Picco, P.; Caorsi, R.; Candotti, F.; Gattorno, M. Type I Interferonopathies in Pediatric Rheumatology. *Pediatric Rheumatol.* **2016**, *14*, 35. [CrossRef] [PubMed]
8. De Andrea, M.; Ravera, R.; Gioia, D.; Gariglio, M.; Landolfo, S. The Interferon System: An Overview. *Eur. J. Paediatr. Neurol.* **2002**, *6*, A41–A46. [CrossRef] [PubMed]
9. Ivashkiv, L.B.; Donlin, L.T. Regulation of Type I Interferon Responses. *Nat. Rev. Immunol.* **2014**, *14*, 36–49. [CrossRef]

10. Rice, G.I.; Melki, I.; Frémond, M.-L.; Briggs, T.A.; Rodero, M.P.; Kitabayashi, N.; Oojageer, A.; Bader-Meunier, B.; Belot, A.; Bodemer, C.; et al. Assessment of Type I Interferon Signaling in Pediatric Inflammatory Disease. *J. Clin. Immunol.* **2017**, *37*, 123–132. [CrossRef] [PubMed]
11. Rönnblom, L.; Eloranta, M.-L. The Interferon Signature in Autoimmune Diseases. *Curr. Opin. Rheumatol.* **2013**, *25*, 248–253. [CrossRef] [PubMed]
12. Morand, E.F.; Furie, R.; Tanaka, Y.; Bruce, I.N.; Askanase, A.D.; Richez, C.; Bae, S.-C.; Brohawn, P.Z.; Pineda, L.; Berglind, A.; et al. Trial of Anifrolumab in Active Systemic Lupus Erythematosus. *N. Engl. J. Med.* **2020**, *382*, 211–221. [CrossRef] [PubMed]
13. Moghaddas, F.; Masters, S.L. The Classification, Genetic Diagnosis and Modelling of Monogenic Autoinflammatory Disorders. *Clin. Sci.* **2018**, *132*, 1901–1924. [CrossRef] [PubMed]
14. Ferraro, R.M.; Lanzi, G.; Masneri, S.; Barisani, C.; Piovani, G.; Savio, G.; Cattalini, M.; Galli, J.; Cereda, C.; Muzi-Falconi, M.; et al. Generation of Three IPSC Lines from Fibroblasts of a Patient with Aicardi Goutières Syndrome Mutated in TREX1. *Stem Cell Res.* **2019**, *41*, 101580. [CrossRef] [PubMed]
15. Bienias, M.; Brück, N.; Griep, C.; Wolf, C.; Kretschmer, S.; Kind, B.; Tüngler, V.; Berner, R.; Lee-Kirsch, M.A. Therapeutic Approaches to Type I Interferonopathies. *Curr. Rheumatol. Rep.* **2018**, *20*, 32. [CrossRef] [PubMed]
16. Nasri, H.; Baradaran, A.; Shirzad, H.; Rafieian-Kopaei, M. New Concepts in Nutraceuticals as Alternative for Pharmaceuticals. *Int. J. Prev. Med.* **2014**, *5*, 1487–1499.
17. Houghton, C.A. Sulforaphane: Its "Coming of Age" as a Clinically Relevant Nutraceutical in the Prevention and Treatment of Chronic Disease. Available online: https://www.hindawi.com/journals/omcl/2019/2716870/ (accessed on 8 April 2020).
18. Kim, J.K.; Park, S.U. Current Potential Health Benefits of Sulforaphane. *EXCLI J.* **2016**, *15*, 571–577. [CrossRef]
19. Wardyn, J.D.; Ponsford, A.H.; Sanderson, C.M. Dissecting Molecular Cross-Talk between Nrf2 and NF-KB Response Pathways. *Biochem. Soc. Trans.* **2015**, *43*, 621–626. [CrossRef] [PubMed]
20. Olagnier, D.; Brandtoft, A.M.; Gunderstofte, C.; Villadsen, N.L.; Krapp, C.; Thielke, A.L.; Laustsen, A.; Peri, S.; Hansen, A.L.; Bonefeld, L.; et al. Nrf2 Negatively Regulates STING Indicating a Link between Antiviral Sensing and Metabolic Reprogramming. *Nat. Commun.* **2018**, *9*, 3506. [CrossRef]
21. Su, X.; Jiang, X.; Meng, L.; Dong, X.; Shen, Y.; Xin, Y. Anticancer Activity of Sulforaphane: The Epigenetic Mechanisms and the Nrf2 Signaling Pathway. Available online: https://www.hindawi.com/journals/omcl/2018/5438179/ (accessed on 8 April 2020).
22. Gao, S.S.; Chen, X.Y.; Zhu, R.Z.; Choi, B.-M.; Kim, B.-R. Sulforaphane Induces Glutathione S-Transferase Isozymes Which Detoxify Aflatoxin B(1)-8,9-Epoxide in AML 12 Cells. *Biofactors* **2010**, *36*, 289–296. [CrossRef]
23. Egner, P.A.; Chen, J.G.; Wang, J.B.; Wu, Y.; Sun, Y.; Lu, J.H.; Zhu, J.; Zhang, Y.H.; Chen, Y.S.; Friesen, M.D.; et al. Bioavailability of Sulforaphane from Two Broccoli Sprout Beverages: Results of a Short Term, Cross-over Clinical Trial in Qidong, China. *Cancer Prev. Res.* **2011**, *4*, 384–395. [CrossRef] [PubMed]
24. Atwell, L.L.; Hsu, A.; Wong, C.P.; Stevens, J.F.; Bella, D.; Yu, T.-W.; Pereira, C.B.; Löhr, C.V.; Christensen, J.M.; Dashwood, R.H.; et al. Absorption and Chemopreventive Targets of Sulforaphane in Humans Following Consumption of Broccoli Sprouts or a Myrosinase-Treated Broccoli Sprout Extract. *Mol. Nutr. Food Res.* **2015**, *59*, 424–433. [CrossRef]
25. Gasper, A.V.; Al-Janobi, A.; Smith, J.A.; Bacon, J.R.; Fortun, P.; Atherton, C.; Taylor, M.A.; Hawkey, C.J.; Barrett, D.A.; Mithen, R.F. Glutathione S-Transferase M1 Polymorphism and Metabolism of Sulforaphane from Standard and High-Glucosinolate Broccoli. *Am. J. Clin. Nutr.* **2005**, *82*, 1283–1291. [CrossRef] [PubMed]
26. Harry, O.; Yasin, S.; Brunner, H. Childhood-Onset Systemic Lupus Erythematosus: A Review and Update. *J. Pediatr.* **2018**, *196*, 22–30. [CrossRef]
27. Lee, Y.-J.; Lee, S.-H. Sulforaphane Induces Antioxidative and Antiproliferative Responses by Generating Reactive Oxygen Species in Human Bronchial Epithelial BEAS-2B Cells. *J. Korean Med. Sci.* **2011**, *26*, 1474–1482. [CrossRef]
28. Vermeulen, M.; Klöpping-Ketelaars, I.W.A.A.; van den Berg, R.; Vaes, W.H.J. Bioavailability and kinetics of sulforaphane in humans after consumption of cooked versus raw broccoli. *J. Agric. Food Chem.* **2008**, *56*, 10505–10509. [CrossRef] [PubMed]
29. Houghton, C.A.; Fassett, R.G.; Coombes, J.S. Sulforaphane and Other Nutrigenomic Nrf2 Activators: Can the Clinician's Expectation Be Matched by the Reality? *Oxid. Med. Cell. Longev.* **2016**, *2016*, 7857186. [CrossRef] [PubMed]

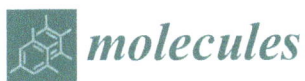

Article

Lycopene Inhibits Toll-Like Receptor 4-Mediated Expression of Inflammatory Cytokines in House Dust Mite-Stimulated Respiratory Epithelial Cells

Jiyeon Choi, Jooweon Lim and Hyeyoung Kim *

Department of Food and Nutrition, College of Human Ecology, Yonsei University, Seoul 03722, Korea; chlwldus6204@hanmail.net (J.C.); jwlim11@yonsei.ac.kr (J.L.)
* Correspondence: kim626@yonsei.ac.kr; Tel.: +82-2-2123-3125; Fax: +82-2-364-5781

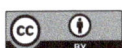

Citation: Choi, J.; Lim, J.; Kim, H. Lycopene Inhibits Toll-Like Receptor 4-Mediated Expression of Inflammatory Cytokines in House Dust Mite-Stimulated Respiratory Epithelial Cells. *Molecules* **2021**, *26*, 3127. https://doi.org/10.3390/molecules26113127

Academic Editors: Sokcheon Pak and Soo Liang Ooi

Received: 16 April 2021
Accepted: 17 May 2021
Published: 24 May 2021

Publisher's Note: MDPI stays neutral with regard to jurisdictional claims in published maps and institutional affiliations.

Copyright: © 2021 by the authors. Licensee MDPI, Basel, Switzerland. This article is an open access article distributed under the terms and conditions of the Creative Commons Attribution (CC BY) license (https://creativecommons.org/licenses/by/4.0/).

Abstract: House dust mites (HDM) are critical factors in airway inflammation. They activate respiratory epithelial cells to produce reactive oxygen species (ROS) and activate Toll-like receptor 4 (TLR4). ROS induce the expression of inflammatory cytokines in respiratory epithelial cells. Lycopene is a potent antioxidant nutrient with anti-inflammatory activity. The present study aimed to investigate whether HDM induce intracellular and mitochondrial ROS production, TLR4 activation, and pro-inflammatory cytokine expression (IL-6 and IL-8) in respiratory epithelial A549 cells. Additionally, we examined whether lycopene inhibits HDM-induced alterations in A549 cells. The treatment of A549 cells with HDM activated TLR4, induced the expression of IL-6 and IL-8, and increased intracellular and mitochondrial ROS levels. TAK242, a TLR4 inhibitor, suppressed both HDM-induced ROS production and cytokine expression. Furthermore, lycopene inhibited the HDM-induced TLR4 activation and cytokine expression, along with reducing the intracellular and mitochondrial ROS levels in HDM-treated cells. These results collectively indicated that the HDM induced TLR4 activation and increased intracellular and mitochondrial ROS levels, thus resulting in the induction of cytokine expression in respiratory epithelial cells. The antioxidant lycopene could inhibit HDM-induced cytokine expression, possibly by suppressing TLR4 activation and reducing the intracellular and mitochondrial ROS levels in respiratory epithelial cells.

Keywords: cytokines; house dust mite; lycopene; Toll-like receptor 4; reactive oxygen species; respiratory epithelial cells

1. Introduction

House dust mites (HDM) are recognized as a critical cause of allergic disorders [1,2]. Among HDM, *Dermatophagoides farinae*, *Dermatophagoides pteronyssinus*, and *Euroglyphus maynei* are the most abundant mites responsible for the production of HDM allergens, which is a common cause of allergic rhinitis and asthma. The predominant species of HDM differ by location, and *D. farinae*, the American house dust mite, is the dominant species in Korea [3]. Recently, we showed that the extract of *D. farinae* increases the levels of reactive oxygen species (ROS), the activation of nuclear factor κB (NF-κB), and IL-8 expression in respiratory epithelial H292 cells [4].

The protease activities of HDM allergens target tight junction proteins such as occludin and claudins and thus, increase the barrier permeability of the airway mucosa [5] and subsequent influx of allergens [5,6]. HDM cleaved tight junction protein ocludin and thus, increased transepithelial influx after 2 h, which continued until 7 h-incubation [5]. These studies show that HDM directly enter into airway epithelium and affect cell organelles. In addition to increasing epithelial cell permeability, HDM proteases trigger and stimulate Toll-like receptor 4 (TLR4) in epithelial cells [7–9]. Moreover, HDM increase NADPH oxidase dual oxidase 1 (DUOX1) and increase ROS production in airway epithelium [10].

Reactive oxygen species (ROS) activate the signaling of TLR4 in non-small cell lung cancer (NSCLC) cells induced by lipopolysaccharide (LPS) stimulation [11]. ROS regulate TLR4-mediated activation of NF-κB κ and IL-8 expression in the monocyte-like cell line THP-1 [12]. TLR4 is a membrane-bound member of the TLR family of pattern-recognition receptor [13]. TLR4 induces an innate immune response through transcriptional regulation, leading to the production of pro-inflammatory cytokines [14–16]. Taken together, we can postulate that HDMs activate NADPH oxidase and produce ROS, which stimulates TLR4 signaling, leading to activation of NF-κB and cytokine expression

Interleukin-6 (IL-6) is a pro-inflammatory cytokine that plays a key role in acute-phase response and the transition from acute to chronic inflammation [17,18]. Several studies have shown that the dysregulation of IL-6 production is a major contributor to the pathogenesis of chronic inflammatory and autoimmune diseases [19,20]. Interleukin-8 (IL-8) is a chemokine that is induced by diverse inflammatory stimuli in various cells, including monocytes, macrophages, fibroblasts, and endothelial cells [21]. IL-8 is known as a key factor in localized inflammation, as its secretion can be increased by oxidative stress, thereby leading to the recruitment of inflammatory cells and a further increase in oxidative stress mediators [22]. The increased expression of selected cytokines, such as IL-6 and IL-8, can eventually promote inflammation in the body, including respiratory epithelium [23].

Lycopene is a lipid-soluble antioxidant and a member of the carotenoid family of phytochemicals. It can be synthesized by many plants and microorganisms, but not by animals or humans, and is found in some red-colored vegetables and fruits, such as tomatoes [24,25]. Lycopene has a highly unsaturated open straight-chain hydrocarbon structure consisting of eleven conjugated and two unconjugated double bonds [26–28]. Lycopene has shown potent antioxidant capacity and protective effect on cells by the suppression of oxidative damage [25]. It can also reduce the levels of inflammatory biomarkers in cells through its antioxidant activity [29]. Lycopene reportedly inhibits LPS-induced liver injury by reducing the serum levels of cytokines (IL-6 and tumor necrosis factor (TNF)-α) and increasing superoxide dismutase activity in mice [30]. Zou et al. [31] showed that lycopene suppresses IL-6 expression in LPS-stimulated macrophages by inhibiting the ROS-induced trafficking of TLR4 to lipid raft-like domains. Recently, we showed that lycopene inhibits NADPH oxidase activity and thus reduces ROS levels, leading to inhibition of NF-kB activation, IL-6 expression in pancreatic acinar cells stimulated with ethanol and palmitoleic acid [32]. Jhou et al. [33] demonstrated that lycopene downregulates NADPH oxidase 4 protein expression of human liver adenocarcinoma SKHep-1 cells. Lycopene decreased oxidative stress partly by downregulation of the expression of NADPH oxidase subunits in hepatic stellate cells [34]. Therefore, lycopene may have an inhibitory effect against HDM-induced inflammation by suppressing ROS production and TRL4 activation in respiratory epithelial cells.

The current study aimed to investigate whether HDM induce the expression of IL-6 and IL-8 through TLR4 signaling and intracellular and mitochondrial ROS production, and whether lycopene inhibits HDM-induced IL-6 and IL-8 production by suppressing TLR4 activation and reducing ROS levels in A549 cells.

2. Results
2.1. HDM Induce IL-6 and IL-8 Expression and Increase ROS in A549 Cells

To investigate whether HDM induce IL-6 and IL-8 mRNA expression, cells were incubated with 20 µg/mL HDM for the indicated time periods (Figure 1A). As shown in Figure 1A, both IL-6 and IL-8 mRNA expression increased the most at 8 h. To determine whether the increase in IL-6 and IL-8 mRNA levels was followed by increased IL-6 and IL-8 protein production due to stimulation by HDM, their levels in the culture medium were determined following the treatment of cells with HDM for the indicated time periods. As shown in Figure 1B, the release of IL-6 and IL-8 showed the highest increase at 16 h of HDM treatment compared to that in cells at 0 h. The results indicated that HDM induced

IL-6 and IL-8 production at both mRNA and protein levels in human respiratory epithelial A549 cells.

For time-course experiment on intracellular and mitochondrial ROS levels, the cells were incubated with 20 μg/mL HDM for the indicated time periods (Figure 1C,D). Both intracellular and mitochondrial ROS levels increased time-dependently and are the most at 2 h. Thus, for the studies on the effect of lycopene on ROS levels, the cells were pretreated with lycopene and stimulated with HDM for 2 h.

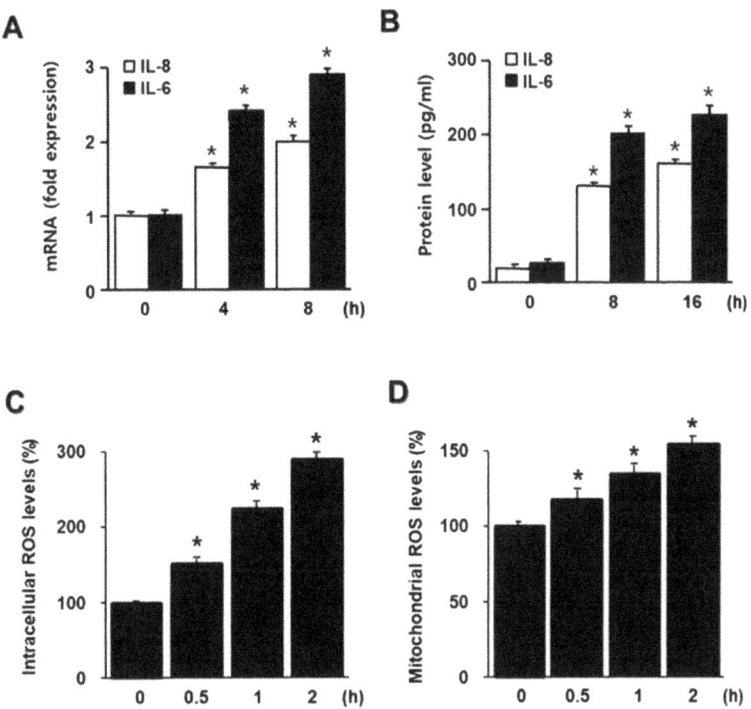

Figure 1. IL-6 and IL-8 mRNA and protein expression and intracellular and mitochondrial levels of ROS upon treatment with house dust mites (HDM). Cells were treated with 20 μg/mL HDM for the indicated time periods. (**A**) mRNA expression of IL-6 and IL-8 was determined with reverse transcription-polymerase chain reaction (RT-PCR) analysis. The mRNA levels at 0 h were set as 1. (**B**) IL-6 and IL-8 protein levels in the medium were determined with enzyme-linked immunosorbent assay (ELISA). (**C**) The intracellular ROS levels were determined using DCF-DA. ROS levels of the cells at 0 h were set as 100%. (**D**) The mitochondrial ROS levels were determined using MitoSOX. ROS levels of the cells at 0 h were set as 100%. All data are shown as the mean ± S.E. of three independent experiments. * $p < 0.05$ versus 0 h.

2.2. Lycopene Inhibits HDM-Induced Expression of IL-6 and IL-8 in A549 Cells

To determine its appropriate concentration, four concentrations of lycopene (0.1, 0.2, 0.5, and 1 μM) were used. As shown in Figure 2A,B, the HDM-induced mRNA expression of IL-6 and IL-8 was suppressed by lycopene. The inhibitory effect of 0.2 μM lycopene on cytokine mRNA expression was higher than that of 0.1 μM lycopene. The effect of 0.2 μM lycopene on cytokine mRNA expression was similar to that of 0.5 μM and 1.0 μM lycopene. Thus, for the studies on the effects of lycopene on cytokine protein levels, ROS levels, and TLR4 activity, HDM-stimulated cells were treated with 0.1 and 0.2 μM lycopene.

To investigate whether lycopene inhibits HDM-induced IL-6 and IL-8 protein expression, cells were pretreated with lycopene (0.1, 0.2 μM) and then with HDM. As shown in Figure 2C,D, the HDM-induced IL-6 and IL-8 protein expression was suppressed by lycopene treatment.

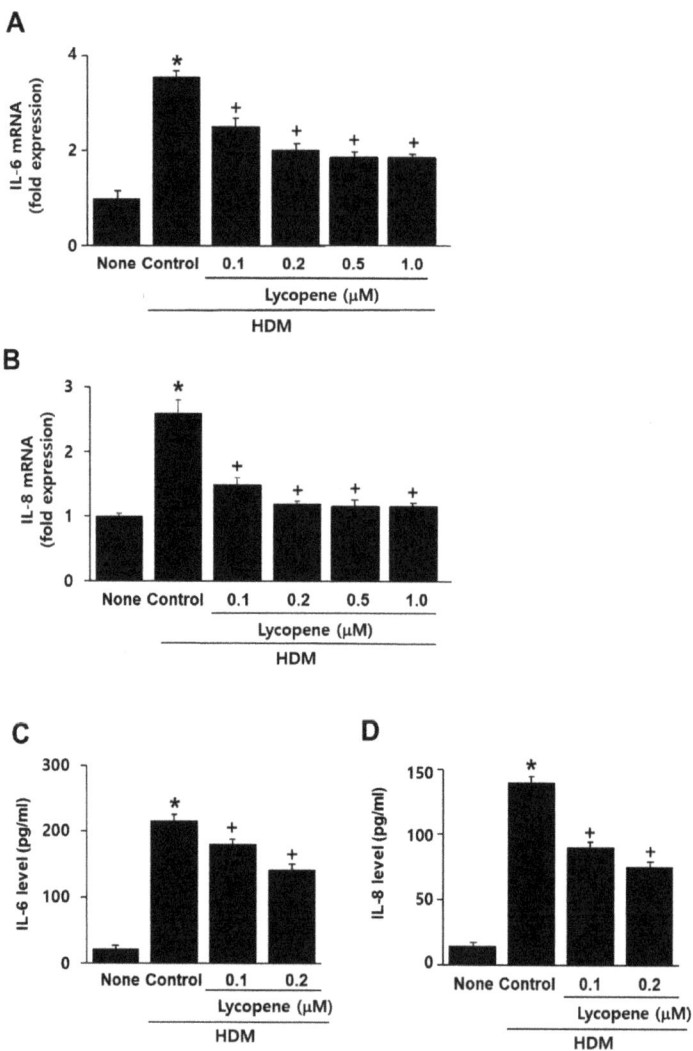

Figure 2. Effects of lycopene on the expression of IL-6 and IL-8 in house dust mite (HDM)-stimulated A549 cells. Cells were pretreated with lycopene (at the indicated concentrations) for 1 h, and then with HDM (20 μg/mL) for 8 h (for determination of mRNA expression) or 16 h (for determination of protein levels). (**A,B**) mRNA expression was determined with reverse transcription-polymerase chain reaction (RT-PCR) analysis. mRNA levels of the cells without any treatment (none) were set as 1. (**C,D**) The protein levels of IL-6 and IL-8 in the medium were determined using enzyme-linked immunosorbent assay (ELISA). All data are shown as the mean ± S.E. of three independent experiments. * $p < 0.05$ vs. none (cells without any treatment); + $p < 0.05$ vs. control (cells with HDM alone).

2.3. Lycopene Inhibits HDM-Induced Production of Intracellular and Mitochodrial ROS in A549 Cells

To determine whether lycopene inhibits the HDM-induced production of intracellular ROS and mitochondrial ROS, cells were pretreated with lycopene and then with HDM. The results obtained from the dichlorofluorescein diacetate- and MitoSOX-based assays are shown in Figure 3A,B. The intracellular ROS levels in the cells treated with HDM ("Control") were increased by 150% compared to those of untreated cells ("None"), whereas the levels of ROS in the mitochondria were increased by 40%. Pre-incubation of the cells with lycopene reduced the HDM-induced increase in ROS, which at 0.2 µM lycopene corresponded to a 40% reduction in intracellular ROS (Figure 3A) and a 30% reduction in mitochondrial ROS levels (Figure 3B).

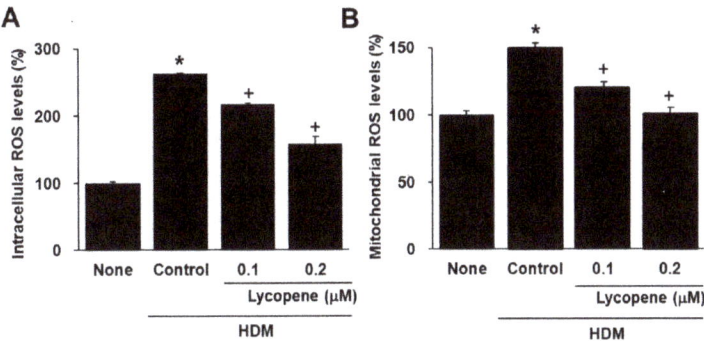

Figure 3. Effects of lycopene on the intracellular and mitochondrial levels of ROS in house dust mite (HDM)-stimulated A549 cells. Cells were pretreated with lycopene (0.1, 0.2 µM) for 1 h and then with HDM (20 µg/mL) for 2 h. (**A**) The intracellular ROS levels were determined using DCF-DA. ROS levels of the cells without any treatment (none) were set as 100%. (**B**) The mitochondrial ROS levels were determined using MitoSOX. ROS levels of the cells without any treatment (none) were set as 100% All data are shown as the mean ± S.E. of three independent experiments. * $p < 0.05$ vs. none (cells without any treatment); + $p < 0.05$ vs. control (cells with HDM alone).

2.4. Lycopene Inhibits HDM-Induced Toll Like Receptor 4 (TLR4) Activation in A549 Cells

Next, we investigated whether HDM-induced TLR4 activation is inhibited following pretreatment with lycopene. A459 cells were treated with HDM and the level of TLR4 was examined by immunofluorescence using a polyclonal antibody for TLR4. and a rhodamine-conjugated mouse anti-rabbit IgG antibody with DAPI counter-staining. As shown in Figure 4A, HDM-treatment increased the level of TLR4 and this effect was significantly inhibited in cells pretreated with lycopene. The results show that HDM may interact with TLR4. TLR4 is associated with the adapto protein myeloid differentiation protein 2 (MD-2). Thus, we examined the effect of HDM and lycopene on the cell surface level of TLR4 by measuring the monoclonal anti-TLR4-MD-2 antibody conjugated with phycoerythrin (PE), using flow cytometry (Figure 4B). Fluorescence analysis show that HDM stimulation increased surface TLR4 levels; this increase was prevented by lycopene treatment in A549 cells. These results indicate that HDM stimulation induces TLR4 activation, which is eventually inhibited by lycopene.

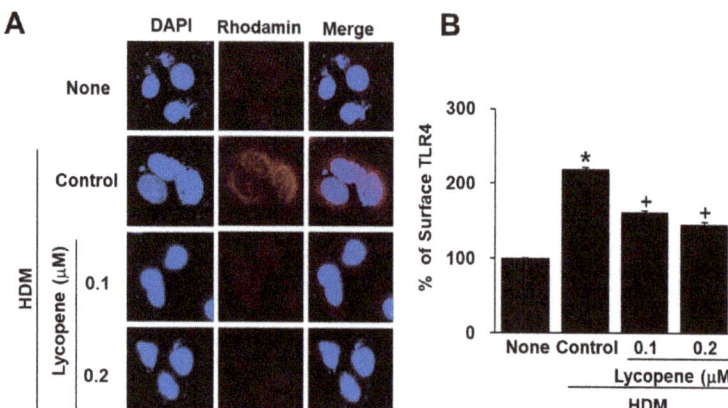

Figure 4. Effect of lycopene on TLR4 Activation in house dust mite (HDM)-stimulated A549 Cells. Cells were pretreated with lycopene (0.1 and 0.2 μM) for 1 h and then with HDMs (20 μg/mL) for 2 h. (**A**) The cells in slides were immunostained with a polyclonal antibody for TLR4. The immunoreactive proteins were visualized using a rhodamine-conjugated mouse anti-rabbit IgG antibody with DAPI counter-staining of the same field. (**B**) Surface TLR4 levels were examined by measuring the monoclonal anti-TLR4-MD-2 antibody conjugated with phycoerythrin (PE), using flow cytometry, and the mean fluorescence intensity was calculated thereafter. Surface TLR4 levels of the cells without any treatment (none) were set as 100%. All data are shown as the mean ± S.E. of three independent experiments. * $p < 0.05$ vs. none (cells without any treatment); + $p < 0.05$ vs. control (cells with HDM alone).

2.5. TAK242 Inhibits the HDM-Induced mRNA Expression of IL-6 and IL-8 and Intracellular and Mitochondrial ROS Increase in A549 Cells

To investigate whether the effect of HDM on IL-6 and IL-8 mRNA expression are mediated through the TLR4 receptor, cells were pretreated with TAK242, a TLR4 inhibitor, and then treated with HDM. TAK242 suppressed HDM-induced IL-6 and IL-8 mRNA expression (Figure 5A,B). This indicates that TLR4 mediates HDM-induced IL-6 and IL-8 mRNA expression.

To investigate whether TLR4 mediates HDM-induced intracellular and mitochondrial ROS production, the cells were pretreated with TAK242 and then treated with HDM. As shown in Figure 5C,D, HDM induced an increase in intracellular and mitochondrial ROS levels, which were subsequently suppressed by treatment with TAK242. These results indicated that TLR4 mediated HDM-induced increase in intracellular and mitochondrial ROS.

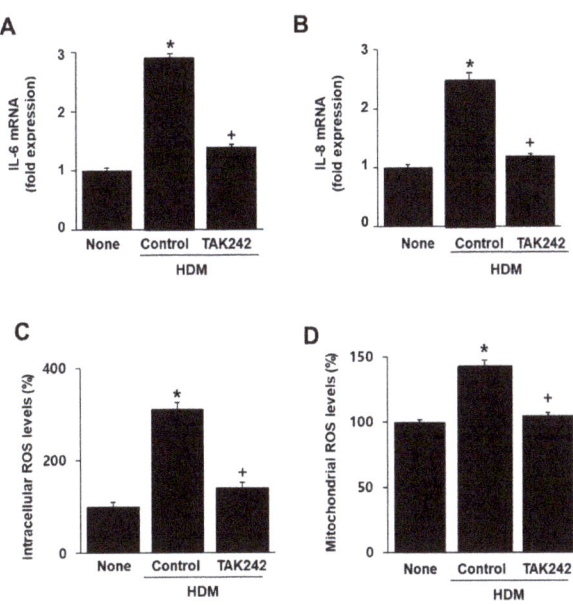

Figure 5. Effects of TAK242 on the mRNA expression of IL-6 and IL-8 and intracellular and mitochondrial ROS levels in human dust mite (HDM)-stimulated A549 cells. (**A,B**) Cells were pretreated with TAK242 (0.5 µM) for 1 h and then treated with HDM (20 µg/mL) for 8 h. mRNA expression of IL-6 and IL-8 was determined with RT-PCR analysis. The mRNA levels in cells without any treatment (none) were set as 1. (**C,D**) Cells were pretreated with TAK242 (0.5 µM) for 1 h and then treated with HDMs (20 µg/mL) for 2 h. (**C**) Intracellular ROS levels were determined using DCF-DA. ROS levels in the cells without any treatment (none) were set as 100%. (**D**) Mitocondrial ROS levels were determined using MitoSOX. ROS levels in the cells without any treatment (none) were set as 100%. All data are shown as the mean ± S.E. of three independent experiments. * $p < 0.05$ vs. none (cells without any treatment); + $p < 0.05$ vs. control (cells with HDM alone).

3. Discussion

Exposure to HDM-allergens induced ROS production in the respiratory epithelial cells of patients with asthma [35]. In airway inflammation, ROS, generated by several inflammatory cells and oxygen metabolites, contributed to epithelial damage. ROS are considered the primary cause of bronchoconstriction, mucus secretion, and increased airway responsiveness [36].

Wang et al. [37] showed that the HDM allergen Der f 1 (Group 1 allergen of *D. farinae*) induces the release of cytokines (IL-25 and IL-33) in airway epithelial cells. Der f 1 increases ROS production and activates mitogen-activated protein kinases (MAPKs) to induce IL-8 expression in human basophilic cells [38]. Der f1 increased ROS production in neutrophils isolated from asthmatic versus non-asthmatic subjects [35]. In a previous study, the intratracheal administration of the HDM allergen Der p 2 (Group 2 allergen of *D. pteronyssinus*) to mice led to inflammatory cell infiltration, mucus gland hyperplasia in the bronchial epithelium, and elevated ROS in bronchoalveolar lavage fluids [39]. Der p2 induced nerve growth factor release and increases ROS levels in LA4 lung epithelial cells [40]. Although the HDM allergens were different, these studies demonstrate the critical role of ROS in HDM-induced respiratory inflammation.

In the present study, we used a standardized extract of *D. farinae* from the Arthropods of Medical Importance Resource Bank (AMIB), Yonsei University (Seoul, Korea). Major allergens are present at a concentration of 17.0 µg/mg (5.0 µg/mg of Der f 1 and 12.0 µg/mg of Der f 2), with the allergy unit (AU) of 12.5 AU/µg for the *D. farinae* extract [41]. Further studies should be performed to determine the effect of lycopene on TLR4 signaling and inflammatory cytokine expression in respiratory epithelial cells exposed to different allergens from HDM, such as Der f 1, Der f 2, Der p 1, and Der p 2, rather than the extract.

Regarding cytokine expression, Jang et al. [42] found that HDM (Der p1) induced the mRNA expression of IL-6 and IL-8 ten times more than TNF-α in THP-1 human monocytic cells. Shi et al. [43] examined the effect of HDM allergen Der p1 on proinflammatory cytokine production (TNF-α, IL-1β, IL-6, IL-8) in cultured primary nasal epithelial cells (NECs) from patients with allergic rhinitis (AR) and control NECs. They found significantly elevated IL-6 and IL-8 production in both NECs after Der p1 stimulation. The levels of IL-6 and IL-8 were 20–100 times higher than that of IL-1β in Der p1-stimulated cells at 24 h-culture. The level of TNF-α was six times higher than that of IL-1β after 24 h-stimulation of HDM. Wong et al. [44] showed that HDM induced the release of IL-6, IL-8, and TNF-α in eosinophils and bronchial epithelial BEAS-2B cells. After 18 h of stimulation with HDM, the levels of IL-6 and IL-8 were seven to eight times higher than that of TNF-α These studies suggest that IL-6 and IL-8 may have critical roles in HDM-associated inflammation compared to TNF-α and IL-1β. Therefore, we assayed for the levels of IL-6 and IL-8 in HDM-stimulated respiratory cells to determine the effects of lycopene. Future studies should determine the expression of various inflammatory cytokines, including TNF-α, MCP-1, and IL-1, β, in cells stimulated with different allergens of HDM.

For the role of the redox-sensitive transcription factor in cytokine expression, Wong et al. [44] demonstrated that the Der p1-induced expression of cytokines is mediated by NF-κB in eosinophils and BEAS-2B cells. We recently showed that the HDM extracts induce the activation of mitogen-activated protein kinases (MAPKs), NF-κB κ, and activator protein-1 in human respiratory epithelial H292 cells [4]. Ascorbic acid suppresses the ROS-mediated activation of MAPKs and transcription factors (NF-κB κ and AP-1) by reducing ROS levels in H292 cells. Therefore, we postulate that lycopene may inhibit these inflammatory signaling pathways and NF-κB, since it decreases ROS levels in HDM-stimulated cells. The anti-inflammatory mechanisms of lycopene should be further examined in HDM-stimulated cells by examining the activities of NF-κB, AP-1, and MAPKs.

Regarding the role of intracellular and mitochondrial ROS in airway inflammation, direct exposure of the human bronchial epithelial cells BEAS-2B to HDM extracts resulted in increased cellular ROS production, mitochondrial oxidative stress, and nitrosative stress [45]. Lowe et al. [46] showed that the mitochondria-targeted antioxidant SS31 reduced airway inflammation in HDM-stimulated mice. They suggested that mitochondrial oxidative stress may contribute to airway hyperresponsiveness and inflammation. These studies support the present findings that HDM (extract of D. farinae) increased both intracellular and mitochondrial ROS levels as well as the expression of IL-6 and IL-8 in respiratory epithelial A549 cells.

HDM induced TRL4 activation and subsequently increased the levels of innate pro-allergic cytokines, granulocyte-macrophage colony stimulating factor, IL-25, and IL-33 in airway structural cells [7]. Additionally, HDM increased TLR 4-mediated infiltration of eosinophils and neutrophils into the lungs of mice [47]. The HDM allergen Derp 2 activated TLR4 and induced IL-6, IL-8, and MCP-1 in THP-1 cells and lymphocytes [48]. These studies demonstrate the relationship between TLR4 and cytokine expression in HDM-stimulated cells.

Upon stimulation, TLR4 is recruited to lipid rafts and subsequently interacts with its adaptor molecules, leading to the activation of downstream targets, such as MAPKs and NF-κB, and the production of pro-inflammatory cytokines in RAW264.7 macrophages [49,50]. This process occurs in an ROS-dependent manner because the inhibition of NADPH oxidase suppresses TLR4 recruitment to lipid rafts [51]. As previously mentioned, Hristova et al. [10] demonstrated that NADPH oxidase DUOX 1 has important role to produce ROS and activate TLR4 in HDM-stimulated airway epithelium. These studies suggest that NADPH oxidase-mediated ROS may be important to recruit TLR4 to lipid rafts and interact with its adaptor proteins for TLR4 signaling.

Zou et al. [31] suggested that lycopene may prevent LPS-induced TLR4 assembly into lipid rafts by reducing intracellular ROS levels in macrophages. Thus, reducing ROS through lycopene may suppress TLR 4 recruitment into lipid rafts and inhibit the activation of downstream signaling pathways, such as MAPKs and NF-κB. Previously, we and others showed that lycopene inhibits NADPH oxidase activity in various cells [32–34]. Therefore, lycopene may inhibit NADPH oxidase in HDM-stimulated cells. Further studies are required to determine whether lycopene suppresses NADPH oxidase and TLR4 recruitment into lipid rafts in the HDM-stimulated cells.

Jiang et al. [34,52] demonstrated that TLR4 is upstream signaling for ROS production and expression of inflammatory cytokines (IL-1β, IL-6 and TNF-α) in lung tissues of LPS-stimulated mice and LPS-stimulated RAW 264.7 macrophages.

Here, we found that lycopene inhibited the activation of TLR4 by reducing the surface levels of TLR4, which increased by HDM stimulation of the cells. TAK242, a TLR4 inhibitor, which disrupts the interaction of TLR4 with adaptor molecules [53], suppressed both intracellular and mitochondrial ROS production and the expression of IL-6 and IL-8 in HDM-stimulated A549 cells. The previous studies and the present finding suggest that ROS activate TLR4 and TLR4 activation increases ROS levels. Therefore, inhibitory effect of TLR4 activation may be caused by antioxidant activity of lycopene in the present study.

Lipid rafts are cell-membrane microdomains composed of cholesterol and sphingolipids, such as monosialotetrahexosylgangliside (GM1), which form a separate liquid-ordered phase in the liquid-disordered matrix of the cell membrane lipid layer [54,55]. Thus, it is essential to determine whether lycopene affects TLR4 localization within membrane lipid rafts by regulating the levels of GM1 in lipid rafts. In addition, it may be necessary to determine the effect of lycopene in the absence or presence of TAK242 to evaluate the synergistic effect of the co-treatment with lycopene and TAK242 in the present system.

Anathy et al. [56] demonstrated that HDM induced mitochondrial fission by increasing fission protein dynamin related protein 1 in human bronchial epithelial cells at 80 min-culture. They showed that HDM exposure increased endoplasmic reticulum-mitochondrial interactions and subsequent mitochondrial fission in bronchial epithelial cells. Therefore, HDM may directly attack mitochondria and mitochondrial dysfunction, which increases mitochondrial ROS.

Lycopene is a potent antioxidant carotenoid that can efficiently quench singlet oxygen species [57]. Tomato and tomato-based products account for 80% of lycopene intake in western countries. Watermelon, pink grapefruit, apricot, and papaya also significantly contribute to lycopene intake [58]. Regarding its anti-inflammatory mechanism, lycopene can neutralize intracellular ROS, as well as reduce the secretion of pro-inflammatory cytokines by macrophages [59]. It decreases monocyte proliferation [60]. In addition, lycopene inhibits mitochondrial ROS production by protecting against stress-induced mitochondrial dysfunction nerve cells [61] and cardiomyocytes [62]. In particular, Zou et al. [31] demonstrated that lycopene suppresses the LPS-stimulated, TLR4-mediated induction of IL-6 expression in macrophages.

Regarding ROS levels and cell viability, we previously showed that treatment with lycopene (0.25 µM) for 24 h reduces the viability (20% reduction in viable cell numbers) and intracellular ROS levels (50% reduction) of pancreatic cancer PANC-1 cells [63]. After 24 h of incubation, lycopene (0.5 µM) did not affect cell viability, but 1 µM lycopene induced apoptosis in gastric cancer AGS cells [64]; 0.5 µM lycopene slightly decreased ROS levels, while 1 µM lycopene significantly decreased ROS levels in AGS cells after 24 h of incubation [64].

Teodoro et al. [65] showed that lycopene (1, 3, and 5 µM) did not affect the viability of A549 cells after 48 h of incubation, but decreased the number of viable cells in three cancer cell lines, including breast, colon, and prostate cell lines (HT-29, T84, and MCF-7), after 48 h. These results showed that the effect of lycopene on cell viability is cell-type specific. Trejo-Solís et al. [66] demonstrated that lycopene treatment could selectively arrest cell growth and induce apoptosis in cancer cells without affecting normal cells. Based on these studies, we postulated that lycopene (0.1 and 0.2 µM) treatment for 16 h, which was used in the present study, may not affect cell viability in A549 cells. Further study should be performed to determine whether the treatment of A549 cells for different time periods with lycopene alone (0.1 and 0.2 µM) affects ROS levels and cell viability (2 h for ROS levels, 8 h for cytokine mRNA level, and 16 h for cytokine protein levels).

Regarding the time point for the determination of ROS levels and TLR4 activity, Zhang et al. [67] demonstrated that mixed HDM allergens increased ROS levels in Calu-3 human airway epithelial cells treated for 2.5 h, which was inhibited by TAK242. Ryu et al. [68] showed that HDM extracts increased the surface TLR4 levels and dual oxidase 2-mediated ROS production in nasal and bronchial epithelial cells after 1 h of incubation. The TLR4 activator CL 097 (2-(ethoxymethyl)-1H-imidazo(4,5-c)quinolin-4-amine) increased the intracellular ROS levels of airway epithelial cells following a 2.5 h incubation. These studies show that increases in ROS are parallel with TLR4 activation in HDM-stimulated respiratory epithelium. In the present study, both intracellular and mitochondrial ROS levels are the most at 2 h. Thus, TRL4 activity was determined after 2 h of stimulation with HDM. For further study, the time-course experiment on TLR4 activity in HDM-stimulated respiratory epithelial cells should be performed.

In the present study, lycopene reduced ROS levels and suppressed TLR4 activation in HDM-stimulated respiratory epithelial A549 cells. Since TLR4 activation leads to increases in intracellular ROS, lycopene may inhibit ROS-mediated inflammatory signaling to induce expression of IL-6 and IL-8 in HDM-stimulated cells. In addition, lycopene reduce mitochondrial ROS and prevents expression of IL-6 and IL-8 which induced by HDM stimulation (Figure 6).

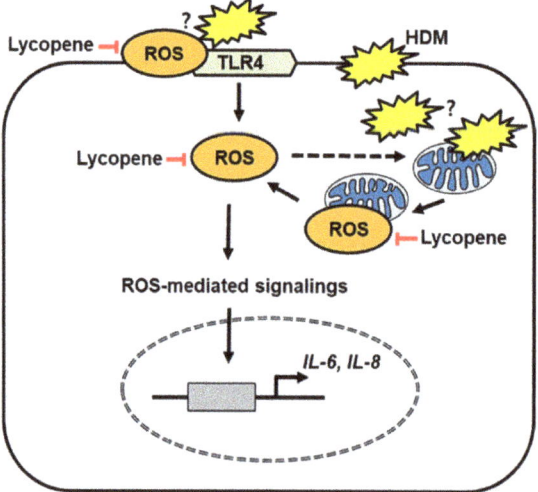

Figure 6. The proposed mechanism by which lycopene inhibits Toll like receptor 4 (TLR4)-mediated expression of inflammatory cytokines in house dust mites (HDM)-stimulated respiratory epithelial cells. HDM may increase the production of reactive oxygen species (ROS) and subsequent TLR4 activation, leading to increasing intracellular ROS levels in the cells. High amounts of ROS may cause mitochondrial dysfunction (dotted line) and increase mitochondrial ROS. In addition, HDM may directly attack mitochondria and increase mitochondrial ROS levels. ROS mediate inflammatory signalings, which induces expression of IL-6 and IL-8. Lycopene reduces ROS levels and inhibits TLR4 activation for cytokine expression. Lycopene scavenges mitochondrial ROS and subsequently suppresses expression of IL-6 and IL-8 in HDM-stimulated respiratory epithelial cells.

Based on the previous studies [6,56] showing that HDM enter the airway epithelium and induce mitochondrial fission, it is necessary to determine whether HDM induce mitochondrial dysfunction by directly interacting with mitochondria for further study. Since HDM stimulate NADPH oxidase in airway epithelial cells [10] and lycopene inhibits NADPH oxidase in various cells [32–34], it should be performed to determine whether lycopene inhibits NADPH oxidase in HDM-stimulated cells.

In conclusion, lycopene inhibits proinflammatory cytokine expression by suppressing HDM-induced increases in intracellular and mitochondrial ROS levels and TLR4 activation. Therefore, it may be considered beneficial for the prevention of respiratory airway inflammation caused by HDM.

4. Materials and Methods

4.1. Reagents

The house dust mite *D. farinae* extract was purchased from the Arthropods of Medical Importance Resource Bank (AMIB), Yonsei University (Seoul, Korea). It was dissolved in PBS and stored at $-80\ °C$. Lycopene (L9879, Sigma-Aldrich, St. Louis, MO, USA) was dissolved in tetrahydrofuran (THF). For the lycopene experiment, cells incubated with THF (less than 0.5%) alone served as the control. The TLR4 inhibitor, TAK242 (614316, Millipore, Burlington, MA, USA) was dissolved in dimethyl sulfoxide (DMSO). For the TAK242 experiment, cells incubated with DMSO (less than 0.3%) alone served as the control.

4.2. Cell Line and Culture Conditions

Human respiratory epithelial (A549) cells were cultured in RPMI-1640 medium (Gibco, Grand Island, NY, USA) supplemented with 10% heat-inactivated fetal bovine serum (Gibco, Grand Island, NY, USA), 100 units/mL penicillin, and 100 μg/mL streptomycin (Sigma-Aldrich). The cells were cultured at $37\ °C$ in a humidified atmosphere of 5% CO_2 and 95% air.

4.3. Quantitative Reverse Transcription-Polymerase Chain Reaction (qRT-PCR) Analysis for IL-6 and IL-8

The cells (6×10^4 cells/well in 6 well plates) were cultured in the absence or presence of HDM for different durations or at different doses of HDM for 8 h. For the effect of lycopene, the cells were pretreated with lycopene (0.1, 0.2, 0.5, and 1.0 μM) or TAK242 (0.5 μM) for 1 h. The mRNA expression of IL-6 and IL-8 was assessed using qRT-PCR. Total RNA was isolated from the cells using TRI reagent (RNA/DNA/Protein isolation reagent, Molecular Research Center Inc., Cincinnati, OH, USA), and converted into cDNA by reverse transcription using a random hexamer and virus reverse transcriptase (Promega, Madison, WI, USA) at $23\ °C$ for 10 min, $37\ °C$ for 60 min, and $95\ °C$ for 5 min. The cDNA was incubated with SYBR Green Real-time PCR Master Mix (Toyobo, Osaka, Japan) that contained 10 pg/mL of forward and reverse primers, and amplified using a Light Cycler PCR system (Roche Applied Sciences, Indianapolis, IN, USA). Real-time PCR was conducted with the following specific primers for IL-6, IL-8, and GAPDH. The sequences of IL-6 primers were: 5-ACAAAT TCG GTACATCCTC-3 for the forward primer and 5-GCAGAATGAGATGAG TTGT-3 for the reverse primer. The sequences of IL-8 primers were: 5-ATGACTTCCAAGCTGGCCGTGGCT-3 for the forward primer and 5-TCTCAG CCCTCTTCAAAAACTTCT-3 for the reverse primer. For GAPDH, the forward primer was 5-GAAGGTGAAGGTCGGAGT-3 and the reverse primer was 5-GAAGATGGTGATGGGATT-3′. The cDNA was amplified by 40 cycles of denaturation at $95\ °C$ for 30 s, annealing at $56\ °C$ for 20 s, and extension at $72\ °C$ for 30 s.

4.4. Enzyme-Linked Immunosorbent Assay (ELISA)

The cells (6×10^4 cells/well in 6 well plates) were pretreated with lycopene (0.1, 0.2 μM) or TAK242 (0.5 μM) and stimulated with HDM (20 μg/mL) for 16 h. The culture supernatants were centrifuged at $10,000 \times g$ for 5 min and then collected to measure IL-6 and IL-8 levels. The latter were determined using an enzyme-linked immunosorbent assay (ELISA) kit (R&D Systems, Inc., Minneapolis, MN, USA) following the manufacturer's instructions.

4.5. Determination of Intracellular ROS and Mitochondrial ROS Levels

For time-course experiment, the cells were treated with HDM (20 µg/mL) and culture for 2 h. For the effect of lycopene or TAK242, the cells were pretreated with lycopene or TAK242 for 1 h and treated with HDM (20 µg/mL) for 2 h. For the determination of intracellular ROS levels, the cells were loaded with 10 µg/mL dichlorofluorescein diacetate (DCF-DA; Sigma-Aldrich) for 30 min. The cells were then washed and scraped off with PBS. The fluorescence intensity of dichlorofluorescein (DCF) was measured using a Victor5 multi-label counter (PerkinElmer Life and Analytical Sciences, Boston, MA, USA) with excitation at 488 nm and emission at 525 nm. ROS trapped in the cells were expressed in terms of a relative increase.

For the determination of mitochondrial ROS levels, the cells were treated with 10 µM MitoSOX (Life Technologies, Grand Island, NY, USA) for 30 min, before being washed and scraped into phosphate-buffered saline (PBS). The intensity of MitoSOX fluorescence at 585 nm (excitation at 524 nm) was measured with a Victor 5 multi-label counter (PerkinElmer Life and Analytical Sciences, Boston, MA, USA).

4.6. Measurement of Surface TLR4 Level

Cells (4×10^5 cells/10-cm dish) were pretreated with lycopene (0.1 and 0.2 µM) for 1 h and then with HDM (20 µg/mL) for 2 h. The cells were washed, scraped off into 1 mL of PBS, and centrifuged at $3000 \times g$ for 5 min. After discarding the supernatants, the cells were resuspended in an ice-cold fluorescence-activated cell sorting (FACS) staining solution (2% FBS; 30 mL of PBS, 0.6 mL of FBS), treated with monoclonal anti-TLR4-MD-2 antibody conjugated with PE (12-9924, Bioscience, San Diego, CA, USA) at 4°C for 30 min, and then centrifuged at $3000 \times g$ for 10 min. This antibody recognizes the complex, but neither TLR4 nor MD-2 alone. After discarding the supernatants, the cells were washed with 500 µL of ice-cold FACS staining solution for 10 min and resuspended in 1 mL of PBS. The fluorescence of PE was measured (488-nm excitation/561-nm emission) using a flow cytometer (FACSVerse, Becton Dickinson and Company, Franklin Lakes, NJ, USA). TLR4 staining represents the surface TLR4 levels.

4.7. Immunofluorescence Staining

To investigate the effect of lycopene on the HDM-induced TLR4 activation, cells were pretreated with lycopene for 1 h, before treatment with HDM for 2 h on glass slides, and then fixed with cold 100% methanol. The fixed cells were blocked for 1 h in a blocking solution and then incubated at 20–22 °C for 1 h with a primary antibody against TLR4 (1:100; SC-10741, Santa Cruz Biotechnology, Dallas, TX, USA). After washing with PBS, the cells were allowed to react with a rhodamine-conjugated mouse anti-rabbit IgG antibody (1:200; SC-2492, Santa Cruz Biotechnology) for 1 h. After removal of the excess of secondary antibody, the cells were washed with PBS and covered with Vectashield antifade mounting medium containing 4,6-diamidino-2-phenylindole (DAPI). The preparations were incubated for 30 min to allow for saturation with DAPI. The cells were stained with rhodamine-conjugated antibody and subsequently examined under a laser scanning confocal microscope (Zeiss LSM700, Carl Zeiss Inc., Thornwood, NY, USA) and photographed.

4.8. Statistical Analysis

One-way analysis of variance followed by the Newman–Keuls post hoc test was used for statistical analysis. All data are reported as the mean ± standard error of three independent experiments. For each experiment, the number of patients in each group was four ($n = 4$ per group). Statistical significance was set at $p < 0.05$.

Author Contributions: Conceptualization: H.K.; investigation, writing, and original draft preparation: J.C.; new reagents and analytical tools: J.L.; writing, review, and editing: H.K. All authors have read and agreed to the published version of the manuscript.

Funding: This research received no external funding.

Institutional Review Board Statement: Not applicable.

Informed Consent Statement: Not applicable.

Data Availability Statement: The data used to support the findings of this study are included in this article.

Acknowledgments: Part of this study was presented at the Joint Conference of the Society for Free Radical Research and the Society of Nutrition and Food Science (SFRR-Europe/SNFS Conference), held at the University of Hohenheim, Stuttgart, Germany, 2–4 September 2015. The abstract of the presentation was published in Free Radical Biology and Medicine 86 (Supplement 1) S21, 2015 (Abstract Number PP7).

Conflicts of Interest: The authors declare no conflict of interest.

Abbreviations

AU	Allergy unit
HDM	House dust mites
DAPI	4′,6-Diamidino-2-phenylindole
DCF	Dichlorofluorescein
DCF-DA	Dichlorofluorescein diacetate
DMSO	Dimethyl sulfoxide
ELISA	Enzyme-linked immunosorbent assay
FACS	Fluorescence-activated single cell sorting
LPS	Lipopolysaccharide
MCP-1	Monocyte chemoattractant protein-1
MD-2	Myeloid differentiation protein 2
NECs	Nasal epithelial cells
PAR-2	Protease activated receptor-2
PE	Phycoerythrin
qRT-PCR	Quantitative reverse transcription-polymerase chain reaction
ROS	Reactive oxygen species
TLR4	Toll-like receptor 4
THF	Tetrahydrofuran
TNF-α	Tumor necrosis factor-α

References

1. Platts-Mills, T.A.; Vervloet, D.; Thomas, W.R.; Aalberse, R.C.; Chapman, M.D. Indoor allergens and asthma: Report of the Third International Workshop. *J. Allergy Clin. Immunol.* **1997**, *100*, S2–S24. [CrossRef]
2. Platts-Mills, T.A.; Carter, M.C. Asthma and Indoor Exposure to Allergens. *N. Engl. J. Med.* **1997**, *336*, 1382–1384. [CrossRef]
3. Ree, H.; Jeon, S.H.; Lee, I.Y.; Hong, C.S.; Lee, D.K. Fauna and geographical distribution of house dust mites in Korea. *Korean J. Parasitol.* **1997**, *35*, 9–17. [CrossRef] [PubMed]
4. Lee, A.J.; Lim, J.W.; Kim, H. Ascorbic Acid Suppresses House Dust Mite-Induced Expression of Interleukin-8 in Human Respiratory Epithelial Cells. *J. Cancer Prev.* **2021**, *26*, 64–70. [CrossRef]
5. Wan, H.; Winton, H.L.; Soeller, C.; Tovey, E.R.; Gruenert, D.C.; Thompson, P.J.; Stewart, G.A.; Taylor, G.W.; Garrod, D.R.; Cannell, M.B.; et al. Der p 1 facilitates transepithelial allergen delivery by disruption of tight junctions. *J. Clin. Investig.* **1999**, *104*, 123–133. [CrossRef] [PubMed]
6. Kim, E.; Joldrichsen, M.R.; Amer, A.O.; Boyaka, P.N. Insights into mucosal innate immune responses in house dust mite-mediated allergic asthma. *Front. Immunol.* **2020**, *11*, 534501.
7. Hammad, H.; Chieppa, M.; Perros, F.; Willart, M.A.; Germain, R.N.; Lambrecht, B.N. House dust mite allergen induces asthma via Toll-like receptor 4 triggering of airway structural cells. *Nat. Med.* **2009**, *15*, 410–416. [CrossRef] [PubMed]
8. Willart, M.A.; Deswarte, K.; Pouliot, P.; Braun, H.; Beyaert, R.; Lambrecht, B.N.; Hammad, H. Interleukin-1alpha controls allergic sensitization to inhaled house dust mite via the epithelial release of GM-CSF and IL-33. *J. Exp. Med.* **2012**, *209*, 1505–1517. [CrossRef]

9. McAlees, J.W.; Whitehead, G.S.; Harley, I.T.; Cappelletti, M.; Rewerts, C.L.; Holdcroft, A.M. Distinct Tlr4-expressing cell compartments control neutrophilic and eosinophilic airway inflammation. *Mucosal Immunol.* **2015**, *8*, 863–873. [CrossRef] [PubMed]
10. Hristova, M.; Habibovic, A.; Veith, C.; Janssen-Heininger, Y.M.; Dixon, A.E.; Geiszt, M.; van der Vliet, A. Airway epithelial dual oxidase 1 mediates allergen-induced IL-33 secretion and activation of type 2 immune responses. *J. Allergy Clin. Immunol.* **2016**, *137*, 1545–1556. [CrossRef] [PubMed]
11. Liu, X.; Pei, C.; Yan, S.; Liu, G.; Liu, G.; Chen, W.; Cui, Y.; Liu, Y. NADPH oxidase 1-dependent ROS is crucial for TLR4 signaling to promote tumor metastasis of non-small cell lung cancer. *Tumor Biol.* **2015**, *36*, 1493–1502. [CrossRef] [PubMed]
12. . Ryan, K.A.; Smith, M.F., Jr.; Sanders, M.K.; Ernst, P.E. Reactive oxygen and nitrogen species differentially regulate Toll-like receptor 4-mediated activation of NF-kappa B and interleukin-8 expression. *IInfect. mmun.* **2004**, *72*, 2123–2130. [CrossRef] [PubMed]
13. Brubaker, S.W.; Bonham, K.S.; Zanoni, I.; Kagan, J.C. Innate immune pattern recognition: A cell biological perspective. *Annu. Rev. Immunol.* **2015**, *33*, 257–290. [CrossRef] [PubMed]
14. Drummond, R.A.; Brown, G.D. The role of Dectin-1 in the host defence against fungal infections. *Curr. Opin. Microbiol.* **2011**, *14*, 392–399. [CrossRef]
15. Deretic, V.; Saitoh, T.; Akira, S. Autophagy in infection, inflammation and immunity. *Nat. Rev. Immunol.* **2013**, *13*, 722–737. [CrossRef]
16. Lamkanfi, M.; Dixit, V.M. Mechanisms and functions of inflammasomes. *Cell* **2014**, *157*, 1013–1022. [CrossRef]
17. Heinrich, P.C.; Castell, J.V.; Andus, T. Interleukin-6 and the acute phase response. *Biochem. J.* **1990**, *265*, 621–636. [CrossRef]
18. Kaplanski, G.; Marin, V.; Montero-Julian, F.; Mantovani, A.; Farnarier, C. IL-6: A regulator of the transition from neutrophil to monocyte recruitment during inflammation. *Trends Immunol.* **2003**, *24*, 25–29. [CrossRef]
19. Tanaka, T.; Kishimoto, T. The biology and medical implications of interleukin-6. *Cancer Immunol. Res.* **2014**, *2*, 288–294. [CrossRef]
20. Atreya, R.; Mudter, J.; Finotto, S.; Müllberg, J.; Jostock, T.; Wirtz, S.; Schütz, M.; Bartsch, B.; Holtmann, M.; Becker, C.; et al. Blockade of interleukin 6 trans signaling suppresses T-cell resistance against apoptosis in chronic intestinal inflammation: Evidence in Crohn disease and experimental colitis in vivo. *Nat. Med.* **2000**, *6*, 583–588. [CrossRef]
21. Roux, J.; McNicholas, C.M.; Carles, M.; Goolaerts, A.; Houseman, B.T.; Dickinson, D.A.; Iles, K.E.; Ware, L.B.; Matthay, M.A.; Pittet, J.-F. IL-8 inhibits cAMP-stimulated alveolar epithelial fluid transport via a GRK2/PI3K-dependent mechanism. *FASEB J.* **2013**, *27*, 1095–1106. [CrossRef]
22. Vlahopoulos, S.; Boldoghm, I.; Casola, A.; Brasierm, A.R. Nuclear factor-kappaB-dependent induction of interleukin-8 gene expression by tumor necrosis factor alpha: Evidence for an antioxidant sensitive activating pathway distinct from nuclear translocation. *Blood* **1999**, *94*, 1878–1889. [CrossRef] [PubMed]
23. Kim, G.Y.; Kim, J.H.; Ahn, S.C.; Lee, H.J.; Moon, D.O.; Lee, C.M.; Park, Y.M. Lycopene suppresses the lipopolysaccharide-induced phenotypic and functional maturation of murine dendritic cells through inhibition of mitogen-activated protein kinases and nuclear factor-κB. *Immunology* **2004**, *113*, 203–211. [CrossRef] [PubMed]
24. Imran, M.; Ghorat, F.; Ul-Haq, I.; Ur-Rehman, H.; Aslam, F.; Heydari, M.; Shariati, M.A.; Okuskhanova, E.; Yessimbekov, Z.; Thiruvengadam, M.; et al. Lycopene as a natural antioxidant used to prevent human health disorders. *Antioxidants* **2020**, *9*, 706. [CrossRef] [PubMed]
25. .Rao, A.V.; Rao, L.G. Carotenoids and human health. *Pharmacol. Res.* **2007**, *55*, 207–216. [CrossRef]
26. Khachik, F.; Carvalho, L.; Bernstein, P.S.; Muir, G.J.; Zhao, D.Y.; Katz, N.B. Chemistry, distribution and metabolism of tomato carotenoids and their impact on human health. *Exp. Biol. Med.* **2002**, *227*, 845–851. [CrossRef]
27. Rao, A.V.; Ray, M.R.; Rao, L.G. Lycopene. *Adv. Food Nutr. Res.* **2006**, *51*, 99–164.
28. Stahl, W.; Schwarz, W.; Sundquist, A.R.; Sies, H. Cis-trans isomers of lycopene and beta-carotene in human serum and tissues. *Arch. Biochem. Biophys.* **1992**, *294*, 173–177. [CrossRef]
29. Saedisomeolia, A.; Moghadam, A.M. Does lycopene decrease the inflammation in airway epithelial cells? *JABS* **2011**, *5*, 81–84.
30. Dong, J.; Li, W.; Cheng, L.-M.; Wang, G.-G. Lycopene attenuates LPS-induced liver injury by inactivation of NF-κB/COX-2 signaling. *Int. J. Clin. Exp. Pathol.* **2019**, *12*, 817–825.
31. Zou, J.; Feng, D.; Ling, W.-H.; Duan, R.-D. Lycopene suppresses proinflammatory response in lipopolysaccharide-stimulated macrophages by inhibiting ROS-induced trafficking of TLR4 to lipid raft-like domains. *J. Nutr. Biochem.* **2013**, *24*, 1117–1122. [CrossRef]
32. Lee, J.; Lim, J.W.; Kim, H. Lycopene inhibits oxidative stress-mediated inflammatory responses in ethanol/palmitoleic acid-stimulated pancreatic acinar AR42J cells. *Int. J. Mol. Sci.* **2021**, *22*, 2101. [CrossRef] [PubMed]
33. Jhou, B.-Y.; Song, T.-Y.; Lee, I.; Hu, M.-L.; Yang, N.-C. Lycopene inhibits metastasis of human liver adenocarcinoma SKHep-1 cells by downregulation of NADPH oxidase 4 protein expression. *J. Agric. Food Chem.* **2017**, *65*, 6893–6903. [CrossRef] [PubMed]
34. Ni, Y.; Zhuge, F.; Nagashimada, M.; Nagata, N.; Xu, L.; Yamamoto, S.; Fuke, N.; Ushida, Y.; Suganuma, H.; Kaneko, S.; et al. Lycopene prevents the progression of lipotoxicity-induced nonalcoholic steatohepatitis by decreasing oxidative stress in mice. *Free Radic. Biol. Med.* **2020**, *152*, 571–582. [CrossRef]
35. Fukunaga, M.; Gon, Y.; Nunomura, S.; Inoue, T.; Yoshioka, M.; Hashimoto, S.; Ra, C. Protease-mediated house dust mite allergen-induced reactive oxygen species production by neutrophils. *Int. Arch. Allergy Immunol.* **2011**, *155*, 104–109. [CrossRef]
36. Barnes, P.J. Reactive oxygen species and airway inflammation. *Free Radic. Biol. Med.* **1990**, *9*, 235–243. [CrossRef]

37. Wang, E.; Liu, X.; Tu, W.; Do, D.C.; Yu, H.; Yang, L.; Zhou, Y.; Xu, D.; Huang, S.-K.; Yang, P.; et al. Benzo(a)pyrene facilitates dermatophagoides group 1 (Der f 1)-induced epithelial cytokine release through aryl hydrocarbon receptor in asthma. *Allergy* **2019**, *74*, 1675–1690. [CrossRef] [PubMed]
38. Yi, M.H.; Kim, H.-P.; Jeong, K.Y.; Kim, C.-R.; Kim, T.Y.; Yong, T.-S. House dust mite allergen Der f 1 induces IL-8 in human basophilic cells via ROS-ERK and p38 signal pathways. *Cytokine* **2015**, *75*, 356–364. [CrossRef]
39. Osterlund, C.; Grönlund, H.; Polovic, N.; Sundström, S.; Gafvelin, G.; Bucht, A. The non-proteolytic house dust mite allergen Der p 2 induce NF-kB and MAPK dependent activation of bronchial epithelial cells. *Clin. Exp. Allergy.* **2009**, *39*, 1199–1208. [CrossRef]
40. Ye, Y.L.; Wu, H.T.; Lin, C.F.; Hsieh, C.Y.; Wang, J.Y.; Liu, F.H.; Ma, C.T.; Bei, C.H.; Cheng, Y.L.; Chen, C.C.; et al. Dermatophagoides pteronyssinus 2 regulates nerve growth factor release to induce airway inflammation via a reactive oxygen species-dependent pathway. *Am. J. Physiol Lung Cell Mol. Physiol.* **2011**, *300*, 216–224. [CrossRef]
41. Jeong, K.Y.; Choi, S.-Y.; Lee, J.-H.; Lee, I.-Y.; Yong, T.-S.; Lee, J.-S.; Hong, C.-S.; Park, J.-W. Standardization of house dust mite extracts in Korea. *Allergy Asthma Immunol. Res.* **2012**, *4*, 346–350. [CrossRef] [PubMed]
42. Jang, J.; Ha, J.-H.; Kim, S.-M.; Kim, W.; Kim, K.; Chung, S.-I.; Yoon, Y. β-catenin mediates the inflammatory cytokine expression induced by the Der p 1 house dust mite allergen. *Mol. Med. Rep.* **2014**, *9*, 633–638. [CrossRef] [PubMed]
43. Shi, J.; Luo, Q.; Chen, F.; Chen, D.; Xu, G.; Li, H. Induction of IL-6 and IL-8 by house dust mite allergen Der p1 in cultured human nasal epithelial cells is associated with PAR/PI3K/NF B signaling. *ORL* **2010**, *72*, 256–265. [CrossRef]
44. Wong, C.K.; Li, M.L.Y.; Wang, C.B.; Ip, W.K.; Tian, Y.P.; Lam, C.W.K. House dust mite allergen Der p 1 elevates the release of inflammatory cytokines and expression of adhesion molecules in co-culture of human eosinophils and bronchial epithelial cells. *Int. Immunol.* **2006**, *18*, 1327–1335. [CrossRef] [PubMed]
45. Chan, T.K.; Tan, W.S.D.; Peh, H.Y.; Wong, W.S.F. Aeroallergens induce reactive oxygen species production and DNA damage and dampen antioxidant responses in bronchial epithelial cells. *J. Immunol.* **2017**, *199*, 39–47. [CrossRef]
46. Lowe, J.; Adcock, I.; Wiegman, C. Oxidative stress and mitochondrial dysfunction in a novel in vivo exacerbation model of severe asthma. *Eur. Res. J.* **2020**, *56*, 4083.
47. Ishii, T.; Niikura, Y.; Kurata, K.; Muroi, M.; Tanamoto, K.; Nagase, T.; Sakaguchi, M.; Yamashita, N. Time-dependent distinct roles of Toll-like receptor 4 in a house dust mite-induced asthma mouse model. *Scand. J. Immunol.* **2018**, *87*, e12641. [CrossRef]
48. Park, B.S.; Lee, N.R.; Kim, M.J.; Kim, S.Y.; Kim, I.S. Interaction of Der p 2 with Toll-like receptor 4 and its effect on cytokine secretion. *Biomed. Sci. Lett.* **2015**, *21*, 152–159. [CrossRef]
49. Akira, S.; Takeda, K. Toll-like receptor signalling. *Nat. Rev. Immunol.* **2004**, *4*, 499–511. [CrossRef] [PubMed]
50. Triantafilou, M.; Miyake, K.; Golenbock, D.T.; Triantafilou, K. Mediators of innate immune recognition of bacteria concentrate in lipid rafts and facilitate lipopolysaccharide-induced cell activation. *J. Cell Sci.* **2002**, *115*, 2603–2611. [CrossRef] [PubMed]
51. Nakahira, K.; Kim, H.P.; Geng, X.H.; Nakao, A.; Wang, X.; Murase, N.; Drain, P.F.; Wang, X.; Sasidhar, M.; Nabel, E.G.; et al. Carbon monoxide differentially inhibits TLR signaling pathways by regulating ROS-induced trafficking of TLRs to lipid rafts. *J. Exp. Med.* **2006**, *203*, 2377–2389. [CrossRef] [PubMed]
52. Jiang, K.; Guo, S.; Zhang, T.; Yang, Y.; Zhao, G.; Shaukat, A.; Wu, H.; Deng, G. Downregulation of TLR4 by miR-181a provides negative feedback regulation to lipopolysaccharide-induced inflammation. *Front. Pharmacol.* **2018**, *9*, 142. [CrossRef] [PubMed]
53. Matsunaga, N.; Tsuchimori, N.; Matsumoto, T.; Ii, M. TAK-242 (resatorvid), a small-molecule inhibitor of Toll-like receptor (TLR) 4 signaling, binds selectively to TLR4 and interferes with interactions between TLR4 and its adaptor molecules. *Mol. Pharmacol.* **2011**, *79*, 34–41. [CrossRef]
54. Sezgin, E.; Levental, I.; Mayor, S.; Eggeling, C. The mystery of membrane organization: Composition, regulation and physiological relevance of lipid rafts. *Nat. Rev. Mol. Cell Biol.* **2017**, *18*, 361–374. [CrossRef] [PubMed]
55. Rissanen, S.; Grzybek, M.; Orłowski, A.; Róg, T.; Cramariuc, O.; Levental, I.; Eggeling, C.; Sezgin, E.; Vattulainen, I. Phase partitioning of GM1 and its bodipy-labeled analog determine their different binding to cholera toxin. *Front. Physiol.* **2017**, *8*, 252. [CrossRef]
56. Anathy, V.; Cunniff, B.; Cahoon, J.M.; Hoffman, S.M.; Taatjes, D.J.; Bouffard, N.A.; Dixon, A.E.; Poynter, M.E.; Heintz, N.H. Endoplasmic reticulum (ER) and mitochondrial interactions modulate house dust mite induced pro-inflammatory response. *Am. J. Res. Crit. Care Med.* **2015**, *191*, A5356.
57. Di Mascio, P.; Kaiser, S.; Sies, H. Lycopene as the most efficient biological carotenoid singlet oxygen quencher. *Arch. Biochem. Biophys.* **1989**, *274*, 532–538. [CrossRef]
58. Maiani, G.; Casto´n, M.J.; Catasta, G.; Toti, E.; Cambrodón, I.G.; Bysted, A.; Granado-Lorencio, F.; Olmedilla-Alonso, B.; Knuthsen, P.; Valoti, M.; et al. Carotenoids: Actual knowledge on food sources, intakes, stability and bioavailability and their protective role in humans. *Mol. Nutr. Food Res.* **2009**, *53*, S194–S218. [CrossRef]
59. Marcotorchino, J.; Romier, B.; Gouranton, E.; Riollet, C.; Gleize, B.; Malezet-Desmoulins, C.; Landrier, J.-F. Lycopene attenuates LPS-induced TNF-α secretion in macrophages and inflammatory markers in adipocytes exposed to macrophage-conditioned media. *Mol. Nutr. Food Res.* **2012**, *56*, 725–732. [CrossRef]
60. McDevitt, T.M.; Tchao, R.; Harrison, E.H.; Morel, D.W. Carotenoids normally present in serum inhibit proliferation and induce differentiation of a human monocyte/macrophage cell line (U937). *J. Nutr.* **2005**, *135*, 160–164. [CrossRef]
61. Sandhir, R.; Mehrotra, A.; Kamboj, S.S. Lycopene prevents 3-nitropropionic acid-induced mitochondrial oxidative stress and dysfunctions in nervous system. *Neurochem. Int.* **2010**, *57*, 579–587. [CrossRef] [PubMed]

62. Yue, R.; Hu, H.; Yiu, K.H.; Luo, T.; Zhou, Z.; Xu, L.; Zhang, S.; Li, K.; Yu, Z. Lycopene protects against hypoxia/reoxygenation-induced apoptosis by preventing mitochondrial dysfunction in primary neonatal mouse cardiomyocytes. *PLoS ONE* **2012**, *7*, e50778. [CrossRef] [PubMed]
63. Jeong, Y.; Lim, J.W.; Kim, H. Lycopene inhibits reactive oxygen species-mediated NF-κB signaling and induces apoptosis in pancreatic cancer cells. *Nutrients.* **2019**, *11*, 762. [CrossRef] [PubMed]
64. Han, H.; Lim, J.W.; Kim, H. Lycopene inhibits activation of epidermal growth factor receptor and expression of cyclooxygenase-2 in gastric cancer cells. *Nutrients.* **2019**, *11*, 2113. [CrossRef] [PubMed]
65. Teodoro, A.J.; Oliveira, F.L.; Martins, N.B.; de Azevedo Maia, G.; Martucci, R.B.; Borojevic, R. Effect of lycopene on cell viability and cell cycle progression in human cancer cell lines. *Cancer Cell Int.* **2012**, *12*, 36. [CrossRef]
66. Trejo-Solís, C.; Chaverri, J.P.; Ramos, M.T.; Farfán, D.; Salgado, A.-C.; Serrano-García, N.; Rico, L.O.; Sotelo, J. Multiple molecular and cellular mechanisms of action of lycopene in cancer inhibition. *Evid-Based-Comp. Alt. Med.* **2013**, *2013*, 705121. [CrossRef]
67. Zhang, J.; Chen, J.; Mangat, S.C.; Perera Baruhupolage, C.; Garrod, D.R.; Robinson, C. Pathways of airway oxidant formation by house dust mite allergens and viral RNA converge through myosin motors, pannexons and Toll-like receptor 4. *Immun. Inflamm. Dis.* **2018**, *6*, 276–296. [CrossRef]
68. Ryu, J.H.; Yoo, J.Y.; Kim, M.J.; Hwang, S.G.; Ahn, K.C.; Ryu, J.C.; Choi, M.K.; Joom, J.H.; Kim, C.H.; Lee, S.N.; et al. Distinct TLR-mediated pathways regulate house dust mite-induced allergic disease in the upper and lower airways. *J. Allergy Clin. Immunol.* **2013**, *131*, 549–561. [CrossRef]

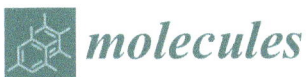

Article

Effect of Korean Red Ginseng and Rg3 on Asian Sand Dust-Induced MUC5AC, MUC5B, and MUC8 Expression in Bronchial Epithelial Cells

Seung-Heon Shin *, Mi-Kyung Ye, Dong-Won Lee, Byung-Jun Kang and Mi-Hyun Chae

Department of Otolaryngology-Head and Neck Surgery, School of Medicine, Catholic University of Daegu, Daegu 42472, Korea; miky@cu.ac.kr (M.-K.Y.); neck@cu.ac.kr (D.-W.L.); rkdqudwns03@naver.com (B.-J.K.); leonen@hanmail.net (M.-H.C.)
* Correspondence: hsseung@cu.ac.kr; Tel.: +82-53-650-4530

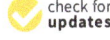

Citation: Shin, S.-H.; Ye, M.-K.; Lee, D.-W.; Kang, B.-J.; Chae, M.-H. Effect of Korean Red Ginseng and Rg3 on Asian Sand Dust-Induced MUC5AC, MUC5B, and MUC8 Expression in Bronchial Epithelial Cells. *Molecules* **2021**, *26*, 2002. https://doi.org/10.3390/molecules26072002

Academic Editors: Sokcheon Pak, Soo Liang Ooi and Carmen Cuadrado

Received: 19 February 2021
Accepted: 25 March 2021
Published: 1 April 2021

Publisher's Note: MDPI stays neutral with regard to jurisdictional claims in published maps and institutional affiliations.

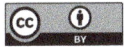

Copyright: © 2021 by the authors. Licensee MDPI, Basel, Switzerland. This article is an open access article distributed under the terms and conditions of the Creative Commons Attribution (CC BY) license (https://creativecommons.org/licenses/by/4.0/).

Abstract: Korean Red ginseng (KRG), commonly used in traditional medicine, has anti-inflammatory, anti- oxidative, and anti-tumorigenic properties. Asian sand dust (ASD) is known to aggravate upper and lower airway inflammatory responses. BEAS-2B cells were exposed to ASD with or without KRG or ginsenoside Rg3. Mucin 5AC (MUC5AC), MUC5B, and MUC8 mRNA and protein expression levels were determined using quantitative RT-PCR and enzyme-linked immunosorbent assay. Nuclear factor kappa B (NF-κB), activator protein 1, and mitogen-activated protein kinase expression and activity were determined using western blot analysis. ASD induced MUC5AC, MUC5B, and MUC8 mRNA and protein expression in BEAS-2B cells, which was significantly inhibited by KRG and Rg3. Although ASD-induced mucin expression was associated with NF-κB and p38 mitogen-activated protein kinase (MAPK) activity, KRG and Rg3 significantly suppressed only ASD-induced NF-κB expression and activity. KRG and Rg3 inhibited ASD-induced mucin gene expression and protein production from bronchial epithelial cells. These results suggest that KRG and Rg3 have potential for treating mucus-producing airway inflammatory diseases.

Keywords: Korean red ginseng; ginsenoside Rg3; bronchial epithelial cell; mucin; transcription factor

1. Introduction

Asian sand dust (ASD), originating from sandstorms in the Gobi Desert and the Ocher Plateau, is inhaled and comes into contact with respiratory epithelial cells, thereby inducing neutrophilic or eosinophilic lung inflammation by stimulating the production of inflammatory mediators [1,2]. The organic and inorganic compounds of ASD, such as SiO_2, Al_2O_3, Fe_2O_3, et al., influence the development of upper and lower airway inflammation, and increased concentration of ASD in the air correlates with asthma severity and adverse respiratory health effects [3]. Particulate matter less than 10 μm (PM10)-main components of ASD- is associated with pulmonary dysfunction, cardiovascular disease, and hepatic fibrogenesis [4,5]. Daily mortality and hospital admission rate increase due to the deterioration of respiratory function during the ASD season [3,6]. ASD influences morbidity and mortality in inflammatory airway diseases by increasing mucin gene expression in upper and lower airway epithelial cells, which causes mucus production, aggravation of respiratory symptoms and severity [7,8].

Mucus overproduction and hypersecretion are frequently observed in several airway diseases. Mucins comprise about 2% of mucus with MUC2, MUC4, MUC5AC, MUC5B, and MUC8 commonly found in airway mucosa. MUC5AC and MUC5B constitute an important component of secretory mucin in airway diseases and are the subjects of frequent study [9,10]. MUC8 mRNA and protein levels were increased in sinus mucosa in chronic rhinosinusitis and in lung of cystic fibrosis, but the physiological functions of MUC8 remain unclear [11,12].

Heat-processing Panax ginseng Meyer converts ginsenoside compounds within the root to yield Korean Red ginseng (KRG). Since red ginseng has higher biological effects and fewer side effects than fresh ginseng, KRG is commonly used in traditional medicine throughout East Asia for its immunomodulatory, anti-allergic, anti-inflammatory, anti-oxidative, and anti-tumorigenic properties [13–15]. Various ginsenosides regulate inflammatory reactions through the regulation of cytokine, chemokine, and cyclooxygenase-2 production [16,17]. KRG is composed of more than 40 ginsenosides, although not all of them significantly affect airway inflammatory responses [17]. Traditional usage suggests that KRG or ginsenosides have therapeutic potential for treating airway inflammatory diseases. Ginsenoside Rg3 (Rg3), a member of protopanaxadiols, is the main component of KRG with anti-inflammatory and anti-cancer properties. Anti-inflammatory effects of Rg3 suppress nitric oxide, reactive oxygen species, prostaglandin E2 and proinflammatory cytokine production [18]. This anti-cancer effect is associated with induction of apoptosis, induction of autophagy, and inhibition of angiogenesis [19]. However, the effects of KRG and Rg3 on mucin production in airway epithelial cells are not commonly studied. In this study, we investigated the effects of KRG and ginsenoside Rg3 on ASD-induced mucin production in bronchial epithelial cells.

2. Results

2.1. The Effects of ASD, KRG, and Rg3 on Cell Viability

To determine the optimal dose of ASD, KRG, and Rg3 and optimal treatment time, we performed a cell proliferation assay. BEAS-2B cells were treated with various concentrations of ASD, KRG, and Rg3 for 24, 48, and 72 h. Cell viability was significantly decreased at 500 and 1000 µg/mL of Rg3 (Figure 1B) and 250 and 500 µg/mL of ASD (Figure 1C) over 24 h incubation, but concentrations less than 500 µg/mL of KRG did not affect the survival (Figure 1A) of BEAS-2B cells. When treated with 50 µg/mL of ASD and 500 µg/mL of KRG or 50 µg/mL of Rg3, bronchial epithelial cells' survival was not significantly affected over 72 h (Figure 1D). Therefore, we used 50 and 100 µg/mL of ASD, 500 µg/mL of KRG, and 50 µg/mL of Rg3 for further experiments. The IC50 values of ASD, KRG, and Rg3 were derived from dose-response curves (24 h: KRG: 995 µg/mL, Rg3 210 µg/mL, and ASD 282 µg/mL; 48 h: KRG 1130 µg/mL, Rg3 148 µg/mL, and ASD 186 µg/mL; 72 h: KRG 613 µg/mL, Rg3 139 µg/mL, and ASD 172 µg/mL, respectively).

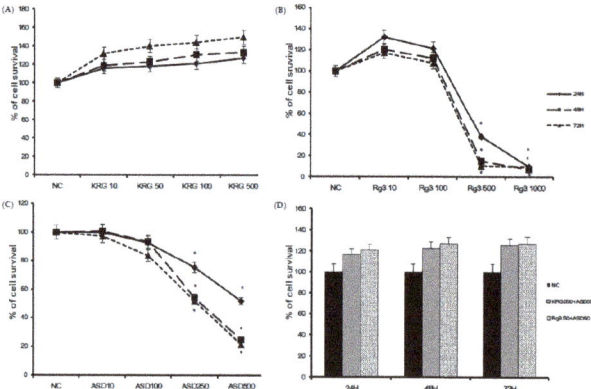

Figure 1. Cell viability of Korean red ginseng (KRG), Rg3, and Asian sand dust (ASD) on bronchial epithelial cells (BEAS-2B) at various concentrations and times using the CellTiter-96® aqueous cell proliferation assay. Cell survival was significantly decreased at 500 µg/mL Rg3 (**B**) and 250 µg/mL ASD (**C**). However, less than 500 µg/mL of KRG (**A**) or 50 µg/mL of ASD and 500 µg/mL of KRG or 50 µg/mL of Rg3 (**D**) did not affect the survival of BEAS-2B cells. *: $p < 0.05$ compared with negative control (NC), $n = 5$.

2.2. The Effects of KRG and Rg3 on ASD Induced MUC5AC, MUC5B, and MUC8 mRNA Expression

When BEAS-2B cells were treated with 100 μg/mL of ASD, MUC5AC, MUC5B, and MUC8 mRNA expression was significantly increased compared to unstimulated cells. In contrast, 50 μg/mL of ASD had no effect on mRNA expression. When the BEAS-2B cells were pretreated with 500 μg/mL of KRG or 50 μg/mL of Rg3, ASD-induced MUC5AC and MUC5B mRNA expression was significantly inhibited (MUC5AC; KRG, 45.9 ± 13.7%, Rg3 42.1 ± 21.4% and MUC5B; KRG 65.6 ± 17.4%, Rg3 56.2 ± 23.2%, respectively). However, KRG and Rg3 did not influence ASD induced MUC8 mRNA expression (Figure 2).

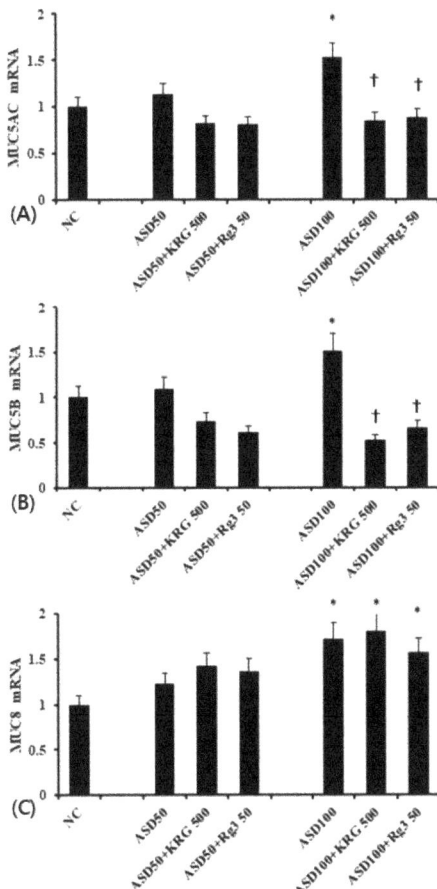

Figure 2. Effects of Korean red ginseng (KRG) and Rg3 on mucin gene expression in bronchial epithelial cells (BEAS-2B). 100 μg/mL Asian sand dust (ASD) significantly enhanced MUC5AC (**A**), MUC5B (**B**), and MUC5B (**C**) mRNA expression in BEAS-2B cells, which was suppressed by Korean red ginseng (KRG) and Rg3. NC; negative control, *; $p < 0.05$ compared with NC, †; $p < 0.05$ compared with ASD stimulated group, $n = 7$.

2.3. The Effects of KRG and Rg3 on ASD Induced MUC5AC, MUC5B, and MUC8 Protein Expression

As with mRNA levels, cells treated with 100 μg/mL of ASD expressed significantly higher levels of MUC5AC, MUC5B, and MUC8 protein than unstimulated cells. 50 μg/mL of ASD again had no effect. When the cells were pretreated with 500 μg/mL of KRG or

50 µg/mL of Rg3, ASD-induced MUC5AC and MUC5B protein levels were significantly decreased (MUC5AC; KRG 25.0 ± 7.3%, Rg3 20.2 ± 6.4%, MUC5B; KRG 22.2 ± 6.7%, Rg3 24.0 ±13.5%, and MUC8; KRG: 23.8 ± 12.1%, Rg3 29.5 ± 9.2%, respectively) (Figure 3).

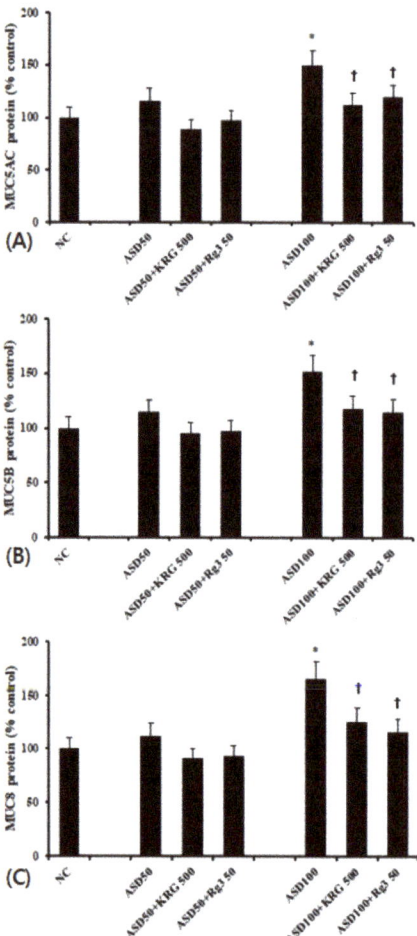

Figure 3. Effects of Korean red ginseng (KRG) and Rg3 on mucin protein expression in bronchial epithelial cells (BEAS-2B). 100 µg/mL Asian sand dust (ASD) significantly enhanced MUC5AC (**A**), MUC5B (**B**), and MUC8 (**C**) protein expression in BEAS-2B cells, which was suppressed by KRG and Rg3. NC; negative control, *; $p < 0.05$ compared with NC, †; $p < 0.05$ compared with ASD stimulated group, $n = 5$.

2.4. The Effects of KRG and Rg3 on ASD-Induced Transcription Factors Expression

Using western blot analysis, we determined the effect of ASD on NF-κB, AP-1, and MAPK transcription factor expression. We found that while ASD enhanced NF-κB and phosphorylated-NF-κB expressions (Figure 4B), it did not affect AP-1 (Figure 4C) and MAPK (Figure 4D) expression. When cells were pretreated with KRG and RG3, ASD-induced increases in NF-κB and phosphorylated-NF-κB expressions were suppressed (Figure 4B).

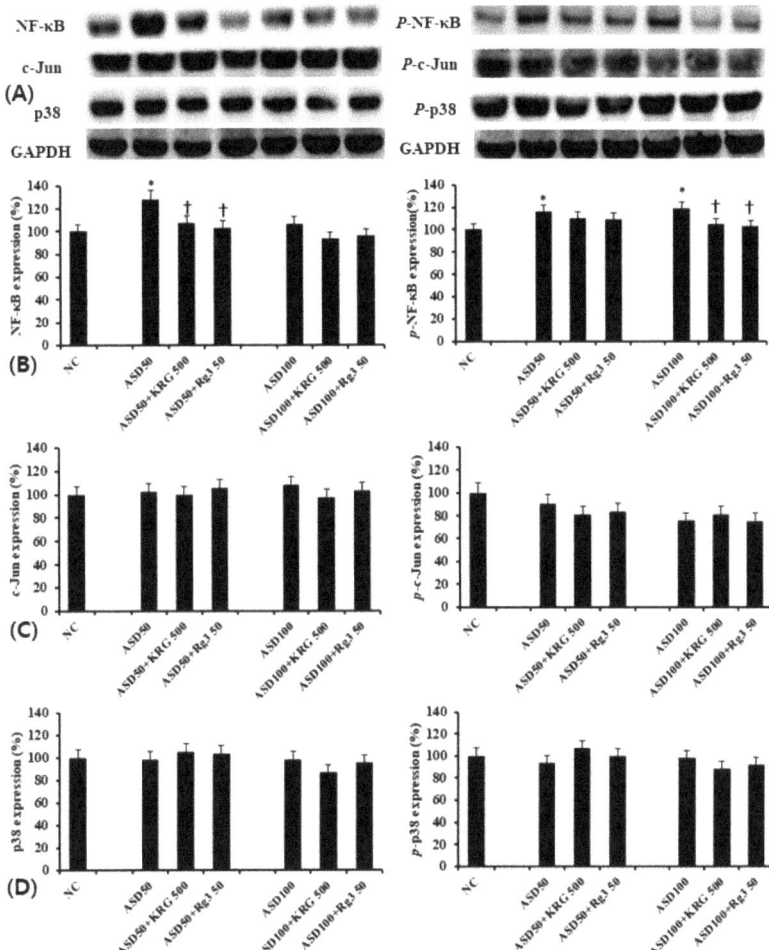

Figure 4. Effects of Korean red ginseng (KRG) and Rg3 on the transcription factor expression in bronchial epithelial cells (BEAS-2B). (**A**) shows representative results of western blot analysis of transcription factors. Asian sand dust (ASD) induced NF-κB and phosphorylated-NF-κB expression, which was significantly inhibited by KRG and Rg3 (**B**). However, KRG and Rg3 did not affect c-Jun (**C**) and p38 (**D**) expressions. NC; negative control, *; $p < 0.05$ compared with NC, †; $p < 0.05$ compared with ASD stimulated group, $n = 5$.

When BEAS-2B cells were pretreated with transcription factor inhibitors, MUC5AC, MUC5B, and MUC8 protein production was significantly and selectively inhibited by NF-κB and p38 MAPK inhibitors (Figure 5).

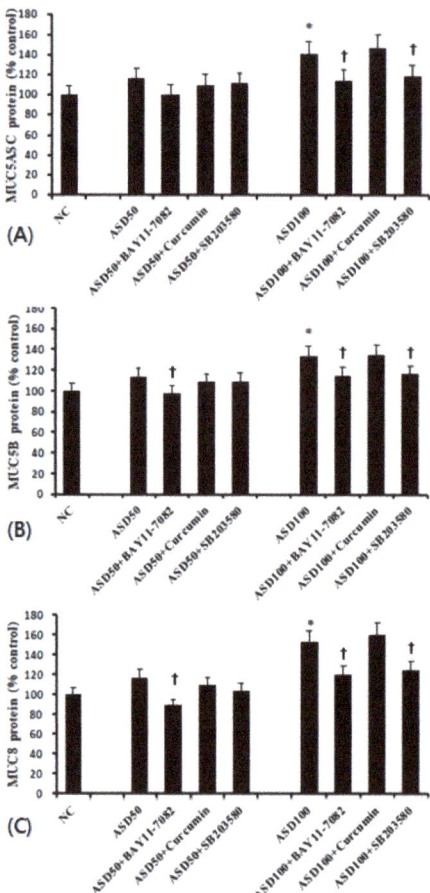

Figure 5. Effects of transcription factor inhibitors on the expression of mucin protein in bronchial epithelial cells (BEAS-2B). ASD-induced MUC5AC (**A**), MUC5B (**B**), and MUC8 (**C**) protein production was significantly inhibited by NF-κB (BAY 11-7082) and p38 MAPK (SB203580) inhibitors. *; $p < 0.05$ compared with NC, †; $p < 0.05$ compared with ASD stimulated group, $n = 5$.

3. Discussion

ASD contains various sizes (0.1–20 μm in diameter) of particles and PM10, fine, and ultrafine particles may influence respiratory inflammatory diseases, such as bronchial asthma, rhinosinusitis, and allergic rhinitis. Mucus hypersecretion is a major pathognomonic finding in both upper and lower airway inflammation. Among the mucin genes, MUC5AC, MUC5B, and MUC8 are the major secretory mucin genes implicated in inflammatory airway diseases [20]. In this study, we found that ASD treatment induced increases in MUC5AC, MUC5B, and MUC8 mRNA and protein expression in bronchial epithelial cells and that these increases were associated with the NF-κB and p38 MAPK pathway. We tested whether KRG and the ginsenoside Rg3 could suppress ASD-induced mucin gene and protein expression in bronchial epithelial cells, finding that they did so through the downregulation of NF-κB.

KRG is known to possess various biological and immunological activities including anti-inflammatory, anti-oxidative, and anti-tumorigenic properties [13–15]. Ginsenosides, the primary active constituents of ginseng, are saponins with steroid-like hydrophobic backbones connected to sugar moieties. Treating fresh ginseng with heat converts it into red ginseng and increases the concentrations of ginsenosides Rg2, Rg3, and Rh1 [21]. KRG and various pure ginsenosides inhibited lung inflammatory responses through the inhibition of MAPK, NF-κB, and c-Fos activation [17]. Although, not all of the ginsenosides isolated from KRG influenced inflammatory responses, Rg3 has an anti-inflammatory effect via the reduction of COX-2, inducible nitric oxide synthase, and proinflammatory cytokines [22,23].Ginsenoside Rb1 was found to inhibit lipopolysaccharide-induced MUC5AC expression in human airway epithelial cells [24]. We evaluated the optimal concentration for the inhibition of mucin gene expression by pretreatment of BEAS-2B cells with various concentrations of KRG (50 to 500 μg/mL) and Rg3 (5 to 50 μg/mL). KRG and RG3 inhibited MUC5AC, MUC5B and MUC8 mRNA expression in a dose dependent manner (data not shown), with 500 μg/mL of KRG and 50 μg/mL of Rg3 used as an optimal dose in this study. ASD-induced MUC MUC5 AC, MUC5B, and MUC8 mRNA and protein expression through NF-κB and p38 MAPK signaling pathways. Inhibition of the ERK, JNK, and AP-1 transcription factors did not influence the production of mucin proteins in these cells. Choi et al. previously reported that ASD-induced MUC5B and MUC8 expression via TLR4-dependent ERK2 and p38 MAPK pathways in NCI-H292 cells and primary nasal epithelial cells [8]. Moreover, ASD-induced the production of ROS and proinflammatory cytokines via the MAPK signaling pathway in nasal fibroblasts [25]. Lipopolysaccharide induced mucus hypersecretion was associated with TLR4 and NF-κB signaling pathway in bronchial epithelial cells [26]. It is thus apparent that ASD leads to the production of chemical mediators or mucus hypersecretion using different pathophysiologic mechanisms dependent on the type of cells studied. Various transcription factors such as NF-κB, AP-1, and ERK2 are responsible for regulation of mucin gene and protein expression in different airway epithelial cells in response to various stimuli [8,24,26]. NF-κB sites on MUC promoters in particular perform a crucial function in regulating MUC expression in bronchial epithelial cells [22]. KRG and ginsenosides show a wide range of anti-inflammatory action, and the mechanisms of action include inhibition of kinase phosphorylation, NF-κB induction, NF-κB translocation, and chemical mediator production [16]. Rg3 exerts an anti-inflammatory effect through the attenuation of the NF-κB signaling pathways in airway epithelial cell and asthmatic airway tissues [22]. This study demonstrates that KRG and Rg3 inhibit ASD-induced MUC5AC, MUC5B, and MUC8 mRNA and protein expression through the inhibition of NF-κB expression and activation independent of P38 MAPK.

KRG contains approximately 40 types of ginsenosides, and other active pharmaceutical constituents. Some ginsenosides are transformed into active metabolites by gut microbiota and are absorbed into the blood before they can exert pharmacological effects, while others have no effect on inflammatory responses of airway epithelial cells [17,27]. Upper and lower airway inflammatory diseases are commonly treated with topical spray or inhalation agents, which make direct contact with airway mucosa to exert pharmacological action. Although we only studied Rg3, the data suggest that it could be a good candidate ginsenoside as a topical treatment to control mucus producing airway diseases.

4. Materials and Methods

4.1. Preparation of KRG and ASD

The standardized water extract of KRG and Rg3 were supplied by the KT&G Corporation (Daejeon, Korea). Panax ginseng Meyer was cultivated for six years in the Korean peninsula. Ginseng roots were collected and dried. KRG was manufactured by steaming and drying white ginseng, and the hot water extract was prepared and provided by KT&G. Ginsenoside Rg3 content was determined by high-performance liquid chromatography. Chemical structure of Rg3 is proposed in Figure 6.

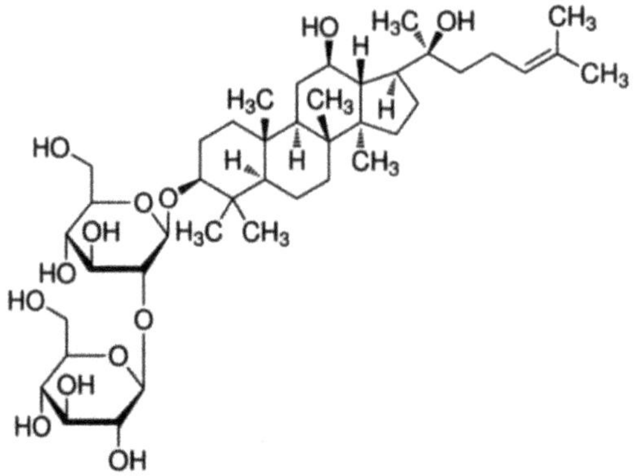

Figure 6. Structure of Rg3.

ASD was collected from air dust using a high-volume air sampler (HV-500F, Sibata, Japan), during an ASD warning period in Incheon. After the dust was collected, the filter paper was washed with 10 mL of phosphate buffer solution (PBS). The fluid was filtered and the particulate matter were collected and then centrifuged. The collected ASD material was placed in a 1.5-mL tube and sterilized at 121 °C for 15 min. The sterilized ASD was stored in a −20 °C freezer.

4.2. Bronchial Epithelial Cell Culture and Cytotoxic Effect of ASD

Human bronchial epithelial BEAS-2B cells, transformed by adenovirus, were purchased from American Type Culture Collection (Rockville, MD, USA). Epithelial cells were cultured with DMEM/F12 medium supplemented with 100 international units of penicillin, 100 μg/mL streptomycin, 2 μg/mL of amphotericin B, and heat-inactivated 10% fetal bovine serum (Invitrogen, Carlsbad, CA, USA) at 37 °C and 5% CO_2. Cell suspensions at 5×10^4 cells/well were grown to 80% confluence for further studies.

To determine the cytotoxic effects of ASD, BEAS-2B cells were incubated with 0, 10, 100, or 500 μg/mL of ASD for 72 h. Cell cytotoxicity was determined using a CellTiter-96® aqueous one solution cell proliferation assay kit (Promega, Madison, WI, USA). For this assay, tetrazolium compound and phenazine etho-sulfate were added to each well and incubated for 4 h at 37 °C in a 5% CO_2 chamber. Color intensities were assessed using a microplate reader at wavelength of 490 nm. The cytotoxic effects of KRG (0 to 500 μg/mL) and Rg3 (0 to 1000 μg/mL) were also determined using a CellTiter-96® aqueous one solution cell proliferation assay kit (Promega).

4.3. The Effect of KRG and Rg3 on ASD-Induced MUC5AC, MUC5B, and MUC8 mRNA Expression

MUC5AC, MUC5B, and MUC8 mRNA expression was measured after stimulation with 50 or 100 μg/mL of ASD for 48 h. To determine the effects of KRG and Rg3 on mucin gene expression, BEAS-2B cells were pretreated with 500 μg/mL of KRG or 50 μg/mL of Rg3 for 1 h. The cells were treated with 1 mL of TRIzole reagent (Roche Diagnostics, Mannheim, Germany), and RNA was extracted. Then RNA was treated with DNase to remove any contamination of DNA. RNA purity and concentration were measured using a spectrophotometer (Beckman, Mountain View, CA, USA). From amplified cDNA, quantitative polymerase chain reaction (PCR) of MUC5AC, MUC5B, MUC8 and β-actin in the same 96 well plate using a SYBR green PCR core kit (PE Applied Biosystems, Foster, CA, USA) was performed with the GeneAmp 5700 system (PE Applied Biosystems). The primer sequences and amplified products were as follows: MUC5AC sense 5′-TCA TCA TCC AGC AGG GCT-3′ and antisense 5′-CCG AGC TCA GAG GAC ATA TGG G-3′ (103 bp), MUC5B sense 5′-TGC CCC TTG TTC TGT GAC TT-3′ and antisense 5′-ACG CAC TTC ATC TGG

TCC TC-3' (194 bp), MUC8 sense 5'-GAC AGG GTT TCT CCT CAT TG-3' and antisense 5'-CGT TTA TTC CAG CAC TGT TC-3' (240 bp), and β-actin sense 5'-ACA GGA AGT CCC TTG CCA TC-3' and antisense 5'-AGG GAG ACC AAA AGC CTT CA-3' (248 bp). The annealing temperature was 54 °C for MUC5B, 60 °C for MUC5AC, and 56 °C for MUC8.

All samples were amplified in triplicate. mRNA expression levels were normalized to the median value of the endogenous control β-actin. The relative quantitation of mRNA levels was determined using the relative quantification 2-delta delta CT method.

4.4. The Effect of KRG and Rg3 on ASD Induced MUC5AC, MUC5B, and MUC8 Protein Production

MUC5AC, MUC5B, and MUC8 protein levels were determined using an enzyme linked immunosorbent assay (ELISA). BEAS-2B cell lysates were prepared at multiple dilutions and incubated at 40 °C until dry. Plates were washed with PBS and blocked with 2% bovine serum albumin. Thereafter, plates were incubated with 1:200 diluted MUC5AC, MUC5B, and MUC8 primary antibodies (Santa Cruz Biotechnology, Santa Cruz, CA, USA) in PBS containing 0.05% Tween 20 for 1 h. The wells were washed with PBS, and then incubated horseradish peroxidase-conjugated secondary antibodies for 4 h. Color was developed with a 3, 3', 5, 5'-tetramethylbenzidine peroxidase solution and stopped with 2N H2SO4. Optical densities were measured for absorbance at 450 nm. Results were expressed as the ratio of baseline controls.

4.5. The Effect of KRG and Rg3 on ASD Induced Transcription Factor Expression

After 1 h exposure with ASD and KRG or Rg3, BEAS-2B cells were harvested and lysed in an ice-cold lysis buffer (Thermo Scientific, Rockford, IL USA). Collected whole cell lysates were subjected to sodium dodecyl sulfate polyacrylamide gel electrophoresis to separate protein and transferred onto a nitrocellulose membrane (Bio-Rad, Berkeley, CA, USA). The membranes were blocked with 5% skim milk solution and incubated with the following antibodies against nuclear factor kappa B (NF-κB): phosphorylated NF-κB, C-Jun, phosphorylated C-Jun, p38, phosphorylated p38, ERK, phosphorylated ERK, JNK, phosphorylated JNK, and GAPDH (Santa Cruz Biotechnology). After 1 h incubation, membranes were washed with Tris-buffered saline with 0.1% Tween 20 and then treated with peroxidase-conjugated anti-rabbit immunoglobulin G (Santa Cruz Biotechnology). Bands were visualized using horseradish peroxidase conjugated secondary antibodies and an enhanced chemiluminescence system (Pierce, Rockford, IL, USA). Band densities were measured using the multi Gauge v.2.02 software (Fujifilm, Tokyo, Japan) and expressed as a percentage of treated versus untreated cells.

4.6. Effects of Transcription Factor Inhibitors on MUC5AC, MUC5B, and MUC8 Protein Expression

BEAS-2B cells were pretreated with the NF-κB inhibitor BAY 11-7082, the activator protein-1 (AP-1) inhibitor curcumin, the p38 inhibitor SB203580, the ERK inhibitor PD98059, and the JNK inhibitor SP600125 to interrogate the MAPK pathway (Calbiochem, San Diego, CA, USA). After a 1-h treatment, cells were stimulated with ASD for 48 h and then MUC5AC, MUC5B, and MUC8 protein expression determined using an ELISA method.

4.7. Statistical Analysis

All experiments were performed in triplicate and repeated at least five times with comparable results. Results are presented as mean ± standard deviation. Statistical significance to determine the cytotoxic effects of ASD and KRG or Rg3 was determined using single-factor repeated measure analysis. Student's t-test was used for comparisons between two groups, while data comparisons between several groups were made using one-way analysis of variance (ANOVA) followed by Turkey's test (SPSS ver. 21.0; IBM Corp., Armonk, NY, USA). A p-value of 0.05 or less was considered statistically significant.

5. Conclusions

This study demonstrated that KRG and Rg3 suppressed ASD-induced MUC5AC, MUC5B, and MUC8 mRNA and protein expression in BEAS2B bronchial epithelial cells through the inhibition of NF-κB. These results provide basic mechanistic information about the inhibition of mucus production by KRG and Rg3 associated with ASD-induced mucus hypersecretion. These results suggest that KRG and Rg3 could be used as a treatment strategy in patients with ASD-related mucus producing airway inflammatory diseases.

Author Contributions: Conceptualization, S.-H.S.; methodology, S.-H.S., and M.-H.C.; formal analysis, M.-K.Y.; investigation, B.-J.K. and M.-H.C.; data curation, S.-H.S.; writing—original draft preparation, D.-W.L.; writing—review and editing, S.-H.S.; visualization, M.-K.Y. and B.-J.K.; supervision, S.-H.S.; project administration, M.-K.Y.; funding acquisition, S.-H.S. All authors have read and agreed to the published version of the manuscript.

Funding: This work was supported by (2019) grant from Korea Society of Ginseng.

Institutional Review Board Statement: Not applicable.

Informed Consent Statement: Not applicable.

Data Availability Statement: The data presented in this study are available on request from the corresponding author.

Conflicts of Interest: The authors declare no conflict of interest.

Sample Availability: Samples of the compounds are not available from the authors.

References

1. Lei, Y.C.; Chan, C.C.; Wang, P.Y.; Lee, C.T.; Cheng, T.J. Effects of Asian dust event particles on inflammation markers in peripheral blood and bronchoalveolar lavage in pulmonary hypertensive rats. *Environ. Res.* **2004**, *95*, 71–76. [CrossRef]
2. Shin, S.H.; Ye, M.K.; Hwang, Y.J.; Kim, S.T. The effect of Asian sand dust-activated respiratory epithelial cells on activation and migration of eosinophils. *Inhal. Toxicol.* **2013**, *25*, 633–639. [CrossRef]
3. Hasunuma, H.; Takeuchi, A.; Ono, R.; Amimoto, Y.; Hwang, Y.H.; Uno, I.; Shimizu, A.; Nishiwaki, Y.; Hashizume, M.; Askew, D.J.; et al. Effect of Asian dust on respiratory symptoms among children with and without asthma, and their sensitivity. *Sci. Total Environ.* **2020**, *753*, 141585. [CrossRef]
4. Rosenlund, M.; Forastiere, F.; Porta, D.; De Sario, M.; Badaloni, C.; Perucci, C.A. Traffic-related air pollution in relation to respiratory symptoms, allergic sensitisation and lung function in schoolchildren. *Thorax* **2009**, *64*, 573–580. [CrossRef]
5. Zheng, Z.; Zhang, X.; Wang, J.; Dandekar, A.; Kim, H.; Qiu, Y.; Xu, X.; Cui, Y.; Wang, A.; Chen, L.C.; et al. Exposure to fine airborne particulate matters induces hepatic fibrosis in murine models. *J. Hepatol.* **2015**, *63*, 1397–1404. [CrossRef]
6. Chen, Y.S.; Sheen, P.C.; Chen, E.R.; Liu, Y.K.; Wu, T.N.; Yang, C.Y. Effects of Asian dust storm events on daily mortality in Taipei, Taiwan. *Environ. Res.* **2004**, *95*, 151–155. [CrossRef] [PubMed]
7. Kim, S.T.; Ye, M.K.; Shin, S.H. Effects of Asian sand dust on mucin gene expression and activation of nasal polyp epithelial cells. *Am. J. Rhinol. Allergy* **2011**, *25*, 303–306. [CrossRef] [PubMed]
8. Choi, Y.S.; Bae, C.H.; Song, S.Y.; Kim, Y.D. Asian sand dust increases MUC8 and MUC5B expressions via TLR4-dependent ERK2 and p38 MAPK in human airway epithelial cells. *Am. J. Rhinol. Allergy* **2015**, *29*, 161–165. [CrossRef] [PubMed]
9. Bonser, L.R.; Erle, D.J. Airway Mucus and Asthma: The Role of MUC5AC and MUC5B. *J. Clin. Med.* **2017**, *6*, 112. [CrossRef]
10. Tong, J.; Gu, Q. Expression and Clinical Significance of Mucin Gene in Chronic Rhinosinusitis. *Curr. Allergy Asthma Rep.* **2020**, *20*, 63. [CrossRef]
11. Lee, H.M.; Kim, D.H.; Kim, J.M.; Lee, S.H.; Hwang, S.J. MUC8 mucin gene up-regulation in chronic rhinosinusitis. *Ann. Otol. Rhinol. Laryngol.* **2004**, *113*, 662–666. [CrossRef]
12. Finkbeiner, W.E.; Zlock, L.T.; Morikawa, M.; Lao, A.Y.; Dasari, V.; Widdicombe, J.H. Cystic fibrosis and the relationship between mucin and chloride secretion by cultures of human airway gland mucous cells. *Am. J. Physiol. Lung Cell. Mol. Physiol.* **2011**, *301*, L402–L414. [CrossRef] [PubMed]
13. Kee, J.Y.; Jeon, Y.D.; Kim, D.S.; Han, Y.H.; Park, J.; Youn, D.H.; Kim, S.J.; Ahn, K.S.; Um, J.Y.; Hong, S.H. Korean Red Ginseng improves atopic dermatitis-like skin lesions by suppressing expression of proinflammatory cytokines and chemokines in vivo and in vitro. *J. Ginseng Res.* **2017**, *41*, 134–143. [CrossRef] [PubMed]
14. Kang, S.W.; Park, J.H.; Seok, H.; Park, H.J.; Chung, J.H.; Kim, C.J.; Kim, Y.O.; Han, Y.R.; Hong, D.; Kim, Y.S.; et al. The Effects of Korea Red Ginseng on Inflammatory Cytokines and Apoptosis in Rat Model with Chronic Nonbacterial Prostatitis. *Biomed. Res. Int.* **2019**, *2019*, 2462561. [CrossRef] [PubMed]

15. Kee, J.Y.; Han, Y.H.; Mun, J.G.; Park, S.H.; Jeon, H.D.; Hong, S.H. Effect of Korean Red Ginseng extract on colorectal lung metastasis through inhibiting the epithelial-mesenchymal transition via transforming growth factor-beta1/Smad-signaling-mediated Snail/E-cadherin expression. *J. Ginseng Res.* 2019, 43, 68–76. [CrossRef] [PubMed]
16. Shergis, J.L.; Di, Y.M.; Zhang, A.L.; Vlahos, R.; Helliwell, R.; Ye, J.M.; Xue, C.C. Therapeutic potential of Panax ginseng and ginsenosides in the treatment of chronic obstructive pulmonary disease. *Complement. Ther. Med.* 2014, 22, 944–953. [CrossRef] [PubMed]
17. Lee, J.H.; Min, D.S.; Lee, C.W.; Song, K.H.; Kim, Y.S.; Kim, H.P. Ginsenosides from Korean Red Ginseng ameliorate lung inflammatory responses: Inhibition of the MAPKs/NF-kappaB/c-Fos pathways. *J. Ginseng Res.* 2018, 42, 476–484. [CrossRef]
18. Im, D.S. Pro-Resolving Effect of Ginsenosides as an Anti-Inflammatory Mechanism of Panax ginseng. *Biomolecules* 2020, 10, 444. [CrossRef]
19. Nakhjavani, M.; Hardingham, J.E.; Palethorpe, H.M.; Tomita, Y.; Smith, E.; Price, T.J.; Townsend, A.R. Ginsenoside Rg3: Potential Molecular Targets and Therapeutic Indication in Metastatic Breast Cancer. *Medicines* 2019, 6, 17. [CrossRef]
20. Turner, J.; Jones, C.E. Regulation of mucin expression in respiratory diseases. *Biochem. Soc. Trans.* 2009, 37, 877–881. [CrossRef]
21. Lee, S.M.; Bae, B.S.; Park, H.W.; Ahn, N.G.; Cho, B.G.; Cho, Y.L.; Kwak, Y.S. Characterization of Korean Red Ginseng (Panax ginseng Meyer): History, preparation method, and chemical composition. *J. Ginseng Res.* 2015, 39, 384–391. [CrossRef] [PubMed]
22. Lee, I.S.; Uh, I.; Kim, K.S.; Kim, K.H.; Park, J.; Kim, Y.; Jung, J.H.; Jung, H.J.; Jang, H.J. Anti-Inflammatory Effects of Ginsenoside Rg3 via NF-kappaB Pathway in A549 Cells and Human Asthmatic Lung Tissue. *J. Immunol. Res.* 2016, 2016, 7521601. [CrossRef] [PubMed]
23. Lee, B.; Sur, B.; Park, J.; Kim, S.H.; Kwon, S.; Yeom, M.; Shim, I.; Lee, H.; Hahm, D.H. Ginsenoside rg3 alleviates lipopolysaccharide-induced learning and memory impairments by anti-inflammatory activity in rats. *Biomol. Ther.* 2013, 21, 381–390. [CrossRef] [PubMed]
24. Kim, Y.D.; Choi, Y.S.; Na, H.G.; Song, S.Y.; Bae, C.H. Ginsenoside Rb1 attenuates LPS-induced MUC5AC expression via the TLR4-mediated ERK1/2 and NF-kappaB pathway in human airway epithelial NCI-H292 cells. *J. Biol. Regul. Homeost. Agents* 2020, 34, 613–618. [CrossRef]
25. Yang, H.W.; Park, J.H.; Shin, J.M.; Lee, H.M.; Park, I.H. Asian Sand Dust Upregulates IL-6 and IL-8 via ROS, JNK, ERK, and CREB Signaling in Human Nasal Fibroblasts. *Am. J. Rhinol. Allergy* 2020, 34, 249–261. [CrossRef] [PubMed]
26. Shang, J.; Liu, W.; Yin, C.; Chu, H.; Zhang, M. Cucurbitacin E ameliorates lipopolysaccharide-evoked injury, inflammation and MUC5AC expression in bronchial epithelial cells by restraining the HMGB1-TLR4-NF-kappaB signaling. *Mol. Immunol.* 2019, 114, 571–577. [CrossRef] [PubMed]
27. Kim, J.K.; Choi, M.S.; Jeung, W.; Ra, J.; Yoo, H.H.; Kim, D.H. Effects of gut microbiota on the pharmacokinetics of protopanaxadiol ginsenosides Rd, Rg3, F2, and compound K in healthy volunteers treated orally with red ginseng. *J. Ginseng Res.* 2020, 44, 611–618. [CrossRef]

Article

β-Carotene Inhibits Expression of Matrix Metalloproteinase-10 and Invasion in *Helicobacter pylori*-Infected Gastric Epithelial Cells

Suji Bae, Joo Weon Lim and Hyeyoung Kim *

Department of Food and Nutrition, BK21 FOUR, College of Human Ecology, Yonsei University, Seoul 03722, Korea; sestnwlrk@naver.com (S.B.); jwlim11@yonsei.ac.kr (J.W.L.)
* Correspondence: kim626@yonsei.ac.kr; Tel.: +82-2-2123-3125; Fax: +82-2-364-5781

Abstract: Matrix metalloproteinases (MMPs), key molecules of cancer invasion and metastasis, degrade the extracellular matrix and cell–cell adhesion molecules. MMP-10 plays a crucial role in *Helicobacter pylori*-induced cell-invasion. The mitogen-activated protein kinase (MAPK) signaling pathway, which activates activator protein-1 (AP-1), is known to mediate MMP expression. Infection with *H. pylori*, a Gram-negative bacterium, is associated with gastric cancer development. A toxic factor induced by *H. pylori* infection is reactive oxygen species (ROS), which activate MAPK signaling in gastric epithelial cells. Peroxisome proliferator-activated receptor γ (PPAR-γ) mediates the expression of antioxidant enzymes including catalase. β-Carotene, a red-orange pigment, exerts antioxidant and anti-inflammatory properties. We aimed to investigate whether β-carotene inhibits *H. pylori*-induced MMP expression and cell invasion in gastric epithelial AGS (gastric adenocarcinoma) cells. We found that *H. pylori* induced MMP-10 expression and increased cell invasion via the activation of MAPKs and AP-1 in gastric epithelial cells. Specific inhibitors of MAPKs suppressed *H. pylori*-induced MMP-10 expression, suggesting that *H. pylori* induces MMP-10 expression through MAPKs. β-Carotene inhibited the *H. pylori*-induced activation of MAPKs and AP-1, expression of MMP-10, and cell invasion. Additionally, it promoted the expression of PPAR-γ and catalase, which reduced ROS levels in *H. pylori*-infected cells. In conclusion, β-carotene exerts an inhibitory effect on MAPK-mediated MMP-10 expression and cell invasion by increasing PPAR-γ-mediated catalase expression and reducing ROS levels in *H. pylori*-infected gastric epithelial cells.

Keywords: β-carotene; gastric epithelial cells; *Helicobacter pylori*; invasion; matrix metalloproteinases; peroxisome-proliferator activator receptor-γ; reactive oxygen species

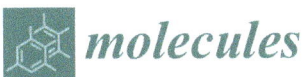

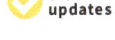

Citation: Bae, S.; Lim, J.W.; Kim, H. β-Carotene Inhibits Expression of Matrix Metalloproteinase-10 and Invasion in *Helicobacter pylori*-Infected Gastric Epithelial Cells. *Molecules* 2021, 26, 1567. https://doi.org/10.3390/molecules26061567

Academic Editor: Sokcheon Pak

Received: 4 February 2021
Accepted: 10 March 2021
Published: 12 March 2021

Publisher's Note: MDPI stays neutral with regard to jurisdictional claims in published maps and institutional affiliations.

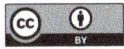

Copyright: © 2021 by the authors. Licensee MDPI, Basel, Switzerland. This article is an open access article distributed under the terms and conditions of the Creative Commons Attribution (CC BY) license (https://creativecommons.org/licenses/by/4.0/).

1. Introduction

Helicobacter pylori (*H. pylori*) is a Gram-negative bacterium that infects nearly half of the world's population. It is a human pathogen that causes stomach diseases such as gastric inflammation, ulcers, and gastric cancer [1]. *H. pylori* infection enhances the migration and invasion of gastric cells, which is closely associated with gastric cancer development [2]. Matrix metalloproteinases (MMPs) are zinc-dependent proteinases that can degrade the extracellular matrix (ECM) and cell–cell adhesion molecules [3]. They can promote cancer progression by increasing cancer-cell growth, migration, invasion, and metastasis. Among these, invasion is an important feature of malignant cancer progression [4]. *H. pylori* infection increases the expression and secretion of various MMPs, including MMP-1 [5,6], MMP-9 [7,8], MMP-7 [9], and MMP-10 [6,10], in the gastric epithelial cells or gastric cancer cells.

Among the MMPs, MMP-10 cleaves numerous ECM components, including fibronectin, proteoglycans, gelatins, and collagens [11]. Since MMPs are synthesized as inactive zymogens (proMMP) and subsequently activated by many factors to degrade the ECM, the activation of pro-MMP is linked to cancer development. MMP-10 cleaves pro-MMPs, including proMMP-1, proMMP-7, and proMMP-9 [12–14]. Therefore, the expression of MMP-10 has a critical role in cancer cell invasion. As signaling pathways for MMP expression, *H. pylori* infection induces MMP-1 expression via c-Jun N-terminal kinase (JNK) and extracellular-signal-regulated kinase (ERK) pathways in gastric cancer cells [5] and MMP-10 expression via the ERK pathway in gastric epithelial cells. [10].

H. pylori increases the production of reactive oxygen species (ROS) in gastric epithelial cells, which affects signal transduction in the gastric epithelia, resulting in gastric carcinogenesis [15–17]. ROS mediate *H. pylori*-induced activation of mitogen-activated protein kinases (MAPKs). Activated MAPKs (JNK, p38, and ERK) translocate to the nucleus, where they regulate the activity of transcription factors, including activator protein-1 (AP-1) [18–20]. As one of the MMP inducers, ROS upregulate MMPs by regulating both gene expression and proenzyme activation [21,22]. In cancer cells, ROS increase MMP activity by growth factor stimulation [21]. The AP-1 plays a dominant role in the transcriptional activation of MMP promoters [23]. These studies suggest the ROS-MAPKs-AP-1 MMPs axis in *H. pylori*-infected gastric epithelial cells. Therefore, reducing ROS levels in the infected tissues/cells may prevent *H. pylori*-induced MMP expression which leads to cell invasion.

Peroxisome-proliferator activator receptor gamma (PPAR-γ) is a ligand-activated nuclear receptor transcription factor that modulates inflammatory activity [24]. PPAR-γ is expressed and functionally active in gastric epithelial cells. Previously, we showed that PPAR-γ regulates the oxidative stress-induced inflammatory response by inducing the expression of antioxidant enzymes, such as catalase, in *H. pylori*-infected gastric epithelial cells [25]. Several studies have demonstrated the inhibitory effect of PPAR-γ ligands or activators on MMP-2 and MMP-9 expression in human myeloid leukemia cells [26] and human bronchial epithelial cells [27]. Taken together, decreasing ROS may be caused by the activation and expression of PPAR-γ-target gene catalase, which may reduce MMP expression in *H. pylori*-infected gastric epithelial cells.

β-Carotene is a red-orange pigment, which is abundant in fungi, plants, and fruits. It is a tetra-terpenoid consisting of a C40 structure including two β-ionone rings. It is among the most frequently consumed dietary carotenoids in human subjects [28,29] and ranking among the highest in serum concentrations [29,30]. Dietary β-carotene is cleaved at its central double bond to yield retinal by β-carotene 15,15′-dioxygenase. Retinal can be converted to retinol (the main active form of vitamin A in the blood). Retinol is oxidized to the biologically active hormone all-trans retinoic acid after delivery to peripheral cells via two steps: first, retinol dehydrogenase (which catalyzes oxidation of retinol to retinal), and second, retinal dehydrogenase (which oxidizes retinal to retinoic acid), respectively [31]. In addition to the conversion to retinal, β-carotene shows potent antioxidant activity by directly quenching singlet oxygen and lipid peroxides [32,33].

β-Carotene inhibits lung metastasis in mice by scavenging free radicals [34]. We previously demonstrated that β-carotene inhibits *H. pylori*-induced hyper-proliferation of gastric epithelial cells by suppressing β-catenin signaling and oncogene expression [35] and inducible nitric oxide synthase and cyclooxygenase-2 by reducing ROS levels [36]. Since ROS activate MAPKs and AP-1, the antioxidant effect of β-carotene may suppress *H. pylori*-induced MAPK and AP-1 signaling in AGS cells.

It has been shown that β-carotene upregulates the PPAR-γ-mediated expression of antioxidant enzymes [37,38]. Therefore, we hypothesized that β-carotene may suppress *H. pylori*-induced ROS generation and MAPK-mediated MMP-10 expression by activating PPAR-γ in gastric epithelial cells.

This study aimed to determine whether (a) β-carotene inhibits MMP-10 expression by suppressing the ROS-mediated activation of MAPKs and AP-1 and (b) whether β-carotene induces PPAR-γ-mediated catalase expression in *H. pylori*-infected AGS cells.

2. Results

2.1. H. pylori Activates MAPKs and Expression of MMP-10 in AGS Cells

First, we wanted to investigate whether *H. pylori* induces mRNA and MMP-10 protein expression by real-time polymerase chain reaction (PCR) and Western blot analysis, respectively. AGS cells were infected with *H. pylori* at the indicated ratios. At 24 h, the MMP-10 mRNA was upregulated by *H. pylori* in a density-dependent manner (Figure 1A). At a 50:1 bacteria/cell ratio, *H. pylori* increased the mRNA and protein levels of MMP-10 in a time-dependent manner. The maximum induction of MMP-10 in *H. pylori*-infected cells was observed at 24 h (Figure 1B,C). To determine whether *H. pylori* activates the MAPK signaling pathway, phosphorylated and total forms of MAPKs were detected by Western blotting. *H. pylori* increased the levels of phosphorylated MAPKs (p-JNK1/2, p-p38, and p-ERK1/2) in AGS cells at 30 min, while the total levels were not changed (Figure 1D). Levels of both p-JNK1/2 and p-38 steadily increased till 60 min but p-ERK1/2 decreased after 30 min.

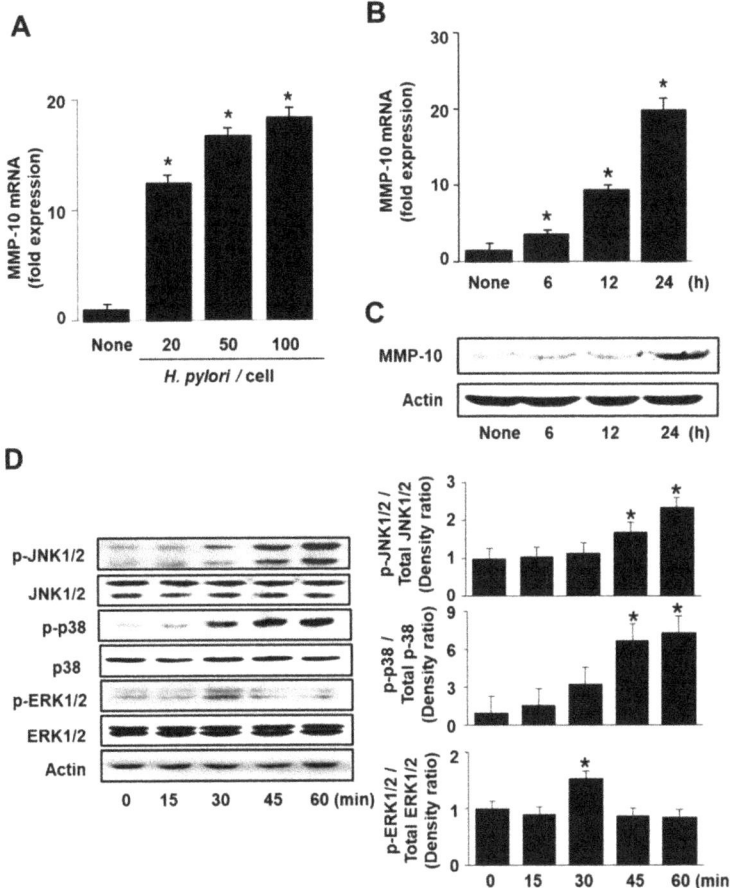

Figure 1. *H. pylori* induces the expression of MMP-10 and activation of MAPKs in AGS cells. (**A**) Cells were infected with *H. pylori* at the indicated ratios (*H. pylori*/cells) for 24 h. (**B–D**) Cells were infected with *H. pylori* at a 1:50 ratio for the indicated time periods. (**A,B**) The expression of MMP-10 mRNA was analyzed by real-time PCR and normalized to β-actin mRNA. All data are shown as the

mean ± standard error (S.E.) of three independent experiments. * $p < 0.05$ vs. none (cells without any treatment or infection). (**C**) Protein levels of MMP-10 were determined by Western blot analysis, using actin as the loading control. (**D**) Protein levels of phosphorylated or total form of JNK1/2, p38 and ERK1/2 were determined by Western blot analysis. Actin served as a loading control (left panel). Right panel: the densitometry data represent means ± S.E. from three immunoblots and are shown as relative density of phosphorylated protein band normalized to total form of protein level. * $p < 0.05$ vs. 0 min.

2.2. MAPK Inhibitors Prevent H. pylori-Induced Expression of MMP-10 in AGS Cells

To confirm the involvement of MAPKs in the *H. pylori*-induced expression of MMP-10, we used MAPK inhibitors SB600125 (JNK inhibitor), SB203580 (p38 inhibitor), and U0126 (ERK inhibitor). AGS cells were pretreated with SB600125 for 60 min, SB203580 for 60 min, and U0126 for 30 min, and infected with *H. pylori* for 24 h. All three MAPK inhibitors suppressed *H. pylori*-induced MMP-10 expression in AGS cells (Figure 2). These results indicate that *H. pylori* induces MMP-10 expression through JNK, p38, and ERK signaling in AGS cells.

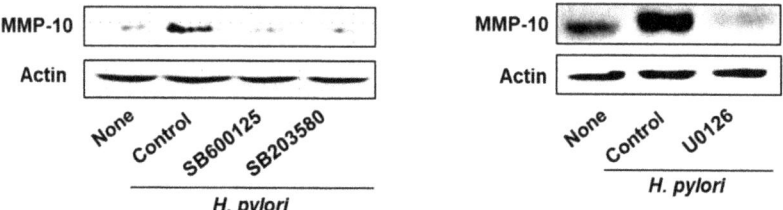

Figure 2. JNK, p38, and ERK inhibitors reduced *H. pylori*-induced MMP-10 expression in AGS cells. The cells were pretreated with SB600125 (a JNK inhibitor, 20 µM) or SB203580 (a p38 inhibitor, 20 µM) for 60 min, or U0126 (an ERK inhibitor, 10 µM) for 30 min, and then infected with *H. pylori* for 24 h. MMP-10 levels were determined by Western blot analysis. Actin was used as a loading control.

2.3. β-Carotene Inhibits H. pylori-Induced Activation of MAPKs and AP-1, and Expression of MMP-10 in AGS Cells

Next, we examined the effect of β-carotene on the *H. pylori*-induced expression of MMP-10. AGS cells were infected with *H. pylori* in the presence or absence of β-carotene. β-Carotene inhibited *H. pylori*-induced mRNA and the protein expression of MMP-10 at 24 h (Figure 3A,B). This prompted us to examine whether the inhibitory effect of β-carotene is mediated by suppressing MAPK activation. Levels of phosphorylated and total forms of MAPKs were determined in cells treated with or without β-carotene and infected with *H. pylori*. As shown in Figure 3C, β-carotene markedly reduced the phosphorylation of JNK1/2, p38, and ERK1/2 in a dose-dependent manner. Since MAPK induction is an upstream signaling event in AP-1-mediated MMP-10 expression, AP-1 DNA-binding activity was determined in the nuclear extracts of cells treated with or without β-carotene and infected with *H. pylori* (Figure 3D). β-Carotene inhibited *H. pylori*-induced AP-1 activation in AGS cells These results suggest that β-carotene inhibits the activation of MAPKs and AP-1 and thus, MMP-10 expression in *H. pylori*-infected AGS cells.

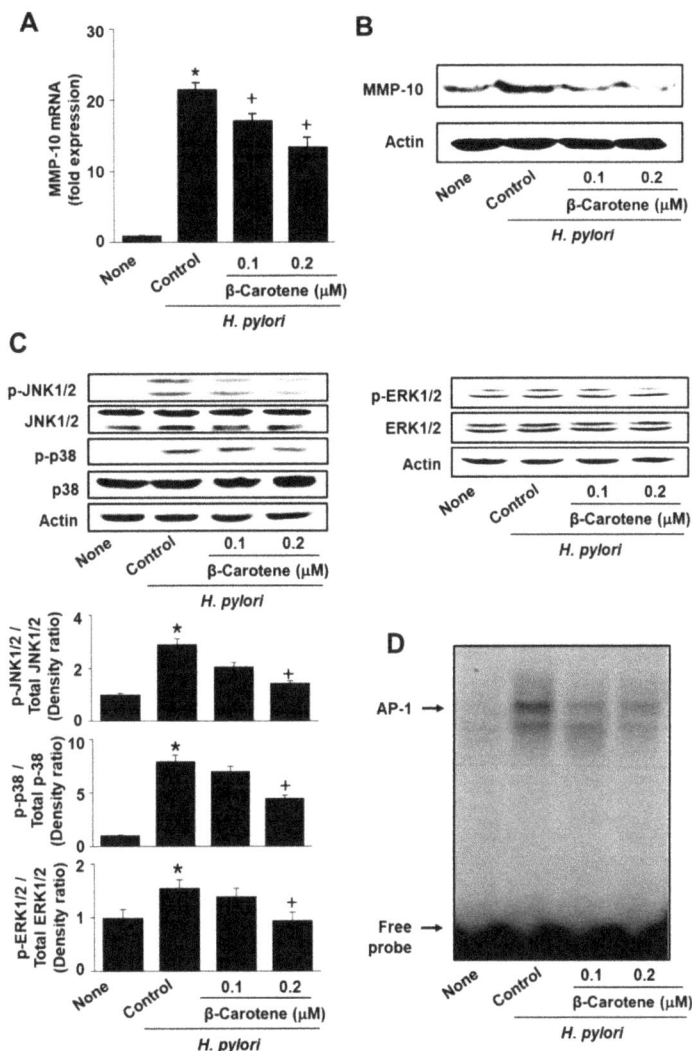

Figure 3. β-Carotene inhibits *H. pylori*-induced activation of MAPKs and AP-1, and expression of MMP-10 in AGS cells. Cells were pretreated with the indicated concentrations of β-carotene for 2 h and then infected with *H. pylori* for 24 h (**A**,**B**), 1 h (**C**, left panel), 30 min (**C**, right panel), and 1 h (**D**). (**A**) MMP-10 mRNA expression was analyzed by real-time PCR and normalized to β-actin mRNA. All data are shown as the mean ± S.E. of three independent experiments. * $p < 0.05$ vs. none (cells without any treatment or infection); + $p < 0.05$ vs. control (cells with *H. pylori* infection alone). (**B**) The level of MMP-10 was determined by Western blot analysis, using actin as the loading control. (**C**) Protein levels of phosphorylated or total form of JNK1/2, p38, and ERK1/2 were determined by Western blot analysis. Actin served as a loading control (upper panel). Lower panel: The densitometry data represent means ± S.E. from three immunoblots and are shown as relative density of phosphorylated protein band normalized to total form of protein level. * $p < 0.05$ vs. none (cells without any treatment or infection); + $p < 0.05$ vs. control (cells with *H. pylori* infection alone). (**D**) The DNA binding activity of AP-1 was measured by an electrophoretic mobility shift assay (EMSA).

2.4. β-Carotene Inhibits Cell Invasion Induced by H. pylori in AGS Cells

To determine whether β-carotene inhibits cell invasion in *H. pylori*-infected cells, AGS cells were infected with *H. pylori* in the presence or absence of β-carotene and analyzed using a cell-invasion assay. *H. pylori* significantly increased cell invasion, which was inhibited by β-carotene (Figure 4). These results demonstrate that β-carotene inhibits cell invasion induced by *H. pylori* infection.

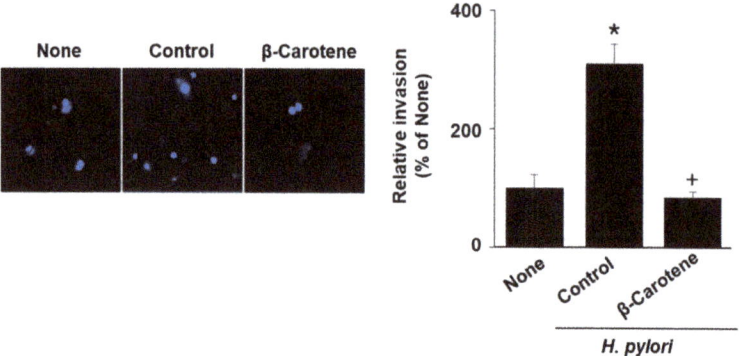

Figure 4. β-Carotene inhibits cell invasion induced by *H. pylori* in AGS cells. AGS cells were pretreated with β-carotene (0.2 μM) for 2 h and then infected with *H. pylori* for 24 h. Invasive cells were measured by staining them on Matrigel-coated filters with 4′,6-diamidino-2-phenylindole (DAPI) and visualizing them under a confocal laser scanning microscope (left panel). The graph represents the relative percentage of invasive cells (right panel). All data are shown as the mean ± S.E. of three independent experiments. The percentage of invasive cells in none (the cells without any treatment or infection) was set as 100%. * $p < 0.05$ vs. none (cells without any treatment or infection); + $p < 0.05$ vs. control (cells with *H. pylori* infection alone).

2.5. β-Carotene Upregulates PPAR-γ and Catalase and Reduces ROS Levels in H. pylori-Infected AGS Cells

Finally, we determined the antioxidant effect and the mechanisms underlying β-carotene in *H. pylori*-infected cells. Intracellular ROS levels and the expression of PPAR-γ and catalase were measured in cells treated with or without β-carotene (0.2 μM), and infected with *H. pylori*. As shown in Figure 5A, β-carotene reduced ROS levels, which were increased by *H. pylori* infection in AGS cells. Treatment with β-carotene (0.2 μM) increased the expression of PPAR-γ at 1 h, but increased the expression of catalase, a PPAR-γ target gene, till 3 h, in the absence of *H. pylori* (Figure 5B). *H. pylori* infection reduced the expression of PPAR-γ, which was prevented by β-carotene (Figure 5C). Additionally, *H. pylori* infection reduced the nuclear levels of PPAR-γ, which was restored by β-carotene treatment (Figure 5D).

To scrutinize the involvement of PPAR-γ in the antioxidant mechanisms of β-carotene, *H. pylori*-infected cells were treated with the PPAR-γ antagonist GW9662 and β-carotene. Co-treatment with GW9662 reversed the effect of β-carotene on *H. pylori*-induced intracellular ROS production (Figure 5E). These results indicate that β-carotene reduces ROS levels by activating PPAR-γ and inducing the expression of catalase in *H. pylori*-infected cells.

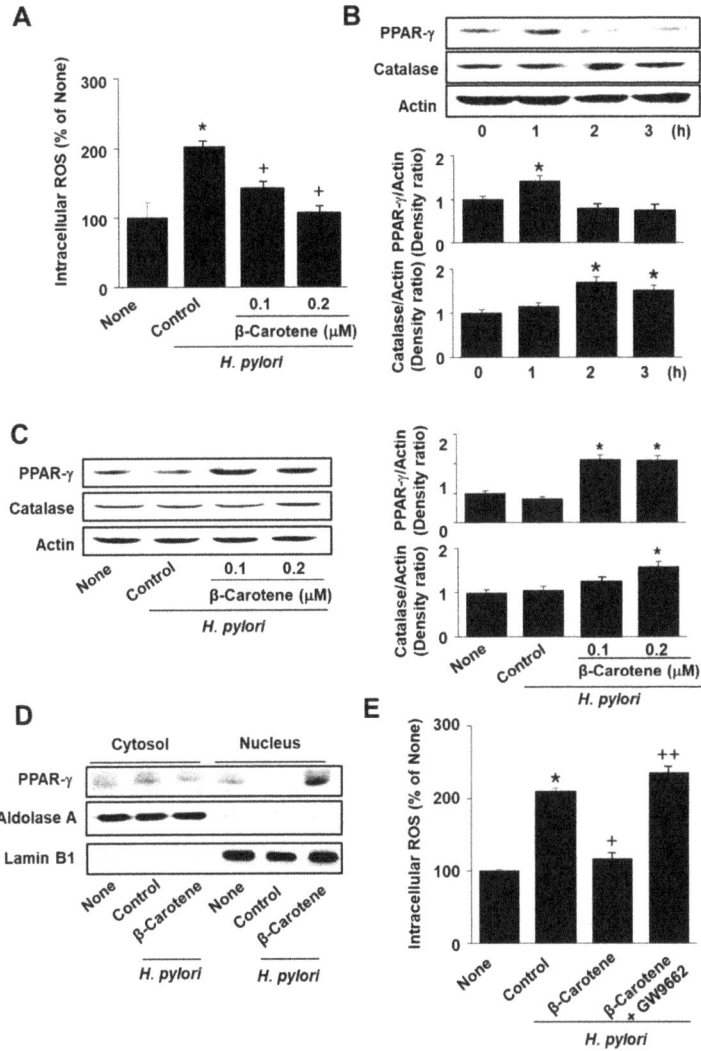

Figure 5. β-Carotene reduces intracellular ROS levels and induces expression of PPAR-γ and catalase in *H. pylori*-infected AGS cells. (**A,C**) Cells were pretreated with the indicated concentrations of β-carotene for 2 h and then infected with *H. pylori* for 30 min. (**B**) Cells were treated with β-carotene (0.2 μM) for the indicated time period without *H. pylori* infection. (**D**) Cells were pretreated with β-carotene (0.2 μM) for 2 h and then infected with *H. pylori* for 30 min. (**E**) Cells were co-treated with the PPAR-γ antagonist GW9662 (5 μM) and β-carotene (0.2 μM) for 2 h and then infected with *H. pylori* for 30 min. (**A,E**) Intracellular ROS levels were measured by dichlorofluorescein (DCF) fluorescence. All data are shown as the mean ± S.E. of three independent experiments. ROS levels in none (the cells without any treatment or infection) were set as 100%. * $p < 0.05$ vs. none (cells without any treatment or infection); + $p < 0.05$ vs. control (cells with *H. pylori* infection alone); ++ $p < 0.05$ vs. cells with β-carotene treatment and *H. pylori* infection. (**B,C**) Protein levels of PPAR-γ and catalase in whole-cell extracts were determined by Western blot analysis, using actin as the loading control. The densitometry data represent means ± S.E. from three immunoblots and are shown as relative density of protein band normalized to actin level. * $p < 0.05$ vs. 0 h (**B**) or control (cells with *H. pylori* infection alone) (**C**). (**D**) Levels of PPAR-γ were measured by Western blot analysis. Aldolase was used as a marker of cytosol, while lamin B was used as a nuclear marker.

3. Discussion

Gastric cancer is the fourth leading cause of cancer. Infection with *H. pylori* is a significant risk factor for chronic gastritis, peptic ulcers, and gastric carcinogenesis. MMP expression is involved in the invasion and metastasis of malignant tumors, and is induced in *H. pylori*-infected gastric epithelial cells [5–10]. High levels of plasma MMPs were found in gastric cancer patients and, therefore, MMPs could serve as important diagnostic markers of gastric cancer [39]. MMP-10 is upregulated via ERK signaling in *H. pylori*-infected AGS cells [10]. Consistent with this study, we observed higher MMP-10 expression in AGS cells following *H. pylori* infection. In addition to ERK, JNK and p38 are activated, which induces MMP-10 expression in *H. pylori*-infected cells.

Cytokines, growth factors, and phorbol esters activate a group of protein kinases (MAPK kinase kinases (MAPKKKs)) that phosphorylate other kinases (MAPK kinases (MAPKKs)), which in turn are responsible for the phosphorylation and activation of MAPK. Upon activation by MAPKKs, MAPKs translocate to the nucleus to phosphorylate and activate various transcription factors [40,41]. Of particular relevance to MMP transcription, JNKs and ERKs phosphorylate and activate AP-1 family member c-Jun [42,43], which dimerizes with c-Fos to drive the transcription of multiple MMP genes. In the present study, we found that the *H. pylori*-induced activation of MAPKs mediates AP-1 activation and MMP-10 expression in AGS cells.

ROS have been implicated in the development of gastric cancer. The overproduction of ROS, which leads to the activation of pro-survival signaling pathways, including cancer cell proliferation and invasion, is induced by *H. pylori* infection [16]. Higher ROS levels activate MAPK signal transduction and the transcription factor, AP-1, in *H. pylori*-infected cells [18,19]. AP-1 transcription factor is important in regulating MMP family members and is sensitive to regulation by redox conditions [21]. Even though ROS generally increase the AP-1 level for the activation of MMP gene expression, ROS can also reduce the transcriptional activity of AP-1-through direct oxidation of cysteine residues contained within the DNA-binding domain [44]. Therefore, the cycling of cysteinyl residues is among the oxidant-dependent mechanisms that regulate the activity of AP-1. In fact, AP-1 DNA-binding activity increases after the reducing agent thioredoxin treatment in monocytes. When the conserved cysteine in the basic binding motif of both Fos and Jun is oxidized, the binding of these proteins to AP-1 sequences is diminished. On the other hand, if Fos/Jun heterodimers are bound to an AP-1 site, they cannot be oxidized [45]. In the present study, *H. pylori* infection increased both ROS levels and AP-1-DNA binding activity in gastric epithelial cells. Therefore, cysteine residues in the DNA-binding domain may not be affected nor oxidized by *H. pylori* infection at the infection ratio of 1:50 (cells: bacterium). On the other hand, Fos/Jun heterodimers may be bound directly to the AP-1 site by MAPK activation in *H. pylori*-infected cells. Further study should be performed to investigate whether a high infection ratio (more than 1:50, cells: bacterium) causes the oxidation of critical cysteine residues in the DNA-binding domain for AP-1 in gastric epithelial cells.

β-Carotene is the most frequently found carotenoid in the human diet. In the human body, β-carotene is absorbed, distributed, and metabolized by enzymatic and/or non-enzymatic oxidant cleavage into several metabolites. Despite the broadly accepted biological value of β-carotene, it is a double-edged sword, due to its potential antioxidant versus pro-oxidant behavior. Regarding the pharmacological role of β-carotene, a high concentration (50 and 100 µM) of β-carotene increases ROS levels and caspase-3 activity, which results in a reduction in DNA rapier protein Ku protein and apoptosis in gastric cancer AGS cells [46]. Furthermore, 100 µM of β-carotene induces apoptosis by increasing apoptotic protein p53 and decreasing anti-apoptotic Bcl-2 as well as nuclear ataxia-telangiectasia mutated (ATM), a sensor for DNA-damaging agents, in AGS cells [47]. Cui et al. [37] suggested that the chemopreventive activity of a high concentration of β-carotene (>20 µM) is associated with ROS production, which results in mitochondrial dysfunction, cytochrome c release, and apoptosis in human breast cancer MCF-7 cells. Palozza et al. [48] demonstrated that β-carotene (>10 µM) induced ROS production and apoptosis in human leukemic HL-60 cells. In addition, β-carotene (50–100 μM) increases ROS levels and inhibits cell growth with the expression of c-myc in colon adenocarcinoma WiDr cells. Thus, a high concentration of β-carotene may exert pro-oxidant activity, which contributes to anti-cancer effects.

However, our previous study showed that a low concentration (0.5 and 1 μM) of β-carotene reduced ROS levels and inhibited NF-B activation, NF-B-regulated expression of tumor necrosis factor receptor associated factor (TRAF), and hyper-proliferation in *H. pylori*-infected gastric epithelial cells [49]. A low concentration of β-carotene (0.15 and 0.3 μM) inhibited peroxynitrite anion-induced lipid peroxide production in rat brain synaptosomes [50]. Therefore, we used 0.1 and 0.2 μM of β-carotene to determine the antioxidant mechanism of β-carotene in relation to MMP expression in *H. pylori*-infected gastric epithelial cells in the present study.

In the present study, we found that β-carotene reduced ROS levels, which was increased by *H. pylori* infection. β-Carotene reduced cell invasion as well as MMP-10 expression in *H. pylori*-infected cells. The *H. pylori*-induced activation of MAPKs and AP-1 was inhibited by β-carotene. The JNK, p38, and ERK inhibitors suppressed *H. pylori*-induced MMP-10 expression. These results indicate that β-carotene inhibits *H. pylori*-induced invasion by downregulating the MAPK-mediated activation of AP-1, which in turn reduces MMP-10 expression in gastric epithelial cells.

Regarding the studies on β-carotene and MMP expression and invasion, β-carotene attenuates invasion and metastasis in neuroblastoma cells in vitro and in vivo [51]. Dietary β-carotene inhibits peroxidized cholesterol-induced MMP-9 activation in hairless mouse skin [52]. In keratinocytes, β-carotene dose-dependently quenches the singlet oxygen-mediated induction of MMP-1 and MMP-10 [53]. β-Carotene treatment downregulates the expression of MMP-2 and MMP-9 by suppressing the nuclear translocation of p65, p50, c-Rel subunits of nuclear factor-kappa B, and other transcription factors, such as c-fos, a component of AP-1, in B16F-10 melanoma cells [54]. β-Carotene reduces invasiveness with a decreased expression of MMP-7 and MMP-28 in colorectal carcinoma cells [55].

For the antioxidant mechanism of β-carotene, we found that β-carotene induces the expression and nuclear translocation of PPAR-γ, which promotes catalase expression in *H. pylori*-infected AGS cells. These data demonstrate that β-carotene reduces ROS levels through the upregulation of the PPAR-γ–mediated expression of the antioxidant enzyme, catalase. Cui et al. [37] demonstrated that β-carotene upregulates PPAR-γ expression, but increases ROS production in MCF-7 breast cancer cells. Kaliappan et al. [56] demonstrated that dietary β carotene inhibits Angiotensin II-induced renal damage by repressing PPARγ and renin 1 in apo E knockout mice. Therefore, the effect of β-carotene on PPAR-γ expression and activation may be different depending on the tissues, stimuli, and environmental and genetic factors. Further studies should be performed to determine the interaction of PPAR-γ, ROS, and antioxidant enzyme expression on *H. pylori*-associated gastric cancer development.

Recently, Mao et al. [57] screened epidemiological studies and demonstrated that increased intake of phytochemicals in fruits and vegetables could reduce the risk of gastric cancer. They suggested that phytochemicals have the potential for the prevention and management of gastric cancer in humans. This study supports the present finding showing that dietary β-carotene, which is abundant in fruits and vegetables, may reduce *H. pylori*-associated gastric cancer incidence by reducing the oxidative stress-mediated MMP-10 expression and invasive property of gastric epithelial cells.

In conclusion, β-carotene activates PPAR-γ and induces its downstream target, catalase, which leads to a reduction in ROS levels and the inhibition of JNK/p38/ERK signaling in *H. pylori*-infected gastric epithelial cells. Through this mechanism, β-carotene significantly suppressed *H. pylori*-induced MMP-10 expression and reduced the invasive phenotype of infected gastric epithelial cells.

4. Materials and Methods

4.1. Cell Line and Culture Conditions

Human gastric epithelial AGS cells were purchased from the American Type Culture Collection (Rockville, MD, USA). The cells were cultured in complete medium consisting of Roswell Park Memorial Institute (RPMI) 1640 medium (GIBCO, Grand Island, NY, USA) with 10% fetal bovine serum (FBS), 2 mM glutamine, 100 units/mL penicillin, and 100 μg/mL streptomycin (Sigma-Aldrich, St. Louis, MO, USA). The cells were cultured at 37 °C and maintained in a humidified atmosphere containing 5% CO_2.

4.2. Bacterial Strain and Growth Conditions

All experiments were performed with *H. pylori*, cag A positive strain 60190 (ATCC 49503). Chocolate agar plates (Becton Dickinson Microbiology Systems, Cockeysvile, MD, USA) were used to grow the bacteria at 37 °C under microaerophilic conditions using an anaerobic chamber (BBL Campy Pouch® System, Becton Dickinson Microbiology Systems, Franklin Lakes, NJ, USA).

4.3. Reagents

β-Carotene (Sigma-Aldrich, St. Louis, MO, USA) was dissolved in THF (final concentration 10 mM) and diluted in media to the desired concentrations. The PPAR-γ antagonist GW9662 (Sigma-Aldrich) was dissolved in DMSO. The MAPK inhibitors, U0126 (an ERK inhibitor; Catalog #9903, Cell Signaling Technology, Inc., Beverly, MA, USA), SB203580 (a p38 inhibitor; Catalog #559389, Calbiochem Biochemicals, San Diego, CA, USA), and SB600125 (a JNK inhibitor; Catalog #10010466, Cayman Chemical, Ann Arbor, MI, USA), were dissolved in DMSO.

4.4. Infection of AGS Cells with H. pylori

AGS cells were seeded and cultivated overnight to reach 80% confluency. *H. pylori* were harvested from the chocolate agar plates and resuspended in antibiotic-free RPMI 1640 medium supplemented with 10% FBS. Subsequently, AGS cells were infected with *H. pylori* at multiplicity-of-infection of 50:1.

4.5. Experimental Protocols

To investigate the effect of β-carotene, AGS cells (1.5×10^5/2 mL, 7.0×10^5/10 mL) were pretreated with β-carotene (0.1 or 0.2 μM) for 2 h and then infected with *H. pylori* for 30 min (for ROS levels, PPAR-γ DNA binding activity, protein levels of PPAR-γ and catalase), 1 h (for protein expression of JNK/p38/ERK and DNA binding activity of AP-1), and 24 h (for mRNA expression and protein levels of MMP-10, and invasion assay). To determine the involvement of MAPKs, the MAPK inhibitors SB203580 and SP600125 were added to the culture medium 1 h before infection with *H. pylori*. In the case of U0126, the cells were pretreated with U0126 for 30 min before infection with *H. pylori*.

4.6. Preparation of Cell Extracts

The cells were collected by treatment with trypsin-ethylenediaminetetraacetic acid (EDTA), followed by centrifugation at $1000 \times g$ for 5 min. The cell pellets were resuspended in lysis buffer, including 10 mM Tris pH 7.4, 15 mM NaCl, 1% NP-40, and protease inhibitor cocktail (Complete; Roche, Mannheim, Germany), and lysed by passing the cells through a 1 mL syringe several times. The resulting mixture was incubated on ice for 30 min and centrifuged at $13,000 \times g$ for 15 min. The supernatants were collected and used as whole-cell extracts. The cytosolic and nuclear extracts were prepared using a NE-PER® nuclear and cytoplasmic extraction kit (Thermo Fisher, Waltham, MA, USA) according to the manufacturer's instructions. In brief, cells were resuspended in the cytoplasmic extraction reagent containing protease inhibitors and vortexed for 15 s, followed by centrifugation at $13,000 \times g$ for 10 min. The supernatants were used as cytosolic extracts. The nuclear pellet was resuspended in nuclear extraction reagent on ice, and then centrifuged at $13,000 \times g$

for 10 min. The supernatants were collected and used as nuclear extracts. The specificity of the nuclear extracts was confirmed by the predominant presence of lamin B1 in the nuclear fraction. A Bradford assay (Bio-Rad Laboratories, Hercules, CA, USA) was used to determine the protein concentrations.

4.7. Real-Time PCR Analysis

Total RNA was isolated using TRI reagent (Molecular Research Center, Inc., Cincinnati, OH, USA). The isolated RNA was reverse transcribed into cDNA using random hexamers and MuLV reverse transcriptase (Promega, Madison, WI, USA) at 23 °C for 10 min, 37 °C for 60 min, and 95 °C for 5 min. For real-time PCR, the cDNA was amplified with specific primers for human MMP-10 and β-actin. For the MMP-10 PCR product, 5′-CATTCCTTGTGCTGTTGTGTC-3′ (forward primer) and 5′-TGTCTAGCTTCCCGTTCACC-3′ (reverse primer) were used. The sequence of β-actin primers was the following: 5′-ACCAACTGGGACGACATGGAG-3′ (forward primer) and 5′-GTGAGGATCTTCATGAGG TAGTC-3 (reverse primer). The cDNA was amplified by 45 cycles including denaturation at 95 °C for 30 s, annealing at 55 °C for 30 s, and extension at 72 °C for 30 s. During the first cycle, the 95 °C step was extended to 3 min. Amplification of the β-actin gene was performed in the same reaction and served as the reference gene.

4.8. Invasion Assay

Invasion of AGS cells infected with *H. pylori* was evaluated in Matrigel-coated 24-well invasion chambers (#354480, Corning Life Sciences, Teterboro, NJ, USA). The upper and lower compartments were separated by Matrigel-coated filters with 8 μm pore size. AGS cells (4.0×10^4 cells/well) were seeded on the reconstituted basement membrane in RPMI 1640 supplemented with 0.01% FBS. Following infection with *H. pylori*, the cells were incubated for 24 h in the upper chamber with or without β-carotene. Cells which crossed the filter and attached to the lower surface of the Matrigel-coated membrane (invasive cells) were washed with PBS and fixed in 4% formaldehyde for 30 min at room temperature. The cells were rinsed twice with PBS and then stained using 4′,6-diamidino-2-phenylindole (DAPI) for 30 min. The number of cells that had migrated to the lower surface was counted in twelve random fields using a laser scanning confocal microscope (Zeiss LSM 880, Carl Zeiss Inc., Thornwood, NY, USA) (10×).

4.9. Measurement of Intracellular ROS Levels

For the measurement of intracellular ROS, cells were treated with 10 μg/mL of dichlorofluorescein diacetate (DCF-DA; Sigma-Aldrich, St. Louis, MO, USA) and incubated at 37 °C for 30 min. DCF fluorescence (excitation 495 nm and emission 535 nm) was measured using a Victor5 multi-label counter (PerkinElmer Life and Analytical Sciences, Boston, MA, USA). ROS levels were quantified based on the relative increase in fluorescence.

4.10. Electrophoretic Mobility Shift Assay (EMSA)

The PPAR-γ gel-shift oligonucleotide (5′-CAAAACTAGGTCAAAGCTCA-3′; sc-2587, Santa Cruz Biotechnology, Dallas, TX, USA) and AP-1 gel-shift oligonucleotide (5′-CGCTT GATAGTCAGCCGGAA-3′; Promega) were radiolabeled using [^{32}P]-dATP (Amersham Biosciences, Piscataway, NJ, USA) and T4 polynucleotide kinase (GIBCO, Grand Island, NY, USA). The radiolabeled oligonucleotides were separated from free [^{32}P]-dATP using Bio-Rad purification columns (Bio-Rad Laboratories, Hercules, CA, USA). Nuclear extracts were incubated at room temperature for 30 min under the following conditions: [^{32}P]-labeled oligonucleotide in buffer containing 12% glycerol, 12 mM HEPES (pH 7.9), 1 mM EDTA, 1 mM DTT, 25 mM KCl, 5 mM $MgCl_2$, and 0.04 μg/mL poly[d(I-C)]. The samples were electrophoretically separated in a nondenaturing 5% acrylamide gel. The gel was dried at 80 °C for 2 h and exposed to a radiography film at −80 °C with intensifying screens.

4.11. Western Blot Analysis

Whole-cell extracts (10–40 μg) were separated using 7–13% SDS polyacrylamide gel electrophoresis under reducing conditions and transferred to nitrocellulose membranes (Amersham, Inc., Arlington Heights, IL, USA) by electroblotting. The transfer of protein was verified using reversible staining with Ponceau S. Membranes were blocked with 3% non-fat dry milk in Tris-buffered saline and 0.2% Tween 20 (Santa Cruz Biotechnology, Dallas, TX, USA) (TBS-T) for 1 h at 15–25 °C. Antibodies against MMP-10 (sc-80197, Santa Cruz Biotechnology), p-ERK (sc-7383, Santa Cruz Biotechnology), ERK (#9102, Cell Signaling Technology, Danvers, MA, USA), p-JNK(#9251S, Cell Signaling Technology), JNK (#9252, Cell Signaling Technology), p-p38 (#9211S, Cell Signaling Technology), p38 (#9212, Cell Signaling Technology), PPAR-γ (sc-7273, Santa Cruz Biotechnology), catalase (ab16731, Abcam, Cambridge, UK), lamin B1 (ab16048, Abcam, Cambridge, UK), aldolase A (sc-390733, Santa Cruz Biotechnology), and actin (sc-47778, Santa Cruz Biotechnology) were diluted in TBS-T containing 3% non-fat dry milk and incubated overnight at 4 °C. Membranes were washed with TBS-T, followed by detection with horseradish peroxidase-conjugated secondary antibodies (anti-mouse or anti-rabbit). Proteins were visualized using an enhanced chemiluminescence detection system (Santa Cruz Biotechnology) through exposure to BioMax MR films (Kodak, Rochester, NY, USA).

Protein level was compared to that of the loading control actin or total form of MAPK (ERK1/2, JNK1/2, p-38). Intensity of each protein band was densitometrically quantified by using the software Image J (National Institutes of Health, USA). The densitometry data represent means ± S.E. from three immunoblots and are shown as relative density of protein band normalized to actin or total form of MAPK.

4.12. Statistical Analysis

One-way analysis of variance followed by the Newman–Keuls post-hoc test was used for statistical analysis. All data are reported as the mean ± S.E. of three independent experiments. For each experiment, the number of each group was 4 ($n = 4$ per each group). A p-value less than 0.05 was considered statistically significant.

Author Contributions: Conceptualization: H.K.; investigation, writing, and original draft preparation: S.B.; new reagents and analytical tools: J.W.L.; writing, review, and editing: H.K. All authors have read and agreed to the published version of the manuscript.

Funding: This research received no external funding.

Data Availability Statement: The data used to support the findings of this study are included within the article.

Conflicts of Interest: The authors declare no conflict of interest.

Abbreviations

AP-1	Activator protein-1
Cag A	Cytotoxin-associated gene A
DCF-DA	Dichlorofluorescein diacetate
ECM	Extracellular matrix
EMSA	Electrophoretic mobility shift assay
JNK	c-Jun N-terminal kinase
ERK	Extracellular signal-regulated kinase
MAPK	Mitogen-activated protein kinase
MAPKKs	MAPK kinases
MAPKKKs	MAPK kinase kinases
MMP	Matrix metalloproteinase
PARγ	Peroxisome proliferator-activated receptor-γ
ROS	Reactive oxygen species

References

1. Hooi, J.K.Y.; Lai, W.Y.; Ng, W.K.; Suen, M.M.Y.; Underwood, F.E.; Tanyingoh, D.; Malfertheiner, P.; Graham, D.Y.; Wong, V.W.S.; Wu, J.C.Y.; et al. Global prevalence of *Helicobacter pylori* infection: Systematic review and meta-analysis. *Gastroenterology* **2017**, *153*, 420–429. [CrossRef]
2. Song, Y.; Liu, G.; Liu, S.; Chen, R.; Wang, N.; Liu, Z.; Zhang, X.; Xiao, Z.; Liu, L. *Helicobacter pylori* upregulates TRPC6 via Wnt/β-catenin signaling to promote gastric cancer migration and invasion. *OncoTargets Ther.* **2019**, *12*, 5269–5279. [CrossRef]
3. Kessenbrock, K.; Plaks, V.; Werb, Z. Matrix metalloproteinases: Regulators of the tumor microenvironment. *Cell* **2010**, *141*, 52–67. [CrossRef]
4. Page-McCaw, A.; Ewald, A.J.; Werb, Z. Matrix metalloproteinases and the regulation of tissue remodelling. *Nat. Rev. Mol. Cell Biol.* **2007**, *8*, 221–233. [CrossRef]
5. Krueger, S.; Hundertmark, T.; Kalinski, T.; Ulrich Peitz, U.; Wex, T.; Malfertheiner, P.; Naumann, M.; Roessner, A. *Helicobacter pylori* encoding the pathogenicity island activates matrix metalloproteinase 1 in gastric epithelial cells via JNK and ERK. *J. Biol. Chem.* **2006**, *281*, 2868–2875. [CrossRef] [PubMed]
6. Jiang, H.; Zhou, Y.; Liao, Q.; Ouyang, H. *Helicobacter pylori* infection promotes the invasion and metastasis of gastric cancer through increasing the expression of matrix metalloproteinase-1 and matrix metalloproteinase-10. *Exp. Ther. Med.* **2014**, *8*, 769–774. [CrossRef] [PubMed]
7. Mori, N.; Sato, H.; Hayashibara, T.; Senba, M.; Geleziunas, R.; Wada, A.; Hirayama, T.; Yamamoto, N. *Helicobacter pylori* induces matrix metalloproteinase-9 through activation of nuclear factor κB. *Gastroenterology* **2003**, *124*, 983–992. [CrossRef]
8. Nam, Y.H.; Ryu, E.; Lee, D.; Shim, H.J.; Lee, Y.C.; Lee, S.T. CagA phosphorylation-dependent MMP-9 expression in gastric epithelial cells. *Helicobacter* **2011**, *16*, 276–283. [CrossRef] [PubMed]
9. Wroblewski, L.E.; Noble, P.J.; Pagliocca, A.; Pritchard, D.M.; Hart, C.A.; Campbell, F.; Dodson, A.R.; Dockray, G.J.; Varro, A. Stimulation of MMP-7 (matrilysin) by *Helicobacter pylori* in human gastric epithelial cells: Role in epithelial cell migration. *J. Cell Sci.* **2003**, *116*, 3017–3026. [CrossRef] [PubMed]
10. Costa, A.M.; Ferreira, R.M.; Pinto-Ribeiro, I.; Sougleri, J.S.; Oliveira, M.J.; Carreto, L.; Santos, M.A.; Sgouras, D.N.; Carneiro, F.; Leite, M. *Helicobacter pylori* activates matrix metalloproteinase 10 in gastric epithelial cells via EGFR and ERK-mediated pathways. *J. Infect. Dis.* **2016**, *213*, 1767–1776. [CrossRef]
11. Frederick, L.A.; Matthews, J.A.; Jamieson, L.; Justilien, V.; Thompson, E.A.; Radisky, D.C.; Fields, A.P. Matrix metalloproteinase-10 is a critical effector of protein kinase Cι-Par6α-mediated lung cancer. *Oncogene* **2008**, *27*, 4841–4853. [CrossRef]
12. Nakamura, H.; Fujii, Y.; Ohuchi, E.; Yamamoto, E.; Okada, Y. Activation of the precursor of human stromelysin 2 and its interactions with other matrix metalloproteinases. *Eur. J. Biochem.* **1998**, *253*, 67–75. [CrossRef]
13. Scheau, C.; Badarau, I.A.; Costache, R.; Caruntu, C.; Mihai, G.L.; Didilescu, A.C.; Constantin, C.; Neagu, M. The role of matrix metalloproteinases in the epithelial-mesenchymal transition of hepatocellular carcinoma. *Anal. Cell. Pathol.* **2019**, *2019*, 9423907. [CrossRef] [PubMed]
14. Gobin, E.; Bagwell, K.; Wagner, J.; Mysona, D.; Sandirasegarane, S.; Smith, N.; Bai, S.; Sharma, A.; Schleifer, R.; She, J.-X. A pan-cancer perspective of matrix metalloproteases (MMP) gene expression profile and their diagnostic/prognostic potential. *BMC Cancer* **2019**, *19*, 581. [CrossRef] [PubMed]
15. Kim, H. Oxidative stress in *Helicobacter pylori*-induced gastric cell injury. *Inflammopharmacology* **2005**, *13*, 63–74. [CrossRef] [PubMed]
16. Handa, O.; Naito, Y.; Yoshikawa, T. *Helicobacter pylori*: A ROS-inducing bacterial species in the stomach. *Inflamm. Res.* **2010**, *59*, 997–1003. [CrossRef]
17. Baek, H.Y.; Lim, J.W.; Kim, H.; Kim, J.M.; Kim, J.S.; Jung, H.C.; Kim, K.H. Oxidative-stress-related proteome changes in *Helicobacter pylori*-infected human gastric mucosa. *Biochem. J.* **2004**, *379 Pt 2*, 291–299. [CrossRef]
18. Seo, J.H.; Lim, J.W.; Kim, H.; Kim, K.H. *Helicobacter pylori* in a Korean isolate activates mitogen-activated protein kinases, AP-1, and NF-κB and induces chemokine expression in gastric epithelial AGS cells. *Lab. Investig.* **2004**, *84*, 49–62. [CrossRef]
19. Allison, C.C.; Kufer, T.A.; Kremmer, E.; Kaparakis, M.; Ferrero, R.L. *Helicobacter pylori* induces MAPK phosphorylation and AP-1 activation via a NOD1-dependent mechanism. *J. Immunol.* **2009**, *183*, 8099–8109. [CrossRef] [PubMed]
20. Choi, J.H.; Cho, S.O.; Kim, H. α-Lipoic acid inhibits expression of IL-8 by suppressing activation of MAPK, Jak/Stat, and NF-κB in *H. pylori*-infected gastric epithelial AGS cells. *Yonsei Med. J.* **2016**, *57*, 260–264. [CrossRef] [PubMed]
21. Nelson, K.K.; Melendez, J.A. Mitochondrial redox control of matrix metalloproteinases. *Free Radic. Biol. Med.* **2004**, *37*, 768–784. [CrossRef] [PubMed]
22. Mori, K.; Shibanuma, M.; Nose, K. Invasive potential induced under long-term oxidative stress in mammary epithelial cells. *Cancer Res.* **2004**, *64*, 7464–7472. [CrossRef] [PubMed]
23. Benbow, U.; Brinckerhoff, C.E. The AP-1 site and MMP gene regulation: What is all the fuss about? *Matrix Biol.* **1997**, *15*, 519–526. [CrossRef]
24. Polvani, S.; Tarocchi, M.; Galli, A. PPARγ and oxidative stress: Con(β) catenating NRF2 and FOXO. *PPAR Res.* **2012**, *2012*, 641087. [CrossRef]
25. Kim, S.H.; Lim, J.W.; Kim, H. Astaxanthin inhibits mitochondrial dysfunction and interleukin-8 expression in *Helicobacter pylori*-infected gastric epithelial cells. *Nutrients* **2018**, *10*, 1320. [CrossRef]

26. Liu, J.; Lu, H.; Huang, R.; Lin, D.; Wu, X.; Lin, Q.; Wu, X.; Zheng, J.; Pan, X.; Peng, J.; et al. Peroxisome proliferator activated receptor-gamma ligands induced cell growth inhibition and its influence on matrix metalloproteinase activity in human myeloid leukemia cells. *Cancer Chemother. Pharmacol.* **2005**, *56*, 400–408. [CrossRef]
27. Hetzel, M.; Walcher, D.; Grüb, M.; Bach, H.; Hombach, V.; Marx, N. Inhibition of MMP-9 expression by PPARγ activators in human bronchial epithelial cells. *Thorax* **2003**, *58*, 778–783. [CrossRef]
28. Biehler, E.; Alkerwi, A.; Hoffmann, L.; Krause, E.; Guillaume, M.; Lair, M.-L.; Bohn, T. Contribution of violaxanthin, neoxanthin, phytoene and phytofluene to total carotenoid intake: Assessment in Luxembourg. *J. Food Compos. Anal.* **2012**, *25*, 56–65. [CrossRef]
29. Wawrzyniak, A.; Hamulka, J.; Friberg, E.; Wolk, A. Dietary, anthropometric, and lifestyle correlates of serum carotenoids in postmenopausal women. *Eur. J. Nutr.* **2013**, *52*, 1919–1926. [CrossRef] [PubMed]
30. Fraser, G.E.; Jaceldo-Siegl, K.; Henning, S.M.; Fan, J.; Knutsen, S.F.; Haddad, E.H.; Sabaté, J.; Beeson, W.L.; Bennett, H. Biomarkers of dietary intake are correlated with corresponding measures from repeated dietary recalls and food-frequency questionnaires in the adventist health study-2. *J. Nutr.* **2016**, *146*, 586–594. [CrossRef] [PubMed]
31. Eroglu, A.; Harrison, E.H. Carotenoid metabolism in mammals, including man: Formation, occurrence, and function of apocarotenoids. *J. Lipid Res.* **2013**, *54*, 1719–1730. [CrossRef] [PubMed]
32. Krinsky, N.I.; Johnson, E.J. Carotenoid actions and their relation to health and disease. *Mol. Aspects Med.* **2005**, *26*, 459–516. [CrossRef]
33. Krinsky, N.I.; Yeum, K.-J. Carotenoid-radical interactions. *Biochem. Biophys. Res. Commun.* **2003**, *305*, 754–760. [CrossRef]
34. Pradeep, C.R.; Kuttan, G. Effect of β-Carotene on the inhibition of lung metastasis in mice. *Phytomedicine* **2003**, *10*, 159–164. [CrossRef] [PubMed]
35. Kim, D.; Lim, J.W.; Kim, H. β-Carotene inhibits expression of c-myc and cyclin E in *Helicobacter pylori*-infected gastric epithelial cells. *J. Cancer Prev.* **2019**, *24*, 192–196. [CrossRef] [PubMed]
36. Jang, S.H.; Lim, J.W.; Kim, H. Beta-carotene inhibits *Helicobacter pylori*-induced expression of inducible nitric oxide synthase and cyclooxygenase-2 in human gastric epithelial AGS cells. *J. Physiol. Pharmacol.* **2009**, *60*, 131–137.
37. Cui, Y.; Lu, Z.; Bai, L.; Shi, Z.; Zhao, W.-E.; Zhao, B. β-Carotene induces apoptosis and up-regulates peroxisome proliferator-activated receptor gamma expression and reactive oxygen species production in MCF-7 cancer cells. *Eur. J. Cancer* **2007**, *43*, 2590–2601. [CrossRef]
38. Ngoc, N.B.; Lv, P.; Zhao, W.E. Suppressive effects of lycopene and β-carotene on the viability of the human esophageal squamous carcinoma cell line EC109. *Oncol. Lett.* **2018**, *15*, 6727–6732.
39. Kushlinskii, N.E.; Gershtein, E.S.; Ivannikov, A.A.; Davydov, M.M.; Chang, V.L.; Ognerubov, N.A.; Stilidi, I.S. Clinical Significance of Matrix Metalloproteinases in Blood Plasma of Patients with Gastric Cancer. *Bull. Exp. Biol. Med.* **2019**, *166*, 373–376. [CrossRef] [PubMed]
40. Garrington, T.P.; Johnson, G.L. Organization and regulation of mitogen-activated protein kinase signaling pathways. *Curr. Opin. Cell Biol.* **1999**, *11*, 211–218. [CrossRef]
41. Kolch, W. Meaningful relationships: The regulation of the Ras/Raf/MEK/ERK pathway by protein interactions. *Biochem. J.* **2000**, *351*, 289–305. [CrossRef] [PubMed]
42. Karin, M. The regulation of AP-1 activity by mitogen-activated protein kinases. *J. Biol. Chem.* **1995**, *270*, 16483–16486. [CrossRef]
43. Leppa, S.; Saffrich, R.; Ansorge, W.; Bohmann, D. Differential regulation of c-Jun by ERK and JNK during PC12 cell differentiation. *EMBO J.* **1998**, *17*, 4404–4413. [CrossRef]
44. Finkel, T.; Holbrook, N.J. Oxidants, oxidative stress and the biology of ageing. *Nature* **2000**, *408*, 239–247. [CrossRef] [PubMed]
45. Clerk, A.; Michael, A.; Sugden, P.H. Stimulation of multiple mitogen-activated protein kinase sub-families by oxidative stress and phosphorylation of the small heat shock protein, HSP25/27, in neonatal ventricular myocytes. *Biochem. J.* **1998**, *333*, 581–589. [CrossRef]
46. Park, Y.; Choi, J.Y.; Lim, J.W.; Kim, H. β-Carotene-induced apoptosis is mediated with loss of Ku proteins in gastric cancer AGS cells. *Genes Nutr.* **2015**, *10*, 467. [CrossRef] [PubMed]
47. Jang, S.H.; Lim, J.W.; Kim, H. Mechanism of β-carotene induced apoptosis of gastric cancer cells: Involvement of Ataxia-Telangiectasia-Mutated. *Ann. N. Y. Acad. Sci.* **2009**, *1171*, 156–162. [CrossRef]
48. Palozza, P.; Serini, S.; Torsello, A.; Di Nicuolo, F.; Piccioni, E.; Ubaldi, V.; Pioli, C.; Wolf, F.I.; Calviello, G. β-carotene regulates NF-κB DNA-binding activity by a redox mechanism in human leukemia and colon adenocarcinoma cells. *J. Nutr.* **2003**, *133*, 381–388. [CrossRef] [PubMed]
49. Park, Y.; Lee, H.; Lim, J.W.; Kim, H. Inhibitory Effect of β-carotene on *Helicobacter pylori*-induced TRAF expression and hyper-proliferation in gastric epithelial cells. *Antioxidants* **2019**, *8*, 637. [CrossRef]
50. Ribeiro, D.; Sousa, A.; Nicola, P.; Ferreira de Oliveira, J.M.P.; Rufino, A.T.; Silva, M.; Freitas, M.; Carvalho, F.; Fernandes, E. β-Carotene and its physiological metabolites: Effects on oxidative status regulation and genotoxicity in in vitro models. *Food Chem. Toxicol.* **2020**, *141*, 111392. [CrossRef] [PubMed]
51. Kim, Y.S.; Lee, H.A.; Lim, J.Y.; Kim, Y.; Jung, C.H.; Yoo, S.H.; Kim, Y. β-Carotene inhibits neuroblastoma cell invasion and metastasis in vitro and in vivo by decreasing level of hypoxia-inducible factor-1α. *J. Nutr. Biochem.* **2014**, *25*, 655–664. [CrossRef] [PubMed]

52. Minami, Y.; Kawabata, K.; Kubo, Y.; Arase, S.; Hirasaka, K.; Nikawa, T.; Bando, N.; Kawai, Y.; Terao, J. Peroxidized cholesterol-induced matrix metalloproteinase-9 activation and its suppression by dietary β-carotene in photoaging of hairless mouse skin. *J. Nutr. Biochem.* **2009**, *20*, 389–398. [CrossRef] [PubMed]
53. Wertz, K.; Seifert, N.; Hunziker, P.B.; Riss, G.; Wyss, A.; Lankin, C.; Goralczyk, R. β-carotene inhibits UVA-induced matrix metalloprotease 1 and 10 expression in keratinocytes by a singlet oxygen-dependent mechanism. *Free Radic. Biol. Med.* **2004**, *37*, 654–670. [CrossRef]
54. Guruvayoorappan, C.; Kuttan, G. β-Carotene inhibits tumor-specific angiogenesis by altering the cytokine profile and inhibits the nuclear translocation of transcription factors in B16F-10 melanoma cells. *Integr. Cancer Ther.* **2007**, *6*, 258–270. [CrossRef] [PubMed]
55. Pham, D.N.T.; Leclerc, D.; Lévesque, N.; Deng, L.; Rozen, R. β, β-Carotene 15,15′-monooxygenase and its substrate β-carotene modulate migration and invasion in colorectal carcinoma cells. *Am. J. Clin. Nutr.* **2013**, *98*, 413–422. [CrossRef] [PubMed]
56. Kaliappan, G.; Nagarajan, P.; Moorthy, R.; Selvi, S.K.G.; Raj, T.A.; Kumar, J.M. Ang II induce kidney damage by recruiting inflammatory cells and up regulates PPAR gamma and Renin 1 gene: Effect of β-carotene on chronic renal damage. *J. Thromb. Thrombolysis* **2013**, *36*, 277–285. [CrossRef] [PubMed]
57. Mao, Q.-Q.; Xu, X.-Y.; Shang, A.; Gan, R.-Y.; Wu, D.-T.; Atanasov, A.G.; Li, H.-B. Phytochemicals for the prevention and treatment of gastric cancer: Effects and mechanisms. *Int. J. Mol. Sci.* **2020**, *21*, 570. [CrossRef] [PubMed]

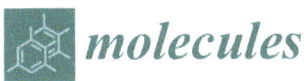

Article

Resveratrol Promotes Hypertrophy in Wildtype Skeletal Muscle and Reduces Muscle Necrosis and Gene Expression of Inflammatory Markers in *Mdx* Mice

Keryn G. Woodman [1,2,3,*], Chantal A. Coles [1,*], Shireen R. Lamandé [1,4] and Jason D. White [2,5]

1. Murdoch Children's Research Institute, Royal Children's Hospital, Parkville, VIC 3052, Australia; Shireen.lamande@mcri.edu.au
2. Faculty of Veterinary and Agricultural Science, The University of Melbourne, Parkville, VIC 3010, Australia; jwhite@csu.edu.au
3. Department of Genetics, Yale University, New Haven, CT 06510, USA
4. Department of Paediatrics, The University of Melbourne, Parkville, VIC 3010, Australia
5. Office of the Pro Vice Chancellor Research and Innovation, Charles Sturt University, Wagga, NSW 2678, Australia
* Correspondence: keryn.woodman@yale.edu (K.G.W.); chantal.coles@mcri.edu.au (C.A.C.); Tel.: +1-203-737-1091 (K.G.W.); +61-3-9936-6021(C.A.C.)

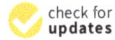

Citation: Woodman, K.G.; Coles, C.A.; Lamandé, S.R.; White, J.D. Resveratrol Promotes Hypertrophy in Wildtype Skeletal Muscle and Reduces Muscle Necrosis and Gene Expression of Inflammatory Markers in *Mdx* Mice. *Molecules* **2021**, *26*, 853. https://doi.org/10.3390/molecules26040853

Academic Editors: Sokcheon Pak and Soo Liang Ooi

Received: 23 December 2020
Accepted: 3 February 2021
Published: 6 February 2021

Publisher's Note: MDPI stays neutral with regard to jurisdictional claims in published maps and institutional affiliations.

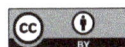

Copyright: © 2021 by the authors. Licensee MDPI, Basel, Switzerland. This article is an open access article distributed under the terms and conditions of the Creative Commons Attribution (CC BY) license (https://creativecommons.org/licenses/by/4.0/).

Abstract: Duchenne muscular dystrophy (DMD) is a progressive fatal neuromuscular disorder with no cure. Therapies to restore dystrophin deficiency have been approved in some jurisdictions but long-term effectiveness is yet to be established. There is a need to develop alternative strategies to treat DMD. Resveratrol is a nutraceutical with anti-inflammatory properties. Previous studies have shown high doses (100–400 mg/kg bodyweight/day) benefit *mdx* mice. We treated 4-week-old *mdx* and wildtype mice with a lower dose of resveratrol (5 mg/kg bodyweight/day) for 15 weeks. Voluntary exercise was used to test if a lower dosage than previously tested could reduce exercise-induced damage where a greater inflammatory infiltrate is present. We found resveratrol promoted skeletal muscle hypertrophy in wildtype mice. In dystrophic muscle, resveratrol reduced exercise-induced muscle necrosis. Gene expression of immune cell markers, CD86 and CD163 were reduced; however, signalling targets associated with resveratrol's mechanism of action including Sirt1 and NF-κB were unchanged. In conclusion, a lower dose of resveratrol compared to the dosage used by other studies reduced necrosis and gene expression of inflammatory cell markers in dystrophic muscle suggesting it as a therapeutic candidate for treating DMD.

Keywords: muscle; muscular dystrophy; mdx; resveratrol; nutraceuticals; duchenne; inflammation

1. Introduction

Duchenne muscular dystrophy (DMD) is a progressive neuromuscular disorder, that arises from mutations in the dystrophin gene [1] and leads to the absence or severe deficiency of the dystrophin protein [2]. Corticosteroids are used in DMD patients to prolong ambulation and maintain respiratory health; however, they have adverse side effects [3,4]. Many types of therapeutics are in development for DMD and include gene correction strategies, exon skipping and utrophin upregulation; some of these therapies are in the initial stages of clinical use [5]. Despite these advances, there is still a need to develop alternative strategies to treat DMD which could be implemented in the short term, especially for patients with mutations not amenable to current trials; or in the longer term as an adjunct to corticosteroids and gene correction strategies.

Nutraceutical use is increasingly popular and this trend has not escaped the DMD community [6]. Whilst nutraceuticals are not able to correct the genetic defect in DMD, many have anti-inflammatory or antioxidant properties which could help dampen the chronic inflammation in DMD patients alongside corticosteroids. Some nutraceuticals with antioxidant or anti-inflammatory properties that have been trialled clinically in DMD include co-enzyme Q10 and green tea extract (reviewed in [6]). Whilst these trials were small in terms of the number of patients the co-enzyme Q10 study showed some encouraging results in terms of muscle performance measured by quantitative muscle testing (QMT). Other pharmacological drugs such as vamorolone have been shown to reduce inflammation and cardiomyopathy in DMD mouse models [7]. Given that many nutraceuticals have documented safety profiles, are already routinely used for other health issues and are available over the counter, they can be readily implemented into a clinical setting for DMD.

Resveratrol (3,5,4-trihydroxy-trans-stilbene), a phytoalexin found in numerous plant species, exerts its beneficial effects on many pathways and targets such as glucose homeostasis, lipid metabolism, insulin sensitivity, reactive oxygen species (ROS), carcinogenicity, inflammation, mitochondrial biogenesis, cell cycle regulation and apoptosis [6,8,9]. Many of resveratrol's actions are due to the activation of sirtuin 1 (Sirt1). Resveratrol allosterically binds to the N terminus of Sirt1 thus activating it [10]. Sirt1 subsequently deacetylates a range of downstream signalling targets in a variety of tissue types.

A series of studies have considered the effect of resveratrol on the myogenic C2C12 cell line [11–13]. Resveratrol increased myoblast elongation and differentiation and this was associated with increased expression of the myogenic regulatory factors (MRFs) *Myod* and *Myog* [11]. In another study, resveratrol increased the expression of *Myf5* and *Myod* during the proliferation phase and *Myog* and *Myhc* during the differentiation phase [12]. Studies using the Sirt1 inhibitor, nicotinamide, directly link the effect of resveratrol on C2C12 cells with Sirt1 expression; proliferation was decreased with nicotinamide treatment [13].

The in vitro effects of resveratrol on myogenesis led to a series of studies in the *mdx* mouse, which is a widely used mouse model of human DMD. The studies used different resveratrol doses at varying ages and duration of treatment. Delivery of 100mg/kg/day for eight weeks resulted in a significant reduction in bodyweight and extensor digitorum longus (EDL), soleus and tibialis anterior (TA) muscle weights, oxidative damage and fibrotic tissue in 41-week old mice [14]. In the same study, fatigue resistance was increased by approximately 20% in the soleus muscle and the EDL and soleus muscles were protected from contraction-induced injury. A high mortality rate is seen with high doses of resveratrol (400 mg/kg/day) [14]. Another study delivered resveratrol to *mdx* mice via oral gavage for 10 days at 10, 100 or 500 mg/kg/day; only the 100 mg/kg dose significantly increased *Sirt1* gene expression and thus was the only dose considered in subsequent analysis [15]. This was associated with decreased immune cell infiltration in the gastrocnemius muscle but no reduction in gene expression of the pro-inflammatory cytokine *TNF-α*. In a later study 100 mg/kg resveratrol treatment did not improve grip strength or fatigue in the *mdx* mice but produced a significant improvement in rotarod performance and in situ peak tension [16].

Overall, the effect of resveratrol administration in the *mdx* mouse investigated in these four studies shows resveratrol improves muscle function, decreases inflammatory infiltrate and reduces fibrotic tissue. However, there are some inconsistencies between the studies. Whilst all of the studies showed improvements in dystrophic pathology; only one study showed reduced inflammatory infiltrate [16]. This could be due to sampling after resveratrol treatment occurring after peak inflammation timing in the *mdx* mice [14,17]. Considering improvements in muscle function and muscle pathology seen in these studies, we wanted to investigate if inducing greater damage in *mdx* mice would more rigorously test resveratrol's anti-inflammatory properties when using a lower dose of 5 mg/kg/day. We have previously shown voluntary exercise induces greater damage in *mdx* mouse muscle and thus is more representative of the human pathology [18,19]. In this study, we treated *mdx* mice with a lower dose of resveratrol (5 mg/kg bodyweight/day) than previously tested [14–17] and used voluntary exercise to induce more dystrophic damage to better assess resveratrol's anti-inflammatory properties.

2. Results

2.1. Resveratrol Increased Hypertrophy in Wildtype Mice

We first investigated the effect of the resveratrol diet on healthy muscle. The average myofibre diameter was larger in the resveratrol treated wildtype mice compared to the mice on the control diet ($p < 0.001$) (Figure 1a–c). In resveratrol treated wildtype mice there was a shift to larger myofibre diameters with more myofibres ranging from 50 to 70 μm in diameter when compared to the wildtype mice on the control diet ($p < 0.05$) (Figure 1d).

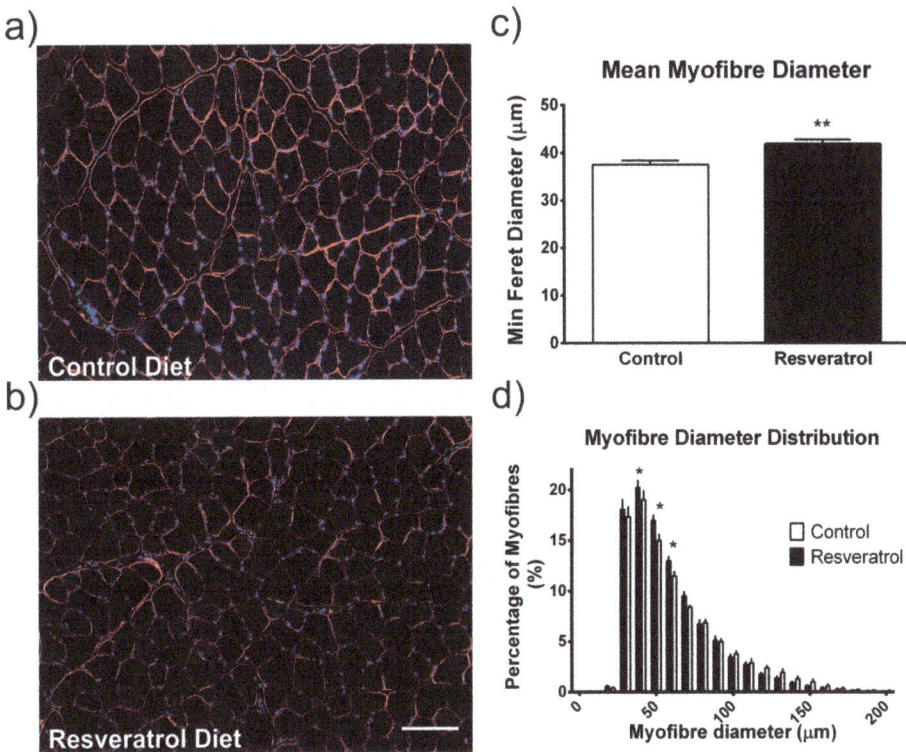

Figure 1. Frozen quadriceps sections were stained with laminin α2 (red) which outlines the individual myofibres and Hoechst (blue) which stains the nuclei. (**a**) Representative image of a stained quadriceps from a mouse on the control diet. (**b**) Representative image of a resveratrol treated mouse quadriceps. (**c**) The average myofibre diameter within the quadriceps muscle is significantly larger in the resveratrol treated cohort in comparison to the control cohort. (**d**) The myofibres were grouped into 10 μm intervals and the proportion of myofibres in each interval was plotted in a histogram. There were more myofibres measuring between 50 and 70 μm in the resveratrol treated group in comparison to the control group. The white scale bar indicates 200 μm. Graphs show mean ± SEM. * indicates $p < 0.05$, ** indicates $p < 0.001$. n = 5 for each treatment group.

2.2. Exercise-Induced Necrosis is Reduced in Mdx Mice with Resveratrol Treatment

Despite an increase in myofibre diameter in wildtype mice, resveratrol did not change the average myofibre diameter or the myofibre size distribution in *mdx* mice (Figure 2a–d). We next examined the muscle for pathological features. Necrosis is a measure of damage in dystrophic muscle and includes areas of mononuclear cells predominantly representing inflammatory infiltrate, myofibres with fragmented sarcoplasm and areas of regenerating myofibres. To determine if resveratrol administration reduced skeletal muscle necrosis in the *mdx* quadriceps muscle, the frozen transverse sections were stained with haematoxylin and eosin (representative images in Figure 3a–d) and necrotic areas were quantitated. The resveratrol treatment did not alter necrosis in the quadriceps of the sedentary *mdx* mice when compared to the control diet cohort (Figure 3e). As in previous studies [18,19], voluntary exercise increased necrosis and damage in *mdx* mice (Figure 3e). Resveratrol treatment protected the muscle from this increase in exercise-induced damage (Figure 3e).

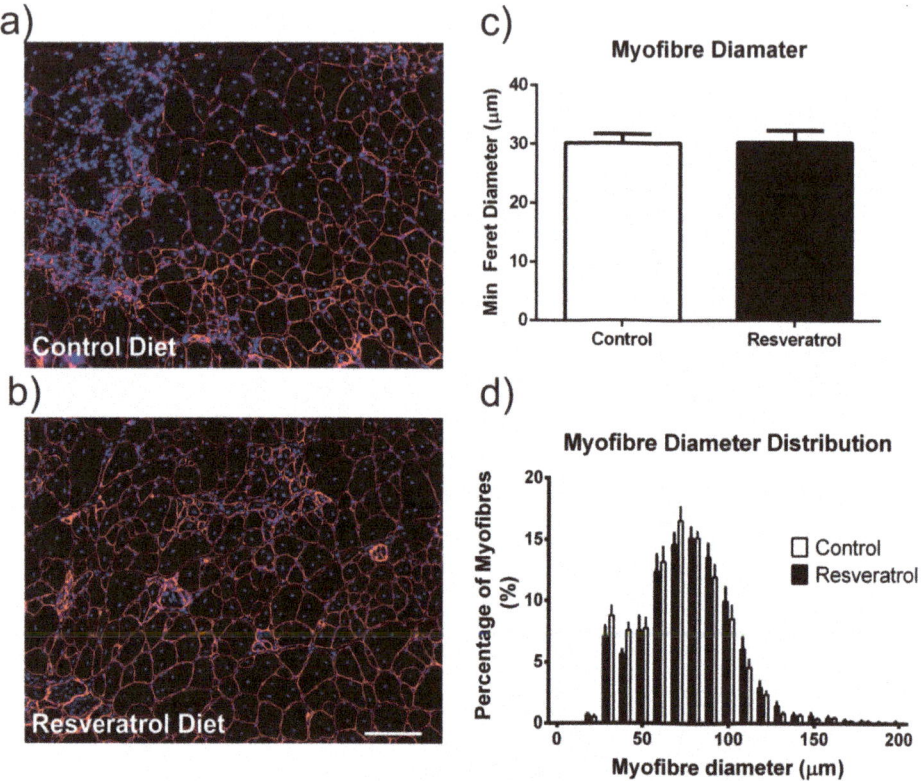

Figure 2. Frozen *mdx* quadriceps sections were stained with laminin α2 (red) and Hoechst (blue). (**a**) Representative image of a stained quadriceps from an *mdx* mouse on the control diet. (**b**) Representative image of a resveratrol treated *mdx* mouse quadriceps. (**c**) The average myofibre diameter within the *mdx* quadriceps muscle is unchanged with resveratrol treatment when compared to the controls. (**d**) The myofibres were grouped into 10 μm intervals and the proportion of myofibres in each interval was plotted in a histogram. There was no change in myofibre distribution with resveratrol treatment. The white scale bar indicates 200 μm. Graphs show mean ± SEM. n = 5 for each treatment group.

2.3. Resveratrol Treatment did not Reduce Damaged Myofibres Mdx Mice

To determine if resveratrol treatment reduced damaged myofibres in the quadriceps of the mdx mice, transverse frozen sections were stained with anti-α2 laminin, Hoechst and anti-IgG (Figure 4a–d). In mdx mice on the control diet, voluntary exercise did not increase the percentage of myofibres positive for anti-IgG (Figure 4e). There was no difference in the percentage of myofibres staining positive for anti-IgG with the resveratrol treatment in either the sedentary or exercised groups compared with mdx on the control diet (Figure 4e). Serum CK activity was also not reduced with resveratrol treatment in either the sedentary or exercise groups when compared to the respective control diet cohorts (Figure 4f).

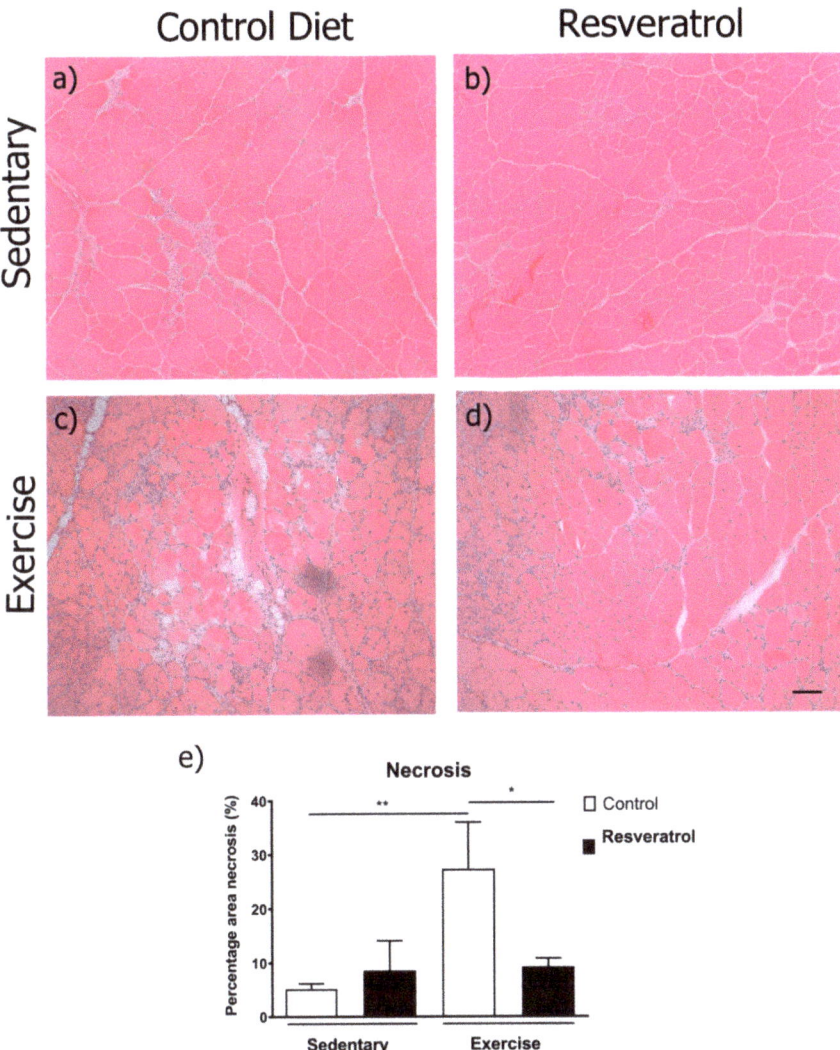

Figure 3. Transverse quadriceps sections were stained with haemotoxylin and eosin to illustrate muscle architecture, areas of inflammation and fibrosis. (**a**) Representative image of an *mdx* control diet sedentary quadriceps, (**c**) an *mdx* control diet exercise quadriceps, (**b**) a resveratrol treated sedentary *mdx* quadriceps and (**d**) an *mdx* resveratrol treated exercised quadriceps. (**e**) Areas of necrosis were quantified and expressed as a percentage of the total quadriceps area. Necrosis was not different with resveratrol treatment in the sedentary *mdx*. Voluntary exercise significantly increased necrosis. This effect is not observed in the resveratrol treated mice when comparing sedentary with exercised resveratrol treated mice. The black scale bars represent 100 μm. Graphs show mean ± SEM. * indicates $p < 0.05$, ** $p < 0.01$. n = 5 for each treatment group.

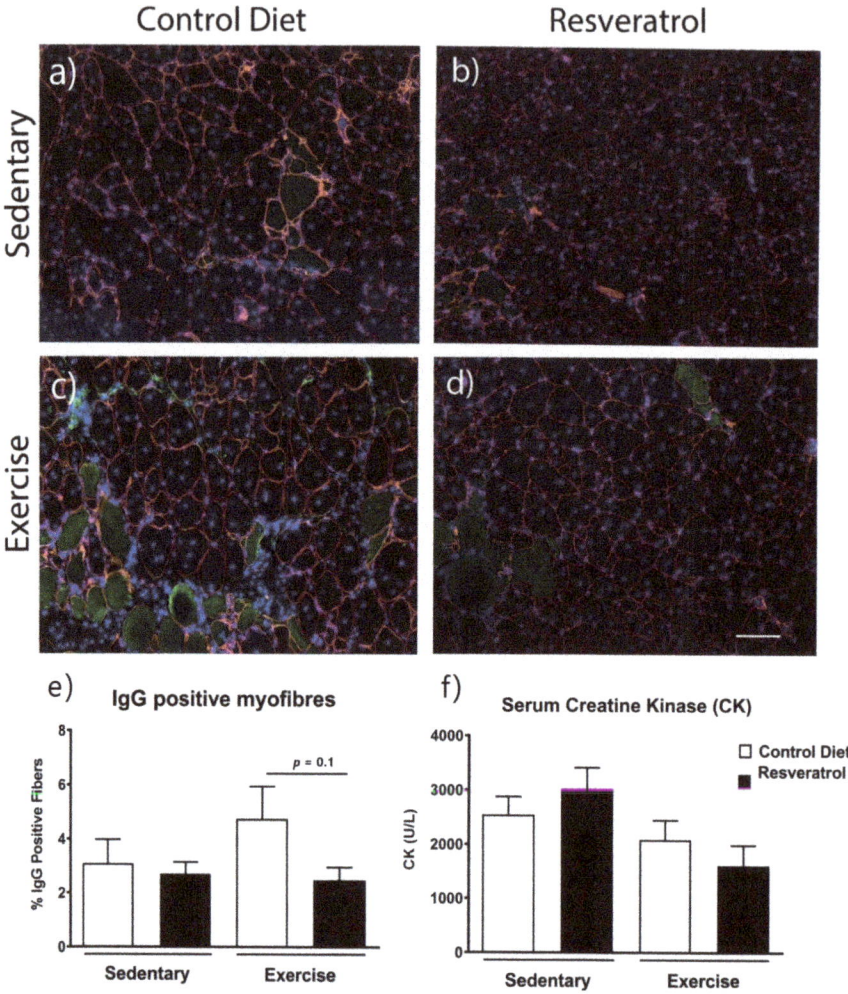

Figure 4. Quadriceps muscles were stained with laminin α2 (red), nuclei with Hoechst (blue) and IgG (green) which enters fibres with impaired sarcolemma. Representative image of (**a**) an *mdx* control diet sedentary quadriceps, (**c**) a control diet exercise *mdx* quadriceps, (**b**) a resveratrol treated sedentary *mdx* quadriceps and a (**d**) resveratrol treated exercise *mdx* quadriceps. (**e**) Quantitative assessment of the quadriceps muscle shows the percentage of damaged IgG positive fibres is unchanged with resveratrol treatment in both exercise and sedentary groups. (**f**) Serum CK activity was similar in all cohorts. The white scale bars represent 200 µm. Graphs show mean ± SEM. n = 5 for each treatment group.

2.4. Resveratrol Administration Decreases Gene Expression of Immune Cell Markers

Since necrosis was decreased with resveratrol treatment in exercised mdx muscle we investigated the gene expression of inflammatory cell markers. Expression of the pan-macrophage marker F4/80 (Emr1) was not changed by resveratrol treatment in either the sedentary or exercised mdx quadriceps (Figure 5a). However, when we assessed Cd86, a cell surface marker for cytotoxic M1 macrophages (Figure 5b) and Cd163 a marker for M2 macrophages (Figure 5c) we found both were downregulated in resveratrol treated sedentary and exercised mice. In addition, gene expression of both these inflammatory markers was increased with voluntary exercise in the control *mdx* suggesting greater numbers of these cells are involved in the exercise-induced inflammatory infiltrate found in necrotic dystrophic muscle. Neutrophils are also present in necrotic dystrophic muscle; however, we found no difference in expression of the neutrophil marker lymphocyte antigen 6 complex, locus G (*Ly6G*) gene with resveratrol treatment in either sedentary or exercise groups (Figure 5d). These data suggest resveratrol exerts its anti-inflammatory effects in dystrophic muscle on macrophage sub-types that are predominant during muscle repair [20].

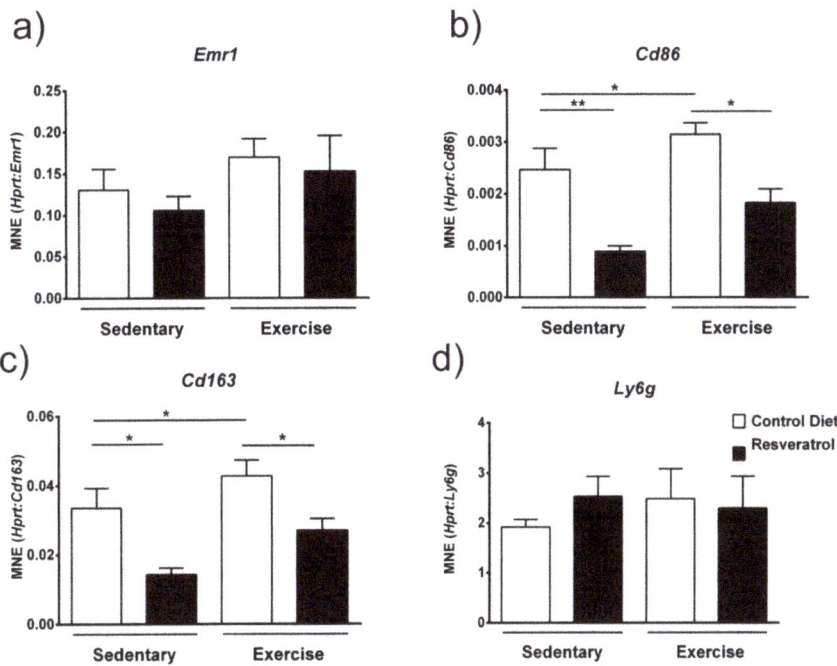

Figure 5. (a) Expression of *Emr1* a marker for (F4/80 positive) macrophages was unchanged with resveratrol treatment. (b) Expression of *Cd86*, a marker for M1 macrophages and (c) Cd163, a marker for M2 macrophages was downregulated with resveratrol treatment in sedentary *mdx*. Voluntary exercise resulted in increased expression of M1 (b) (*Cd86*) and M2 (c) (*Cd163*) gene expression. Resveratrol treatment was effective in preventing this increase in exercised *mdx*. (d) Expression of the neutrophil marker *Ly6g* was unchanged with resveratrol administration in both sedentary and exercise *mdx*. Graphs show mean ± SEM. * $p < 0.05$, ** $p < 0.01$. n = 5 for each treatment group.

2.5. Resveratrol Treatment Increased Gene Expression of Il6 and Tnf

As gene expression of an M1 macrophage marker Cd86 was downregulated with resveratrol treatment, we assessed if this was accompanied by a decrease in inflammatory cytokine expression. Gene expression of interleukin 10 (*Il-10*) remained unchanged with resveratrol administration (Figure 6a) in both sedentary and exercised *mdx*. Interestingly, expression of two cytokines, interleukin 6 (*Il6*) (Figure 6b) and tumour necrosis factor (*Tnf*) (Figure 6c) were significantly increased with resveratrol treatment in the sedentary mice ($p < 0.05$) yet remained unchanged in the exercised mice (Figure 6b–c). Resveratrol treatment did not change the expression of transforming growth factor-beta (*TGF-β*) in either the sedentary or control groups when compared to the controls (Figure 6d).

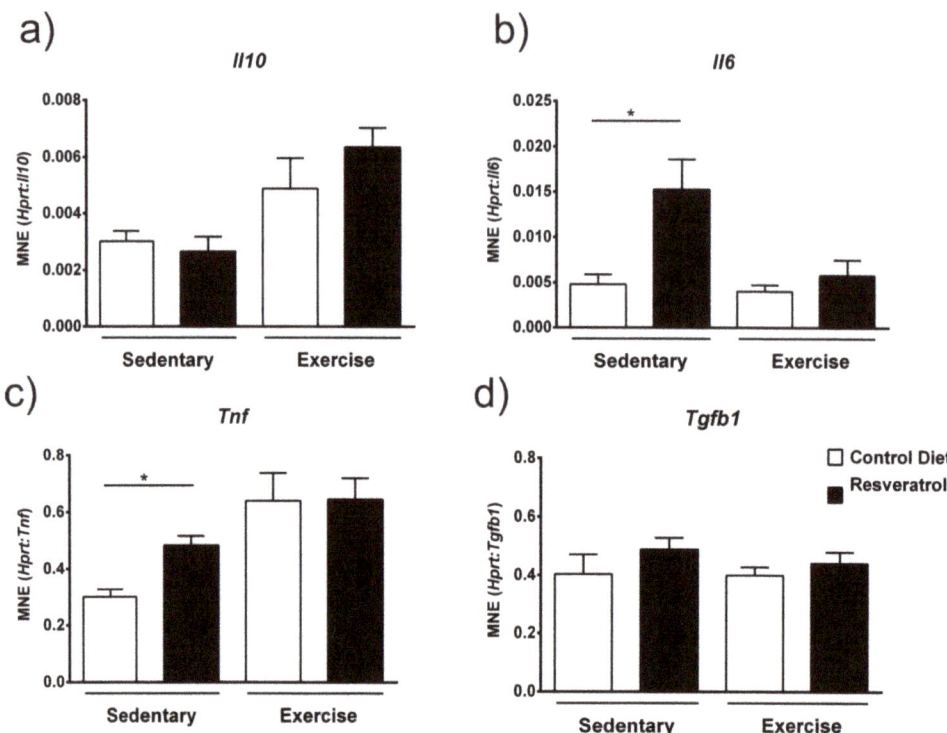

Figure 6. (a) *Il-10* gene expression is unchanged with resveratrol treatment. (b) *Il-6* gene expression was up-regulated with resveratrol treatment in the sedentary *mdx* mice but remained unchanged in the exercised group. (c) Gene expression of TNF-α was up-regulated with resveratrol treatment in the sedentary *mdx* mice, yet remained unchanged in the exercised group. (d) Gene expression of *Tgf-β* was unchanged with resveratrol treatment. There was also no effect of exercise on gene expression of these pro-inflammatory cytokines. Graphs show mean ± SEM. * $p < 0.05$. n = 5 for each treatment group.

2.6. Resveratrol Treatment does not Alter Sirt1 or Nfb gene Expression in Mdx Mice

Resveratrol is thought to elicit its anti-inflammatory and antioxidant effects through downstream signalling targets such as Sirt1 and NF-κB. Sirt1 belongs to the NAD+-dependent protein deacetylase family or sirtuins, which have key roles in many cellular processes including inflammation and oxidative stress. Resveratrol can regulate Sirt1 expression [21,22]. The NF-κβ pathway is another target of resveratrol and has critical roles in inflammation, immunity, cell proliferation, differentiation and survival [23]. We assessed if resveratrol altered gene expression of these signalling targets. Sirt1 (Figure 7a), *Nfkb1* (Figure 7b) or *Nfb2* (Figure 7c) gene expression was unchanged with resveratrol administration in both the sedentary and exercise mdx.

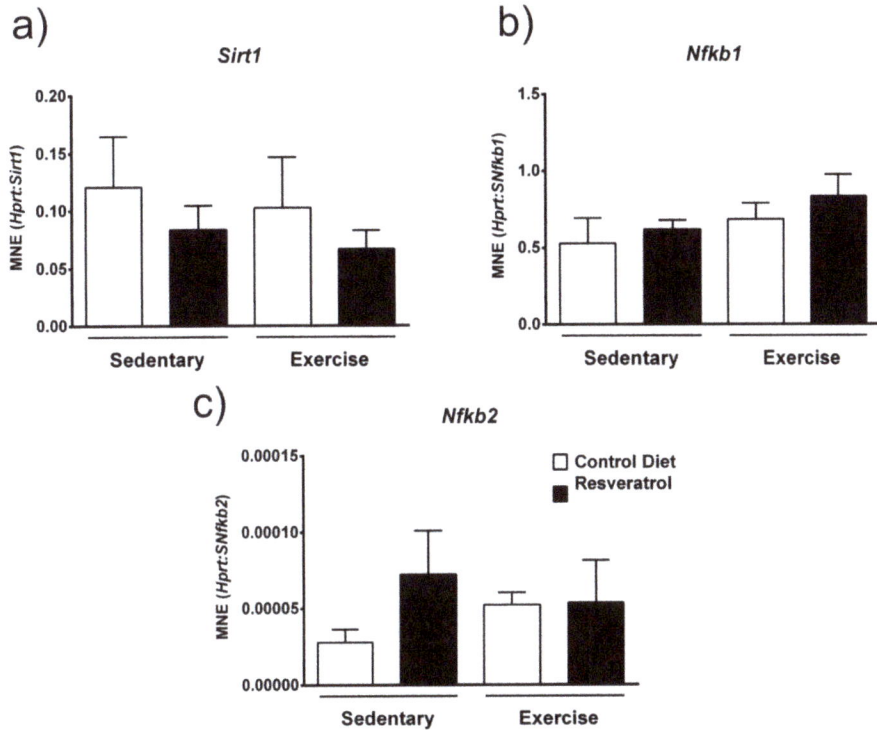

Figure 7. (**a**) *Sirt1* gene expression is unchanged with resveratrol treatment in both sedentary and exercise groups when compared to respective controls. (**b**) Gene expression of *NF-κB1* is unchanged with resveratrol treatment in both the sedentary and exercise cohorts. (**c**) Likewise, *NF-κB2* gene expression is not significantly altered with resveratrol administration in either sedentary or exercised *mdx* mice. Graphs show mean ± SEM. n = 5 per treatment group.

3. Discussion

Whilst previous studies have shown that treating *mdx* mice with resveratrol has beneficial effects on muscle pathology and performance, only one study showed a positive effect on immune infiltration [14–17]. This inconsistency could be explained by the fact that the *mdx* mouse has a milder disease pathology than the human condition with peak inflammation occurring between 6 and 12 weeks of age [24]. The age at which muscles were harvested for immune cell analysis and therefore the amount of immune infiltration could be a major factor in determining resveratrol's ability to suppress inflammation. When tissues were harvested around the time of peak inflammation, resveratrol treated samples had fewer muscle leukocytes (CD45+ cells) and F4/80 positive macrophages [15]. By contrast, when the tissue was harvested well beyond the period of peak inflammation no differences in immune infiltration were seen in the resveratrol treated mice [16]. Another group also found no change in total immune infiltration (CD45+ cells) after treating *mdx* mice with resveratrol for 32 weeks from 9 weeks of age [17]. Based on this we used voluntary exercise to increase muscle damage and necrosis and thus immune infiltration in mdx and tested if administration of resveratrol at a much lower dose would protect against exercise-induced damage. We found where there is greater necrotic tissue in *mdx* mice due to exercise-induced damage, resveratrol is able to protect the dystrophic muscle from contraction-induced injury at a much lower dose (5 mg/kg bodyweight/day) than previously shown to be beneficial (100–400 mg/kg bodyweight/day). This suggests there needs to be a certain amount of inflammation present in the muscle tissue for the effects of resveratrol to be clearly seen and thus timing in the *mdx* mouse is critical to ensure this.

In necrotic *mdx* tissue, the immune infiltrate is comprised of macrophages, T-cells, neutrophils, eosinophils and mast cells; however, the number of macrophages greatly outnumbers the other immune cells [25]. Due to resveratrol's effects on reducing exercise-induced necrosis in this study, we investigated the gene expression of immune cell markers expressed by macrophages and neutrophils. There are two distinct populations of macrophages; the M1 "cytotoxic" population release pro-inflammatory cytokines, and can promote cell lysis and phagocytosis of necrotic myofibres, clearing the way for muscle regeneration [26], whilst the M2 anti-inflammatory macrophages release anti-inflammatory cytokines and factors which attenuate tissue repair, such as IL-10 and TGF-β [27]. In *mdx* mice; however, the normal inflammation and regeneration process is disrupted and the normally well-coordinated inflammatory process and muscle repair is impaired and M1 macrophages continue to be present in the muscle. The shift from M1 to M2 macrophages is instead replaced with co-invasion of M2 macrophages with M1 macrophages and neutrophils [28]. The M2 macrophages produce IL-10 in an immunomodulation attempt to deactivate the M1 macrophages. IL-10 and IL-4 are able to modulate macrophage polarisation from the M1 to M2 phenotype and thus reduce inflammation and damage in *mdx* mice [28]. We show that exercise increased the gene expression of *Cd86*, a marker of cytotoxic M1 macrophages and *Cd163*, a marker of anti-inflammatory M2 macrophages. This increase was dampened with resveratrol treatment. The gene expression of these inflammatory markers was also decreased in sedentary *mdx* with resveratrol treatment suggesting these macrophage subsets are directly impacted by resveratrol irrespective of the magnitude of an inflammatory infiltrate. In a murine myocardial infarction model, resveratrol treatment reduced damage and fibrosis and that resveratrol was cardioprotective by suppressing inflammation [29]. They also showed via flow cytometry that CD11c+ M1 macrophages were significantly decreased with resveratrol treatment [29]. Overall, these data highlight resveratrol's anti-inflammatory role and suggests that it could potentially have a role in macrophage polarisation during muscle injury.

Another recent study investigated resveratrol's actions on human THP-1 monocytes and macrophages in vitro [30]. They first showed that the addition of resveratrol at a concentration of 5 μmol/L inhibited proliferation of THP-1 monocytes and at >10 μmol/L concentrations resveratrol induced cell apoptosis and caused G0/G1 phase arrest in vitro [30]. The reduced necrosis and decreased gene expression of M1 and M2 inflammatory macrophages found in our treated exercised *mdx* mice and the reduced immune cell infiltration with resveratrol treatment [15] is consistent with this study [30] and suggests that resveratrol has effects on macrophage proliferation/polarisation. Future studies could use flow cytometry to explore the effect of resveratrol on macrophages and other immune cell populations as well as to further elucidate which cell type is responsible for increases in cytokine production such as Il6 and Tnf.

The anti-inflammatory and anti-apoptotic effects of resveratrol are thought to be due to effects on Sirt1 activation and NF-κB inhibition [31–33]. Previous research assessed Sirt1 activation with different resveratrol doses and found 100 mg/kg was the most effective in up-regulating Sirt1 mRNA [15]. We, therefore, conclude that our low dose of 5 mg/kg was not sufficient to increase gene expression of *Sirt1* and therefore the results seen in our cohort are likely attributed to effects on inflammation and are therefore not mediated by Sirt1. This effect was also observed for *NF-κB1* and *NF-κB2* which were unchanged by resveratrol treatment in the *mdx* mice again suggesting that resveratrol's effects in *mdx* mice are due to its ability to suppress inflammation, perhaps through its effects on other signalling targets such as the p38 MAPK pathways [34]. Overall resveratrol has shown potential to reduce pathology in the *mdx* mouse model of DMD and highlights the need for this to be tested clinically. A recent 2020 study tested resveratrol supplementation in an open-label, single-arm, phase IIa trial in 11 patients with Duchenne, Becker or Fukuyama muscular dystrophies [35]. Whilst this study was quite small, they were able to show a significant reduction in creatine kinase levels and improved motor function measurements [35]. These results are highly encouraging and open the door for trials with increased patient numbers.

Whilst we have shown beneficial effects in *mdx* mice, we also investigated resveratrol's ability to affect healthy muscle. Previous in vitro studies demonstrate that resveratrol increases myoblast differentiation in C2C12 cells and in primary myoblasts [11,12,36]. Here we show a significant increase in the average myofibre diameter, particularly in fibres which are larger than average, in the quadriceps muscle of resveratrol treated wildtype mice. These findings correlate with a study that found increased myofibre hypertrophy in resveratrol treated mice (25 mg/kg for 4 weeks) that underwent a repetitive ladder-climbing protocol [37]. Whilst changes in muscle mass and metabolic markers were seen, the underlying mechanism behind the increased hypertrophy was not explored [37]. Together these data suggest that resveratrol treatment promotes muscle hypertrophy in wildtype mice and this could have direct applications to the livestock industry, sports medicine or potentially for treating cachexia.

4. Materials and Methods

4.1. Mice and Trial Design

All animal experiments were approved by the University of Melbourne Animal Ethics Committee (AEC) and the Murdoch Children's Research Institute AEC. Male C57BL10/ScSn (wildtype) and C57Bl10/mdx (*mdx*) mice were obtained from Animal Resources Centre (Perth, WA, Australia). At 4 weeks of age (after weaning and prior to the peak period of inflammation in *mdx* mice [24]), 12 mice received either a control diet or resveratrol diet (5 mg/kg bodyweight/day) for 12 weeks. After 12 weeks the groups were divided into sedentary and exercised groups. Mice were housed singly with running wheels for three weeks, with wheel rotation data being recorded as described [18]. The trial design included treatment of sedentary mice for 12 weeks followed by 3 weeks of further treatment with voluntary exercise. Peak inflammation occurs at 6–12 weeks of age [24] and is exacerbated by adding the voluntary exercise protocol. The trial design thus ensured robust testing of resveratrol's anti-inflammatory properties. The mice continued to receive their specified diet over the exercise period. The quadriceps were chosen for further analyses as they are highly susceptible to exercise-induced damage [18]. At trial completion blood was obtained via cardiac puncture and the quadriceps muscles were harvested and snap-frozen. The contralateral quadriceps muscles from the remaining hindlimb were mounted in 5% tragacanth (*w/v*) (Sigma, St Louis, MO, USA) and frozen in liquid nitrogen-cooled isopentane (Sigma, St Louis, MO, USA) and stored at −80 °C for histological analyses.

4.2. Immunostaining

The quadriceps muscle was cryosectioned (10 µm) and blocked in 10% (*v/v*) donkey serum (Millipore, Billerica, MA, USA) in wash buffer (0.1% Tween, 0.5% Bovine albumin serum in PBS) before immunodetection of rat anti-laminin α-2 (Santa Cruz Biotechnology, Dallas, TX, USA) to identify myofibre boundary. Sections were imaged on a Zeiss Axio Imager M1 upright fluorescent microscope with an AxioCam MRm camera running AxioVision software V4.8.2.0 (Carl Zeiss, Oberkochen, Germany, 2015).

4.3. Histology and Morphometric Analysis

4.3.1. Minimum Feret's Diameter

Image J version 1.48G (U. S. National Institutes of Health, Bethesda, MD, USA) was used to calculate minimum Feret's diameter as described in Treat-NMD standard operating procedure "Quantitative determination of muscle fibre diameter" (http://www.treat-nmd.eu/downloads/file/sops/dmd/MDX/DMD_M.1.2.001.pdf (accessed on 12 December 2020)).

4.3.2. Damaged Myofibres

To determine the percentage of damaged myofibres, muscles were stained for intracellular IgG using AlexaFluor donkey anti-mouse IgG 488 (Thermofisher Scientific, Waltham, MA, USA), Anti-IgG positive myofibres in the entire muscle cross-section were counted manually and expressed as a percentage of the total myofibre number.

4.3.3. Central Nuclei and Necrosis

Quadriceps were cryosectioned (10 μm) and stained with hematoxylin and eosin. The necrotic area and percentage of central nuclei were calculated for entire muscle cross-sections as previously described [18].

4.3.4. Creatine Kinase Enzyme Activity

Blood was centrifuged at 12,000 g for 15 min to separate the serum. To measure CK activity, the serum was thawed and 5 μL was aliquoted into a 96 well plate in triplicate, followed by CK-NAC reagent (Thermofisher Scientific, Waltham, MA, USA). The change in absorbance was recorded at 340 nm over three minutes (measured in 20 s intervals) at 37 °C using a Paradigm Detection Platform (Beckman Coulter, Brea, CA, USA) [38].

4.3.5. RNA Extraction, cDNA Synthesis, qPCR and Oligonucleotide Primer Design

RNA was extracted from snap-frozen quadriceps and reverse transcribed to cDNA as previously described [38]. Each qPCR reaction contained 25 ng of cDNA added to "Go Taq Sybr Green" qPCR master mix (Promega, Madison, WI, USA) as per manufacturer's instructions. All qPCR reactions were performed using a LightCycler480 (Roche Applied Bioscience, Basel, Switzerland).

4.3.6. Statistical Analyses

Where data was normally distributed GraphPad Prism 5 (GraphPad Software, La Jolla, CA, USA) was used to assess statistical significance. Where there was a direct comparison between two groups or two data points, a Student's t-test was used. RT-qPCR data and data that were not normally distributed, such as myofibre diameter, were assessed using a non-parametric Mann–Whitney U test in GraphPad Prism [39].

5. Conclusions

Treating healthy wildtype mice with 5 mg/kg/day of resveratrol increased myofibre diameter and the proportion of larger myofibres. This finding supports in vitro experiments and could have particular relevance to the livestock, sports medicine fields or cachexia fields where increased muscle mass would be beneficial.

Voluntary exercise increased muscle pathology and immune infiltration in the *mdx* mouse and provided a greater therapeutic challenge for the anti-inflammatory resveratrol supplementation. Low dose resveratrol dampened exercise-induced necrosis. Expression of a cytotoxic M1 macrophage marker was reduced as was an M2 macrophage marker, suggesting there were fewer inflammatory cells and highlighting resveratrol's anti-inflammatory properties. Overall, we show that resveratrol could be beneficial for treating DMD and future experiments could focus on optimising the dose and treatment duration in exercised mice. Combined administration of resveratrol and corticosteroids could have synergistic therapeutic benefits.

Author Contributions: K.G.W. assisted with the conceptualisation of the study, performed the methodology and formal analysis and prepared and edited the manuscript. C.A.C. provided technical advice, assisted in data interpretation and edited the manuscript. S.R.L. interpreted data and edited the manuscript. J.D.W. conceptualised and supervised the study and data interpretation and edited the manuscript. All authors have read and agreed to the published version of the manuscript.

Funding: This work was supported by Muscular Dystrophy Australia, Murdoch Children's Research Institute and the Victorian Government's Operational Infrastructure Support Program. S.R.L. was supported by a National Health and Medical Research Council of Australia research fellowship (GNT1043837).

Institutional Review Board Statement: Not applicable.

Informed Consent Statement: Not applicable.

Conflicts of Interest: The authors declare no conflict of interest.

Sample Availability: Samples of the compounds are not available from the authors.

References

1. Koenig, M.; Monaco, A.P.; Kunkel, L.M. The complete sequence of dystrophin predicts a rod-shaped cytoskeletal protein. *Cell* **1988**, *53*, 219–228. [CrossRef]
2. Hoffman, E.P.; Brown, R.H.J.; Kunkel, L.M. Dystrophin: The protein product of the Duchenne muscular dystrophy locus. *Cell* **1987**, *51*, 919–928. [CrossRef]
3. Biggar, W.D. Deflazacort in Duchenne muscular dystrophy: A comparison of two different protocols. *Neuromuscul. Disord.* **2004**, *14*, 476–482. [CrossRef] [PubMed]
4. Bushby, K.; Muntoni, F.; Urtizberea, A.; Hughes, R.; Griggs, R. Report on the 124th ENMC International Workshop. Treatment of Duchenne muscular dystrophy; defining the gold standards of management in the use of corticosteroids. 2–4 April 2004, Naarden, The Netherlands. *Neuromuscul. Disord.* **2004**, *14*, 526–534. [CrossRef]
5. Chamberlain, J.R.; Chamberlain, J.S. Progress toward Gene Therapy for Duchenne Muscular Dystrophy. *Mol. Ther.* **2017**, *25*, 1125–1131. [CrossRef] [PubMed]
6. Woodman, K.G.; Coles, C.A.; Lamande, S.R.; White, J.D. Nutraceuticals and Their Potential to Treat Duchenne Muscular Dystrophy: Separating the Credible from the Conjecture. *Nutrients* **2016**, *8*, 731. [CrossRef]
7. Heier, C.R.; Yu, Q.; Fiorillo, A.A.; Tully, C.B.; Tucker, A.; Mazala, D.A.; Uaesoontrachoon, K.; Srinivassane, S.; Damsker, J.M.; Hoffman, E.P.; et al. Vamorolone targets dual nuclear receptors to treat inflammation and dystrophic cardiomyopathy. *Life Sci. Alliance* **2019**, *2*, e201800186. [CrossRef] [PubMed]
8. Oshaghi, E.A.; Goodarzi, M.T.; Higgins, V.; Adeli, K. Role of resveratrol in the management of insulin resistance and related conditions: Mechanism of action. *Crit. Rev. Clin. Lab. Sci.* **2017**, *54*, 267–293. [CrossRef]
9. Szkudelski, T.; Szkudelska, K. Resveratrol and diabetes: From animal to human studies. *Biochim. Biophys. Acta* **2015**, *1852*, 1145–1154. [CrossRef] [PubMed]
10. Hubbard, B.P.; Gomes, A.P.; Dai, H.; Li, J.; Case, A.W.; Considine, T.; Riera, T.V.; Lee, J.E.; Yen E, S.; Lamming, D.W.; et al. Evidence for a common mechanism of SIRT1 regulation by allosteric activators. *Science* **2013**, *339*, 1216–1219. [CrossRef]
11. Kaminski, J.; Lançon, A.; Aires, V.; Limagne, E.; Tili, E.; Michaille, J.-J.; Latruffe, N. Resveratrol initiates differentiation of mouse skeletal muscle-derived C2C12 myoblasts. *Biochem. Pharmacol.* **2012**, *84*, 1251–1259. [CrossRef]
12. Montesano, A.; Luzi, L.; Senesi, P.; Mazzocchi, N.; Terruzzi, I. Resveratrol promotes myogenesis and hypertrophy in murine myoblasts. *J. Transl. Med.* **2013**, *11*, 310. [CrossRef] [PubMed]
13. Wang, L.; Zhang, T.; Xi, Y.; Yang, C.; Sun, C.; Li, D. Sirtuin 1 promotes the proliferation of C2C12 myoblast cells via the myostatin signaling pathway. *Mol. Med. Rep.* **2016**, *14*, 1309–1315. [CrossRef] [PubMed]
14. Selsby, J.T.; Morine, K.J.; Pendrak, K.; Barton, E.R.; Sweeney, H.L. Rescue of dystrophic skeletal muscle by PGC-1α involves a fast to slow fiber type shift in the mdx mouse. *PLoS ONE* **2012**, *7*, e30063. [CrossRef]
15. Gordon, B.S.; Díaz, D.C.D.; Kostek, M.C. Resveratrol decreases inflammation and increases utrophin gene expression in the mdx mouse model of Duchenne muscular dystrophy. *Clin. Nutr.* **2013**, *32*, 104–111. [CrossRef]
16. Gordon, B.S.; Delgado-Diaz, D.C.; Carson, J.; Fayad, R.; Wilson, L.B.; Kostek, M.C. Resveratrol improves muscle function but not oxidative capacity in young mdx mice. *Can. J. Physiol. Pharmacol.* **2014**, *92*, 243–251. [CrossRef] [PubMed]
17. Hori, Y.S.; Kuno, A.; Hosoda, R.; Tanno, M.; Miura, T.; Shimamoto, K.; Horio, Y. Resveratrol ameliorates muscular pathology in the dystrophic mdx mouse, a model for Duchenne muscular dystrophy. *J. Pharmacol. Exp. Ther.* **2011**, *338*, 784–794. [CrossRef]
18. Smythe, G.M.; White, J.D. Voluntary wheel running in dystrophin-deficient (mdx) mice: Relationships between exercise parameters and exacerbation of the dystrophic phenotype. *PLoS Curr.* **2011**, *3*, RRN1295. [CrossRef]
19. Coles, C.A.; Gordon, L.; Hunt, L.C.; Webster, T.; Piers, A.T.; Kintakas, C.; Woodman, K.; Touslon, S.L.; Smythe, G.M.; White, J.D.; et al. Expression profiling in exercised mdx suggests a role for extracellular proteins in the dystrophic muscle immune response. *Hum. Mol. Genet.* **2020**, *29*, 353–368. [CrossRef]
20. Tidball, J.G.; Villalta, S.A. Regulatory interactions between muscle and the immune system during muscle regeneration. *Am. J. Physiol. Regul. Integr. Comp. Physiol.* **2010**, *298*, R1173–R1187. [CrossRef]
21. Borra, M.T.; Smith, B.C.; Denu, J.M. Mechanism of human SIRT1 activation by resveratrol. *J. Biol. Chem.* **2005**, *280*, 17187–17195. [CrossRef] [PubMed]
22. Kaeberlein, M.; McDonagh, T.; Heltweg, B.; Hixon, J.; Westman, E.A.; Caldwell, S.D.; Napper, A.; Curtis, R.; Distefano, P.S.; Fields, S.; et al. Substrate-specific activation of sirtuins by resveratrol. *J. Biol. Chem.* **2005**, *280*, 17038–17045. [CrossRef]

23. Sadeghi, A.; Ebrahimi, S.S.S.; Golestani, A.; Meshkani, R. Resveratrol Ameliorates Palmitate-Induced Inflammation in Skeletal Muscle Cells by Attenuating Oxidative Stress and JNK/NF-κB Pathway in a SIRT1-Independent Mechanism. *J. Cell. Biochem.* **2017**, *118*, 2654–2663. [CrossRef]
24. McGeachie, J.K.; Grounds, M.D.; Partridge, T.A.; Morgan, J.E. Age-related changes in replication of myogenic cells in mdx mice: Quantitative autoradiographic studies. *J. Neurol. Sci.* **1993**, *119*, 169–179. [CrossRef]
25. Villalta, S.A.; Rinaldi, C.; Deng, B.; Liu, G.; Fedor, B.; Tidball, J.G. Interleukin-10 reduces the pathology of mdx muscular dystrophy by deactivating M1 macrophages and modulating macrophage phenotype. *Hum. Mol. Genet.* **2011**, *20*, 790–805. [CrossRef]
26. Villalta, S.A.; Nguyen, H.X.; Deng, B.; Gotoh, T.; Tidball, J.G. Shifts in macrophage phenotypes and macrophage competition for arginine metabolism affect the severity of muscle pathology in muscular dystrophy. *Hum. Mol. Genet.* **2009**, *18*, 482–496. [CrossRef]
27. Gordon, S.; Martinez, F.O. Alternative activation of macrophages: Mechanism and functions. *Immunity* **2010**, *32*, 593–604. [CrossRef]
28. Tidball, J.G. Mechanisms of muscle injury, repair, and regeneration. *Compr. Physiol.* **2011**, *1*, 2029–2062. [CrossRef] [PubMed]
29. Liu, S.; Du, Y.; Shi, K.; Yang, Y.; Yang, Z. Resveratrol improves cardiac function by promoting M2-like polarization of macrophages in mice with myocardial infarction. *Am. J. Transl. Res.* **2019**, *11*, 5212–5226.
30. Feng, L.; Yasmeen, R.; Schoene, N.W.; Lei, K.Y.; Wang, T.T.Y. Resveratrol differentially modulates immune responses in human THP-1 monocytes and macrophages. *Nutr. Res.* **2019**, *72*, 57–69. [CrossRef] [PubMed]
31. Chávez, E.; Reyes-Gordillo, K.; Segovia, J.; Shibayama, M.; Tsutsumi, V.; Vergara, P.; Moreno, M.G.; Muriel, P. Resveratrol prevents fibrosis, NF-kappaB activation and TGF-beta increases induced by chronic CCl4 treatment in rats. *J. Appl. Toxicol.* **2008**, *28*, 35–43. [CrossRef]
32. Howitz, K.T.; Bitterman, K.J.; Cohen, H.Y.; Lamming, D.W.; Lavu, S.; Wood, J.G.; Zipkin, R.E.; Chung, P.; Kisielewski, A.; Zhang, L.-L.; et al. Small molecule activators of sirtuins extend Saccharomyces cerevisiae lifespan. *Nature* **2003**, *425*, 191–196. [CrossRef]
33. Lagouge, M.; Argmann, C.; Gerhart-Hines, Z.; Meziane, H.; Lerin, C.; Daussin, F.; Messadeq, N.; Milne, J.; Lambert, P.; Elliott, P.; et al. Resveratrol improves mitochondrial function and protects against metabolic disease by activating SIRT1 and PGC-1alpha. *Cell* **2006**, *127*, 1109–1122. [CrossRef]
34. Meng, T.; Xiao, D.; Muhammed, A.; Deng, J.; Chen, L.; He, J. Anti-Inflammatory Action and Mechanisms of Resveratrol. *Molecules* **2020**, *26*, 229. [CrossRef]
35. Kawamura, K.; Fukumura, S.; Nikaido, K.; Tachi, N.; Kozuka, N.; Seino, T.; Hatakeyama, K.; Mori, M.; Ito, Y.M.; Takami, A.; et al. Resveratrol improves motor function in patients with muscular dystrophies: An open-label, single-arm, phase IIa study. *Sci. Rep.* **2020**, *10*, 20585. [CrossRef]
36. Saini, A.; Al-Shanti, N.; Sharples, A.P.; Stewart, C.E. Sirtuin 1 regulates skeletal myoblast survival and enhances differentiation in the presence of resveratrol. *Exp. Physiol.* **2012**, *97*, 400–418. [CrossRef]
37. Kan, N.-W.; Lee, M.-C.; Tung, Y.-T.; Chiu, C.-C.; Huang, C.-C.; Huang, W.-C. The Synergistic Effects of Resveratrol combined with Resistant Training on Exercise Performance and Physiological Adaption. *Nutrients* **2018**, *10*, 1360. [CrossRef]
38. Hunt, L.C.; Upadhyay, A.; Jazayeri, J.A.; Tudor, E.M.; White, J.D. Caspase-3, myogenic transcription factors and cell cycle inhibitors are regulated by leukemia inhibitory factor to mediate inhibition of myogenic differentiation. *Skelet. Muscle* **2011**, *1*, 17. [CrossRef]
39. Pfaffl, M.W.; Tichopad, A.; Prgomet, C.; Neuvians, T.P. Determination of stable housekeeping genes, differentially regulated target genes and sample integrity: BestKeeper—Excel-based tool using pair-wise correlations. *Biotechnol. Lett.* **2004**, *26*, 509–515. [CrossRef]

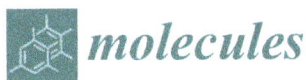

Article

Micellar Casein and Whey Powder Hold a TGF-β Activity and Regulate ID Genes In Vitro

Layla Panahipour [1], Selma Husejnovic [1], Jila Nasirzade [1], Stephan Semelmayer [1] and Reinhard Gruber [1,2,3,*]

1. Department of Oral Biology, Medical University of Vienna, Sensengasse 2a, 1090 Vienna, Austria; layla.panahipour@meduniwien.ac.at (L.P.); n1350960@students.meduniwien.ac.at (S.H.); jila.nasirzaderajiri@meduniwien.ac.at (J.N.); n01629942@students.meduniwien.ac.at (S.S.)
2. Department of Periodontology, School of Dental Medicine, University of Bern, Freiburgstrasse 7, 3010 Bern, Switzerland
3. Austrian Cluster for Tissue Regeneration, Donaueschingenstraße 13, 1200 Vienna, Austria
* Correspondence: reinhard.gruber@meduniwien.ac.at

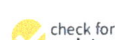

Citation: Panahipour, L.; Husejnovic, S.; Nasirzade, J.; Semelmayer, S.; Gruber, R. Micellar Casein and Whey Powder Hold a TGF-β Activity and Regulate ID Genes In Vitro. *Molecules* **2021**, *26*, 507. https://doi.org/10.3390/molecules26020507

Academic Editor: Sokcheon Pak
Received: 31 December 2020
Accepted: 14 January 2021
Published: 19 January 2021

Publisher's Note: MDPI stays neutral with regard to jurisdictional claims in published maps and institutional affiliations.

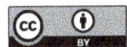

Copyright: © 2021 by the authors. Licensee MDPI, Basel, Switzerland. This article is an open access article distributed under the terms and conditions of the Creative Commons Attribution (CC BY) license (https://creativecommons.org/licenses/by/4.0/).

Abstract: Casein and whey being food supplements have been considered to be used in oral health care products. However, the response of oral cells to micellar casein and whey powder remains unclear. Considering that milk contains the growth factor TGF-β, and lactoperoxidase was recently reported to decrease the expression of inhibitor of DNA-binding (ID) proteins, there is a rationale to assume that casein and whey can also provoke these responses in oral cells. To examine the TGF-β activity, gingival fibroblasts were exposed to reconstituted casein and whey powder from food supplement before the expression of TGF-β target genes were analyzed by reverse transcription-quantitative polymerase chain reaction. Immunoassays were performed for interleukin11 (IL11) in the cell culture supernatant and for TGF-β in the reconstituted casein and whey. We blocked TGF-β by neutralizing the antibody and the TGF-β receptor type I kinase with the inhibitor SB431542. We also showed smad3 phosphorylation and smad2/3 nuclear translocation by Western blot and immunostaining, respectively. Moreover, with reconstituted casein and whey powder, ID1 and ID3 expression analysis was evaluated in HSC2 human oral squamous carcinoma cells. We report here that casein and whey powder caused a robust increase of TGF-β target genes interleukin11 (IL11), NADPH oxidase 4 (NOX4) and proteoglycan4 (PRG4) in gingival fibroblasts that was blocked by SB431542 and the neutralizing antibody. Moreover, casein and whey powder increased the phosphorylation of smad3 and nuclear translocation of smad2/3. No changes of proliferation markers Ki67 and cyclinD1 were observed. Furthermore, reconstituted casein and whey powder decreased ID1 and ID3 expression in the HSC2 oral squamous carcinoma cells. These findings suggest that the processing of milk into casein and whey powder maintains the TGF-β activity and its capacity to regulate ID1 and ID3 genes in oral fibroblasts and oral squamous carcinoma cells, respectively. These data increase the scientific knowledge on the biological activity of casein and whey with a special emphasis on oral health.

Keywords: casein; whey; TGF-β; fibroblasts; epithelial cells; oral health; nutrition

1. Introduction

Milk, being a hallmark of mammalian evolution, exerts its beneficial effects in newborns undergoing breastfeeding serving as a nutritional supply for milk proteins casein and whey, in addition to carbohydrates, lipids and minerals [1]. Milk should not be restricted to its nutritional aspects being a rich source of the TGF-β [2]. Milk TGF-β is supposed to exert at least part of the beneficial activity of milk in vivo, for example to reduce the allergic reactions in ovalbumin-tolerized mice [3] and to ameliorate tissue damage and mortality in colitis and endotoxemia murine models [4]. In vitro, TGF-β activity is identified by its ability to regulate target genes, most notably interleukin11 (IL11), NADPH oxidase 4 (NOX4) and proteoglycan4 (PRG4) based on independent screening approaches [5–7], and some of TGF-β effects in vivo are mediated via IL11 [8,9] and NOX4 [10]. This in vitro bioassay was recently used to confirm that milk [11] but also regular infant formula has a potent TGF-β activity [12]. Nevertheless, casein and whey powder have not been tested for their TGF-β activity. Among the bioactive proteins in milk is also lactoperoxidase with its application in food, cosmetics and medical industries as it exhibits an antimicrobial activity [13]. Lactoperoxidase provokes cellular responses, for example to decrease the expression of DNA-binding protein inhibitor 1 (ID1) and ID3 in HSC2 human oral squamous carcinoma cells [14]. IDs proteins are helix–loop–helix transcription factors regulating cell-cycle progression and cell differentiation [15], also during wound healing [16]. Apart from lactoperoxidase, TGF-β1 can downregulate ID genes in keratinocytes [16]. We want to take advantage of our established bioassays to refine knowledge on how casein and whey may support tissue homeostasis in the oral cavity.

Casein being the major protein in milk [17] and whey remaining as a byproduct in cheese production [18], are processed into powder. The most obvious market for trading micellar casein and whey powder is for athletes seeking to support muscle growth by weight training [19]. Apart from athletes, it is the elderly or even geriatric person who can benefit from milk-based supplements to counteract sarcopenia [20,21]. Preschool children might benefit from milk-based supplements by improved overall nutritional status and psychomotor learning [22]. Even though the consumption of micellar casein and whey powder steadily increase, particularly in athletes and elderly people, the TGF-β activity in oral fibroblasts and the effect of changing ID1 and ID3 in HSC2 oral squamous carcinoma cells has not been reported so far. Finding answers to this question seems relevant as TGF-β [23] as well as lactoperoxidase [24] are rather heat stable molecules.

Casein and whey, apart from serving as food supplements, have received attention in oral health research. For example, the adsorption of bovine milk caseins on the tooth surface was proposed having a positive impact on the prevention of dental diseases by affecting the adhesion of early bacterial colonizers [25–27] and reducing demineralization of hydroxyapatite [28,29]. The possible role of TGF-β activity to contribute to oral health, however, remains at the hypothetic level that is based on findings of the gastrointestinal system [3,4]. It is particularly the mixing of toothpaste with lactoperoxidase that has entered the market of health care products [13]. Thus, there is a demand to better understand the influence of casein and whey on oral cells. Considering that regular infant formula holds a potent TGF-β activity [12] that reduces allergic reactions in ovalbumin-tolerized mice [3], it is likely that this is also true for the main ingredient's casein and whey protein. If, however, casein and whey, similar to milk [14], activate cells of the epithelial cell lineage remains to be studied. The aim of the present study was therefore to investigate casein and whey powder with respect to provoking a TGF-β response in gingival fibroblasts and decreasing ID1 and ID3 expression in HSC2 oral squamous carcinoma cells.

2. Results

2.1. Casein and Whey Powders Do Not Affect Viability and Proliferation of Gingival Fibroblasts

In a first step, the viability of gingival fibroblasts being exposed to aqueous fraction of casein and whey powder was determined. Formazan formation, indicating the presence of NAD(P)H-dependent cellular oxidoreductase enzymes, was maintained at 1% but decreased at 10% casein ($p = 0.019$) and whey ($p = 0.301$), respectively (Figure 1). We therefore performed the downstream experiments with 1% aqueous fraction of casein and whey powder. Under these conditions, the potent mitogen PDGF-BB but not 1% aqueous fraction of casein and whey powder caused a strong Ki67 nuclear signal and an increased expression of the cell cycle regulator cyclin D1 in gingival fibroblasts (Figure 2).

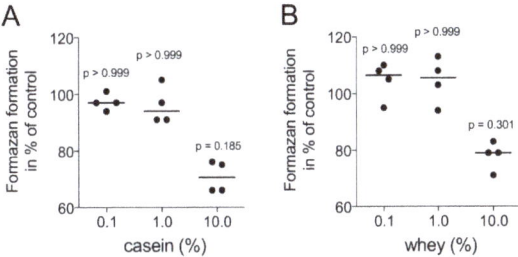

Figure 1. Casein and whey powder at 1% do not affect the viability of gingival fibroblasts. Gingival fibroblasts were incubated for 24 h with 0.1% to 10% (**A**) casein and (**B**) whey. Substrate conversion into solubilized formazan crystals was determined on a photometer. Graphs showing the formation of formazan crystals being expressed as percentage of unstimulated controls (100%). Statistic was based on a Friedmann test.

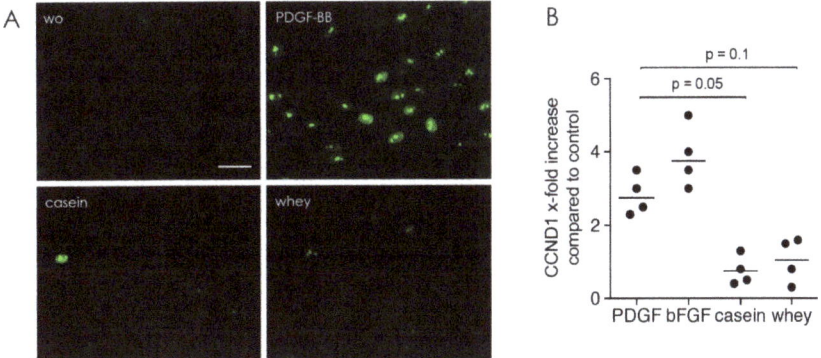

Figure 2. Casein and whey powder at 1% have no impact on cell proliferation. Gingival fibroblasts were incubated for 24 h with 1% casein and whey powder, as well as with 100 ng/mL of the mitogens PDGF-BB and 50 ng/mL bFGF. (**A**) Immunostaining for Ki-67 protein (also known as MKI67), a cellular marker for proliferation and (**B**) the expression of the cell cycle regulator cyclin D1 (CCND1) were determined. Data were normalized for the untreated control being "one". Statistic was based on a Friedmann test. Scale bar indicates 100 µm. "wo" stands for without, indicating the unstimulated cells.

2.2. Casein and Whey Powder Stimulate TGF-β Target Genes Expression in Gingival Fibroblasts

First, the amount of TGF-β1 in the aqueous fraction of 1% casein and whey powder was measured by immunoassay showing median levels of 755.4 pg/mL (min 570.0, max 930.0) and 77.4 pg/mL (min 74.0, max 100.0), respectively. In aqueous fraction of total cow milk, median levels of TGF-β1 were 532.0 pg/mL (min 309.0, max 1161.1). Next, gingival fibroblasts were exposed to the aqueous fraction of casein and whey powder. With 1% casein and whey powder, transcript levels of IL11, NOX4 and PRG4 were increased in gingival fibroblasts using GAPDH for normalization (Figure 3). More insights are provided by showing that the increase of TGF-β target gene is independent of the manufacturer of the casein and whey powder (data not shown).

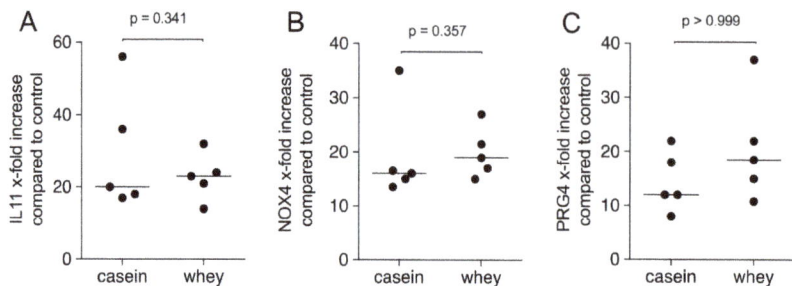

Figure 3. Casein and whey powder enhance TGF-β target genes in gingival fibroblasts. Gingival fibroblasts were exposed to 1% of a pooled reconstituted powder from three providers of casein and whey for 24 h followed by expression analysis of (**A**) IL11, (**B**) NOX4 and (**C**) PRG4. Data points represent fold change of independent experiments compared to the unstimulated controls. Statistical analysis was based on Mann–Whitney U test.

2.3. A TGF-β Neutralizing Antibody Reduce the Whey-Stimulated Gene Expression

We then exposed gingival fibroblasts with the aqueous fraction of whey powder in the presence and absence of a TGF-β pan specific neutralizing antibody. When used at 10 ng/mL, the antibody significantly lowered the response of the fibroblasts to aqueous fraction of whey powder (Figure 4). When using casein, the antibody was not effective, likely because of the known blocking activity of casein (data not shown).

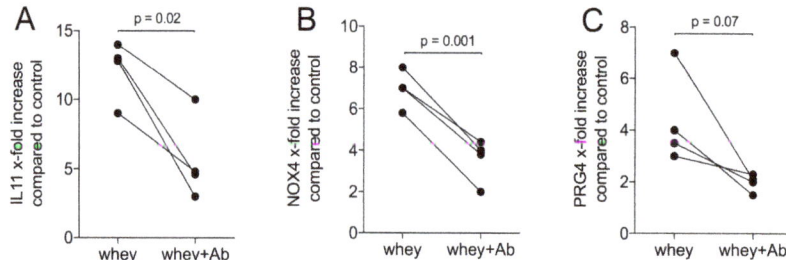

Figure 4. TGF-β pan specific neutralizing antibody reduces whey TGF-β activity. Gingival fibroblasts were exposed to 1% whey powder with and without 10 ng/mL of a TGF-β pan specific neutralizing antibody for 24 h followed by expression analysis of (**A**) IL11, (**B**) NOX4 and (**C**) PRG4. Data points represent fold change of independent experiments compared to the unstimulated controls. Statistical analysis was based on paired T-test.

2.4. Gene Expression Is Suppressed by TGF-β Receptor I Kinase Inhibitor SB431542

We further determined that the TGF-β receptor I kinase inhibitor SB431542 can neutralize the effects of casein and whey powder. Pharmacological inhibition of TGF-β receptor I kinase blocked the response of gingival fibroblasts to processed casein and whey powder based on the expression of IL11, NOX4 and PRG4 (Figure 5). In agreement with the findings based on the transcription, also IL11 protein release into the supernatant was prevented by SB431542 (Figure 6). Moreover, IL11 protein levels in the respective supernatant were increased, again at a similar magnitude between casein and whey (Figure 6).

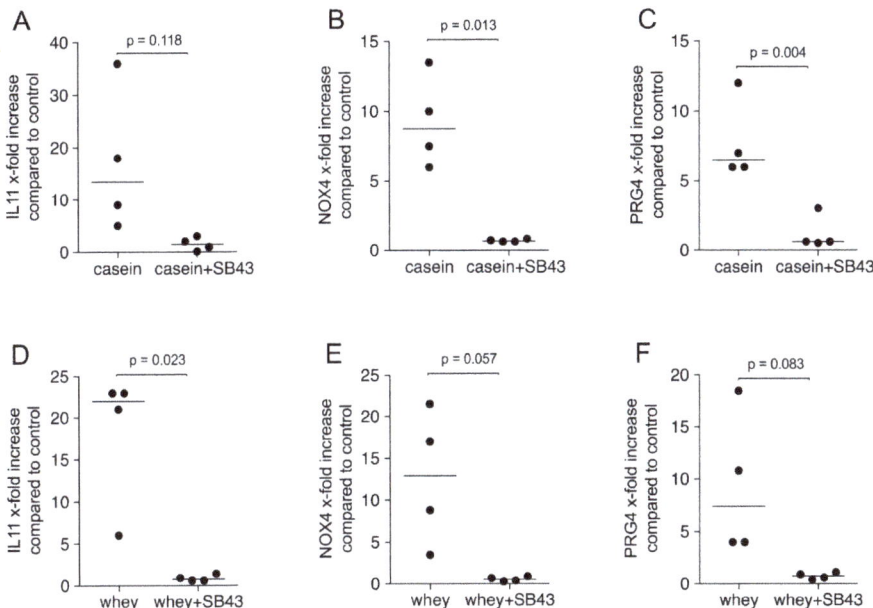

Figure 5. Casein and whey powder formulation enhances TGF-β target genes via TGF-β RI kinase. Gingival fibroblasts were exposed to 1% of a reconstituted pooled casein (**A–C**) and whey (**D–F**) powder with and without the TGF-β RI kinase inhibitor SB431542 (SB43). Expression analysis of (**A,D**) IL11, (**B,E**) NOX4 and (**C,F**) PRG4 was performed with RT-PCR. Data points represent fold change of independent experiments compared to the unstimulated controls. Statistical analysis was based on paired T-test.

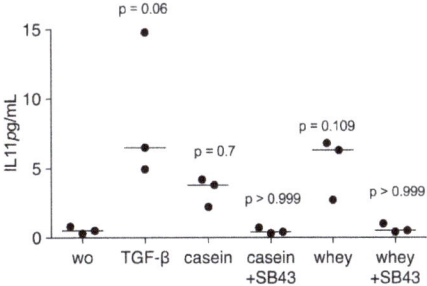

Figure 6. IL11 immunoassay of fibroblasts exposed to cell supernatants. Immunoassay for IL11 was performed with the supernatant of the cells and the data are expressed as pg/mL. TGF-β RI kinase inhibitor SB431542 is marked as SB43. Statistical analysis was based on a Friedman test and Dunn's multiple comparison. "wo" stands for without, indicating the unstimulated cells.

2.5. Casein and Whey Stimulate Phosphorylation and Nuclear Translocation of Smad Proteins

To further confirm the activation of canonical TGF-β receptor signaling, we focused on smad2 and smad3 signaling. In support of the activation of the TGF-β receptor, casein and whey caused the phosphorylation of smad3, as identified by Western blot analysis (Figure 7). Considering that activated smads translocate into the nucleus, we report here that casein and whey caused smad2/3 nuclear translocation in gingival fibroblasts (Figure 8), without any obvious differences in the signaling intensity when comparing casein and whey.

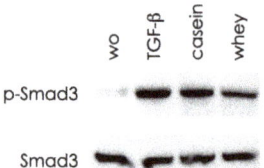

Figure 7. Casein and whey powder enhance phosphorylation of smad3. Serum-starved gingival fibroblasts were exposed to 1% of a reconstituted pooled casein and whey powder for 30 min before being subjected to Western blot analysis of phosphorylation of smad3. Cells exposed to recombinant TGF-β and casein and whey powder caused a strong increase in the phosphorylation of smad3. "wo" stands for without, indicating the unstimulated cells.

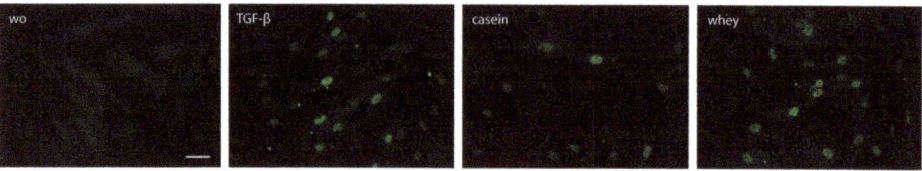

Figure 8. Casein and whey powder enhance smad2/3 nuclear translocation. Serum-starved gingival fibroblasts were exposed to TGF-β (10 ng/mL) and 1% of a casein and whey powder for 30 min before fluorescent labelling of smad2/3. The nuclear signal is visible with cells exposed to recombinant TGF-β and casein and whey powder. Scale bar indicates 100 μm. "wo" stands for without, indicating the unstimulated cells.

2.6. Gene Expression Analysis of HSC2 Exposed to Casein and Whey Powder

To further prove that cells of the oral epithelial cell lineage are responsive, HSC2 cells were exposed to 1% casein and whey powder. Similar to our recent findings obtained with aqueous fractions of pasteurized milk [6], transcript levels of ID1 and ID3 were decreased with GAPDH used for normalization (Figure 9).

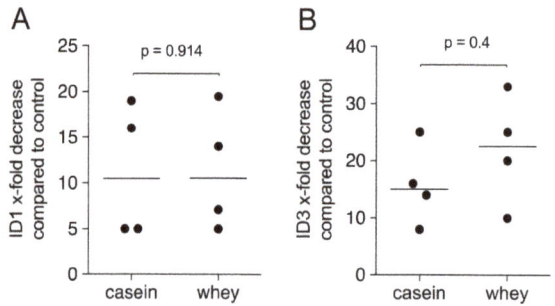

Figure 9. ID1 and ID3 expression in HSC2 exposed to casein and whey powder. HSC2 oral squamous cell carcinoma cells were exposed to 1% casein and whey powder for 24 h, before expression analysis of the target genes (**A**) ID1 and (**B**) ID3 were performed. Data indicate the x-fold decrease compared to unstimulated control cells. Statistical analysis was based on Mann–Whitney U test.

3. Material and Methods

3.1. Aqueous Fractions of Casein and Whey Powder

Three different batches of casein ((i) ESN Micellar Casein, Fitmart Gmbh & Co. Kg, Elmshorn, Germany; (ii) Casein Zero, BioTechUSA, Szada, Hungary; (iii) Sportnahrung Casein, Sporternährung Mitteregger GmbH, Graz)), and whey powder ((i) ESN Isowhey Hardcore, Fitmart Gmbh and Co. Kg, Elmshorn, Germany; (ii) Iso Whey Zero, BioTechUSA,

Szada, Hungary; (iii) Sportnahrung Whey, Sporternährung Mitteregger GmbH, Graz)) were reconstituted with serum-free Dulbecco's Modified Eagle Medium (DMEM) to reach a 2% solution, always prepared fresh for each experiment. Sportnahrung Casein and Whey have been supplemented with papain and bromelain by the manufacturer. To obtain the aqueous fractions, suspended casein and whey were immediately centrifuged at $10,000 \times g$ for 5 min at room temperature. The aqueous fractions were then 0.2 µm filtered (VWR international, Radnor, PA, USA) and either equivolumetricaly pooled or representing the different batches. Prior to cell stimulation, the aqueous fractions were further diluted with DMEM representing a 1% solution of casein and whey.

3.2. Primary Gingival Fibroblasts and Oral Squamous Cells

Human gingival fibroblasts were prepared from explant cultures of three independent donors after approval of the Ethical Committee of the Medical University of Vienna (EK Nr. 631/2007). The oral squamous cell carcinoma cell line HSC2, originally obtained from Health Science Research Resources Bank (Sennan, Japan), was kindly provided by Prof. Rausch-Fan, Department of Periodontology, Medical University of Vienna, Austria. Gingival fibroblasts and HSC2 cells were plated in growth medium at 30,000 and 50,000 cells/cm^2 into culture dishes, respectively. The following day, cells were exposed to the aqueous fractions representing a 1% solution of casein and whey, if not otherwise indicated. Gingival fibroblasts were also exposed to 10 ng/mL recombinant human TGF-β1 (ProSpec-Tany TechnoGene Ltd., Rehovot, Israel) in serum-free medium for 24 h, before gene expression analysis was performed. SB431542, a TGF-β receptor I kinase inhibitor, was used at 10 µM (Calbiochem, Merck Millipore, Darmstadt, Germany). The TGF-β neutralizing pan-specific polyclonal rabbit IgG AB-100-NA (R&D Systems, Minneapolis, MN, USA) was used at 10 ng/mL. Platelet-derived growth factor (PDGF-BB) (R&D Systems, Inc., Minneapolis, MN, USA) was used at 100 ng/mL; and basic fibroblast growth factor (bFGF, FGF2) (50 ng/mL; Strathmann Biotech AG, Hamburg, Germany) was used in indicated experiments. Cell culture supernatant was harvested, centrifuged and stored frozen until subjected to immunoassay. Fibroblasts expanded for less than 10 passages were used for the experiments.

3.3. Viability Assay

For viability experiments, gingival fibroblasts were incubated with aqueous fractions of casein and whey at the indicated concentrations. After 24 h, an MTT (3-[4,5-dimethythiazol-2-yl]-2,5-diphenyltetrazolium bromide; Sigma, St. Louis, MO, USA) solution at a final concentration of 0.5 mg/mL was added to each well of a microtiter plate (CytoOne, Starlab International, Hamburg, Germany) for 2 h at 37 °C. Medium was removed and formazan crystals were solubilized with dimethyl sulfoxide. Optical density was normalized to unstimulated control values.

3.4. qRT-PCR Analysis and Immunoassay

Total RNA was isolated with the ExtractMe total RNA kit (Blirt S.A., Gdańsk, Poland). Reverse transcription was performed with SensiFAST^{TM} cDNA (Bioline, London, UK). Polymerase chain reaction was done with the SensiFAST^{TM} SYBR ROX Kit (Bioline, Luckenwalde, Germany) on a CFX Connect^{TM} Real-Time PCR Detection System (Bio-Rad Laboratories, Hercules, CA, USA). Primer sequences are hPRG4_F CAGTTGCAGGTGGCATCTC, hPRG4_R TCGTGATTCAGCAAGTTTCATC; hNOX4a_F TCTTGGCTTACCTCCAGGA, hNOX4a_R CTCCTGGTTCTCCTGCTTGG; hGAPDH_F AAGCCACATCGCTCAGACAC, hGAPDH_R GCCCAATACGACCAAATCC, hID1_F CCAGAACCGCAAGGTGAG, hID1_R GGTCCCTGATGTAGTCGATGA; hID3_F CATCTCCAACGACAAAAGGAG, hID3_R CTTCCGGCAGGAGAGGTT. hCCND1_F TCGGTGTCCTACTTCAAATGT, hCCND1_R GGGATGGTCTCCTTCATCTTAG. The IL11 primer was from Bio-Rad (qHsaCEP0049951). The mRNA levels were calculated by normalizing to the housekeeping gene GAPDH using the ΔΔCt method. The amount of TGF-β1 in the aqueous fraction of 1% casein and 1% whey powder was measured by TGF-β1 Quantikine ELISA (#DY240; R&D Systems, Minneapolis, MN, USA). For the IL11 immunoassay, gingival fibroblasts were exposed to 1% of a reconstituted pooled casein and whey powder. After 24 h, the cell culture supernatant was harvested and subjected to the human IL11 Quantikine ELISA testing (#DY218; R&D Systems). ELISA data were not normalized to an internal compound.

3.5. Western Blot Analysis

Gingival fibroblasts were serum-starved for 24 h and then preincubated for 30 min with 1% casein and whey powder. Cell extracts containing SDS buffer and protease inhibitors (PhosSTOP with cOmplete; Sigma, St. Louis, MO, USA) were separated by SDS-PAGE and transferred onto nitrocellulose membranes (Whatman, GE Healthcare, General Electric Company, Fairfield, CT, USA). Membranes were blocked and the binding of the first antibody raised against p-smad3 (rabbit; phospho S423 + S425; EP823Y, Abcam, Cambridge, UK) and the smad3 (mouse; Smad3 (38-Q): sc-101154, Santa Cruz Biotechnology, SCBT, Santa Cruz, CA, USA) were detected with the appropriate secondary antibody linked to a peroxidase. Chemiluminescence signals were visualized with the ChemiDoc imaging system (Bio-Rad Laboratories, Inc., Hercules, CA, USA).

3.6. Immunofluorescence

Gingival fibroblasts exposed to reconstituted casein and whey powder for 24 h were incubated with anti-smad2/3 antibody (D7G7 XP® Rabbit mAb, Cell Signaling, Danvers, MA, USA) and with Ki67 (8D5, Mouse mAb antibody, 9449 Cell Signaling Danvers, MA, USA) for 24 h at 4 °C. Following blocking by 1% BSA and permeabilization with 0.1% Triton X, an Alexa Fluor® 488-conjugated secondary antibody (Cell Signaling) was added for 1 h at room temperature. Images were captured under a fluorescent microscope (Axio Imager M2, Carl Zeiss AG, Oberkochen, Germany).

3.7. Statistical Analysis

All experiments were repeated at least three times. Data from individual experiments are shown as dot-blots. Statistical analysis was based on Friedmann test (Figures 1, 2 and 6), Mann–Whitney U test (Figures 3 and 9) and paired T-test (Figures 4 and 5). Data were analyzed by the Prism 8.0e software (GraphPad Software; San Diego, CA, USA). The p-values are indicated in the respective figures.

4. Discussion

This study assumes that micellar casein and whey powder contributes to the biological activity of food supplements and possibly have beneficial effects on oral health. In support of this assumption, we show here that aqueous fraction of micellar casein and whey powder are rich in TGF-β activity as indicated by the increased expression of the respective target genes IL11, NOX4 and PRG4 involving the canonical TGF-β receptor I kinase and smad3 signaling pathway in gingival fibroblasts. The TGF-β activity is not related to changes of the proliferation marker protein Ki-67 and cyclinD1 expression in gingival fibroblasts. Moreover, we provide data that aqueous fraction of micellar casein and whey powder exert the same activity as pasteurized milk in the oral squamous epithelial cell line HSC2 by decreasing the ID1 and ID3 genes [14]. The latter is an indirect evidence for the presence of lactoperoxidase, a heat stable milk enzyme, in casein and whey powder. We thus show that casein and whey maintain the basic in vitro properties of pasteurized milk we have recently reported [11,12,14].

Our data thus confirm the TGF-β activity of milk and dairy products including whey [11] and infant formula [12] based on the activation of TGF-β receptor I kinase expression of IL11 and NOX4 in oral fibroblasts, both genes that mediate the fibrotic activity of TGF-β in cardiovascular and liver fibrosis [8,9] and acute kidney injury and pulmonary fibrosis [10,30], respectively. PRG4 is involved in mediating TGF-β in osteoarthritis in mice [31]. These findings should not be extrapolated to a possible fibrotic activity of micellar casein and whey powder but to support the use of the target genes in a bioassay. Moreover, our observation that the TGF-β pan specific neutralizing antibody blocked TGF-β activity of whey but not casein can be explained by the unspecific cross-reactivity between the casein and antibodies. The TGF-β activity has no effect on fibroblast proliferating as micellar casein and whey powder failed to change Ki-67 and cyclinD1, while PDGF-BB and bFGF, both strong mitogens, greatly increased staining and expression, respectively. This finding is in line with the rather low and biphasic mitogenic activity of TGF-β in periodontal fibroblasts [32]. Whey proteins even prevent the expression of Ki-67 in UV irradiated cells [33]. PDGF-BB and bFGF are strong mitogens for mesenchymal cells [34], thus in line with the increased Ki-67 staining [34] and cyclinD1 expression [35]. Also, in line with our previous data is that aqueous fraction of micellar casein and whey powder decrease the ID1 and ID3 genes in HSC2 cells presumably via lactoperoxidase activity [14]. The present study is thus another piece of evidence that processing of milk into casein and whey powder maintains the TGF-β and presumably also the lactoperoxidase activity.

TGF-β and seemingly also the lactoperoxidase activity survives the processing of milk into the final products. Casein is precipitated by acidification of skim milk, cooked and washed. The acid casein is then neutralized and spray-dried to obtain caseinates and milled to produce casein powder. Whey was originally considered as the soluble serum proteins that remain after precipitation of casein during cheese production. Other methods to gain whey proteins are based on ion exchangers [36] and membrane filtration [37]. TGF-β is heat stable and resists low pH, they are both conditions that can even increase the activity of the preforms of the growth factor [23]. Similarly, lactoperoxidase is among the minor whey proteins that are heat stable and also resist pH changes. Lactoperoxidase is resistant in vitro to acid pH 3 and to human gastric juice [38]. Moreover, the heat stability of lactoperoxidase is used as an index of pasteurization efficiency in milk [24]. Obviously, the manufacturers of casein and whey proteins included do not provide insights into the manufacturing process, thus no conclusions on the impact of the processing of milk into casein and whey on TGF-β and possibly also lactoperoxidase activity can be drawn. The TGF-β activity of Sportnahrung Casein and Whey being supplemented with papain and bromelain by the manufacturer can be explained by the fresh preparation of the aqueous fraction and immediate cell exposure.

The clinical relevance of the finding that micellar casein and whey powder, independent of the manufacturer, strongly increase TGF-β target genes and decrease ID1 and ID3 genes, remains unclear but leaves room for speculations. Considering that milk TGF-β can reduce the allergic reactions in ovalbumin-tolerized mice [3] and ameliorate tissue damage in colitis and endotoxemia murine models [4], some beneficial effects of the TGF-β in micellar casein and whey powder can also be assumed. Particularly in athletes, micellar casein and whey powder support muscle growth upon weight training [19]. Maybe it is also TGF-β that exerts some beneficial effects in the gastrointestinal system in the elderly person taking milk-based supplements [20,21] and even systemic effects of dietary TGF-β should not be ruled out. Support for this assumption comes from preclinical research showing that the oral administration of TGF-β1 can protect against gastrointestinal diseases and lower systemic IL6 and IFN-γ levels based on a necrotizing enterocolitis model [39] and summarized in a review on maternal TGF-β and immunological outcomes [40]. Thus, future research should identify if the in vitro TGF-β activity of micellar casein and whey powder can be translated into a clinically relevant beneficial effect that presumably exceeds the oral health system.

Not so easy to translate is the clinical meaning of decreased ID1 and ID3 genes in oral squamous oral epithelial cell line HSC2 [14]. ID proteins are overexpressed and ID1 may serve as an independent prognostic factor to predict survival time of human oral squamous cell carcinomas [41,42] but also in other squamous cell carcinoma entities [43]. It can be speculated that micellar casein and whey powder might exert some beneficial effect by returning the IDs to normal levels. In addition, ID1 and ID3 are usually known as target genes for BMP4, but in this case ID1 and ID3 are increasingly expressed [44].

Also, TGF-β increased the expression of ID1 and ID3 in prostate cancer cell lines [45] and so far, only lactoperoxidase was reported to decrease ID1 and ID3 expression on oral squamous oral epithelial cell line [14]. Interestingly, ID1 and ID3 can downregulate extracellular components induced by TGF-β, including fibronectin and collagen in various cell types [44]. Apart from the lack of knowledge on the clinical meaning of decreased ID1 and ID3, it remains open if it is lactoperoxidase in micellar casein and whey [46] being responsible or not for the gene expression changes. Considering that toothpaste and mouth rinses with lactoperoxidase are available under the trade names Biotène® Dry Mouth Moisturizing Spray; Zendium™, Orabarrier™, Bioxtra® as summarized recently [13], we might suggest studies, first to determine the amount of lactoperoxidase and then using micellar casein and whey powder as supplements for oral health care products.

In summary, our data provide convincing evidence that micellar casein and whey powder are a rich source of TGF-β based on expression changes of the respective target genes in oral fibroblasts, while the support for the lactoperoxidase activity being responsible for the decreased ID1 and ID3 in oral squamous epithelial cells is indirect. This research might serve as a scientific basis to further investigate the effects of micellar casein and whey powder that go beyond their nutritional aspects.

Author Contributions: Conceptualization, L.P., R.G.; data curation, L.P., S.H., J.N., S.S.; formal analysis, L.P., R.G.; funding acquisition, L.P., R.G.; methodology, L.P., R.G.; project administration, L.P.; resources, R.G.; supervision, L.P., R.G.; validation, L.P., J.N., R.G.; visualization, L.P.; writing—original draft, L.P., R.G.; writing—review and editing, L.P., S.H., J.N., S.S., R.G. All authors have read and agreed to the published version of the manuscript.

Funding: Austrian Science Fund: 4072-B28.

Institutional Review Board Statement: Human gingival fibroblasts were prepared from explant cultures of three independent donors after approval of the Ethical Committee of the Medical University of Vienna (EK Nr. 631/2007).

Informed Consent Statement: Informed consent was obtained from all donors involved in the study.

Data Availability Statement: All raw data are made available on request.

Acknowledgments: Open Access Funding by the Austrian Science Fund (FWF).

Conflicts of Interest: The authors declare no conflict of interest.

References

1. Ogra, P.L.; Walker, W.A. Immunology of Human Milk and Lactation: Historical Overview. In *Milk, Mucosal Immunity and the Microbiome: Impact on the Neonate*; Lönnerdal, B., Ed.; Nestlé Nutr Inst Workshop Ser; Karger: Basel, Switzerland, 2020; Volume 94, pp. 11–26. [CrossRef]
2. Sitarik, A.R.; Bobbitt, K.R.; Havstad, S.L.; Fujimura, K.E.; Levin, A.M.; Zoratti, E.M.; Kim, H.; Woodcroft, K.J.; Wegienka, G.; Ownby, D.R.; et al. Breast Milk Transforming Growth Factor β Is Associated with Neonatal Gut Microbial Composition. *J. Pediatr. Gastroenterol. Nutr.* **2017**, *65*, e60–e67. [CrossRef] [PubMed]
3. Holvoet, S.; Perrot, M.; de Groot, N.; Prioult, G.; Mikogami, T.; Verhasselt, V.; Nutten, S. Oral Tolerance Induction to Newly Introduced Allergen is Favored by a Transforming Growth Factor-beta-Enriched Formula. *Nutrients* **2019**, *11*, 2210. [CrossRef] [PubMed]
4. Ozawa, T.; Miyata, M.; Nishimura, M.; Ando, T.; Ouyang, Y.; Ohba, T.; Shimokawa, N.; Ohnuma, Y.; Katoh, R.; Ogawa, H.; et al. Transforming growth factor-beta activity in commercially available pasteurized cow milk provides protection against inflammation in mice. *J. Nutr.* **2009**, *139*, 69–75. [CrossRef] [PubMed]
5. Stahli, A.; Bosshardt, D.; Sculean, A.; Gruber, R. Emdogain-regulated gene expression in palatal fibroblasts requires TGF-betaRI kinase signaling. *PLoS ONE* **2014**, *9*, e105672. [CrossRef] [PubMed]
6. Zimmermann, M.; Caballe-Serrano, J.; Bosshardt, D.D.; Ankersmit, H.J.; Buser, D.; Gruber, R. Bone-Conditioned Medium Changes Gene Expression in Bone-Derived Fibroblasts. *Int. J. Oral Maxillofac. Implants* **2015**, *30*, 953–958. [CrossRef] [PubMed]
7. Strauss, F.J.; Stahli, A.; Beer, L.; Mitulovic, G.; Gilmozzi, V.; Haspel, N.; Schwab, G.; Gruber, R. Acid bone lysate activates TGFbeta signalling in human oral fibroblasts. *Sci. Rep.* **2018**, *8*, 16065. [CrossRef]
8. Schafer, S.; Viswanathan, S.; Widjaja, A.A.; Lim, W.W.; Moreno-Moral, A.; DeLaughter, D.M.; Ng, B.; Patone, G.; Chow, K.; Khin, E.; et al. IL-11 is a crucial determinant of cardiovascular fibrosis. *Nature* **2017**, *552*, 110–115. [CrossRef]

9. Widjaja, A.A.; Singh, B.K.; Adami, E.; Viswanathan, S.; Dong, J.; D'Agostino, G.A.; Ng, B.; Lim, W.W.; Tan, J.; Paleja, B.S.; et al. Inhibiting Interleukin 11 Signaling Reduces Hepatocyte Death and Liver Fibrosis, Inflammation, and Steatosis in Mouse Models of Nonalcoholic Steatohepatitis. *Gastroenterology* **2019**, *157*, 777–792.e14. [CrossRef]
10. Jeong, B.Y.; Park, S.R.; Cho, S.; Yu, S.L.; Lee, H.Y.; Park, C.G.; Kang, J.; Jung, D.Y.; Park, M.H.; Hwang, W.M.; et al. TGF-beta-mediated NADPH oxidase 4-dependent oxidative stress promotes colistin-induced acute kidney injury. *J. Antimicrob. Chemother.* **2018**, *73*, 962–972. [CrossRef]
11. Panahipour, L.; Stahli, A.; Haiden, N.; Gruber, R. TGF-beta activity in cow milk and fermented milk products: An in vitro bioassay with oral fibroblasts. *Arch. Oral. Biol.* **2018**, *95*, 15–21. [CrossRef]
12. Panahipour, L.; Tabatabaei, A.A.; Gruber, R. Hypoallergenic infant formula lacks transforming growth factor beta activity and has a lower anti-inflammatory activity than regular infant formula. *J. Dairy Sci.* **2020**, *103*, 6771–6781. [CrossRef] [PubMed]
13. Magacz, M.; Kedziora, K.; Sapa, J.; Krzysciak, W. The Significance of Lactoperoxidase System in Oral Health: Application and Efficacy in Oral Hygiene Products. *Int. J. Mol. Sci.* **2019**, *20*, 1443. [CrossRef] [PubMed]
14. Panahipour, L.; Biasi, M.; Bokor, T.S.; Thajer, A.; Haiden, N.; Gruber, R. Milk lactoperoxidase decreases ID1 and ID3 expression in human oral squamous cell carcinoma cell lines. *Sci. Rep.* **2020**, *10*, 5836. [CrossRef] [PubMed]
15. Roschger, C.; Cabrele, C. The Id-protein family in developmental and cancer-associated pathways. *Cell Commun. Signal.* **2017**, *15*, 7. [CrossRef] [PubMed]
16. Rotzer, D.; Krampert, M.; Sulyok, S.; Braun, S.; Stark, H.J.; Boukamp, P.; Werner, S. Id proteins: Novel targets of activin action, which regulate epidermal homeostasis. *Oncogene* **2006**, *25*, 2070–2081. [CrossRef]
17. Caroli, A.M.; Savino, S.; Bulgari, O.; Monti, E. Detecting β-Casein Variation in Bovine Milk. *Molecules* **2016**, *21*, 141. [CrossRef]
18. Abbring, S.; Hols, G.; Garssen, J.; van Esch, B. Raw cow's milk consumption and allergic diseases–The potential role of bioactive whey proteins. *Eur. J. Pharmacol.* **2019**, *843*, 55–65. [CrossRef]
19. Devries, M.C.; Phillips, S.M. Supplemental protein in support of muscle mass and health: Advantage whey. *J. Food. Sci.* **2015**, *80*, A8–A15. [CrossRef]
20. Gade, J.; Beck, A.M.; Bitz, C.; Christensen, B.; Klausen, T.W.; Vinther, A.; Astrup, A. Protein-enriched, milk-based supplement to counteract sarcopenia in acutely ill geriatric patients offered resistance exercise training during and after hospitalisation: Study protocol for a randomised, double-blind, multicentre trial. *BMJ Open* **2018**, *8*, e019210. [CrossRef]
21. Gryson, C.; Ratel, S.; Rance, M.; Penando, S.; Bonhomme, C.; Le Ruyet, P.; Duclos, M.; Boirie, Y.; Walrand, S. Four-month course of soluble milk proteins interacts with exercise to improve muscle strength and delay fatigue in elderly participants. *J. Am. Med. Dir. Assoc.* **2014**, *15*, 958.e1–958.e9. [CrossRef]
22. Cervo, M.M.C.; Mendoza, D.S.; Barrios, E.B.; Panlasigui, L.N. Effects of Nutrient-Fortified Milk-Based Formula on the Nutritional Status and Psychomotor Skills of Preschool Children. *J. Nutr. Metab.* **2017**, *2017*, 6456738. [CrossRef] [PubMed]
23. Miyazono, K.; Hellman, U.; Wernstedt, C.; Heldin, C.H. Latent high molecular weight complex of transforming growth factor beta 1. Purification from human platelets and structural characterization. *J. Biol. Chem.* **1988**, *263*, 6407–6415. [CrossRef]
24. Barrett, N.E.; Grandison, A.S.; Lewis, M.J. Contribution of the lactoperoxidase system to the keeping quality of pasteurized milk. *J. Dairy. Res.* **1999**, *66*, 73–80. [CrossRef] [PubMed]
25. Cassiano, L.P.S.; Ventura, T.M.S.; Silva, C.M.S.; Leite, A.L.; Magalhaes, A.C.; Pessan, J.P.; Buzalaf, M.A.R. Protein Profile of the Acquired Enamel Pellicle after Rinsing with Whole Milk, Fat-Free Milk, and Water: An in vivo Study. *Caries. Res.* **2018**, *52*, 288–296. [CrossRef] [PubMed]
26. Kensche, A.; Durasch, A.; Konig, B.; Henle, T.; Hannig, C.; Hannig, M. Characterization of the in situ pellicle ultrastructure formed under the influence of bovine milk and milk protein isolates. *Arch. Oral Biol.* **2019**, *104*, 133–140. [CrossRef] [PubMed]
27. Cheaib, Z.; Rakmathulina, E.; Lussi, A.; Eick, S. Impact of Acquired Pellicle Modification on Adhesion of Early Colonizers. *Caries. Res.* **2015**, *49*, 626–632. [CrossRef]
28. Barbour, M.E.; Shellis, R.P.; Parker, D.M.; Allen, G.C.; Addy, M. Inhibition of hydroxyapatite dissolution by whole casein: The effects of pH, protein concentration, calcium, and ionic strength. *Eur. J. Oral. Sci.* **2008**, *116*, 473–478. [CrossRef]
29. Romero, M.J.; Nakashima, S.; Nikaido, T.; Ichinose, S.; Sadr, A.; Tagami, J. Inhibition of hydroxyapatite growth by casein, a potential salivary phosphoprotein homologue. *Eur. J. Oral. Sci.* **2015**, *123*, 288–296. [CrossRef]
30. Ghatak, S.; Hascall, V.C.; Markwald, R.R.; Feghali-Bostwick, C.; Artlett, C.M.; Gooz, M.; Bogatkevich, G.S.; Atanelishvili, I.; Silver, R.M.; Wood, J.; et al. Transforming growth factor beta1 (TGFβ1)-induced CD44V6-NOX4 signaling in pathogenesis of idiopathic pulmonary fibrosis. *J. Biol. Chem.* **2017**, *292*, 10490–10519. [CrossRef]
31. Chavez, R.D.; Sohn, P.; Serra, R. Prg4 prevents osteoarthritis induced by dominant-negative interference of TGF-ss signaling in mice. *PLoS ONE* **2019**, *14*, e0210601. [CrossRef]
32. Oates, T.W.; Rouse, C.A.; Cochran, D.L. Mitogenic effects of growth factors on human periodontal ligament cells in vitro. *J. Periodontol.* **1993**, *64*, 142–148. [CrossRef]
33. Kimura, Y.; Sumiyoshi, M.; Kobayashi, T. Whey peptides prevent chronic ultraviolet B radiation-induced skin aging in melanin-possessing male hairless mice. *J. Nutr.* **2014**, *144*, 27–32. [CrossRef]
34. Gruber, R.; Karreth, F.; Frommlet, F.; Fischer, M.B.; Watzek, G. Platelets are mitogenic for periosteum-derived cells. *J. Orthop. Res.* **2003**, *21*, 941–948. [CrossRef]

35. He, S.; Chen, M.; Lin, X.; Lv, Z.; Liang, R.; Huang, L. Triptolide inhibits PDGF-induced proliferation of ASMCs through G0/G1 cell cycle arrest and suppression of the AKT/NF-kappaB/cyclinD1 signaling pathway. *Eur. J. Pharmacol.* **2020**, *867*, 172811. [CrossRef] [PubMed]
36. Heebøll-Nielsen, A.; Justesen, S.F.; Thomas, O.R. Fractionation of whey proteins with high-capacity superparamagnetic ion-exchangers. *J. Biotechnol.* **2004**, *113*, 247–262. [CrossRef] [PubMed]
37. Wen-Qiong, W.; Yun-Chao, W.; Xiao-Feng, Z.; Rui-Xia, G.; Mao-Lin, L. Whey protein membrane processing methods and membrane fouling mechanism analysis. *Food. Chem.* **2019**, *289*, 468–481. [CrossRef] [PubMed]
38. Baat, C.A.; Tortorello, M.-L. *Encyclopedia of Food Microbiology*; Academic Press: Cambridge, MA, USA, 2014.
39. Shiou, S.R.; Yu, Y.; Guo, Y.; Westerhoff, M.; Lu, L.; Petrof, E.O.; Sun, J.; Claud, E.C. Oral administration of transforming growth factor-beta1 (TGF-beta1) protects the immature gut from injury via Smad protein-dependent suppression of epithelial nuclear factor kappaB (NF-kappaB) signaling and proinflammatory cytokine production. *J. Biol. Chem.* **2013**, *288*, 34757–34766. [CrossRef]
40. Oddy, W.H.; McMahon, R.J. Milk-derived or recombinant transforming growth factor-beta has effects on immunological outcomes: A review of evidence from animal experimental studies. *Clin. Exp. Allergy* **2011**, *41*, 783–793. [CrossRef] [PubMed]
41. Nishimine, M.; Nakamura, M.; Mishima, K.; Kishi, M.; Kirita, T.; Sugimura, M.; Konishi, N. Id proteins are overexpressed in human oral squamous cell carcinomas. *J. Oral. Pathol. Med.* **2003**, *32*, 350–357. [CrossRef]
42. Chen, J.; Zhang, F.; Wang, D.; Yang, Z.; Liu, S.; Dong, Z. Prognostic ability of DNA-binding protein inhibitor ID-1 expression in patients with oral squamous cell carcinoma. *Oncol. Lett.* **2020**, *19*, 3917–3922. [CrossRef]
43. Luo, K.J.; Wen, J.; Xie, X.; Fu, J.H.; Luo, R.Z.; Wu, Q.L.; Hu, Y. Prognostic relevance of Id-1 expression in patients with resectable esophageal squamous cell carcinoma. *Ann. Thorac. Surg.* **2012**, *93*, 1682–1688. [CrossRef] [PubMed]
44. Mody, A.A.; Wordinger, R.J.; Clark, A.F. Role of ID Proteins in BMP4 Inhibition of Profibrotic Effects of TGF-beta2 in Human TM Cells. *Invest. Ophthalmol. Vis. Sci.* **2017**, *58*, 849–859. [CrossRef] [PubMed]
45. Strong, N.; Millena, A.C.; Walker, L.; Chaudhary, J.; Khan, S.A. Inhibitor of differentiation 1 (Id1) and Id3 proteins play different roles in TGFbeta effects on cell proliferation and migration in prostate cancer cells. *Prostate* **2013**, *73*, 624–633. [CrossRef]
46. Heidebrecht, H.J.; Kulozik, U. Data concerning the fractionation of individual whey proteins and casein micelles by microfiltration with ceramic gradient membranes. *Data. Brief.* **2019**, *25*, 104102. [CrossRef] [PubMed]

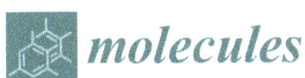

Article

Effect of Vitamin B Complex Treatment on Macrophages to Schwann Cells Association during Neuroinflammation after Peripheral Nerve Injury

Adil Ehmedah [1,†], Predrag Nedeljkovic [2,†], Sanja Dacic [1], Jelena Repac [1], Biljana Draskovic-Pavlovic [3], Dragana Vučević [3], Sanja Pekovic [4] and Biljana Bozic Nedeljkovic [1,3,*]

1. Institute of Physiology and Biochemistry "Ivan Djaja", Faculty of Biology, University of Belgrade, 11000 Belgrade, Serbia; aozhe77@gmail.com (A.E.); sanjas@bio.bg.ac.rs (S.D.); jelenag@bio.bg.ac.rs (J.R.)
2. Institute for Orthopedic Surgery "Banjica", 11000 Belgrade, Serbia; nedeljkovicpredrag@gmail.com
3. Institute for Medical Research, Military Medical Academy, 11000 Belgrade, Serbia; biljadp@gmail.com (B.D.-P.); draganavucevic@yahoo.com (D.V.)
4. Department of Neurobiology, Institute for Biological Research "Sinisa Stankovic", National Institute of Republic of Serbia, University of Belgrade, 11060 Belgrade, Serbia; sanjapekovic@gmail.com
* Correspondence: biljana@bio.bg.ac.rs; Tel.: +381-11-303-23-56
† These authors contributed equally to this study.

Academic Editors: Sokcheon Pak and Soo Liang Ooi
Received: 17 September 2020; Accepted: 6 November 2020; Published: 19 November 2020

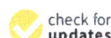

Abstract: Peripheral nerve injury (PNI) triggers a complex multi-cellular response involving the injured neurons, Schwann cells (SCs), and immune cells, often resulting in poor functional recovery. The aim of this study was to investigate the effects of the treatment with vitamin B (B1, B2, B3, B5, B6, and B12) complex on the interaction between macrophages and SCs during the recovery period after PNI. Transection of the motor branch of the femoral nerve followed by reconstruction by termino-terminal anastomosis was used as an experimental model. Isolated nerves from the sham (S), operated (O), and operated groups treated with the B vitamins (OT group) were used for immunofluorescence analysis. The obtained data indicated that PNI modulates interactions between macrophages and SCs in a time-dependent manner. The treatment with B vitamins complex promoted the M1-to M2-macrophage polarization and accelerated the transition from the non-myelin to myelin-forming SCs, an indicative of SCs maturation. The effect of B vitamins complex on both cell types was accompanied with an increase in macrophage/SC interactions, all of which correlated with the regeneration of the injured nerve. Clearly, the capacity of B vitamins to modulate macrophages-SCs interaction may be promising for the treatment of PNI.

Keywords: peripheral nerve injury; vitamin B complex; neuroinflammation; macrophages; Schwann cells

1. Introduction

Peripheral nerve injuries (PNI) represent a considerable health burden and a far-reaching issue of the modern lifestyle, with an estimated incidence of even ~300,000 cases per year in Europe, mostly caused by increasing rates of traffic, industrial and workplace-associated traumatism [1]. Neuroinflammation induced by PNI assumes precise orchestration of interactions between different cells, primarily Schwann cells (SCs) and phagocytic-macrophages. While latter get recruited to the injury site by cytokines released from the denervated-SCs [2–5], the recruited hematogenous macrophages, together with the resident-population, release cytokines necessary for the subsequent SCs' activation and extracellular matrix remodeling [6].

The inflammatory and reparatory roles of macrophages were proven essential for all tissues. Accordingly, it has been shown that the macrophage depletion, following PNI, triggers an impaired process of neuroregeneration, coupled with a very poor outcome [7]. Despite this, unambiguous data about the precise macrophage contribution to neuroregeneration is still missing [8], although the importance of recruited monocytes and resident macrophages in PNI-triggered neuroinflammation has been well acknowledged. Moreover, despite how distinct resident macrophage subsets have been associated to peripheral nerves in various tissues, and linked to protective and deleterious effects on neuroregeneration, a systematic analysis of macrophage type association with peripheral nerves is still lacking [9]. Macrophages exhibit remarkable plasticity and are highly heterogeneous. According to the activation state and functions, they are classified into two polarized phenotypes: "classically activated" pro-inflammatory macrophages (M1) and "alternatively activated" anti-inflammatory macrophages (M2) [10]. So far, M1-macrophages have been recognized as primary phagocytes at the PNI site, whilst M2-macrophages subsequently take over neuroreparation, whose timely activation becomes vital to circumvent the putative M1-subset neurotoxicity [11].

SCs are considered crucial in orchestrating distinct functional modalities between macrophage subsets. Firstly, the resident-SCs, experiencing hyperproliferation, reinforce the initial macrophage activity by secreting cytokines that further recruit monocytes to the injured site [12]. As a result, SCs change the phenotype to the pre-myelinating state. Re-established interactions between SCs with the tissue-macrophages restore the remyelinating-SC phenotype, which behaves indispensable during the axonal regeneration [13]. The layers of novel myelin may stimulate macrophages to finalize the on-going inflammation at the injured nerve, so that the macrophage-SCs interaction enables fine tuning of the reparatory processes, which demands clarification to a greater extent.

Injuries of the peripheral nerves result in long-term disability and conditions characterized by wide-ranging symptoms, depending on the severity and involved nerve types. The principal PNI target is axon where microsurgery represents the first therapeutic method of choice [14]. In the context of enhanced potential for neuroregeneration [15], the development of adjuvant strategies was nowadays recognized as highly needed, transforming quickly into a novel and attractive research field [16]. Hereby, B vitamins might serve as a prominent choice, due to their broad usage in regenerative medicine, as well as in treating injuries of both central and peripheral nervous system [17].

Vitamins of the B complex act as coenzymes in a plethora of enzymatic reactions, critically affecting vital cellular functions. Numerous studies clearly revealed therapeutic potential of the B complex vitamins in peripheral nerve recovery [18–20]. For example, the sciatic nerve injury has been associated to decreased levels of the vitamin B complex and vitamin B12 [18], indicating that the administration of these vitamins may improve the nerve regeneration process. Moreover, a positive effect of the vitamin B12 on SC proliferation and migration has been shown, including also the myelination of axons after end-to-side neurorrhaphy in rats [21]. Further on, vitamins B1, B6, and B12, display analgesic effects in experimental animal models for acute and chronic pain, upon the neuronal injury [22]. In addition, the same vitamins have been found to promote neurite outgrowth and enhance the velocity of nerve conduction in rat acrylamide-induced neuropathy [23]. In our previously published papers we have reported that treatment with vitamin B (B1, B2, B3, B5, B6, and B12) complex could improve the recovery of the motor nerve [19], and this progress was caused by effective transition from M1-proinflammatory to M2-anti-inflammatory/reparatory macrophage phenotype, followed by the inflammatory response suppression [20]. Consistently, the aim of the present study was to demonstrate whether the same B vitamins cocktail (B1, B2, B3, B5, B6, and B12) could affect the relationship between macrophages and SCs, the essential constituents of PNI-triggered processes of neuroinflammation/neuroregeneration; thus, ultimately promoting enhanced nerve repair.

2. Results

2.1. Treatment with Vitamin B Complex Altered Macrophages/Schwann Cells Interaction during the Recovery Period after PNI

To explore the effects of vitamin B complex on the spatiotemporal relationships of macrophages and SCs during the recovery period after PNI, immunohistochemical analyses were performed on the cross sections of the femoral nerve motor branch. Results of the sham control groups (S) were compared to the profiles obtained at different investigated time points (1st, 3rd, 7th, and 14th day post operation (dpo)) in the operated (O) and in the operated groups after the administration of 1, 3, 7, and 14 intraperitoneal (i.p.) injections of vitamin B complex (OT group). We used ED1 (anti-CD68) antibody as a commonly utilized marker of activated macrophages, and S100 antibody as a well-established marker of SCs [24–26]. Double immunofluorescence (IF) staining was performed to visualize the CD68/S100 overlapping. As we have also noticed in our recently published paper [18], only a few ED1$^+$ cells were detected in the sham operated (S) group, and this number was not significantly changed during all of the investigated time points (Figure 1(I)–Figure 4(I) A, D, G, white arrow heads and Figure 6(I) A, D, G, J). Remarkably, most of the SCs, intensively stained with S100 (Figure 1(I)–Figure 4(I) A, D, yellow arrow heads), displayed morphology of myelin-forming SCs and no overlapping of ED1 and S100 immunoreactivity was detected. In the O group, the number of ED1$^+$ cells was increased at the 1st dpo, where these macrophages had round and oval morphology (Figure 1(I) B, E, H, white arrow heads) resembling the M1-type. The observed macrophages were concentrated in clusters surrounding the dark spots (Figure 1(I) B, E, K, red arrow heads), consisting of SCs with very low or without S100 immunoreactivity. Additionally, strongly stained S100$^+$ cells (Figure 1(I) K, yellow arrow heads) with myelinating SCs morphology were also detected, but with no overlapping of ED1 and S100 immunoreactivity. The administration of one vitamin B complex injection was not sufficient to overcome all of the effects of PNI, although the number of ED1$^+$ cells was decreased (Figure 1(I) I, white arrow heads), while the morphology of S100$^+$ SCs was similar to those observed in the S group (Figure 1(I) F and L, yellow arrow heads). The total number of ED1$^+$/S100$^+$ cells was presented in Figure 1(II), as a number of double positive cells/mm^2 and in Figure 1(III) as the percentage of double positive cells in ED1$^+$ cells population. The number of ED1$^+$ macrophages that co-localized with S100$^+$ SCs was negligible in the O group (10.04 ± 0.93/mm^2 and represented only 9.86 ± 0.76% of total ED1$^+$ cells), while in the OT group it was 1.5-fold higher (15.36 ± 1.14/mm^2), but still represented a small fraction (17.72 ± 0.62%) of total ED1$^+$ cells.

Interestingly, at the 3rd dpo in the O, as well as in the OT group, we have noticed ED1$^+$/S100$^+$ cells (yellow fluorescence) (Figure 2(I) E and F, yellow arrows). As depicted in Figure 2(I) H and I, these ED1$^+$ macrophages, found in close association with SCs, had more "foamy" morphology of the M2 type. Anyhow, these ED1$^+$/S100$^+$ cells were more represented in the OT group.

The quantification of ED1$^+$/S100$^+$ cells was presented in Figure 2(II), as a number of double positive cells/mm^2 and in Figure 2(III) as the percentage of double positive cells in the total population of ED1$^+$ cells. The number of ED1$^+$ macrophages that co-localized with S100$^+$ SCs in the O group was 28.29 ± 1.26/mm^2 and represented 21.44 ± 0.91% of total ED1$^+$ cells, while in the OT group, it was 32.56 ± 0.67/mm^2, representing 29.42 ± 0.66% of total ED1$^+$ cells. Besides these ED1$^+$/S100$^+$ cells, in both O and OT group we have noticed macrophages with "foamy" morphology that were only ED1$^+$ (Figure 2(I) H and I, white arrows), and SCs that were only S100$^+$ (Figure 2(I) K and L, yellow arrow heads). In addition, in the O group, some ED1$^+$ macrophages of the M1-type morphology (Figure 2(I) H, white arrow heads), were still detected around SCs with weak S100 immunoreactivity (Figure 2(I) K, red arrow heads).

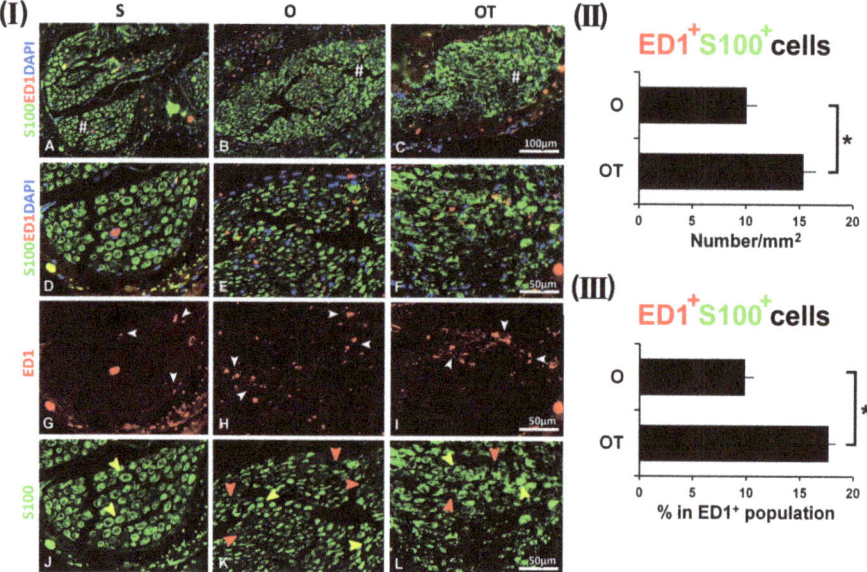

Figure 1. Effect of peripheral nerve injury (PNI) and treatment with B vitamins on Schwann cells (SCs)-macrophages co-localization at the 1st day post operation (dpo). (**I**) Cross sections of femoral nerve obtained from sham (S), operated (O, the transection of the motor branch and immediate reconstruction using termino-terminal anastomosis) and operated and treated with the vitamin B complex (B1, B2, B3, B5, B6, and B12) (OT) groups were stained for ED1 (anti-CD68, red) antibody, a marker of activated macrophages. Anti-S100 antibody (green) was used as a marker of SCs. The sections were counterstained with DAPI (blue) to visualize cell nuclei. The representative images demonstrated that in the S group only a few ED1$^+$ cells were detected (**G**, white arrow heads), most of the SCs had morphology of myelin-forming SCs and were intensively stained with S100 (**J**, yellow arrow heads). There was negligible overlapping of ED1 and S100 immunoreactivity (**A**–**D**). In the O group, ED1$^+$ macrophages with round and oval morphology of the M1 type were abundantly present (**H**, white arrow heads), particularly around the dark spots (**E**, **K**, red arrow heads), consisting of SCs with low S100 immunoreactivity. S100$^+$ cells (**K**, yellow arrow heads) of myelinating SCs morphology were also seen, but without ED1 and S100 immunoreactivity overlapping (**B**, **E**). After one vitamin B complex injection, the number of ED1$^+$ cells was decreased (**I**, white arrow heads). S100$^+$ cells of the myelinating SCs morphology were also present (**F** and **L**, yellow arrow heads). # indicates where the high magnification micrographs were taken from. Scale bars: **A**–**C** = 100 µm, **D**–**L** = 50 µm. (**II**) The quantification of double positive ED1$^+$/S100$^+$ cells from the O and OT experimental groups is depicted in the graphs (black bars) as a number of double positive cells/mm^2 and (**III**) the percentage of double positive cells in the ED1$^+$ cells population. The data are shown as the mean ± SEM of three independent experiments (three images/group/independent experiment were captured). Statistical analysis was done using a two-sided Student's *t*-test (* $p < 0.05$ vs. O group, as indicated at the graphs).

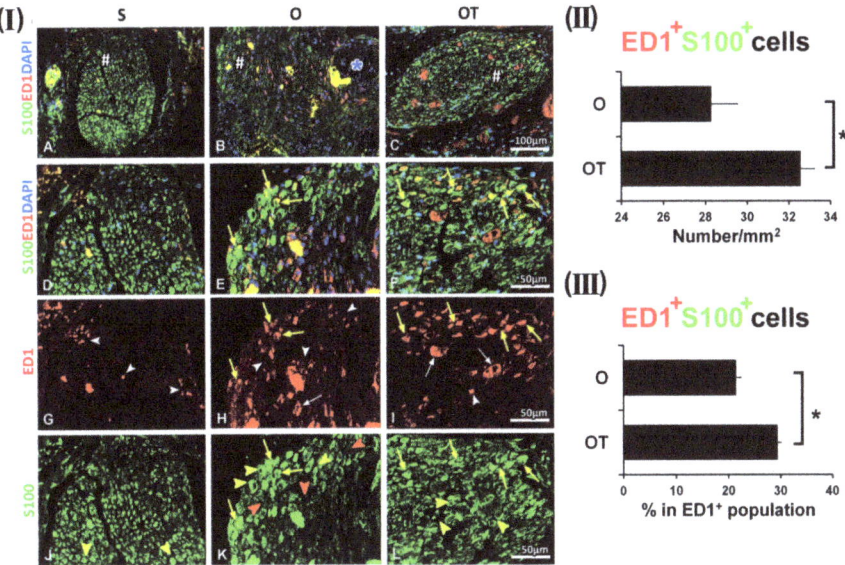

Figure 2. Effect of PNI and the treatment with B vitamins on SCs-macrophages co-localization at the 3rd dpo. (**I**) Cross sections of the femoral nerve obtained from the sham (S), operated (O, the transection of the motor branch) and operated and treated with the vitamin B complex (B1, B2, B3, B5, B6, and B12) (OT) groups were stained for ED1 (red), a marker of activated macrophages, anti-S100 antibody (green) as a marker of SCs, and counterstained with DAPI (blue) for visualizing cell nuclei. In the S group, a paucity of ED1$^+$ cells was detected (**G**, white arrow heads), myelinating, mature SCs were the predominant cell type (**J**, yellow arrow heads) and there was no overlapping of ED1 and S100 immunoreactivity (**A**, **D**). In the O and OT groups ED1$^+$/S100$^+$ cells (**E** and **F**, yellow arrows) were noticed, whereby ED1$^+$ macrophages, closely associated to SCs, had "foamy" morphology of M2 type (**H** and **I**, yellow arrows). In both groups, ED1$^+$ macrophages with the "foamy" morphology (**H** and **I**, white arrows), and SCs that were only S100$^+$ (**K** and **L**, yellow arrow heads) were noticed as well. In the O group some ED1$^+$ macrophages of the M1 type morphology (**H**, white arrow heads), were detected around faintly stained SCs (**K**, red arrow heads). Blue asterisk marks the site of transection and immediate reconstruction by termino-terminal anastomosis, while # indicates where the high magnification micrographs were taken from. Scale bars: **A–C** = 100 µm, **D–L** = 50 µm. (**II**) The quantification of double positive ED1$^+$/S100$^+$ cells from the O and OT experimental groups is depicted in the graphs (black bars) as a number of double positive cells/mm^2 and (**III**) the percentage of double positive cells in the ED1$^+$ cells population. The data are shown as the mean ± SEM of three independent experiments (three images/group/independent experiment were captured). Statistical analysis was done using a two-sided Student's *t*-test (* $p < 0.05$ vs. O group, as indicated at the graphs).

During the recovery period after the PNI, the most interesting interaction pattern between macrophages and SCs was observed at the 7th dpo (Figure 3). Equally, in both the O and OT group, a huge number of ED1$^+$ macrophages, predominantly with the M2-like morphology and only a paucity of ED1$^+$ macrophages with the M1-like morphology were detected (Figure 3(I) H and I, white arrows and white arrow heads, respectively). In the O group we found a wide spread distribution of the dark spots (Figure 3(I) B, E, K), consisting of SCs with low S100 immunoreactivity (Figure 3(I) K, red arrow heads). These spots were surrounded with many ED1$^+$/S100$^+$ macrophages (yellow fluorescence) (Figure 3(I) E and H, yellow arrows), characterized by the transitional morphology (between the M1- and M2-type). These ED1$^+$/S100$^+$ cells were counted and the corresponding quantification was presented in Figure 3(II), as a number of double positive cells/mm^2 and in Figure 3(III) as the percentage of double positive cells in the ED1$^+$ cells population. The number of ED1$^+$ macrophages that co-localized with S100$^+$ SCs in the O group was 24.94 ± 0.72/mm^2 and represented 21.22 ± 0.76% of total ED1$^+$ cells, while in the OT group their number was statistically higher 37.41 ± 1.21/mm^2, comprising 29.23 ± 0.54% of the total ED1$^+$ cell population. In addition, besides these ED1$^+$/S100$^+$ cells, we have also noticed macrophages that were only ED1$^+$, some of them showing the "foamy", M2-type-like morphology (Figure 3(I) H, white arrows), while others displaying the M1-type-like morphology (Figure 3(I) H, white arrow heads). After the administration of seven consecutive injections of the vitamin B complex, we detected increased number of ED1$^+$/S100$^+$ cells (Figure 3(I) F, yellow arrows), with ED1$^+$ macrophages, closely associated to S100$^+$ SCs, exhibiting the "foamy" M2-type-like morphology (Figure 3(I) I, yellow arrows). Importantly, these ED1$^+$ macrophages were closely associated only to S100$^+$ SCs with the non-myelinating morphology (Figure 3(I) L, red arrows), while no co-localization of the ED1 immunoreactivity with the S100$^+$ myelinating SCs was noted (Figure 3(I) L, yellow arrow heads).

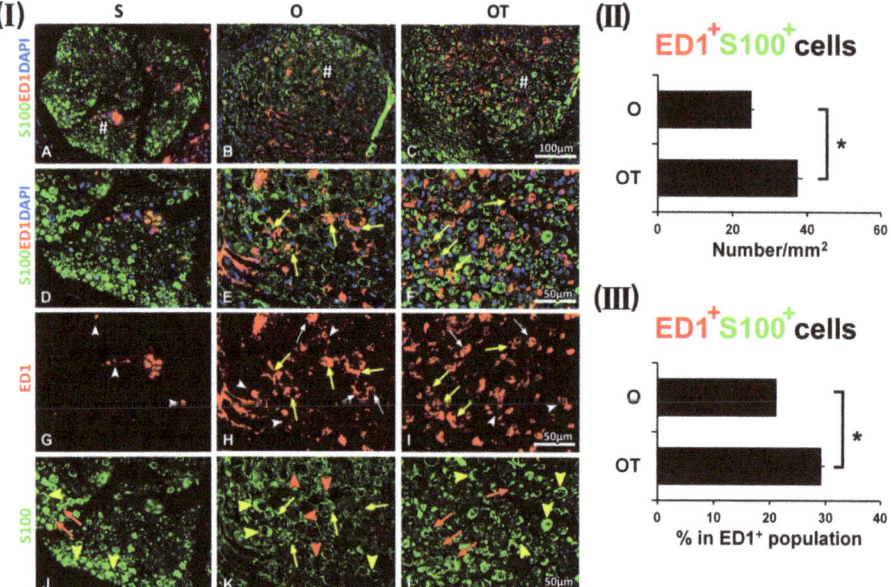

Figure 3. Effect of PNI and the treatment with B vitamins on SCs-macrophages co-localization at the 7th dpo. (**I**) Cross sections of femoral nerve obtained from the sham (S), operated (O, the transection of the motor branch) and operated and treated with the vitamin B complex (B1, B2, B3, B5, B6, and B12) (OT) groups were stained for ED1 (red), a marker of activated macrophages, anti-S100 antibody (green) as a marker of SCs, and counterstained with DAPI (blue) for visualizing cell nuclei. In the S group rare ED1$^+$ cells were detected (**G**, white arrow heads), while besides myelinating, mature SCs (**J**, yellow arrow heads) some S100$^+$ SCs of the non-myelinating morphology (**J**, red arrows) were seen. No overlapping of ED1 and S100 immunoreactivity was noted (**A**, **D**). The representative images of the O and in the OT group revealed a huge number of ED1$^+$ macrophages with the predominantly M2-like morphology and a few ED1$^+$ macrophages with the M1-like morphology (**H** and **I**, white arrows and white arrow heads, respectively). In the O group a widespread distribution of dark spots (**B**, **E**, **K**), consisting of faintly-stained SCs (**K**, red arrow heads) and surrounded with many ED1$^+$/S100$^+$ macrophages (**E** and **H**, yellow arrows), was observed. Some of the macrophages that were only ED1$^+$ had "foamy" morphology of the M2 type (**H**, white arrows), while others were of the M1 type morphology (**H**, white arrow heads). Seven consecutive injections of the vitamin B complex increased the number of ED1$^+$/S100$^+$ cells (**F**, yellow arrows), whereby ED1$^+$ macrophages of the "foamy" morphology resembling the M2

type (**I**, yellow arrows) were tightly associated to S100$^+$ SCs of the non-myelinating morphology (**L**, red arrows). No co-localization of the ED1 immunoreactivity with S100$^+$ myelinating SCs was noted (**F, L**, yellow arrow heads). # indicates where the high magnification micrographs were taken from. Scale bars: **A–C** = 100 µm, **D–L** = 50 µm. (**II**) The quantification of double positive ED1$^+$/S100$^+$ cells from the O and OT experimental groups is given in the graphs (black bars) as a number of double positive cells/mm^2 and (**III**) the percentage of double positive cells in the ED1$^+$ cells population. The data are shown as the mean ± SEM of three independent experiments (three images/group/independent experiment were captured). Statistical analysis was done using a two-sided Student's *t*-test (* $p < 0.05$ vs. O group, as indicated at the graphs).

By day 14, ED1$^+$ macrophages with the M2-type morphology appeared to be prevalent in the both O and OT groups (Figure 4(I) H and I, white arrows), while S100$^+$ SCs were predominantly of the myelin-forming phenotype (Figure 4(I) K and L, yellow arrow heads). Interestingly, ED1$^+$/S100$^+$ cells (Figure 4(I) E, yellow arrows) were mostly detected in the O group, and these ED1$^+$ macrophages with the M2-type morphology were associated (Figure 4(I) E, yellow arrows) to the S100$^+$ non-myelinating SCs (Figure 4(I) K, red arrow) and some myelinating SCs (Figure 4(I) K, yellow arrows). In contrast, in the OT group, reduced co-localization of the ED1 and S100 immunoreactivity was detected (Figure 4(I) F), indicating that following 14 injections of the B vitamin complex the complete transition to mature, myelin-forming SCs occurred. ED1$^+$/S100$^+$ cells were counted and the values obtained are given in Figure 4(II), as a number of double positive cells/mm^2 and in Figure 4(III) as the percentage of double positive cells in the total ED1$^+$ cell population. The number of ED1$^+$ macrophages that co-localized with S100$^+$ SCs in the O group was 21.87 ± 1.38/mm^2 and represented 31.49 ± 1.66% of total ED1$^+$ cells, while in the OT group their number was statistically lower (15.44 ± 0.69/mm^2), and the corresponding fraction in the total ED1$^+$ cell population was only 18.17 ± 0.78%.

To confirm that the S100$^+$ SCs, closely associated to ED1$^+$ macrophages, were the non-myelinating SCs, we performed double immunofluorescence staining with growth associated protein 43 (GAP43), a well-known marker of growing axons [27], but also a marker of non-myelinating SCs [26,28,29]. In sham controls, GAP43 immunostaining was predominantly detected in large-diameter myelinated axons, at both-time points (7th and 14th dpo) (Figure 5A,D, red asterisk). Although the majority of the myelinating S100$^+$ SCs, wrapping these axons, were GAP43$^-$ (Figure 5A,D, yellow arrow heads), some of them were also S100$^+$/GAP43$^+$ (Figure 5A,D, yellow arrows). In addition, rare non-myelinating GAP43$^+$ SCs were observed as well (Figure 5D, red arrows). At the 7th dpo, the nerve tissue was damaged, the major portion of myelin sheaths was degraded and axons destroyed, while most of the SCs underwent degeneration (Figure 5B, red arrow heads). Interestingly, in the OT group, beside myelin-forming SCs (Figure 5C, yellow arrow heads), seven consecutive injections of B vitamins significantly increased the number of non-myelinating S100$^+$/GAP43$^+$ SCs (Figure 5C, red arrows) that wrapped multiple, small-diameter, non-myelinated axons (Figure 5C, white asterisk). Similarly, a vast number of S100$^+$/GAP43$^+$ non-myelinating SCs ensheathing multiple small-caliber axons (Figure 5E, red arrows) together with a paucity of myelin-forming S100$^+$/GAP43$^+$ (Figure 5E, yellow arrows) and S100$^+$/GAP43$^-$ (Figure 5E, yellow arrow heads) SCs, was detected at the 14th dpo in the O group (Figure 5E, arrow head). In contrast, in the OT, as well as in the S group, myelinating, mature S100$^+$/GAP43$^-$ SCs were detected as a predominant cell type (Figure 5F, yellow arrow heads), with only a few S100$^+$/GAP43$^+$ myelinating SCs found (Figure 5F, yellow arrows). Furthermore, strong GAP43 immunostaining was detected in large-diameter myelinated axons (Figure 5F, red asterisk).

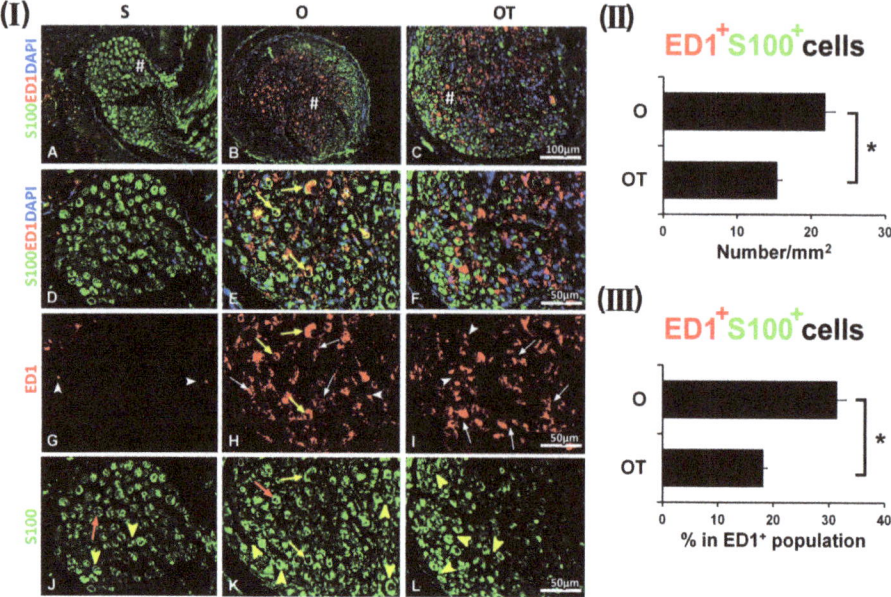

Figure 4. Effect of PNI and the treatment with B vitamins on SCs-macrophages co-localization at the 14th dpo. (**I**) ED1 (red), a common marker of activated macrophages, anti-S100 antibody (green), a marker of SCs and DAPI (blue) for visualizing cell nuclei, were used for immunostaining of the femoral nerve cross sections of the sham (S), operated (O, the transection of the motor branch) and operated and treated with the vitamin B complex (B1, B2, B3, B5, B6, and B12) (OT) groups. Almost no ED1$^+$ cells were detected (**G**, white arrow heads) in the S group. Apart from myelinating SCs (**J**, yellow arrow heads), some S100$^+$ SCs of the non-myelinating morphology (**J**, red arrows) were seen as well. There was no overlapping of ED1 and S100 immunoreactivity (**A**, **D**). ED1$^+$ macrophages with the M2-type morphology were predominant in the both O and OT groups (**H** and **I**, white arrows), while S100$^+$ SCs mostly belong to myelin-forming SCs (**K** and **L**, yellow arrow heads). ED1$^+$/S100$^+$ cells (**E**, yellow arrows) were detected only in the O group. ED1$^+$ macrophages of the M2-type morphology were associated (**E**, yellow arrows) to the S100$^+$ non-myelinating SCs (**K**, red arrow) and some myelinating SCs (**K**, yellow arrows). Minor overlapping of ED1 and S100 immunoreactivity (**C**, **F**) was obtained in the OT group. # indicates where the high magnification micrographs were taken from. Scale bars: **A–C** = 100 μm, **D–L** = 50 μm. (**II**) The quantification of double positive ED1$^+$/S100$^+$ cells from the O and OT experimental groups was depicted in the graphs (black bars) as a number of double positive cells/mm^2 and (**III**) the percentage of double positive cells in the ED1$^+$ cells population. The data are shown as the mean ± SEM of three independent experiments (three images/group/independent experiment were captured). Statistical analysis was done using a two-sided Student's *t*-test (* $p < 0.05$ vs. O group, as indicated at the graphs).

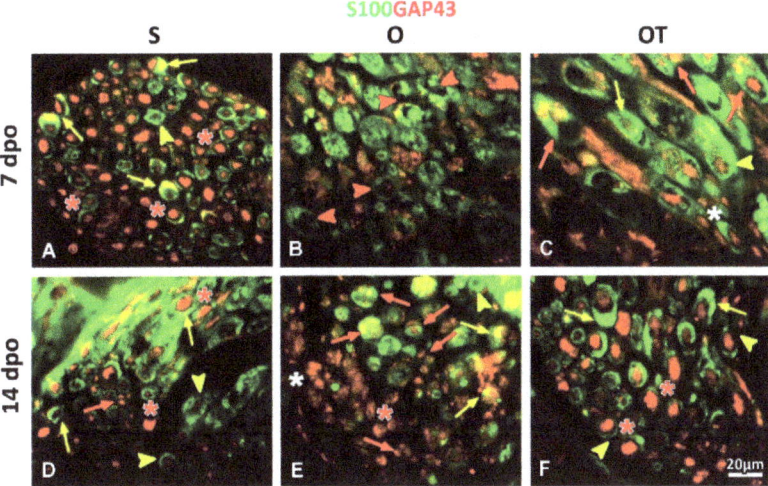

Figure 5. GAP43 (growth associated protein 43) expression in SCs and axons after PNI and the treatment with B vitamins. Expression of GAP43 (red) in SCs was determined in the femoral nerve cross sections obtained from the: sham (S), operated (O) and operated and treated with the vitamin B (B1, B2, B3, B5, B6, and B12) complex (OT) group at the 7th and 14th dpo. Anti-S100 antibody (green) was used as a marker of SCs. In the S group, both at the 7th (**A**) and the 14th (**D**) dpo GAP43 immunostaining was mostly detected in large-diameter myelinated axons (red asterisk), and in a few myelinated S100$^+$/GAP43$^+$ (yellow arrows) and non-myelinated SCs (red arrows), while S100$^+$/GAP43$^-$ (yellow arrow heads) SCs were predominant. (**B**) In the O group, at the 7th dpo most of the axons were destroyed and the majority of SCs degenerated (red arrow heads). (**C**) 7 consecutive injections of B vitamins (OT) increased the number of non-myelinating S100$^+$/GAP43$^+$ SCs (red arrows) wrapping multiple small-diameter GAP43$^+$ non-myelinated axons (white asterisk). Only a few S100$^+$/GAP43$^+$ myelinated SCs (yellow arrows) and S100$^+$/GAP43$^-$ (yellow arrow heads) were seen. (**E**) At the 14th dpo, in the O group, a huge number of S100$^+$/GAP43$^+$ non-myelinated SCs (red arrows) unsheathing multiple small-caliber axons (white asterisk), and a paucity of myelin-forming S100$^+$/GAP43$^+$ (yellow arrows) and S100$^+$/GAP43$^-$ (yellow arrow heads) SCs was detected. (**F**) After 14 treatments with B vitamins myelinating, mature S100$^+$/GAP43$^-$ SCs emerged as the principal cell type (yellow arrow heads), while S100$^+$/GAP43$^+$ myelinating SCs were rarely present (yellow arrows). Strong GAP43 immunostaining was detected in large-diameter myelinated axons (red asterisk). Scale bar: 20 µm.

The comparative presentation of time-dependent changes in macrophages-SCs co-localization within the cross sections of the femoral nerve obtained from the S, O, and OT groups, during the investigated postoperative period (1, 3, 7, and 14 days) and upon the administration of 1, 3, 7, and 14 injections of the B vitamin complex, was depicted in Figure 6(I). As mentioned above, within the cross nerve sections of the S group, only a paucity of ED1$^+$ cells was detected; their number did not undergo significant changes during all of the investigated time points; myelinating, mature SCs were detected as a predominant cell type and no overlapping of the ED1 and S100 immunoreactivity was noted (Figure 6(I) A, D, G and J).

In the O group (Figure 6(I) E, H and K), an intensive overlapping of the ED1/S100 immunoreactivity was seen at the 3rd, 7th, and 14th dpo, whereas in the OT group, the same was noticed after the administration of three and seven vitamin B complex injections (Figure 6(I) F, I). However, close ED1/S100 interactions were detected only between macrophages with the M2-like morphology and non-myelinating SCs, as well as between the macrophages with the M2-like morphology and SCs with low S100 immunoreactivity. In the both O and OT group, no interactions between mature, myelinating SCs and M2- or M1- type macrophages was detected. The temporal pattern of ED1$^+$/S100$^+$

participation in the ED1$^+$ cells population in the femoral nerve cross sections obtained from Figure 6(II) O and Figure 6(III) OT experimental groups is given in the graphs (black bars). The fraction of ED1$^+$/S100$^+$ cells in the total ED1$^+$ population varied over the recovery period. In the O group, the participation of ED1$^+$/S100$^+$ cells in the ED1$^+$ cells population increased over the time post-injury reaching 31.49 ± 1.66% at the 14th dpo. At this post-injury time-point, a 3-fold increase was detected in the O group when compared to the 1st dpo. In the OT group, treatments with vitamin B complex increased the percentage of ED1$^+$/S100$^+$ cells, reaching 30% even after 3 injections and remained at the same level for seven days. However, the vitamin B complex treatment after 14 days reduced the number of ED1$^+$/S100$^+$ cells and their fraction in the total ED1$^+$ cell population was only 18.17 ± 0.78%. Given that interaction between macrophages and mature, myelin-forming SCs was negligible, obtained results indicated that treatment with the B vitamin complex after 14 days triggered the complete transition to mature, myelin-forming SCs. Based on these results, it can be concluded that PNI alters interactions between macrophages and SCs in a time-dependent manner, while the treatment with the B vitamins complex accelerates the transition from the non-myelin to myelin-forming SCs type and from M1- to M2-like macrophage morphology.

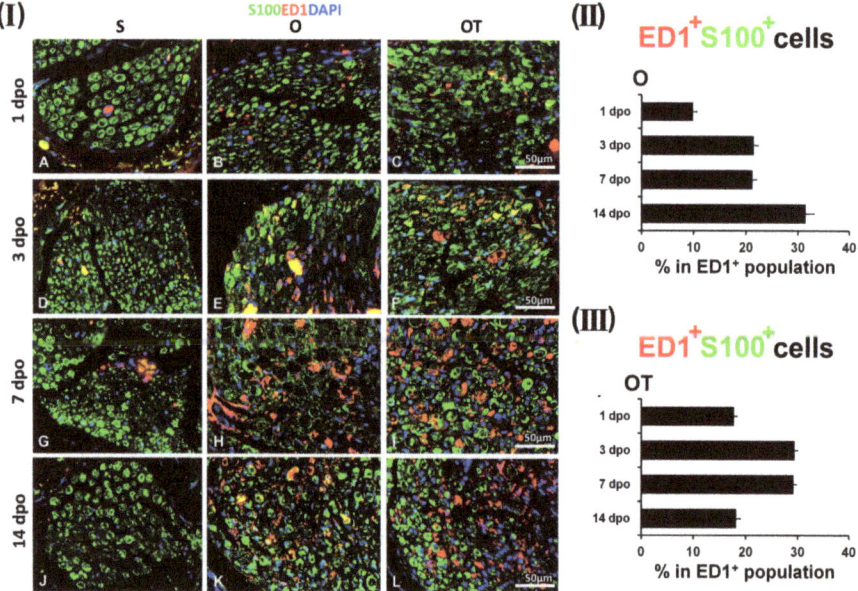

Figure 6. Time course immunohistochemical analysis of macrophages/SCs co-localization after PNI and the treatment with B vitamins. (**I**) Comparative analysis of macrophages/SCs crosstalk in the cross sections of the femoral nerve obtained from the sham (S) group at different time points (**A**—1 dpo; **D**—3 dpo; **G**—7 dpo; **J**—14 dpo). Time course of changes in macrophages/SCs co-localization was analyzed in the operated (O) femoral nerve during the 1, 3, 7, and 14 days of the postoperative period (**B**—1 dpo; **E**—3 dpo; **H**—7 dpo; **K**—14 dpo) and after 1, 3, 7, and 14 injections of the complex of B (B1, B2, B3, B5, B6, and B12) vitamins (OT group) (**C**—1 dpo; **F**—3 dpo; **I**—7 dpo; **L**—14 dpo). ED1 (red) was used as a common marker of activated macrophages, anti-S100 antibody (green) as a marker of SCs and DAPI (blue) for visualizing cell nuclei. Scale bar: 50 µm. Time-dependent changes in the percentage of double positive ED1$^+$/S100$^+$ cells in ED1$^+$ cells population from the (**II**) O and (**III**) OT experimental groups was depicted in the graphs (black bars). The data are shown as the mean ± SEM of three independent experiments (three images/group/independent experiment were captured).

2.2. Administration of the Vitamin B Complex Reduced the Expression of Proinflammatory Cytokine TNF-α in SCs after the PNI

Next, we wanted to investigate how the PNI affects the expression profile of proinflammatory cytokine tumor necrosis factor alpha (TNF-α) in SCs and whether the treatment with B vitamins could modulate this TNF-α expression pattern after the PNI.

In our model of the femoral nerve transection at the 14th dpo we have noted increased expression of TNF-α within cross sections of the operated nerve (O) (Figure 7H) compared to the sham-operated controls (S) (Figure 7G). The administration of 14 injections of the vitamin B complex (OT group) reduced the TNF-α expression (Figure 7I), which was, however, still higher compared to the S group (Figure 7G). Interestingly, besides in macrophages with the M2-like morphology (Figure 7E,F,H,I, white arrows), the TNF-α immunoreactivity was detected in some (Figure 7E,F,H,I, yellow arrows), but not all SCs (Figure 6E,F,H,I, yellow arrow heads).

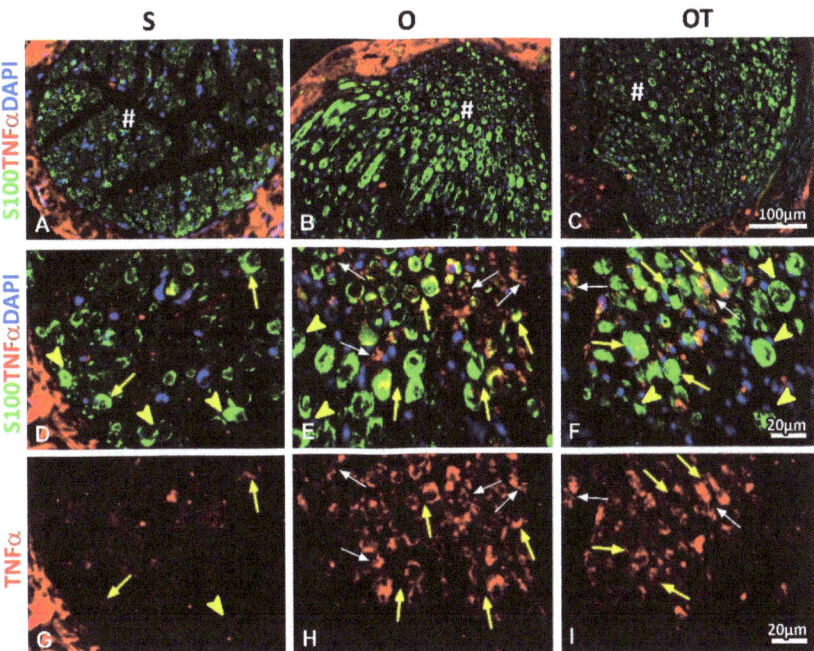

Figure 7. Effects of PNI and the B vitamins treatment on expression of proinflammatory cytokine tumor necrosis factor alpha (TNF-α) in SCs. Femoral nerve cross sections obtained from the: sham (S: **A, D, G**), operated (O: **B, E, H**) and operated and treated with the vitamin B (B1, B2, B3, B5, B6, and B12) complex (OT: **C, F, I**) group immunostained for TNF-α (red) demonstrated strong increase of immunofluorescence intensity in the O group (**H**) compared to the S group (**G**) at the 14th dpo. Immunofluorescence staining for TNF-α protein was observed in some (**E, F, H, I**, yellow arrows), but not all SCs (**E, F, H, I**, yellow arrow heads) as detected by co-localization with S100 immunostaining (green). DAPI (blue) was used for visualizing cell nuclei. Administration of 14 injections of the vitamin B complex (OT group) reduced TNF-α expression (**I**). TNF-α immunoreactivity was detected in some S100$^+$ myelinated SCs (**F**, yellow arrows). In addition, TNF-α immunoreactivity was demonstrated in macrophages with the M2-like morphology (**E, F, H, I**, white arrows). # indicates where the high magnification micrographs were taken from. Scale bars: **A–C** = 100 μm, **D–I** = 20 μm.

2.3. Effect of PNI and the Vitamin B Complex Treatment on the Expression of Anti-Inflammatory Cytokine IL-10 in SCs

Further, we investigated the expression of anti-inflammatory cytokine interleukin 10 (IL-10) in SCs in all of the examined (S, O, and OT) groups. IL-10 immunoreactivity was detected in all of these groups (Figure 8G–I), being mostly pronounced in the O group (Figure 7H). Strikingly, the bulk of IL-10 immunoreactivity was noticed in IL-10$^+$ cells resembling M2-macrophages, although IL-10$^+$/S100$^+$ cells were abundantly present as well (Figure 8E,F, yellow arrows). In the OT group, the overlapping of IL-10/S100 immunoreactivity (Figure 8F,I, yellow arrows) was detected in mature, myelinating SCs, albeit the larger part of S100$^+$ SCs were IL-10$^-$ (Figure 8F, yellow arrow heads). The similar pattern of IL-10 immunoreactivity was seen in the S group, but IL-10$^+$/S100$^+$ cells were less represented (Figure 8D,G, yellow arrows, and yellow arrow heads).

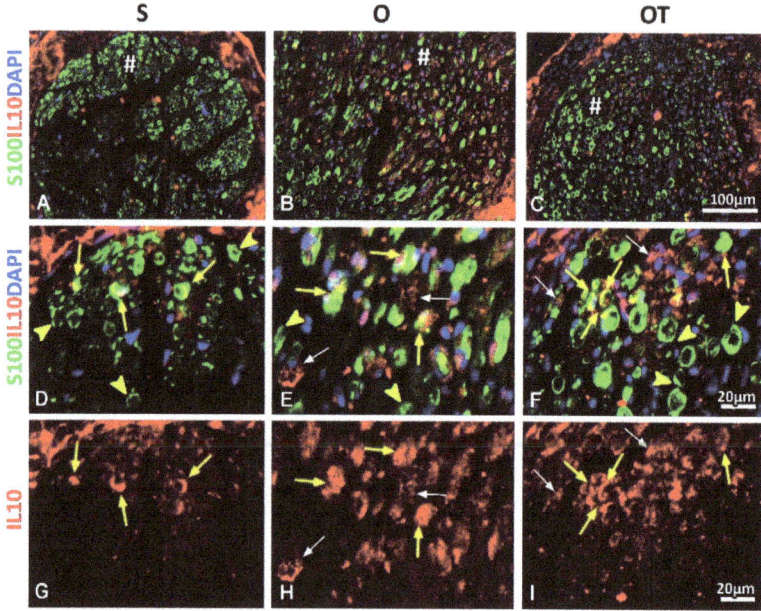

Figure 8. Effects of PNI and the B vitamins treatment on expression of anti-inflammatory cytokine interleukin 10 (IL-10) in SCs. Cross sections of the femoral nerve obtained from the: sham (S), operated (O) and operated and treated with the vitamin B (B1, B2, B3, B5, B6, and B12) complex (OT) group immunostained for IL-10 (red) showed strong IL-10 immunoreactivity in all of the groups (**G**, **H**, and **I**) at the 14th dpo, being the most pronounced in the O group (**H**). Increased IL-10 immunoreactivity was found in S100$^+$ (green) myelinating SCs (**E** and **F**, yellow arrows) and in IL-10$^+$ macrophages with the M2-like morphology (**E**, **F**, **H**, and **I**, white arrows) that were closely associated to them. In the OT group, the larger part of S100$^+$ SCs was IL-10$^-$ (**F**, yellow arrow heads). The similar pattern of IL-10 immunoreactivity was seen in the S group, although IL-10$^+$/S100$^+$ cells were less represented (**D** and **G**, yellow arrows and yellow arrow heads). DAPI (blue) was used to visualize cell nuclei. # indicates where the high magnification micrographs were taken from. Scale bars: **A–C** = 100 μm, **D–I** = 20 μm.

Using serial transversal sections we were able to visualize tight interactions between M2-macrophages and SCs, that were aligned to form bands of Büngner (Figure 9A–C) and were intensively stained with IL-10 (Figure 9D–F).

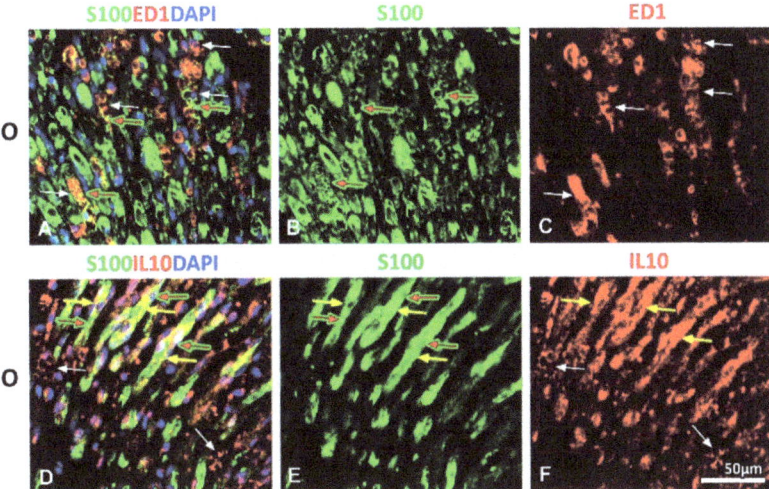

Figure 9. Interactions between M2 macrophages and SCs in injured femoral nerve. (**A–C**) We used double immunofluorescence to visualize the close contact between M2 macrophages and SCs at the 14th dpo. Serial transversal sections obtained from the operated (O) femoral nerve were immunostained for ED1 (anti-CD68, red) antibody, as a marker of activated macrophages (**C**, white arrows), anti-S100 (green) antibody as a marker of SCs (**B**, red arrows) and DAPI (blue) for visualizing cell nuclei. Complete overlapping (**A**, yellow fluorescence) of ED1 (white arrows) and S100 (red arrows) immunoreactivity confirmed tight interactions between M2 macrophages and SCs that were aligned to form bands of Büngner. (**D–F**) Transversal sections of the operated (O) femoral nerve immunostained with S100 (green), IL10 (red) and DAPI (blue) demonstrated that M2 macrophages (**D, F**, white arrows) and S100$^+$ SCs (**E**, red arrows) in bands of Büngner were intensively stained with IL-10 (**D**, yellow arrows).

3. Discussion

The aim of this study was to highlight the molecular mechanism underlying previously detected B vitamins-induced locomotor activity improvement after PNI. Herewith, the macrophages-SCs interaction, following the peripheral nerve controlled transection emerged as an important target of the applied treatment [19,30]. Noteworthy, these macrophages-SCs interactions were modulated in a time-dependent manner either post-PNI alone, or upon B vitamins application. However, the treatment accelerated the transition from the non-myelin- to myelin-forming-SCs phenotype. Furthermore, the stimulation of the M1-to-M2 macrophage phenotype switching consequently altered macrophages-SCs interactions.

Previously, we have shown that the vitamin B complex treatment effectively promotes PNI-induced M1-to-M2 macrophage polarization and suppresses inflammation, by reducing the expression of proinflammatory and up-regulating the expression of anti-inflammatory cytokines [20]. Herewith, we address the relationship between macrophages and SCs, the most fundamental cell-to-cell interaction during the PNI-triggered neuroinflammation. Hereby, Wallerian degeneration affects the nerve stumps distal to the lesion, which are not directly physically traumatized. SCs initiate the elimination of damaged axons by rejecting the myelin and, subsequently, recruit the bone-marrow-derived macrophages together with activated-resident-SCs for tissue debris removal [31]. Our results indicate the copious presence of destructed axon areas in the injured nerve of O animals, at the 1st dpo, concurrently with the dedifferentiation of demyelinated-SCs. Consistent to this, in young rats, such as our animals, the lag period separating the injury and axon degeneration involves the first 24–48 h [32]. The detached axon segments remain intact for days post-PNI, and can still transmit action potentials when stimulated [33,34]. Accordingly, the noted decrease in the number of M1-like-macrophages along with the preserved SCs morphology and myelination in the injured OT animals nerve, led us to hypothesize that the B vitamins treatment may prolong the lag period and reduce the extent of axon degeneration.

After the first period of intensive PNI-induced axon destruction, at the 3rd dpo in both O and OT animals, we noticed ED1$^+$ macrophages closely associated to SCs, displaying more "foamy"-M2-type morphology, particularly in the OT group. Conversely, in the O group, ED1$^+$ macrophages of M1-type-morphology and SCs with low S100 immunoreactivity were still detected. According to a study [8], it was proposed that SCs most likely support the macrophage PNI-functioning via expressing several ligands known to interact with macrophage receptors, thus regulating the M1-to-M2 transition. SCs secrete classical M2-associated cytokines and behave as potent inducers of M2-macrophages. These, in turn, stimulate tissue repair, via promoting remyelination by activating endogenous SCs. Moreover, since macrophages were shown to regulate PNI-triggered SCs maturation, one could not exclude that macrophages-SCs interaction operates vice-versa as well [35].

The most interesting pattern of post-PNI macrophage-SC interaction was noted in our study at the 7th dpo. Regardless of the treatment conditions, we detected an extensive repertoire of ED1$^+$ macrophages and SCs in the injured nerve. M2-like-macrophages appeared predominant, with only a small fraction of M1-like-cells observed. Additionally, in the O group, a widespread distribution of the dark spots representing damaged axons was noted marginal to SCs, with weak S100 immunoreactivity, probably undergoing degeneration/dedifferentiation. The analogous was not observed after the B vitamins treatment. Interestingly, these areas of axonal/SC-degeneration appeared borderline to many ED1$^+$/S100$^+$ macrophages displaying transitional M1-to-M2 morphology. Macrophages with the M1- or M2-morphology were also present. On the other hand, we noticed that B vitamins significantly increased S100$^+$ SCs closely associated to ED1$^+$ cells. Importantly, these ED1$^+$ macrophages displayed the M2-like-morphology and were closely associated to only S100$^+$ SCs of non-myelinating morphology, wrapping multiple small-diameter non-myelinated axons and being GAP43$^+$.

A similar profile of M2-macrophages to non-myelinating-SCs interaction was detected in the O nerve at the 14th dpo. These S100$^+$ SCs were also GAP43$^+$. Considering that GAP43, a marker of growing axons [27], may also represent a marker of the non-myelinating-SCs [26,28,29], the overlapping between S100 and GAP43 immunoreactivity classifies implicated SCs to the non-myelinating class. Contrary, only a paucity of the myelin-forming (S100$^+$/GAP43$^+$ and S100$^+$/GAP43$^-$) SCs was detected in the O group. However, after 14 days of exposure to B vitamins the myelinating, mature SCs, which were GAP43$^-$, appeared as the predominant SC-type in the OT group, while a strong GAP43 immunostaining was detected in the large-diameter myelinated-axons.

As evidenced in our study, PNI causes the destruction of the majority of SCs at the 7th dpo, as well as reprogramming from the myelin to non-myelin-forming (Remak) SCs. This aligns with both SC classes undergoing large-scale gene expression post-PNI, leading to the specialized, repair-promoting phenotype [36]. Given that the Remak SCs unsheathed uninjured fibers and are capable of acting as "sentinels" of injury/disease in proximity [37,38], it is not surprising that exactly this SCs phenotype appears most abundant at the 7th and 14th dpo.

Considering all, we can safely conclude that the B vitamins treatment protects myelin-forming SCs and accelerates the appearance of non-myelin-forming SCs. This preserves the functionality of the injured femoral nerve, as manifested by enhanced recovery of the locomotor performances in rats, which was demonstrated previously by our group [19]. Consistently, some recent publications report positive effects of individual B vitamins application (B12 > B1 > B6) on the damaged sciatic nerve repair by affecting myelination and SCs. Importantly, to obtain an optimal regenerative effect, the usage of B vitamins cocktail was proposed [39]. Moreover, beneficial effects of vitamin B12 were acknowledged in a focal demyelination rat model, in terms of accelerated re-myelination, improved recovery of motor/sensory functions, and stimulation of SCs differentiation [40]. Likewise, folic acid may stimulate the post-PNI repair by promoting SCs proliferation and migration, and secretion of nerve growth factors [41].

As outlined above, during the post-PNI recovery, we observed time-dependent changes in macrophage and SC morphology in terms of transition from the round-shaped, smaller M1-, to the "foamy"-shaped, larger M2-macrophages, and non-myelinating-SCs to the myelinating-mature-SCs. Concerning this, we conclude that the B vitamins treatment balances the macrophages-to-SCs interaction to limit the injured nerve damage by accelerating the transition from indispensable inflammation to neuroreparation right after PNI.

Consistently, we demonstrated that PNI affects the expression profile of TNF-α and IL-10 in SCs, this being modulated through the administration of B vitamins for 14 dpo. Following the sciatic nerve transection a phasic TNF-α mRNA expression pattern was observed, peaking immediately (14 h), after 5 days and also two weeks [42,43]. In our model of the femoral nerve transection, we also noted increased expression of TNF-α at the 14th dpo within O, compared to S animals, while the administration of B vitamins reduced the TNF-α immunoreactivity. Apart in M2-macrophages, the TNF-α immunoreactivity was detected in some, but not all SCs. Interestingly, the B vitamins treatment reduces the TNF-α expression, thus, protecting myelin-forming-SCs that produce IL-10. Hence, the preserved femoral nerve functionality is manifested as increase in GAP-43 expression and improved locomotor recovery.

IL-10, whose up-regulation was shown from 7 up to 28 days post-injury [44,45], was proposed to modulate the proinflammatory cytokines expression and axonal plasticity [46]. In two different PNI models [42,43], the expression of IL-10 mRNA underwent gradual increase during Wallerian degeneration, while the recent results [20] imply the prevalence of macrophages expressing IL-10, which represents the M2-(anti-inflammatory)-phenotype marker [47–50] at the 14th dpo. Remarkably, fractions of ED1$^+$/IL-10$^+$ cells in total ED1$^+$ population were equivalent between O and OT animals. Moreover, some IL-10$^+$ cells lacking ED1 immunoreactivity, with SCs-like morphology were observed as well [20]. In the present study, at the 14th dpo bulk of IL-10 immunoreactivity was detected in ED1$^+$ M2-like-morphology macrophages, and in IL-10$^+$/S100$^+$ cells, which were also abundantly present. We assumed that increased IL-10 expression in "foamy"-M2-macrophages [20] together with the IL-10$^+$/S100$^+$ SCs presence may contribute to the resolution of PNI-triggered inflammation/nerve repair. In contrast, B vitamins treatment diminishes the overlapping of IL-10 and S100 immunoreactivity in myelinating, mature SCs, with larger fraction of S100$^+$ SCs being IL-10$^-$, as seen in the S group. Analogous inflammatory profile of post-PNI SCs was obtained by Dubový et al. [51], who suggested that such a simultaneous induction of proinflammatory and anti-inflammatory cytokines balances PNI-induced inflammation to promote axonal growth.

Accordingly, the main aim of our study was to investigate the association between different types of macrophages and SCs after PNI and to explore whether the treatment with the vitamin B complex could influence this relationship. We have clearly demonstrated that only M2-repair-promoting macrophages were in close-association with SCs, particularly of the non-myelinating type, while no co-localization between macrophages and myelin-forming SCs was observed. Regarding the quantification of ED1$^+$/S100$^+$ cells and their fraction in the total ED1$^+$ cell population, these results gave us the information about the extent of ED1$^+$ macrophages and S100$^+$ SCs interaction during the recovery period after PNI and also how the B vitamin treatment affected the temporal profile of the corresponding interactions, all telling us about the success/extent of the recovery. Thus, in the O group, we have noticed that at the 14th dpo the prevalence of ED1$^+$/S100$^+$ cells in the total population of ED1$^+$ cells was the highest. This suggests that interactions between macrophages and SCs are intense. Most likely, the majority of these SCs belong to the non-myelinating SCs class, while ED1$^+$ macrophages belong to the M2 phenotype, being involved, together with aforementioned non-myelinating S100$^+$ SCs, in the formation of Büngner bands, which are shown to represent the regeneration tracks for directing axons to their targets [19,36]. In contrast, after 14 days of the treatment with the vitamin B complex we have noted significant reduction in the number of ED1$^+$/S100$^+$ cells and their fraction in the total ED1$^+$

cell population. Most of the axons had a renewed myelin sheath and myelin-forming SCs were the predominant type of SCs, as we have also seen in the sham-control nerve sections. Given that the interaction between macrophages and myelin-forming SCs was negligible, obtained results indicated that 14 days of the consecutive B vitamin complex treatment triggered the complete transition to mature, myelin-forming SCs that wrapped large-caliber axons intensively labeled with GAP43, a marker of axonal outgrowth. These results suggested that, by the 14th dpo, the regeneration of injured nerve and the recovery of muscle function gets completed after the treatment with B vitamins, which we have confirmed with behavioral and electromyography testing in our previously published paper [19].

Axon regeneration proceeds at a rate of 1–3 mm/day and depends on the location along the neuron, as well as cytoskeletal materials and proteins, such as actin and tubulin. Further elongation happens through the remaining endoneurial tube, which directs axons back to their original target organs. SCs are essential at this stage of regeneration, as they form Büngner repair bands, which protect and preserve the endoneurial channel. Moreover, together with macrophages, SCs release various neurotrophic factors to stimulate nerve regrowth. After reaching the endoneurial tube, the growth cone has a higher probability of reaching the target organ and triggers the maturation process. This process involves remyelination, axon expansion, and ultimately, functional re-innervation [52]. Related to this, in this study, tight M2-macrophages-to-SCs interactions were confirmed in transversal sections of the injured nerve. Moreover, we clearly demonstrated that the IL-10 immunoreactivity was associated with M2-macrophages, but also with SCs forming the Büngner's bands. Consistent with the literature data [35], our results confirm the role of macrophages as regulators of SCs maturation after PNI.

Versatile effects of the investigated B vitamins treatment stand as an important result, since most compounds that reduce neuroinflammation safeguard the myelin-forming SCs. Importantly, our data show that following PNI, a balance in myelin-forming SCs protection, transition to non-myelin-forming SCs, and vice-versa, can be rapidly established by applying B vitamins during the early recovery period. The underlying molecular and intracellular signaling pathways pave for more thorough clarification. Overall, macrophage/SCs plasticity induced by applying adjuvant to surgery after PNI provides a basis for macrophage/SCs-centered therapeutic strategy, as an alternative repair approach. Concerning this, in the upcoming research, the exact molecular basis of macrophage-SCs interactions in response to the B vitamins, applied hereby, remain to be thoroughly examined.

4. Materials and Methods

4.1. Ethical Approval and Consent to Participate

The study was approved by the Ethics Review Committee for Animal Experimentation of the Military Medical Academy and Ministry of Agriculture and Environmental Protection Republic of Serbia, Veterinary Directorate No. 323-07-7363/2014-05/5.

4.2. Femoral Nerve Injury Rat Model

Irintchev and colleagues described the controlled transection of the peripheral nerve as a widely used model for the examination of peripheral nerve regeneration [30]. In this study, we used adult male Albino Oxford (AO) rats (15 in total), weighing between 250 and 300 g, that were randomly divided into three groups (5 per group). Animals that underwent transection of the femoral nerve motor branch with immediate reconstruction, using a technique of termino-terminal anastomosis, form the first group of so called "operated animals" (O). The second group (OT) included animals that passed the same surgical procedure but were additionally receiving vitamin B complex therapy. The "sham operated" animals (S), which also underwent the dissection of the femoral nerve motor branch but without transection, represent the third experimental group. All of the groups were additionally divided into sub-groups (four per group), based on the post-operation day that (dpo) the animals were sacrificed on (1, 3, 7, and 14 dpo). During the entire period of the study, the animals were kept under the same environmental conditions (laboratory temperature 23 ± 2 °C, humidity between 50% and 60%, 12 h/12 h light/dark cycle with lights on at 07:00 a.m., free availability of water and food).

As anesthesia, intraperitoneal application of ketamine (50 mg/kg; Ketalar, Eczacibasi, Turkey) and xylazine (5 mg/kg; Rompun, Bayer, Turkey) was used on all animals. Following anesthesia, the animals from all investigated groups (S, O, and OT) were appropriately positioned for identification of the femoral nerve motor branch on the rat left hind paw by skin incision in the left groin and femoral region, under aseptic conditions (as previously described [19]). In all experimental groups (S, O, and OT), the motor branch was identified just before entry into the quadriceps muscle. Subsequently, animals from the O and OT groups underwent the transection of the branch, and immediate reconstruction using a 10.0 non-absorbable suture in the form of termino-terminal anastomosis, under the microscope magnification. The skin was sutured using a 4.0 absorbable suture (Peters Surgical, Paris, France). At selected time points, the animals were sacrificed by intravenous injection of a lethal dose of ketamine/xylazine. The motor branches of the femoral nerves (both reconstructed and intact contralateral) were isolated for subsequent immunofluorescence staining. All of the procedures performed in this study were based on the rules and guidelines of the EU Directive 2010/63/EU regarding the protection of animals used for experimental and other scientific purposes.

4.3. Protocol for Vitamin B Complex Treatment

For the investigation of vitamin B complex treatment, ampoules (2 mL) of Beviplex (Beviplex®, Galenika a.d. Belgrade, Serbia), each containing B1 (40 mg), B2 (4 mg), B3 (100 mg), B5 (10 mg), B6 (8 mg), and B12 (4 µg), were used. The given dose was 1.85 mL/kg/day. The complex of B vitamins was injected intraperitoneally immediately (15 min) after the operation and then every 24 h from the day of the operation until the day of sacrifice. Operated, but untreated animals (O) were intraperitoneally injected with the same volume of physiological solution.

4.4. Femoral Nerve Processing Procedure for Immunofluorescence Staining

In the Laboratory for Pathohistology and Cytology HistoLab, Belgrade, all of the isolated motor branches of femoral nerves were prepared for immunohistochemistry in this study. The isolated nerve samples underwent the fixation procedure in the 10% formaldehyde solution to preserve the tissue morphology and antigenicity of target molecules on the dissected nerve. Prior to the addition of melted paraffin wax, the isolated nerves underwent a series of dehydration steps at room temperature (RT): (1) 3 × 30 min in 70% ethanol; (2) 3 × 30 min in 90% ethanol; (3) 3 × 30 min in 100% ethanol; and (4) 3 × 30 min in xylene. Following dehydration, the tissue was immerged into the melted paraffin wax at 58 °C. Microtome sectioning of the paraffin-embedded tissue was next done at a thickness of 5 µm. Sections were then incubated at 56 °C in water bath, mounted onto histological slides, pre-coated with gelatin for better tissue adhesion, and dried overnight at RT.

4.5. Procedure of Immunofluorescence Staining and Digital Image Processing

Immunofluorescence (IF) staining was used for protein localization on nerves slides. For indirect immunofluorescence staining, the fluorescent-dye conjugated secondary antibody, which binds to the unlabeled primary antibody, was used. The all IF staining procedures were done at RT. Only incubation with primary antibody was performed at a temperature of 4 °C. All of the solutions were prepared in 0.01 M Phosphate-Buffered Saline (PBS), pH 7.4, which was also used for washing after certain steps. Double IF staining proceeded according to the following steps:

Deparaffinization and rehydration: Microscope slides with paraffin-embedded sections were deparaffinized and rinsed in xylene 1, xylene 2, absolute alcohol, 95% alcohol, 70% alcohol, and distilled water, for 5 min in each solution. Antigen retrieval: Antigenic epitope unmasking was done by boiling microscope slides in 0.01 M sodium citrate buffer, pH 6, for 8 min at 99 °C–100 °C, followed by cooling at RT for 30 min and 3 × 5 min PBS washing. Blocking solution: after the washing step, microscope slides were incubated for 60 min in 5% blocking serum (originating from the same species as the secondary antibody) to prevent nonspecific binding of the secondary antibody. To enable membrane permeabilization, 0.5% Triton X-100 detergent was added to the blocking serum. Primary antibody, diluted in PBS, was applied onto slides and incubated overnight at 4 °C temperature. Next day, slides were washed out 3 × 5 min in PBS. Secondary antibody, diluted in PBS, was applied onto slides, where it specifically binds to the present primary antibody. Slides were next washed for 3 × 5 min in PBS. In the case of double or triple IF staining, the steps starting from the incubation in the blocking serum were repeated for the following markers. The primary and secondary antibodies used for IF labeling are indicated in the Table 1.

Table 1. List of primary and secondary antibodies used for immunofluorescence labeling.

Antibodies	Dilution	Company
Mouse monoclonal anti-CD68 (Clone ED1)	1:100	Abcam, Cambridge, MA, USA
Goat monoclonal anti-TNF-α	1:100	Santa Cruz Biotechnology, CA, USA
Goat monoclonal anti-IL-10	1:100	Santa Cruz Biotechnology, CA, USA
Mouse monoclonal anti-S100	1:200	Chemicon International, CA, USA
Rabbit monoclonal anti-S100	1:200	Bio-Rad Laboratories, CA, USA
Rabbit monoclonal anti-GAP43	1:200	Millipore, Darmstadt, Germany
Donkey anti-goat IgG (Alexa Fluor 555)	1:200	Invitrogen, Carlsbad, CA, USA
Donkey anti-rabbit IgG (Alexa Fluor 488)	1:200	Invitrogen, Carlsbad, CA, USA
Donkey anti-rabbit IgG (Alexa Flour 555)	1:200	Invitrogen, Carlsbad, CA, USA
Donkey anti-mouse IgG (Alexa Fluor 488)	1:200	Invitrogen, Carlsbad, CA, USA
Donkey anti-mouse IgG (Alexa Fluor 555)	1:200	Invitrogen, Carlsbad, CA, USA

After incubation with the last secondary antibody, slides were incubated in 4′,6-diamidin-2-fenilindolom (DAPI; Invitrogen, Grand Island, NY, USA) for 10 min to counterstain the nuclei and then washed 6 × 5 min in PBS and mounted with Mowiol (Calbiochem, Millipore, Germany). After drying overnight, slides were ready for viewing under the microscope. As a staining control, microscope slides that underwent the same IF procedure, but without the primary antibody application, were used.

The Carl Zeiss Axiovert fluorescent microscope, equipped with the Axiocam monochromatic camera (Axio Observer Microscope Z1, ZEISS, Gottingen, Germany), at the magnifications of 20×, 40×, and 63× was used for image processing of the prepared motor branch of femoral nerve sections and saved in .tiff format. To capture images at 63× magnification ApoTome software was used. Co-localization on the obtained fluorescent images was done using AxioVision Rel. 4.6 program, which represents a standard part of the Zeiss Axiovert microscope equipment, and then assembled and labeled in Photoshop CS6 (Adobe Systems). The quantification of single- and double-stained cells from experimental groups (S, O, OT) was performed for each time point (1, 3, 7, 14 dpo), and obtained from three independent experiments. High resolution digital images (600 pixels/inch) captured at 40× magnification (1388 μm × 1040 μm) (three images/group/independent experiment) were used for cells counting. The total number of single- or double-positive cells was counted manually using Adobe Photoshop Creative Cloud (Version 14.0). Additionally, the percentage of double-positive cells in some investigated cells populations was calculated and presented.

4.6. Statistical Analysis

Statistical comparison between two experimental groups was performed using a two-sided Student's t test and a value of $p < 0.05$ or less was considered significant. Values were shown as mean values with standard error (SEM).

5. Conclusions

In this study we report for the first time that the treatment with the complex of B vitamins (B1, B2, B3, B5, B6, and B12) could effectively promote PNI-induced transition of the non-myelinating to myelin-forming-SCs phenotype and suppress neurodegeneration by reducing the expression of proinflammatory and up-regulating the expression of anti-inflammatory cytokines, produced by macrophages and SCs. This consequently changes interactions between these cells, thereby contributing to the regeneration of the injured nerve. In conclusion, the ability of B vitamins to modulate macrophages-SCs interaction reveals their potential as an additional tool in peripheral nerve regeneration therapies in humans, which requires extensive further research and confirmation in clinical trials.

Author Contributions: Conceptualization, B.B.N. and P.N.; methodology and investigation, A.E., P.N., S.D., B.D.-P., D.V., S.P. and B.B.N.; software, S.D., S.P. and B.B.N.; writing—original draft preparation, A.E., J.R., S.P. and B.B.N.; writing—review and editing, J.R., S.P. and B.B.N.; visualization, J.R., S.P. and B.B.N.; supervision, S.P. and B.B.N.; project administration, B.B.N. All authors have read and agreed to the published version of the manuscript.

Funding: This work was supported by the Ministry of Education, Science and Technological Development of the Republic of Serbia (451-03-68/2020-14/200178) and Ministry of Defense of the Republic of Serbia (MFVMA/10/16-18).

Acknowledgments: Some data sets included in this manuscript were presented as oral presentations at the Meeting of COST Action BM1406: Ion Channels and Immune Response toward a global understanding of immune cell physiology and for new therapeutic approaches (IONCHAN-IMMUNRESPON) (October 2018, Seillac, France).

Conflicts of Interest: The authors declare no conflict of interest.

References

1. Ciardelli, G.; Chiono, V. Materials for peripheral nerve regeneration. *Macromol. Biosci.* **2006**, *6*, 13–26. [CrossRef] [PubMed]
2. Bigbee, J.W.; Yoshino, J.E.; DeVries, G.H. Morphological and proliferative responses of cultured Schwann cells following rapid phagocytosis of a myelin-enriched fraction. *J. Neurocytol.* **1987**, *16*, 487–496. [CrossRef] [PubMed]
3. Stoll, G.; Griffin, J.; Li, C.Y.; Trapp, B. Wallerian degeneration in the peripheral nervous system: Participation of both Schwann cells and macrophages in myelin degradation. *J. Neurocytol.* **1989**, *18*, 671–683. [CrossRef] [PubMed]
4. Hirata, K.; Kawabuchi, M. Myelin phagocytosis by macrophages and nonmacrophages during Wallerian degeneration. *Microsc. Res. Tech.* **2002**, *57*, 541–547. [CrossRef] [PubMed]
5. Tofaris, G.K.; Patterson, P.H.; Jessen, K.R.; Mirsky, R. Denervated Schwann cells attract macrophages by secretion of leukemia inhibitory factor (LIF) and monocyte chemoattractant protein-1 in a process regulated by interleukin-6 and LIF. *J. Neurosci.* **2002**, *22*, 6696–6703. [CrossRef] [PubMed]
6. Fleur, M.L.; Underwood, J.L.; Rappolee, D.A.; Werb, Z. Basement membrane and repair of injury to peripheral nerve: Defining a potential role for macrophages, matrix metalloproteinases, and tissue inhibitor of metalloproteinases-1. *J. Exp. Med.* **1996**, *184*, 2311–2326. [CrossRef]
7. Barrette, B.; Hébert, M.-A.; Filali, M.; Lafortune, K.; Vallieres, N.; Gowing, G.; Julien, J.-P.; Lacroix, S. Requirement of myeloid cells for axon regeneration. *J. Neurosci.* **2008**, *28*, 9363–9376. [CrossRef]
8. Stratton, J.A.; Shah, P.T. Macrophage polarization in nerve injury: Do Schwann cells play a role? *Neural Regen. Res.* **2016**, *11*, 53. [CrossRef]
9. Brown, H.C. Macrophages and the Nervous System. Ph.D. Thesis, University of Oxford, Oxford, UK, 1996.
10. Murray, P.J.; Allen, J.E.; Biswas, S.K.; Fisher, E.A.; Gilroy, D.W.; Goerdt, S.; Gordon, S.; Hamilton, J.A.; Ivashkiv, L.B.; Lawrence, T. Macrophage activation and polarization: Nomenclature and experimental guidelines. *Immunity* **2014**, *41*, 14–20. [CrossRef]
11. Kolter, J.; Kierdorf, K.; Henneke, P. Origin and differentiation of nerve-associated macrophages. *J. Immunol.* **2020**, *204*, 271–279. [CrossRef]
12. Pan, B.; Shi, Z.-J.; Yan, J.-Y.; Li, J.-H.; Feng, S.-Q. Long non-coding RNA NONMMUG014387 promotes Schwann cell proliferation after peripheral nerve injury. *Neural Regen. Res.* **2017**, *12*, 2084. [PubMed]
13. Lutz, A.B.; Barres, B.A. Contrasting the glial response to axon injury in the central and peripheral nervous systems. *Dev. Cell* **2014**, *28*, 7–17.
14. Scholz, T.; Krichevsky, A.; Sumarto, A.; Jaffurs, D.; Wirth, G.A.; Paydar, K.; Evans, G.R. Peripheral nerve injuries: An international survey of current treatments and future perspectives. *J. Reconstr. Microsurg.* **2009**, *25*, 339–344. [CrossRef] [PubMed]

15. Pan, H.-C.; Yang, D.-Y.; Ho, S.-P.; Sheu, M.-L.; Chen, C.-J.; Hwang, S.-M.; Chang, M.-H.; Cheng, F.-C. Escalated regeneration in sciatic nerve crush injury by the combined therapy of human amniotic fluid mesenchymal stem cells and fermented soybean extracts, Natto. *J. Biomed. Sci.* **2009**, *16*, 75. [CrossRef] [PubMed]
16. Wiberg, M.; Terenghi, G. Will it be possible to produce peripheral nerves? *Surg. Technol. Int.* **2003**, *11*, 303–310. [PubMed]
17. Fernández-Villa, D.; Jiménez Gómez-Lavín, M.; Abradelo, C.; San Román, J.; Rojo, L. Tissue engineering therapies based on folic acid and other vitamin B derivatives. Functional mechanisms and current applications in regenerative medicine. *Int. J. Mol. Sci.* **2018**, *19*, 4068. [CrossRef] [PubMed]
18. Altun, I.; Kurutaş, E.B. Vitamin B complex and vitamin B12 levels after peripheral nerve injury. *Neural Regen. Res.* **2016**, *11*, 842. [CrossRef]
19. Nedeljković, P.; Zmijanjac, D.; Drašković-Pavlović, B.; Vasiljevska, M.; Vučević, D.; Božić, B.; Bumbaširević, M. Vitamin B complex treatment improves motor nerve regeneration and recovery of muscle function in a rodent model of peripheral nerve injury. *Arch. Biol. Sci.* **2017**, *69*, 361–368. [CrossRef]
20. Ehmedah, A.; Nedeljkovic, P.; Dacic, S.; Repac, J.; Draskovic Pavlovic, B.; Vucevic, D.; Pekovic, S.; Bozic Nedeljkovic, B. Vitamin B Complex Treatment Attenuates Local Inflammation after Peripheral Nerve Injury. *Molecules* **2019**, *24*, 4615. [CrossRef]
21. Liao, W.-C.; Wang, Y.-J.; Huang, M.-C.; Tseng, G.-F. Methylcobalamin facilitates collateral sprouting of donor axons and innervation of recipient muscle in end-to-side neurorrhaphy in rats. *PLoS ONE* **2013**, *8*, e76302. [CrossRef]
22. Wang, Z.-B.; Gan, Q.; Rupert, R.L.; Zeng, Y.-M.; Song, X.-J. Thiamine, pyridoxine, cyanocobalamin and their combination inhibit thermal, but not mechanical hyperalgesia in rats with primary sensory neuron injury. *Pain* **2005**, *114*, 266–277. [CrossRef] [PubMed]
23. Fujii, A.; Matsumoto, H.; Yamamoto, H. Effect of vitamin B complex on neurotransmission and neurite outgrowth. *Gen. Pharmacol. Vasc. Syst.* **1996**, *27*, 995–1000. [CrossRef]
24. Shearman, J.D.; Franks, A.J. S-100 protein in Schwann cells of the developing human peripheral nerve. *Cell Tissue Res.* **1987**, *249*, 459–463. [CrossRef] [PubMed]
25. Mata, M.; Alessi, D.; Fink, D.J. S100 is preferentially distributed in myelin-forming Schwann cells. *J. Neurocytol.* **1990**, *19*, 432–442. [CrossRef] [PubMed]
26. Liu, Z.; Jin, Y.-Q.; Chen, L.; Wang, Y.; Yang, X.; Cheng, J.; Wu, W.; Qi, Z.; Shen, Z. Specific marker expression and cell state of Schwann cells during culture in vitro. *PLoS ONE* **2015**, *10*, e0123278. [CrossRef]
27. Donnelly, C.J.; Park, M.; Spillane, M.; Yoo, S.; Pacheco, A.; Gomes, C.; Vuppalanchi, D.; McDonald, M.; Kim, H.H.; Merianda, T.T. Axonally synthesized β-actin and GAP-43 proteins support distinct modes of axonal growth. *J. Neurosci.* **2013**, *33*, 3311–3322. [CrossRef]
28. Curtis, R.; Stewart, H.; Hall, S.M.; Wilkin, G.P.; Mirsky, R.; Jessen, K.R. GAP-43 is expressed by nonmyelin-forming Schwann cells of the peripheral nervous system. *J. Cell Biol.* **1992**, *116*, 1455–1464. [CrossRef]
29. Sensenbrenner, M.; Lucas, M.; Deloulme, J.-C. Expression of two neuronal markers, growth-associated protein 43 and neuron-specific enolase, in rat glial cells. *J. Mol. Med.* **1997**, *75*, 653–663. [CrossRef]
30. Irintchev, A. Potentials and limitations of peripheral nerve injury models in rodents with particular reference to the femoral nerve. *Ann. Anat. Anat. Anz.* **2011**, *193*, 276–285. [CrossRef]
31. Rotshenker, S. Wallerian degeneration: The innate-immune response to traumatic nerve injury. *J. Neuroinflamm.* **2011**, *8*, 109. [CrossRef]
32. Lubińska, L. Early course of Wallerian degeneration in myelinated fibres of the rat phrenic nerve. *Brain Res.* **1977**, *130*, 47–63. [CrossRef]
33. Luttges, M.W.; Kelly, P.T.; Gerren, R.A. Degenerative changes in mouse sciatic nerves: Electrophoretic and electrophysiologic characterizations. *Exp. Neurol.* **1976**, *50*, 706–733. [CrossRef]
34. Tsao, J.W.; George, E.B.; Griffin, J.W. Temperature modulation reveals three distinct stages of Wallerian degeneration. *J. Neurosci.* **1999**, *19*, 4718–4726. [CrossRef] [PubMed]
35. Stratton, J.A.; Holmes, A.; Rosin, N.L.; Sinha, S.; Vohra, M.; Burma, N.E.; Trang, T.; Midha, R.; Biernaskie, J. Macrophages regulate Schwann cell maturation after nerve injury. *Cell Rep.* **2018**, *24*, 2561–2572.e6. [CrossRef]
36. Jessen, K.; Mirsky, R. The repair Schwann cell and its function in regenerating nerves. *J. Physiol.* **2016**, *594*, 3521–3531. [CrossRef]

37. Griffin, J.W.; Thompson, W.J. Biology and pathology of nonmyelinating Schwann cells. *Glia* **2008**, *56*, 1518–1531. [CrossRef]
38. Armati, P.J.; Mathey, E.K. An update on Schwann cell biology—immunomodulation, neural regulation and other surprises. *J. Neurol. Sci.* **2013**, *333*, 68–72. [CrossRef]
39. Al-saaeed, S.M.; Al-khalisy, M.H. The Regenerative Role of Vitamins B1, B6, B12 in Treatment of Peripheral Neuropathy. *Int. J. Sci. Res.* **2017**, *6*, 2411–2415.
40. Nishimoto, S.; Tanaka, H.; Okamoto, M.; Okada, K.; Murase, T.; Yoshikawa, H. Methylcobalamin promotes the differentiation of Schwann cells and remyelination in lysophosphatidylcholine-induced demyelination of the rat sciatic nerve. *Front. Cell. Neurosci.* **2015**, *9*, 298. [CrossRef]
41. Kang, W.-B.; Chen, Y.-J.; Lu, D.-Y.; Yan, J.-Z. Folic acid contributes to peripheral nerve injury repair by promoting Schwann cell proliferation, migration, and secretion of nerve growth factor. *Neural Regen. Res.* **2019**, *14*, 132.
42. Taskinen, H.; Olsson, T.; Bucht, A.; Khademi, M.; Svelander, L.; Röyttä, M. Peripheral nerve injury induces endoneurial expression of IFN-γ, IL-10 and TNF-α mRNA. *J. Neuroimmunol.* **2000**, *102*, 17–25. [CrossRef]
43. Okamoto, K.; Martin, D.P.; Schmelzer, J.D.; Mitsui, Y.; Low, P.A. Pro-and anti-inflammatory cytokine gene expression in rat sciatic nerve chronic constriction injury model of neuropathic pain. *Exp. Neurol.* **2001**, *169*, 386–391. [CrossRef] [PubMed]
44. George, A.; Kleinschnitz, C.; Zelenka, M.; Brinkhoff, J.; Stoll, G.; Sommer, C. Wallerian degeneration after crush or chronic constriction injury of rodent sciatic nerve is associated with a depletion of endoneurial interleukin-10 protein. *Exp. Neurol.* **2004**, *188*, 187–191. [CrossRef] [PubMed]
45. Sawada, T.; Sano, M.; Omura, T.; Omura, K.; Hasegawa, T.; Funahashi, S.; Nagano, A. Spatiotemporal quantification of tumor necrosis factor-alpha and interleukin-10 after crush injury in rat sciatic nerve utilizing immunohistochemistry. *Neurosci. Lett.* **2007**, *417*, 55–60. [CrossRef]
46. Vidal, P.M.; Lemmens, E.; Dooley, D.; Hendrix, S. The role of "anti-inflammatory" cytokines in axon regeneration. *Cytokine Growth Factor Rev.* **2013**, *24*, 1–12. [CrossRef]
47. Mantovani, A.; Biswas, S.K.; Galdiero, M.R.; Sica, A.; Locati, M. Macrophage plasticity and polarization in tissue repair and remodelling. *J. Pathol.* **2013**, *229*, 176–185. [CrossRef]
48. Wang, N.; Liang, H.; Zen, K. Molecular mechanisms that influence the macrophage M1–M2 polarization balance. *Front. Immunol.* **2014**, *5*, 614. [CrossRef]
49. Chen, P.; Piao, X.; Bonaldo, P. Role of macrophages in Wallerian degeneration and axonal regeneration after peripheral nerve injury. *Acta Neuropathol.* **2015**, *130*, 605–618. [CrossRef]
50. Rőszer, T. Understanding the mysterious M2 macrophage through activation markers and effector mechanisms. *Mediat. Inflamm.* **2015**, *2015*, 816460. [CrossRef]
51. Dubový, P.; Klusáková, I.; Hradilová Svíženská, I. Inflammatory profiling of Schwann cells in contact with growing axons distal to nerve injury. *Biomed Res. Int.* **2014**, *2014*. [CrossRef]
52. Menorca, R.M.; Fussell, T.S.; Elfar, J.C. Peripheral nerve trauma: Mechanisms of injury and recovery. *Hand Clin.* **2013**, *29*, 317. [CrossRef] [PubMed]

Sample Availability: Samples of the compounds are available from the authors. It is commercial product Beviplex (Beviplex®, Galenika a.d. Belgrade, Serbia) and it is written in the Section 4.3. Protocol for Vitamin B Complex Treatment.

Publisher's Note: MDPI stays neutral with regard to jurisdictional claims in published maps and institutional affiliations.

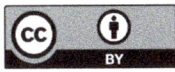

© 2020 by the authors. Licensee MDPI, Basel, Switzerland. This article is an open access article distributed under the terms and conditions of the Creative Commons Attribution (CC BY) license (http://creativecommons.org/licenses/by/4.0/).

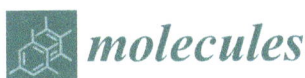

Article

Glucosamine Enhancement of BDNF Expression and Animal Cognitive Function

Lien-Yu Chou [1], Yu-Ming Chao [1], Yen-Chun Peng [2], Hui-Ching Lin [1] and Yuh-Lin Wu [1,*]

[1] Department of Physiology, School of Medicine, National Yang-Ming University, Taipei 11221, Taiwan; jackychou82@yahoo.com.tw (L.-Y.C.), chao.s976827@gmail.com (Y.-M.C.); hclin7@ym.edu.tw (H.-C.L.)
[2] Department of Internal Medicine, Taichung Veterans General Hospital, Taichung 40705, Taiwan; pychunppp@gmail.com
* Correspondence: ylwu@ym.edu.tw; Tel.: +886-2-2826-7081; Fax: +886-2-2826-4049

Received: 22 July 2020; Accepted: 11 August 2020; Published: 12 August 2020

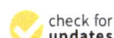

Abstract: Brain-derived neurotrophic factor (BDNF) is an important factor for memory consolidation and cognitive function. Protein kinase A (PKA) signaling interacts significantly with BDNF-provoked downstream signaling. Glucosamine (GLN), a common dietary supplement, has been demonstrated to perform a variety of beneficial physiological functions. In the current study, an in vivo model of 7-week-old C57BL/6 mice receiving daily intraperitoneal injection of GLN (0, 3, 10 and 30 mg/animal) was subjected to the novel object recognition test in order to determine cognitive performance. GLN significantly increased cognitive function. In the hippocampus GLN elevated tissue cAMP concentrations and CREB phosphorylation, and upregulated the expression of BDNF, CREB5 and the BDNF receptor TrkB, but it reduced PDE4B expression. With the in vitro model in the HT22 hippocampal cell line, GLN exposure significantly increased protein and mRNA levels of BDNF and CREB5 and induced cAMP responsive element (CRE) reporter activity; the GLN-mediated BDNF expression and CRE reporter induction were suppressed by PKA inhibitor H89. Our current findings suggest that GLN can exert a cognition-enhancing function and this may act at least in part by upregulating the BDNF levels via a cAMP/PKA/CREB-dependent pathway.

Keywords: glucosamine; cognition; BDNF; PKA

1. Introduction

Learning and memory are two critical functions of the brain and several different regions within the brain have been demonstrated to have involvement in the consolidation of diverse forms of learning/memory, including the cortex, striatum, amygdala and hippocampus [1]. The cortex has involvement with spatial learning; the striatum correlates with motor skills; the amygdala is related to emotional memory; and finally, the hippocampus is involved in spatial learning and working and recognition memory. Many have generally recognized the hippocampus as the most critical region [2,3].

A variety of neurotrophin (NT) polypeptides play important roles in neural activities by regulating cell proliferation, differentiation, maturation and plasticity. Among the NTs, the brain-derived neurotrophic factor (BDNF) in general performs the highest expression in the brain [4]. In the mouse model, BDNF has been shown to be required for neurogenesis in the hippocampus [5] and a declined BDNF level was noted in the ageing adults, indicating a possible connection of low BDNF to reduced memory, neurodegeneration and cognitive impairments [6]. In neurons, activation of the cAMP/PKA/cAMP-responsive element binding (CREB) protein signaling pathway can lead to the induction of an array of genes, including BDNF [7]. It has been proposed that while BDNF interacts with its cognate kinase receptor TrkB, the PKA pathway can activate and cause a positive feedback-like circle to amplify the BDNF-modulated physiological activities [8]. Phosphodiesterase (PDE) is the enzyme capable of degrading cAMP and thus it is able to attenuate the PKA signaling by reducing the availability of the intracellular cAMP. In fact, PDE4 is a cAMP-specific PDE isoform detected in various tissues, including several brain regions [9,10]. Indeed PDE4 has been regarded as a potential therapeutic target, for example for the treatment for the cognitive impairment [11]. All of these studies have pointed out that maintaining the cellular cAMP/PKA/CREB signaling by increasing the cAMP and/or by decreasing the PDE activity appears to be a potential strategy for treating a decline in cognitive functions [11].

Glucosamine (GLN) is a crucial component within glycoproteins and proteoglycans [12]. The clinical value of GLN was not established until it was first suggested for use in treating osteoarthritis [13]. Besides the glycolysis-related events, GLN and its derivatives have been demonstrated to have involvement in a variety of cellular activities in a glycolysis-independent manner [14]. GLN is involved in the O-linked N-acetylglucosaminylation (O-GlcNAcylation) of different proteins and this should lead to a wide range of regulation in cell physiology, such as cellular signal transduction, transcription, protein modification and more [14,15]. Importantly, most GLN administrated orally can be absorbed from the gastrointestinal system and the resultant GLN has been shown to pass the blood–brain barrier (BBB) to reach the brain [16,17], indicating that GLN can possibly reach any tissue of the body.

Previous studies have reported a list of different potential functions of GLN [15]. The involvement of O-GlcNAcylation in the regulation of protein homeostasis has been well-recognized; O-GlcNAcylation modification is highly prevalent in the mammalian brain and errors in this mechanism have been suggested to contribute to many cellular cascades in relation to neurological or neurodegenerative diseases [12,18]. Therefore, this study aimed to disclose the impact of GLN in brain cognitive performance in relation to BDNF production and PKA signaling with in vivo and in vitro approaches.

2. Results

2.1. GLN Enhancement on Animal Cognitive Function

During the 2 weeks of GLN injection (0, 3, 10 and 30 mg/mouse/day), GLN did not cause any change in body weight among different treatment groups (Supplementary Figure S1). To examine the GLN impact on cognitive function, the 7-week-old mice receiving 14 consecutive days of daily GLN intraperitoneal (IP) injection were subjected to the novel object recognition test (NORT) at day 7 and day 14 to evaluate the cognitive performance of the animals. The recorded video analyzed by the software revealed the total time spent and the tracks in relation to the familiar (F) and novel (N) objects (Figure 1A,D). The recognition index was derived from the formula of TN/TN + TF (TN: time spent exploring the novel object and TF: time spent exploring the familiar object). It appeared that the total time was not different among different treatment groups (Figure 1C,F), indicating that GLN did not affect general locomotive activity. Interestingly, there was a significant elevation of the recognition index by GLN at 3, 10 and 30 mg/mouse at day 7 (Figure 1B) and at 10 and 30 mg/mouse at day 14 (Figure 1E).

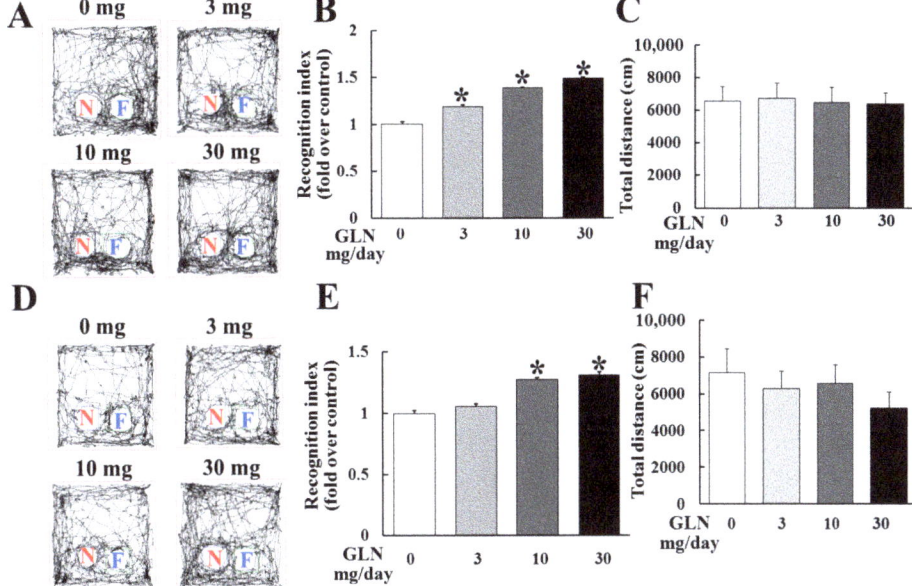

Figure 1. GLN enhancement of animal cognitive performance. The C57BL/6 male mice received a daily intraperitoneal (IP) GLN injection (0, 3, 10 and 30 mg/mouse) for 7 (**A–C**) or 14 days (**D–F**), followed by the novel object recognition test (NORT). A set of objects with a previously presented familiar object (**F**) and a new novel object (**N**) were presented to the trained animals. The moving tracks of the animals were recorded (**A,D**). The recognition index (**B,E**) and total moving distance (**C,F**) were determined. The results represent the means ± S.D. ($n = 8$) *, $p < 0.05$, compared with the 0 mg group.

2.2. GLN Induction of the Genes Potentially Associated with the Brain Cognitive Functions

To examine whether GLN may regulate the genes encoding various NTs, which have been reported as important in brain functions, the hippocampus, striatum and cortex from GLN-treated animals were harvested at day 14, followed by RNA extraction, and the mRNA levels were monitored by a quantitative RT-PCR analysis. All the NTs examined, such as BDNF, NGF, NT-3, NT-4 and CNTF were all induced by GLN in hippocampus (Figure 2A); BDNF and NT-3 were induced in striatum (Figure 2B) and NGF and NT-4 were induced, but CNTF was reduced by GLN in cortex (Figure 2C). In parallel, BDNF protein expression was also examined in all three tissues. GLN was able to increase the mature form BDNF levels in all three tissues and the pro-BDNF levels in the hippocampus and cortex (Figure 1D). Notably, the BDNF cognate receptor TrkB mRNA expression in the hippocampus was also increased by GLN (Supplementary Figure S2).

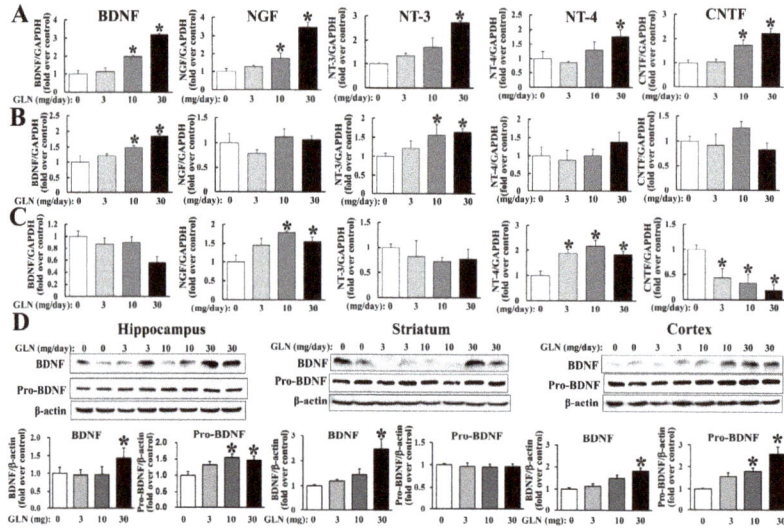

Figure 2. GLN impact on the expression of mRNAs encoding neurotrophins and the BDNF protein in the hippocampus, striatum and cortex. The RNAs were extracted from the hippocampus (**A**), striatum (**B**) and cortex (**C**), followed by the RT-PCR assay to detect the mRNAs of BDNF, NGF, NT-3, NT-4 and CNTF using GAPDH as an internal control. Protein samples were also prepared from the same tissues and the expression of BDNF and pro-BDNF was analyzed by Western blotting with β-actin as an internal control (**D**). The results represent the means ± S.D. ($n = 8$) *, $p < 0.05$, compared with the 0 mg group.

2.3. GLN Impact on Expression of BDNF, CREB5 and PDE4B, and the PKA Signaling in the Hippocampus and HT22 Hippocampal Cells

As the hippocampus is the critical tissue to regulate the cognitive function and as the cAMP/PKA pathway is crucial to brain function [3,11], we therefore looked into GLN's impact on the expression of CREB5 and PDE4B, both of which are involved in regulating cAMP/PKA signaling [9,10]. The GLN treatment (10 and 30 mg/mouse) was able to increase the CREB5 mRNA concentration, but decreased PDE4B mRNA levels in the hippocampus (Figure 3A). The cAMP concentration in the hippocampal tissue elevated after GLN treatment (Figure 3B). Meanwhile, the corresponding downstream signal activation of the cAMP/PKA in terms of CREB phosphorylation in the hippocampus seemed to be promoted by GLN (Figure 3C). In addition, we examined the GLN effect on regulation of the BDNF, CREB5 and PDE4B genes in HT22 cells. The GLN treatment (10 mM) increased the mRNA levels of BDNF, CREB5 and PDE4B (Figure 3D), while both BDNF and CREB5 protein levels were increased by GLN (1 and 10 mM), but the PDE4B protein expression remained unaffected by GLN (Figure 3E,F). To assure that the GLN treatment in HT22 cells does not affect the cellular viability, MTT and alamarBlue assays were used to confirm that GLN at all doses did not result in significant changes in cell viability (Supplementary Figure S3).

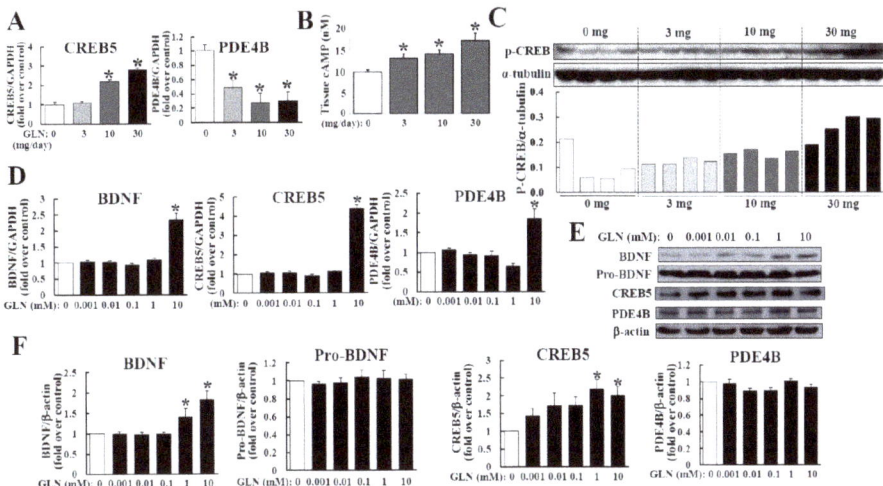

Figure 3. GLN regulation of CREB5 and PDE4B mRNAs, cAMP accumulation and CREB phosphorylation in the hippocampus and the expression of BDNF, CREB5 and PDE4B in the hippocampal cells. The RNA samples prepared from GLN-injected animal's hippocampus (**A**) and from GLN-treated HT22 cells (**D**) were subjected to RT-PCR to analyze the mRNAs of BDNF, CREB5 and PDE4B. The cAMP concentration (**B**) and CREB phosphorylation (**C**) in hippocampal tissues were determined. Protein expression of BDNF, CREB5 and PDE4B in GLN-treated HT22 cells were analyzed by Western blotting (**E,F**). The results represent the means ± S.D. (n = 8). *, $p < 0.05$ compared with the 0 mg (**A–C**) or the 0 mM group (**D,F**).

2.4. Delineation of the GLN Regulation of the cAMP/PKA/CREB Pathway in Relation to BDNF Production

We observed GLN upregulation on BDNF in the hippocampus (Figure 2A,D) and HT22 cells (Figure 3D–F), CREB5 in the hippocampus (Figure 3A) and HT22 cells (Figure 3D–F), and CREB phosphorylation in the hippocampus (Figure 3C), and further, the downregulation on PDE4B in the hippocampus (Figure 3A). The peculiar question emerged as to how these regulatory profiles by GLN would contribute to BDNF production. In HT22 hippocampal cells, we first analyzed the GLN effect on CREB phosphorylation and GLN indeed mediated a significant induction of CREB phosphorylation (Figure 4A). GLN also induced CRE reporter activation and such an induction was suppressed by PKA inhibitor H89 (Figure 4B). More importantly, the GLN-mediated BDNF production was inhibited by H89 (Figure 4C).

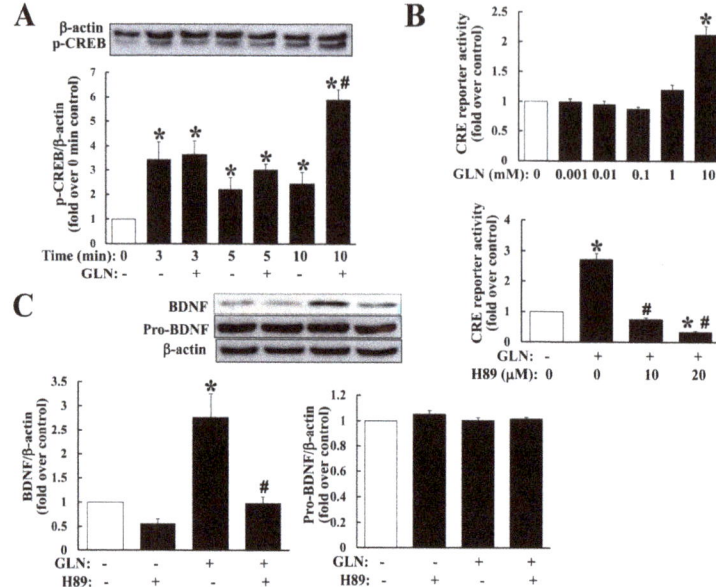

Figure 4. GLN impact on the cAMP/PKA signaling in relation to BDNF production in HT22 cells. HT22 cells were exposed to GLN (10 mM) for indicated times and the CREB phosphorylation manner was analyzed with Western blotting normalized by the β-actin (**A**). To examine the GLN effect on the CRE reporter activity, HT22 cells were cotransfected with a CRE reporter plasmid and a *p*-CMV-β-gal control plasmid, followed by the treatment with GLN (10 mM) alone or in combination with H89 (10 and 20 μM) for 24 h. The luciferase activity in cell lysates was analyzed and normalized against the β-gal activity within the same sample (**B**). To reveal the significance of the GLN-induced cAMP/PKA signaling in BDNF expression, HT22 cells were treated with GLN (10 mM) alone or in combination with H89 (20 μM) for 24 h and BDNF expression was determined (**C**). The results represent the means ± S.D. (*n* = 3–4). *, $p < 0.05$ compared with the 0 mM group (**A–C**); #, $p < 0.05$ compared with the control group within the same time point (**A**) or with the GLN alone group (**B,C**).

3. Discussion

Our current study clearly demonstrated that GLN mediates an enhancement on cognitive performance in mice and an upregulation of BDNF production and the cAMP/PKA/CREB signaling in the hippocampus and hippocampal cell line. The GLN-mediated cAMP/PKA signaling appeared to connect with the induction of BDNF production.

The significance of the superfamily of NTs, including BDNF, NGF, NT-3, NT-4 and CNTF in the proliferation or differentiation of neural cells has been well-recognized [19,20]. Our findings of the upregulation of all or some of these NTs in the hippocampus, striatum or cortex and particularly the BDNF protein induced by GLN in all three tissues (Figure 2D) have strongly suggested that GLN may improve cognitive function by modulating the local production of these NTs in the brain. In fact, whenever BDNF bounds to its cognate receptor TrkB, several genes involved in neuronal survival, differentiation and synaptic plasticity would be induced [21]. The GLN upregulation of TrkB receptor expression in the hippocampus (Supplementary Figure S2) further suggests the potential role of BDNF signaling in such GLN-mediated cognition enhancement.

In the neural system, the cAMP/PKA/CREB signaling is critical in neural functions and memory formation [22]. This is consistent with our findings of increased CREB5, CREB phosphorylation and cAMP accumulation by GLN in vivo and in vitro. Previous studies have noted the importance of BDNF/TrkB and CREB signaling in promoting cognition and memory formation [23–25].

The functioning of PDE4, which presumably reduces the cAMP levels, is significant for attenuating the PKA signaling, and thus the inhibitors for PDE4 have been a therapeutic option to treat different CNS diseases, including memory impairment [11]. Another finding of the GLN downregulation of PD4B mRNA in the hippocampus implies that GLN may act not only by inducing CREB5, but also by suppressing PDE4B expression in the hippocampus and consequently this would lead to the upregulation of cAMP levels and CREB phosphorylation in the hippocampus (Figure 3). This appears to make GLN a potential alternative option for treating cognitive or memory diseases by improving cognitive function.

Similar to our finding of the PKA-dependence for the GLN-mediated BDNF production (Figure 4C), the cAMP/CREB-dependent induction of BDNF in developing neurons was previously reported [26]. A recent study has demonstrated a transcriptional autoregulation of BDNF in the rat hippocampus during a BDNF-induced long-term potentiation, suggesting an important intra-hippocampal transcriptional autoregulation mechanism of BDNF via the CREB activation [27]. In this study, we noted GLN's consistent impact on upregulation of BDNF, CREB5, cAMP accumulation, CREB phosphorylation and also on the downregulation of PDE4B in the hippocampus (Figure 3), as well as the GLN-induced CRE reporter activation and CREB phosphorylation and finally a PKA-dependence of GLN-mediated BDNF production in HT22 cells (Figure 4). These highly suggest that GLN may activate the PKA pathway to first induce BDNF production, and the resultant BDNF may therefore initiate a potential autoregulation of its own expression in the hippocampus.

As a popular supplement with the capability to pass the BBB after consumption or injection, GLN is presumably able to reach the hippocampus, striatum and cortex [16,17]. Meanwhile, several different transporters for glucose or GLN have been detected in the brain [28] and the glucose transporter 2 (GLUT2) indeed performs the highest affinity for GLN and it has been detected in neurons [29,30]. For the brain, conditional GLUT2 knockout would result in a defect in neural functions and increased cell death [31]. These studies highly support the significance of GLN in brain functioning. In addition, previous studies have demonstrated that GLN administration in animals with large doses (5000–15,000 mg/kg) did not result in apparent toxicity and the median lethal dose LD50 in rats and mice was >8000 mg/kg. The subacute and chronic administration in rats, mice, rabbits and dogs receiving doses from 159 to 2700 mg/kg/day for 12–365 days did not cause significant adverse effects [32]. Thus, the daily administration of GLN of 3, 10 and 30 mg/mouse (120–1200 mg/kg) for 14 days in our current study could be regarded as relatively safe. From our current data, the question of whether a higher dose of GLN can mediate an even more potent enhancement on cognitive performance should warrant further investigation.

In addition to its role in energy metabolism, GLN and its derivatives have been demonstrated to involve themselves in a variety of cellular events in a glycolysis-independent manner [14]. For example, the involvement of GLN in the O-GlcNAcylation of a variety of proteins should lead to the modulation of a wide range of regulation in cell physiology, including cellular signal transduction, transcription, protein modification and more [14,15]. Given that the O-GlcNAcylation modification is highly prevalent in the mammalian brain and that O-GlcNAcylation has been suggested to regulate many cellular cascades in relation to neurological or neurodegenerative diseases [12,18], what molecules GLN would target in relation to O-GlcNAcylation to mediate the noted enhancement on cognitive performance certainly calls for further endeavors.

Collectively, this study provides clear evidence that GLN does appear to promote both cognitive function and increases in BDNF production in the hippocampus, striatum and cortex. Specifically, GLN treatment significantly facilitates the cAMP/PKA/CREB signaling by increasing CREB5 levels and by decreasing PDE4B levels in the hippocampus, and this possibly leads to the induction of BDNF production to enhance cognitive function.

4. Materials and Methods

4.1. Chemicals and Reagents

Fetal bovine serum (FBS) was purchased from HyClone (Waltham, MA, USA). Reverse transcriptase and SYBR green reagent were obtained from ThermoFisher (ThermoFisher Scientific, Waltham, MA, USA). Antibodies were purchased from different companies: rabbit monoclonal anti-BDNF (abcam, Cambridge, MA, USA), rabbit polyclonal anti-PDE4B (abcam), mouse monoclonal anti-CREB5 (ThermoFisher Scientific), rabbit monoclonal anti-phospho-CREB antibody (Cell signaling, Danvers, MA, USA) and mouse monoclonal anti-β-actin antibody (Novus, Centennial, CO, USA). Unless otherwise specified, all the other chemicals and reagents used in this study were from Sigma Chemicals (St. Louis, MO, USA).

4.2. Animal Ethics and Experiments

Seven-week-old male C57BL/6 mice were obtained from the National Laboratory Animal Center in Taipei, Taiwan. All the animal procedures were approved by the Institutional Animal Care and Use Committee of the National Yang-Ming University (Permit Number 1080203). After daily intraperitoneal (IP) injection of GLN (0, 3, 10 and 30 mg/mouse) for 7 or 14 days, the mice were subjected to the novel object recognition test (NORT). In brief, each individual animal was habituated to an acrylic chamber (40 cm × 30 cm × 20 cm) on three consecutive days, including habituation (20 min), acquisition trial (20 min), and test trial (15 min). During the training, two randomly selected objects were presented to each animal for 20 min. One day after training, another set of objects (one previously presented familiar object (F) and a new novel object (N)) was presented to the trained animals [33]. The time spent exploring each object (F or N) of each animal was recorded with a video device, followed by software analysis (SMART video tracking software 3.0, Panlab (Holliston, MA, USA)).

4.3. Cell Culture

The mouse hippocampal cell line HT22 was a generous gift from Dr. David Schubert (Salk Institute, La Jolla, CA, USA) [34]. HT22 cells were maintained in DMEM-high glucose medium with 10% fetal bovine serum, 100 units/mL penicillin and 100 μg/mL streptomycin. HT22 cells were seeded the previous night into 6-well plate to reach 70–80% confluence in the following day, and then the cells were treated with serum-free medium containing different compounds for 6 h to determine mRNA concentrations or for 24 h to measure protein levels in cell lysates.

4.4. Determination of Cellular Protein Expression

To extract proteins from treated cells, 200 μL of lysis buffer (50 mM Tris, 5 mM EDTA, 300 mM NaCl, 1% Triton X-100, 5 mM PMSF, 10 μg/mL aprotinin and 10 μg/mL leupeptin-hemisulfate) were used to harvest cells. Cell lysates were scratched down and collected into 1.5 mL eppendorf tubes. Similarly, to collect tissue proteins, 200 μL of lysis buffer was mixed with a tissue of an appropriate size. Then the harvested cells or tissues in lysis buffer were sonicated 2 s for 3 times, followed by centrifugation at 13,500 rpm for 30 min to collect the proteins in the supernatants. Protein concentrations were determined using the Bio-Rad protein assay reagent (Bio-Rad, Hercules, CA, USA). The total protein concentrations were adjusted with 5 × SDS sample loading buffer (312 mM Tris-HCl, 10% SDS, 25% β-mercaptoethanol, 50% glycerol and 0.05% bromophenol blue) and heated to 100 °C for 10 min before regular Western blotting assay. Fifty micrograms of each protein sample was separated on 10% SDS-PAGE, transferred onto a PVDF membrane, blocked with 5% milk at room temperature for 1 h and incubated at 4 °C overnight with various specific antibodies (rabbit monoclonal anti-BDNF (1:1000); rabbit polyclonal anti-PDE4B (1:1000); mouse monoclonal anti-CREB5 (1:1000); rabbit monoclonal anti-phospho-CREB antibody (1:1000); mouse monoclonal anti-β-actin antibody (1:2000) and mouse monoclonal anti-α-tubulin antibody (1:5000), followed by incubation for 2 h with the corresponding horseradish peroxidase-coupled secondary antibodies (1:5000)). After incubation with secondary antibodies, membranes were washed 3 times and the ECL solution (Millipore, Burlington, MA, USA) was added and incubated for 1 min at room temperature. The chemiluminescence signal on the blot was monitored by the GE Amersham Imager 600 (Chicago, IL, USA) and the protein signals were quantified by Multi Gauge 3.0 software (FUJIFILM, Tokyo, Japan).

4.5. Measurement of cAMP by Enzyme-Linked Immunosorbent Assay (ELISA)

The concentration of the cAMP in the hippocampal tissue was determined using a cAMP-Glo™ assay kit from Promega (Madison, WI, USA). The assay was performed according to the manufacturer's instructions.

4.6. Measurement of mRNA Concentration by Quantitative Real-Time Polymerase Chain Reaction (RT-PCR)

Total cellular RNAs were extracted from the harvested tissues and treated cells using Tri-reagent according to the manufacturer's instructions (Sigma). The purified RNA samples were dissolved in RNase-free water and each sample underwent quantitative RT-PCR to measure the levels of mRNAs of various genes. The mouse primer sequences used and the resultant product sizes were: BDNF (75 bp): Forward (F): 5′-TAA ATG AAG TTT ATA CAG TAC AGT GGT TCT ACA-3′, Reverse (R): 5′-AGT TGT GCG CAA ATG ACT GTT T-3′; NGF (nerve growth factor) (212 bp): F: 5′-CAC AGC CAC AGA CAT CAG GGC-3′, R: 5′-CCT GCT TCT CAT CTG TTG TC-3′; NT-3 (79 bp): F: 5′-GGT AGC CAA TAG AAC CTC ACC AC-3′, R: 5′-GTC ACA CAC TGA GTA CTC TCC TC-3′; NT-4 (235 bp); F: 5′-CCC TGC GTC AGT ACT TCT TCG AGA C-3′, R: 5′-CTG GAC GTC AGG CAC GGC CTG TTC-3′; CNTF (ciliary neurotrophic factor) (124 bp): F: 5′-ACA GTG GAC TGT GAG GTC TAT CC-3′, R: 5′-GGA GAC AGA GGC AAG AGT TAA GAG-3′; CREB5 (106 bp): F: 5′-TGT GCC TCC TTG AAA CAA GCC ATT-3′, R: 5′-ACC AGC ATA TGC CCA GAC TG-3′; PDE4B (188 bp): F: 5′-CTG CAG CCT AAC TAC CTG TC-3′, R: 5′-ACA CTT GGT TCC CTG ATC TG-3′ and GAPDH (222 bp): F: 5′-AAG GTC ATC CCA GAG CTG AA-3′, R: 5′-CTG CTT CAC CAC CTT CTT GA-3′. In brief, the reverse transcription was carried out by using 1 μg of total RNAs in RNase-free H_2O (8.5 μL) and 1 μL oligo dT (0.5 μg/μL) and heated at 70 °C for 5 min. Then the denatured RNAs were mixed with 5 μL 5× reaction buffer, 2 μL dNTP (10 mM stock), 2.5 μL dithiothreitol (100 mM stock), 0.5 μL Moloney murine leukemia virus reverse transcriptase (200 U/μL) and 0.5 μL RNase inhibitor to a total 25 μL in volume, and then incubated at 42 °C for 60 min, followed by 70 °C for 10 min (MyCyler™ thermal cycler system, Bio-Rad, Hercules, CA, USA). To perform real-time PCR, 2 μL of cDNAs, 0.16 μL of forward and reverse primers (100 μM stock), 8 μL of SYBR Green and appropriate amounts of H_2O to bring up the total volume to 20 μL were used and transferred into the 8-strip PCR tube. The real-time PCR System (ABI StepOne Plus, ABI QuanStudio 3, Waltham, MA, USA) was used for the PCR reaction. The temperature was set at 95 °C for 2 min for denaturation, followed by the PCR cycle: 2 min at 95 °C for denaturing, 10 s at 60 °C for annealing and 20 s at 72 °C for elongating. The PCR cycle would repeat 40 times to monitor the fluoresce signal of SYBR Green. The threshold cycle (Ct) values for the target genes were normalized with the Ct value of the housekeeping gene GAPDH. Normalization was performed based on the following formula:

$$\text{relative mRNA expression} = 2^{-\Delta Ct} \ (\Delta Ct = Ct^{\text{target gene}} - Ct^{\text{GAPDH}}) \tag{1}$$

4.7. Monitoring the CRE Reporter Activity

To analyze regulation of the CRE-mediated transcription, a minimal promoter sequence bearing a CRE-driven luciferase reporter gene (Addgene, Watertown, MA, USA) was transfected into HT22 cells seeded in 24-well plate and a pCMV-β-Gal plasmid was co-transfected as a control. In brief, a mixture including 1 μg CRE reporter plasmid, 0.1 μg of the pCMV-β-Gal plasmid and 1 μL P3000™ enhancer reagent (Invitrogen, Waltham, MA, USA) in 25 μL serum-free medium were prepared for each well. Meanwhile, 1 μL of Lipofectamine™ 3000 transfection reagent (Invitrogen) was dissolved in 25 μL serum-free medium for each well. Two parts were then mixed and incubated at room temperature for 30 min. Consequently, 50 μL of the resultant mixture and 200 μL of serum-free medium were added to each well. Cells were then incubated at 37 °C for 4 h, followed by various treatments for an additional 24 h. After the cultured medium was removed, 150 µL of Glo lysis buffer (Promega) was added to collect total cell lysates. After the centrifugation at 13,500 rpm for 10 min, 50 µL of the harvested supernatant was mixed with 50 µL of luciferase substrate (Britelite™, PerkinElmer Inc., Waltham, MA, USA) and the luminescence signal was measured by FB12-single tube luminometer (Berthold Detectin Systems, Level Biotechnology Inc., Taipei, Taiwan). To measure β-galactosidase activity, 50 µL supernatant was mixed with 50 µL substrate ONPG (*O*-nitrophenyl-β-*D*-galactopyranoside) in a 96-well plate and incubated at room temperature for 30 min. The readout by measuring the absorbance at 482 nm wavelength was used to provide the transfection efficiency. The luciferase activity determined was then normalized against the β-galactosidase activity within the same sample. There were triplicate wells of each treatment group of each independent experiment and 4 independent experiments were performed.

4.8. Statistical Analysis

Experimental data are expressed as the mean plus/minus the standard deviation (mean ± S.D.) for the indicated number of repeated observations. The results were analyzed using the Student's *t*-test for two-group comparisons or a one-way analysis of variance followed by the Dunnett's test, where appropriate, for multiple-group comparisons. In all cases, $p < 0.05$ was regarded as statistically significant.

Supplementary Materials: The following are available online: Quantitative RT-PCR for TrkB gene in the hippocampus. The purified hippocampal RNA samples from GLN-injected mice underwent quantitative RT-PCR to measure the mRNA levels of TrkB. The mouse primer sequences used and the resultant product sizes were Forward: 5'-CAA GAA CGA GTA TGG GAA GGA TGA G-3' and Reverse: 5'-TTG GCG TGG TCC AGT CTT CAT A-3' to give a 107 bp product. Figure S1: No effect of GLN treatment on body weight (BW) of mice. Seven-week-old C57BL/6 male mice were injected with different doses of GLN (0, 3, 10 and 30 mg) for 14 days. The changes in BW were recorded and compared among different GLN treatment groups. The results represent the means ± S.D. ($n = 8$), Figure S2: GLN induction of TrkB mRNA expression in hippocampus. The RNA samples prepared from GLN-injected animal's hippocampus were subjected to RT-PCR to determine the TrkB mRNA levels using GAPDH as an internal control. The results represent the means ± S.D. ($n = 8$), *, $p < 0.05$ compared with the 0 mg group. Figure S3: No effect of GLN on cell viability of HT22 cells. Plated HT22 cells were treated with GLN (0, 0.001, 0.01, 0.1, 1 and 10 mM) for 24 h and then the 3-(4,5-cimethylthiazol-2-yl)-2,5-diphenyl tetrazolium bromide (MTT) or alamarBlue reagent was included for an additional 4 h. Consequently the readouts were obtained by measuring the OD with a test wavelength at 560 nm and a reference wavelength at 630 nm for MTT, and by monitoring an excitation wavelength at 550 nm and an emission at 590 nm for alamarBlue, respectively. The results represent the means ± S.D. ($n = 4$).

Author Contributions: The study was conceived and designed by L.-Y.C., H.-C.L. and Y.-L.W. Experiments were performed by L.-Y.C. and Y.-M.C. Data analysis and interpretation were performed by L.-Y.C., Y.-M.C., Y.-C.P., H.-C.L. and Y.-L.W. All authors were involved in writing the paper. All authors have read and agreed to the published version of the manuscript.

Funding: This work was supported by grants from the Taiwan Ministry of Science and Technology (MOST 105-2320-B-010-026-MY3; MOST 108-2320-B-010-025) to Y.-L.W., and from the Taiwan Ministry of Education, Aim for the Top University Plan.

Conflicts of Interest: The authors declare no conflict of interest.

References

1. Yavas, E.; Gonzalez, S.; Fanselow, M.S. Interactions between the hippocampus, prefrontal cortex, and amygdala support complex learning and memory. *F1000Research* **2019**, *8*, 1292. [CrossRef]
2. Eriksson, J.; Vogel, E.K.; Lansner, A.; Bergström, F.; Nyberg, L. Neurocognitive Architecture of Working Memory. *Neuron* **2015**, *88*, 33–46. [CrossRef]
3. Zeithamova, D.; Mack, M.L.; Braunlich, K.; Davis, T.; Seger, C.A.; Van Kesteren, M.T.R.; Wutz, A. Brain Mechanisms of Concept Learning. *J. Neurosci.* **2019**, *39*, 8259–8266. [CrossRef]
4. Miranda, M.; Morici, J.F.; Zanoni, M.B.; Bekinschtein, P. Brain-Derived Neurotrophic Factor: A Key Molecule for Memory in the Healthy and the Pathological Brain. *Front. Cell. Neurosci.* **2019**, *13*, 363. [CrossRef] [PubMed]

5. Sairanen, M.; Lucas, G.; Ernfors, P.; Castrén, M.L.; Castren, E. Brain-Derived Neurotrophic Factor and Antidepressant Drugs Have Different But Coordinated Effects on Neuronal Turnover, Proliferation, and Survival in the Adult Dentate Gyrus. *J. Neurosci.* **2005**, *25*, 1089–1094. [CrossRef] [PubMed]
6. Zuccato, C.; Cattaneo, E. Brain-derived neurotrophic factor in neurodegenerative diseases. *Nat. Rev. Neurol.* **2009**, *5*, 311–322. [CrossRef] [PubMed]
7. Hardingham, G.E.; Fukunaga, Y.; Bading, H. Extrasynaptic NMDARs oppose synaptic NMDARs by triggering CREB shut-off and cell death pathways. *Nat. Neurosci.* **2002**, *5*, 405–414. [CrossRef]
8. Yi, B.; Wu, C.; Shi, R.; Han, K.; Sheng, H.; Li, B.; Mei, L.; Wang, X.; Huang, Z.; Wu, H. Long-term Administration of Salicylate-induced Changes in BDNF Expression and CREB Phosphorylation in the Auditory Cortex of Rats. *Otol. Neurotol.* **2018**, *39*, e173–e180. [CrossRef]
9. Olsen, C.M.; Liu, Q.-S. Phosphodiesterase 4 inhibitors and drugs of abuse: Current knowledge and therapeutic opportunities. *Front. Biol.* **2016**, *11*, 376–386. [CrossRef]
10. Nabavi, S.F.; Talarek, S.; Listos, J.; Devi, K.P.; De Oliveira, M.R.; Tewari, D.; Arguelles, S.; Mehrzadi, S.; Hosseinzadeh, A.; D'Onofrio, G.; et al. Phosphodiesterase inhibitors say NO to Alzheimer's disease. *Food Chem. Toxicol.* **2019**, *134*, 110822. [CrossRef]
11. Blokland, A.; Heckman, P.; Vanmierlo, T.; Schreiber, R.; Paes, D.; Prickaerts, J. Phosphodiesterase Type 4 Inhibition in CNS Diseases. *Trends Pharmacol. Sci.* **2019**, *40*, 971–985. [CrossRef] [PubMed]
12. Akan, I.; Stichelen, S.O.-V.; Bond, M.R.; Hanover, J.A. Nutrient-driven O-GlcNAc in proteostasis and neurodegeneration. *J. Neurochem.* **2017**, *144*, 7–34. [CrossRef]
13. Mccarty, M. The neglect of glucosamine as a treatment for osteoarthritis—A personal perspective. *Med. Hypotheses* **1994**, *42*, 323–327. [CrossRef]
14. Ryan, P.; Xu, M.; Davey, A.K.; Danon, J.J.; Mellick, G.D.; Kassiou, M.; Rudrawar, S. O-GlcNAc Modification Protects against Protein Misfolding and Aggregation in Neurodegenerative Disease. *ACS Chem. Neurosci.* **2019**, *10*, 2209–2221. [CrossRef] [PubMed]
15. Hardivillé, S.; Hart, G.W. Nutrient regulation of signaling, transcription, and cell physiology by O-GlcNAcylation. *Cell Metab.* **2014**, *20*, 208–213. [CrossRef] [PubMed]
16. Popov, N. Effects of D-galactosamine and D-glucosamine on retention performance of a brightness discrimination task in rats. *Biomed. Biochim. Acta* **1985**, *44*, 611–622. [PubMed]
17. Setnikar, I.; Rovati, L. Absorption, Distribution, Metabolism and Excretion of Glucosamine Sulfate. *Arzneimittelforschung* **2011**, *51*, 699–725. [CrossRef]
18. Ma, X.; Li, H.; He, Y.; Hao, J. The emerging link between O-GlcNAcylation and neurological disorders. *Cell. Mol. Life Sci.* **2017**, *74*, 3667–3686. [CrossRef]
19. Rocco, M.L.; Soligo, M.; Manni, L.; Aloe, L. Nerve Growth Factor: Early Studies and Recent Clinical Trials. *Curr. Neuropharmacol.* **2018**, *16*, 1455–1465. [CrossRef]
20. Bothwell, M.A. Recent advances in understanding context-dependent mechanisms controlling neurotrophin signaling and function. *F1000Research* **2019**, *8*, 1658. [CrossRef]
21. Park, H.; Poo, M.-M. Neurotrophin regulation of neural circuit development and function. *Nat. Rev. Neurosci.* **2012**, *14*, 7–23. [CrossRef]
22. Kandel, E.R. The molecular biology of memory: cAMP, PKA, CRE, CREB-1, CREB-2, and CPEB. *Mol. Brain* **2012**, *5*, 14. [CrossRef] [PubMed]
23. Andero, R.; Choi, D.C.; Ressler, K.J. BDNF–TrkB Receptor Regulation of Distributed Adult Neural Plasticity, Memory Formation, and Psychiatric Disorders. *Prog. Mol. Biol. Transl. Sci.* **2014**, *122*, 169–192. [CrossRef] [PubMed]
24. Cocco, S.; Podda, M.V.; Grassi, C. Role of BDNF Signaling in Memory Enhancement Induced by Transcranial Direct Current Stimulation. *Front. Mol. Neurosci.* **2018**, *12*, 427. [CrossRef]
25. Kawahata, I.; Yoshida, M.; Sun, W.; Nakajima, A.; Lai, Y.; Osaka, N.; Matsuzaki, K.; Yokosuka, A.; Mimaki, Y.; Naganuma, A.; et al. Potent activity of nobiletin-rich Citrus reticulata peel extract to facilitate cAMP/PKA/ERK/CREB signaling associated with learning and memory in cultured hippocampal neurons: identification of the substances responsible for the pharmacological action. *J. Neural Transm.* **2013**, *120*, 1397–1409. [CrossRef]
26. Obrietan, K.; Gao, X.-B.; Pol, A.N.V.D. Excitatory actions of GABA increase BDNF expression via a MAPK-CREB-dependent mechanism–a positive feedback circuit in developing neurons. *J. Neurophysiol.* **2002**, *88*, 1005–1015. [CrossRef]

27. Esvald, E.-E.; Tuvikene, J.; Sirp, A.; Patil, S.; Bramham, C.R.; Timmusk, T. CREB Family Transcription Factors Are Major Mediators of BDNF Transcriptional Autoregulation in Cortical Neurons. *J. Neurosci.* **2020**, *40*, 1405–1426. [CrossRef] [PubMed]
28. Jurcovicova, J. Glucose transport in brain—Effect of inflammation. *Endocr. Regul.* **2014**, *48*, 35–48. [CrossRef] [PubMed]
29. Mardones, L.; Ormazabal, V.; Romo, X.; Jaña, C.; Binder, P.; Peña, E.; Vergara, M.; Zúñiga, F.A. The glucose transporter-2 (GLUT2) is a low affinity dehydroascorbic acid transporter. *Biochem. Biophys. Res. Commun.* **2011**, *410*, 7–12. [CrossRef]
30. Uldry, M.; Ibberson, M.; Hosokawa, M.; Thorens, B. GLUT2 is a high affinity glucosamine transporter. *FEBS Lett.* **2002**, *524*, 199–203. [CrossRef]
31. Marín-Juez, R.; Rovira, M.; Crespo, D.; Van Der Vaart, M.; Spaink, H.P.; Planas, J.V. GLUT2-Mediated Glucose Uptake and Availability Are Required for Embryonic Brain Development in Zebrafish. *Br. J. Pharmacol.* **2014**, *35*, 74–85. [CrossRef]
32. Anderson, J.; Nicolosi, R.; Borzelleca, J. Glucosamine effects in humans: A review of effects on glucose metabolism, side effects, safety considerations and efficacy. *Food Chem. Toxicol.* **2005**, *43*, 187–201. [CrossRef] [PubMed]
33. Seo, H.-S.; Yang, M.; Song, M.-S.; Kim, J.-S.; Kim, S.-H.; Kim, J.-C.; Kim, H.; Shin, T.; Wang, H.; Moon, C. Toluene inhibits hippocampal neurogenesis in adult mice. *Pharmacol. Biochem. Behav.* **2010**, *94*, 588–594. [CrossRef] [PubMed]
34. Li, Y.; Maher, P.; Schubert, D. Phosphatidylcholine-specific phospholipase C regulates glutamate-induced nerve cell death. *Proc. Natl. Acad. Sci. USA* **1998**, *95*, 7748–7753. [CrossRef] [PubMed]

Sample Availability: Samples and the compounds are not available from the authors.

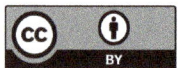

© 2020 by the authors. Licensee MDPI, Basel, Switzerland. This article is an open access article distributed under the terms and conditions of the Creative Commons Attribution (CC BY) license (http://creativecommons.org/licenses/by/4.0/).

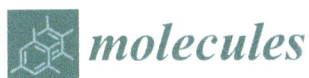

Article

In Vitro Hormetic Effect Investigation of Thymol on Human Fibroblast and Gastric Adenocarcinoma Cells

Ayse Günes-Bayir [1],*, Abdurrahim Kocyigit [2], Eray Metin Guler [2] and Agnes Dadak [3]

1. Department of Nutrition and Dietetics, Faculty of Health Sciences, Bezmialem Vakif University, Silahtaraga Cad., Eyüpsultan 34065, Istanbul, Turkey
2. Department of Medical Biochemistry, Faculty of Medicine, Bezmialem Vakif University, Vatan Cad., Fatih 34093, Istanbul, Turkey; akocyigit@bezmialem.edu.tr (A.K.); emguler@bezmialem.edu.tr (E.M.G.)
3. Institute of Pharmacology, Department for Biomedical Sciences, University of Veterinary Medicine Vienna, Veterinärplatz 1, A-1210 Vienna, Austria; Agnes.Dadak@vetmeduni.ac.at
* Correspondence: agunes@bezmialem.edu.tr; Tel.: +90-212-453-17-00-4596; Fax: +90-212-453-18-83

Received: 25 June 2020; Accepted: 16 July 2020; Published: 17 July 2020

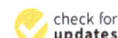

Abstract: The concept of hormesis includes a biphasic cellular dose-response to a xenobiotic stimulus defined by low dose beneficial and high dose inhibitory or toxic effects. In the present study, an attempt has been made to help elucidate the beneficial and detrimental effects of thymol on different cell types by evaluating and comparing the impact of various thymol doses on cancerous (AGS) and healthy (WS-1) cells. Cytotoxic, genotoxic, and apoptotic effects, as well as levels of reactive oxygen species and glutathione were studied in both cell lines exposed to thymol (0–600 µM) for 24 h. The results showed significant differences in cell viability of AGS compared to WS-1 cells exposed to thymol. The differences observed were statistically significant at all doses applied ($P \leq 0.001$) and revealed hormetic thymol effects on WS-1 cells, whereas toxic effects on AGS cells were detectable at all thymol concentrations. Thymol at low concentrations provides antioxidative protection to WS-1 cells in vitro while already inducing toxic effects in AGS cells. In that sense, the findings of the present study suggest that thymol exerts a dose-dependent hormetic impact on different cell types, thereby providing crucial information for future in vivo studies investigating the therapeutic potential of thymol.

Keywords: thymol; hormetic effect; cancerous cells; healthy cells

1. Introduction

The term of hormesis has been widely utilized in the field of biomedical, nutrition and toxicological sciences [1]. The hormetic effect of a substance is described as a biphasic dose-response to an environmental or chemical agent with a low dose stimulation or favorable effect and a high dose inhibitory or toxic effect on the cells or organisms. In a review article, it was reported that a great number of anticancer agents proliferate human cancer cells at low doses based on the hormetic dose-response relationship [2]. In general, natural phenolic compounds have been gaining increasing attention in cancer chemoprevention and anticancer treatment [3]. It has been shown that polyphenols inhibit cell proliferation and induce apoptosis in vitro and in vivo [3,4]. There are two main pathways; the intrinsic and extrinsic pathways that have been linked to phyto-compound induced apoptosis. The intrinsic pathway is mainly activated by the release of the Bcl-2 family proteins from the mitochondria and the extrinsic pathway by the activation of transmembrane death receptors and ligands [5]. Studies provided evidence for the redox status of glutathione (GSH) playing a critical role in cell apoptosis in various cell types [6–8]. It has been revealed that most anticancer or cancer-chemopreventive agents have the potential to induce apoptosis. Although these apoptotic effects are significant for cancer chemoprevention, the cytotoxic and genotoxic activity of such agents in healthy cells are unwanted. Therefore, an ideal anticancer agent should increase apoptosis and inhibit the proliferation of cancer cells while minimally affecting healthy cells.

Thymol, as a phenolic compound is known to possess therapeutic qualities such as antioxidative, antimicrobial, antiinflammatory, and anticancer activities [9]. Therefore, thymol has gained more and more scientific attention in recent years. The cytotoxic, genotoxic, and antioxidative potentials of thymol have been investigated in vitro on various healthy cells: human lymphocytes, V79 Chinese hamster lung fibroblasts, mouse cortical neurons and peripheral-blood mononuclear cells [10–13]. Additionally, the anticancer effect of thymol has been studied in in vitro systems. Various cell lines such as human glioblastoma, promyelocytic cancer, gastric adenocarcinoma, colon carcinoma, hepatoma and lung carcinoma cells [11,14–20] were used, but the clinical significance of the thymol-induced effects remains unknown. To the authors knowledge, only a couple in vivo studies are published, one reporting that 100 mg of thymol per kg of body weight induced genotoxic effects on bone marrow cells in rats [21]. Another study focused on in vivo passage kinetics and has evidenced thymol metabolization in the stomach or intestine after an oral application [22]. Our research recently revealed that human gastric adenocarcinoma (AGS) cells are highly sensitive to thymol in a concentration-dependent manner [14,15]. Given those studies, it is of great interest to elucidate in depth whether thymol may have therapeutic potential against e.g., gastric cancer. On the other hand, the hormetic effect of isothiocyanates depends on the investigated cell types which are healthy or cancer cells [23]. Therefore, we focused first on an in vitro comparison of the proposed thymol activity on human gastric adenocarcinoma (AGS) cells with findings gained from thymol-treated healthy human fibroblasts (WS-1) at different concentrations. The study was designed to gain a more in-depth insight into the thymol-sensitivity of various cell lines in order to disclose potential limitations of this phenolic compound as a natural anticancer drug aspirant.

2. Results

2.1. Cell Viability

The inhibitory effect of thymol on cell viability was assessed in both cell cultures using the ATP cell viability assay. Thymol showed cytotoxic effects by reducing cell viability on AGS and WS-1 cells in a dose-dependent manner (Figure 1). Statistically significant differences were found among thymol (50–600 µM) exposed healthy and cancerous cells ($P \leq 0.001$). However, thymol at the lowest concentration used (10 µM) did not significantly increase the number of healthy cells when it was compared to untreated control cells. In addition, IC_{50} values of thymol were 75.63 ± 4.01 µM and 167 ± 11 µM in cancerous and healthy cells, respectively.

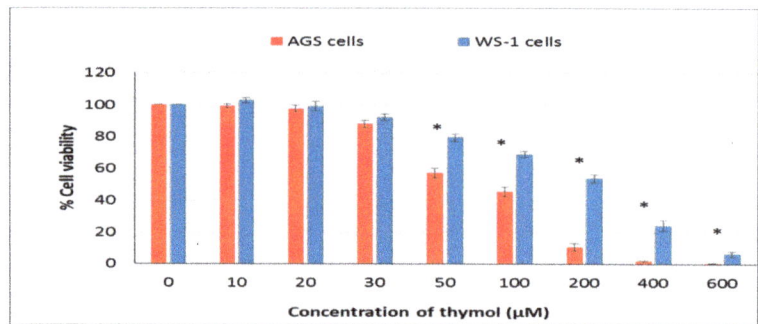

Figure 1. Cytotoxicity effect of thymol (0–600 µM) after 24 h incubation was studied in healthy and cancerous cells. All values are expressed as the mean ± SD. * Differences were considered significant compared to the control group from $P \leq 0.001$. SD: Standard deviation.

2.2. Reactive Oxygen Species (ROS)

The pro-oxidative effect of thymol was studied using the oxidation-sensitive fluorescent dye DCFH-DA. A dose-dependent intracellular reactive oxygen species (ROS) generating effect of thymol was detected in cells. Differences were statistically significant among thymol (20–100 μM) exposed healthy and cancerous cells ($P \leq 0.001$) (Figure 2). An increased thymol concentration and relative ROS levels in AGS cells were positively correlated. However, no statistically significant differences were observed in WS-1 cells treated with thymol (10–100 μM) as compared to ROS levels of control cells.

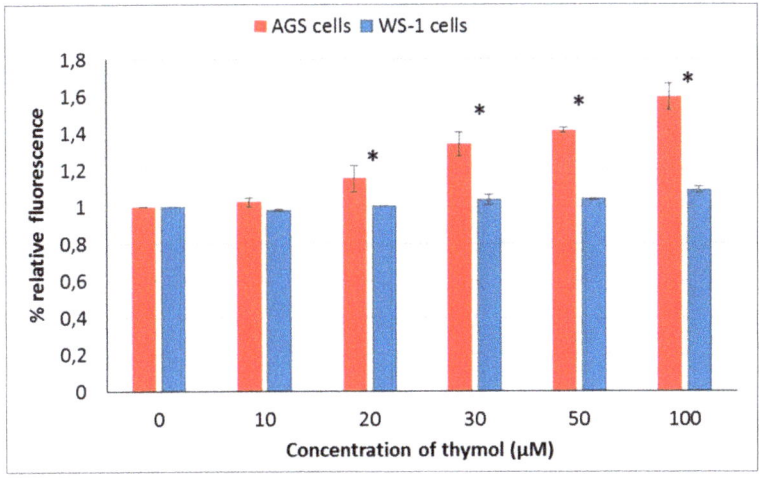

Figure 2. Reactive oxygen species (ROS) levels in healthy and cancerous cells exposed to thymol (0–100 μM) were investigated by DCFH-DA assay after 24 h incubation. All values are expressed as the mean ± SD. * Differences were considered significant compared to the control group from $P \leq 0.001$. SD: Standard deviation.

2.3. Glutathione (GSH) Level

In order to assess the antioxidative effect of thymol, GSH levels were measured using GSH/GSSG-Glo assay. Thymol (20–100 μM) induced a dose-dependent reduction in GSH levels in healthy and cancerous cell lines. An increased concentration of thymol in the range of 20–100 μM and the relative GSH level in both cell types were negatively correlated. At 20 μM, GSH levels of AGS cells were significantly higher than in WS-1 cells ($P \leq 0.001$) (Figure 3). On the other hand, GSH levels in both cell lines at 20–100 μM of thymol were significantly reduced in comparison with their controls ($P \leq 0.001$). At the lowest concentration used (10 μM), healthy cells indicated the same GSH level as unexposed control cells, whereas GSH levels started to decrease in AGS cells exposed to the same concentration.

2.4. Effect of Thymol on Apoptosis Induction

To assess the cytotoxic effect of thymol, whether caused by apoptosis or not, the AO/EB staining was applied to visualize nuclear changes and apoptosis-characteristic body formation. After staining, the cells were observed under a fluorescence microscope and counted to quantify apoptosis. Cell morphology was determined after exposing to thymol (0–100 μM) for 24 h. In both cell lines, the cell viability was decreased significantly at 10–50 μM ($P \leq 0.001$). The number of apoptotic cells at 10–20 μM and 50–100 μM increased significantly in a dose-dependent manner ($P \leq 0.001$) (Figure 4a). A significant difference was also detected for necrotic cells at the highest dose (100 μM) ($P \leq 0.001$) (Figure 4b).

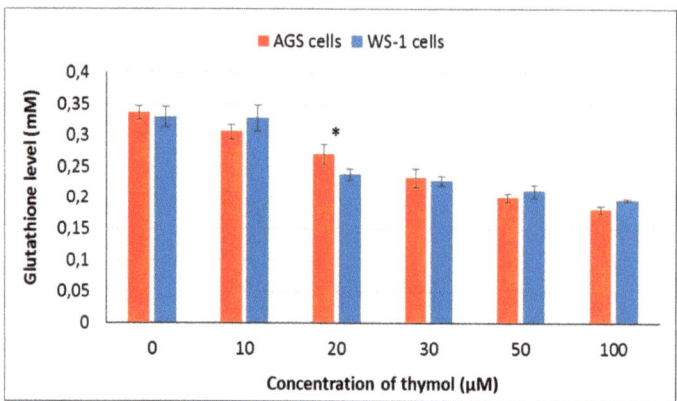

Figure 3. GSH levels in healthy and cancerous cells were shown after 24 h of exposure to thymol (0–100 µM). All values are expressed as the mean ± SD. * Differences were considered significant compared to the control group from $P \leq 0.001$. SD: Standard deviation.

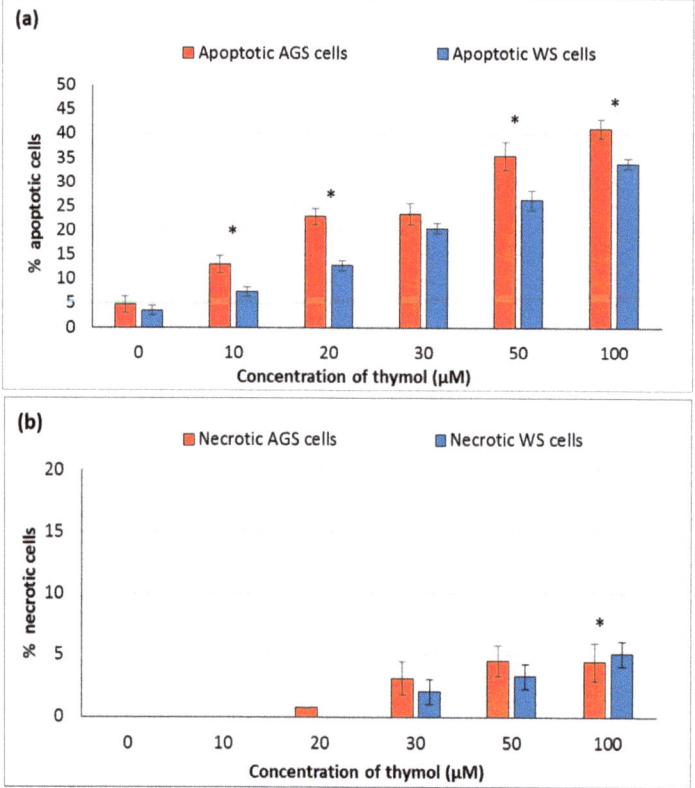

Figure 4. Morphological changes in healthy and cancerous cells were demonstrated, which were exposed to thymol (0–100 µM) after 24h incubation. (**a**) Apoptotic and (**b**) necrotic effects of thymol on both cell cultures are given in comparison with control cells as percentages. All values are expressed as the mean ± SD. * Differences were considered significant compared to the control group from $P \leq 0.001$. SD: Standard deviation.

An expressional analysis of apoptosis proteins was examined in healthy and cancerous cells by Western blot analysis in order to evaluate whether thymol induces apoptosis via caspase activation. Changes were observed in both cell lines when cells were treated with different doses of thymol. Protein expressions for both cell lines are demonstrated in Figure 5a–d. β-actin was used as a control, and was positive in all samples. The results revealed that the expression levels of *Bax*, *Caspase-9*, and *Caspase-3* proteins were significantly increased in both cell lines exposed to 50 μM thymol whereas *Bcl-2* protein was decreased in a dose-dependent manner (Figure 5a–d; $P \leq 0.001$). It was also suggested that thymol induces apoptosis via decreasing the *Bcl-2/Bax* ratio and overexpression of *Caspase-9* and *Caspase-3* proteins. However, *Bcl-2* levels in healthy cells exposed to thymol (30 and 50 μM) were higher than in cancerous cells ($P \leq 0.001$).

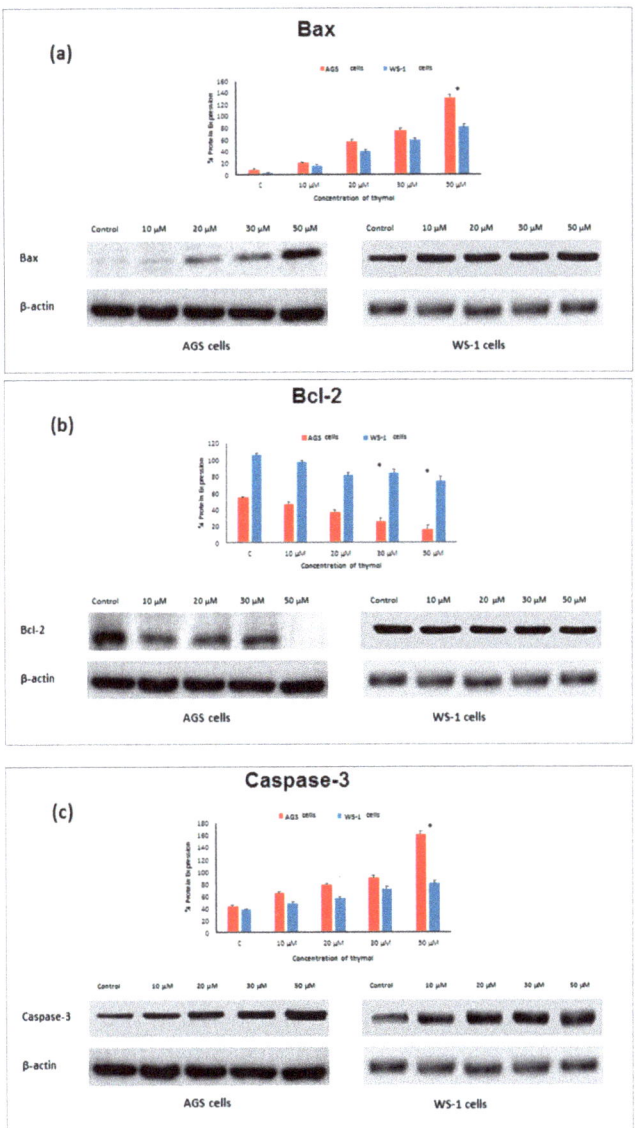

Figure 5. *Cont.*

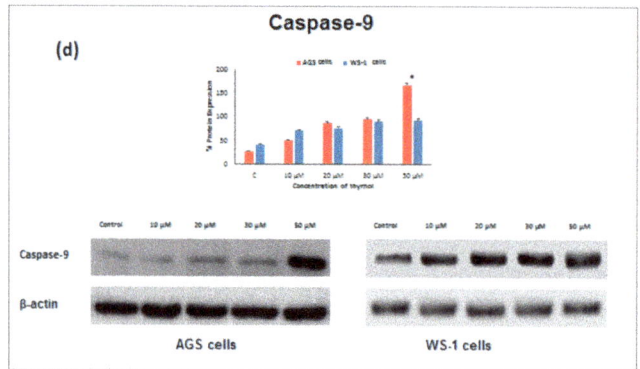

Figure 5. Thymol induced apoptosis was detected by Western blotting. Healthy and cancerous cells were treated with 0–50 µM of thymol. Expressions of *Bax* (**a**), *Bcl-2* (**b**), *Caspase-3* (**c**), and *Caspase-9* (**d**) proteins are presented as percentages as well as on gel. All values are expressed as the mean ± SD. * Differences were considered significant compared to the control group from $P \leq 0.001$. SD: Standard deviation. C: Control.

2.5. DNA Damage

The comet assay was used for the determination of thymol induced DNA damage in this study. Genotoxic effects of thymol on both cell lines were visualized as comet formation. The percentages of DNA in the tail are shown for both cell lines (Figure 6). A positive correlation was detected among the DNA damage and an increased dose of thymol in both cell lines. Differences in the amount of tail DNA were detected statistically significant among healthy and cancerous cells ($P \leq 0.001$).

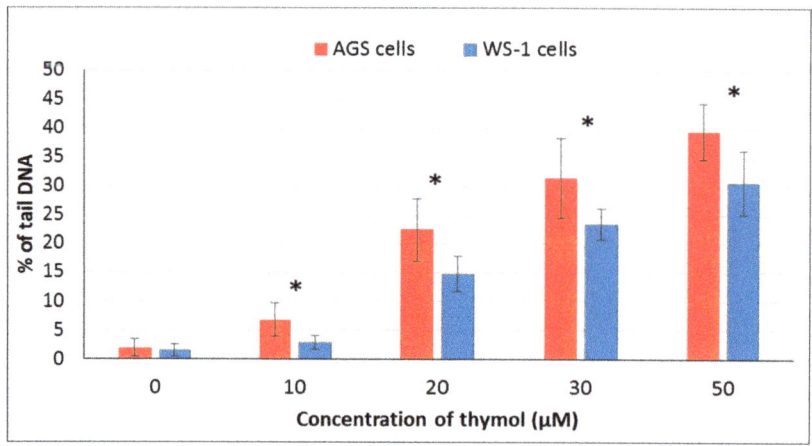

Figure 6. The genotoxic effect of thymol on healthy and cancerous cells was detected by comet assay. Cells exposed to thymol (0–50 µM) were analyzed after 24 h of incubation. All values are expressed as the mean ± SD. * Differences were considered significant compared to the control group from $P \leq 0.001$. SD: Standard deviation.

3. Discussion

Phytochemicals are gaining increasing attention as tentative chemopreventive or anticancer agents. Various natural compounds have been investigated for the use in various types of cancers using in vitro and in vivo models [3]. It seems that polyphenols may have the potential to express anticancer activity by inhibiting the multiplication of cancerous cells and stimulating apoptosis. However, the clinical efficacy and safety of these phytocompounds needs to be carefully evaluated in terms of avoiding toxicological side effects on healthy cells [24]. The hormetic effect of an agent, defined as a biphasic dose-response to an agent characterized by a beneficial effect at low doses and a toxic/inhibitory activity at high doses, depends on the selected endpoint and/or the healthy or cancer cells studied [3]. The present study revealed that thymol exhibits a hormetic dose-response in the sense of antioxidant and pro-oxidant activity on cell viability and DNA genotoxicity. The observed low dose benefit of thymol might be beneficial for cancer chemoprevention whilst the data on its high dose effects provide valuable information for future in vivo studies investigating the therapeutic anticancer potential of this phytocompound. Thymol is one of the major compounds found in members of the *Lamiaceae* family [9] and some other plants. This natural monoterpene phenol has important biological activities; however, its effect on cancer has not yet been fully elucidated [15]. In the present study, the cytotoxic, apoptotic, genotoxic, pro-oxidative and antioxidative effects of thymol were investigated in healthy and cancerous cell lines, and the results from both cell lines were compared. As evident from the present results, thymol induces intracellular ROS generation with the concomitant onset of cytotoxicity, apoptosis, and genotoxicity. The effects on human gastric adenocarcinoma cells were more pronounced than on healthy human fibroblast cells. These findings are in accordance with a report on peripheral blood mononuclear cells (PBMC) and acute promyelocytic cancer cells [11].

In the present study, the hormetic effect of thymol was examined using ATP cell viability and AO/EB staining assays, respectively. Cancerous and healthy cells exposed to thymol for 24 h were evaluated for apoptotic, necrotic, and viable cells by apoptosis assay. The impaired cell functions induced by thymol were in a dose-dependent manner and more pronounced in cancerous cells than healthy cells. To our knowledge, only one study has compared the thymol effect on the cell viability and apoptosis in cancerous (acute promyelocytic cancer HL-60) and healthy (peripheral blood mononuclear) cells [11] so far, and found similar results. Thymol-induced suppression of cell proliferation was observed in a dose-dependent manner in various cancer cell types such as human gastric adenocarcinoma AGS, hepatocellular carcinoma HepG2, lung carcinoma H1299, or glioblastoma cells [15,16,19,20]. However, studies on human colon carcinoma Caco-2 cells and primary cultures of mouse cortical neuron cells exposed to thymol (0–250 μM and 1–1000 μM, respectively) showed no cytotoxicity; but ultrastructural changes and induction of apoptosis were evident in Caco-2 cells [12,18].

Phenolic compounds, such as thymol, are suggested to display either antioxidative or prooxidant activity depending on concentration, cell resistance, and exposing time [25]. In this regard, the cell altering mechanism of thymol has been linked to its capacity of disrupting cytoplasmic membranes, especially mitochondrial membranes, resulting in a prooxidant status and subsequent apoptosis induction [13,19,26]. Recent studies reported that thymol at lower doses protects human colon carcinoma, glioblastoma, acute promyelocytic leukemia and gastric adenocarcinoma cells against ROS, whereas higher doses induce oxidative stress by increasing ROS generation [11,15–17,26]. A study performed on fibroblast cells showed a slight reduction in ROS levels when using thymol at a concentration of 1–100 μM [13]. Although there is essential research data characterizing the apoptotic and antioxidative effects of thymol, limited information is available on its prooxidant activity. In this respect, it is valuable to monitor intracellular levels of reduced glutathione (GSH) which has been shown to be crucial for the regulation of cell proliferation, cell cycle progression, and apoptosis [27]. The main function of GSH is to reduce intracellularly numerous oxidizing compounds, including ROS. With respect to the potential therapeutic use of thymol as a (co)drug in cancer treatment, the effect of thymol on intracellular ROS and GSH levels was investigated at different doses in vitro in AGS versus WS-1 cells. A positive correlation was found among cell death and ROS production after 24 h of exposure to thymol at higher doses, whereas a negative correlation was observed between cell death and GSH levels. These findings are in agreement with earlier reports [11,13–15]. It is noteworthy to mention that in the present study, low doses of thymol induced the increased proliferation of healthy human fibroblasts as compared to unexposed control cells. This activity was accompanied by unaltered

ROS and decreased GSH levels in healthy cells, whereas none of these effects were seen in cancerous cells, which were harmed by thymol even at the lowest concentration. This result might be of special value when selecting doses for in vivo studies.

Apoptosis as the gene-directed and programmed cell death [5] is regulated by different proteins such as *Bax, Bcl-2, Caspase-3,* and *Caspase-9*. In the present study, the apoptotic effect of thymol (0–50 µM) was investigated at the protein expression level in cancerous and healthy cells. Protein levels of *Bcl-2* decreased in both thymol-treated (0–50 µM) cell lines, but *Bcl-2* levels were significantly higher in healthy cells than in cancerous cells. Similarly, one study reported that thymol (0–50 µM) induced apoptosis in human promyelocytic leukemia (HL-60) cells in a concentration-dependent manner, involving both caspase-dependent and caspase-independent pathways [11]. To our knowledge, our study is the first report describing the *Caspase-3* and *Caspase-9* activity of thymol on cancerous cells in comparison to healthy cells. The down-regulation of *Bcl-2* and up-regulation of *Bax, Caspase-9,* and *Caspase-3* protein expression in cancerous cells may draw attention to thymol as a potential candidate for the development of future gastric adenocarcinomas treatment strategies. The observed effect that anti-apoptotic *Bcl-2* remained upregulated in healthy cells seems appealing in this context.

It has been suggested that phenolic compounds induce DNA damage via their pro-oxidative effects on cells [4]. In the present study, the genotoxic effect of thymol (0–50 µM) was assessed via detecting DNA damage by comet assay. Thymol (10–50 µM) showed genotoxic effects on both cell types in a dose-dependent manner, but this effect was more statistically significant in cancerous cells than healthy cells. To our knowledge, the present report is the first study evaluating and comparing genotoxic effects of thymol on cancer and healthy cells. One study was recently published on the apoptotic as well as genotoxic effects of thymol on cancerous human AGS cells [15]. However, genotoxicity tests were included in studies on other cancerous cells such as human non-small lung cancer (H1299) and human hepatoma (HepG2) cells exposed to thymol which showed data similar to our findings [19,20]. Another study reported that thymol (25 µM) induces genotoxicity in the V79 cells [13]. Additionally, a study on Caco-2 and HepG2 cells exposed to thymol up to 600 µM revealed cytotoxicity, but the results were not associated with DNA-damaging effects [28]. Studies mentioned above were conducted exclusively on cancer cells. In an in vivo experiment, thymol caused genotoxicity at all doses used (40, 60, 80, and 100 mg/kg body weight) in rat bone marrow cells. Interestingly, thymol induced numerical chromosome abnormalities at the highest concentration [21]. Further in vivo studies are required to explore whether low doses of thymol can be better tolerated by healthy cells, as observed in our in vitro experiments, while being still effective against cancerous cells.

4. Material and Methods

4.1. Chemicals

Materials purchased from Sigma Chemical Co. (St. Louis, MO, USA) were thymol, DMSO (dimethyl sulfoxide), DCFH-DA (2′,7′- dichlorofluorescein-diacetate), AO/EB (acridine orange/ethidium bromide) stain, SDS polyacrylamide gels, coomassie brilliant-blue-dye, powdered skim milk, trypan blue, comet assays, low-melting agarose, normal melting agarose, and lysis solution. Ham's F-12 culture medium, fetal bovine serum (FBS), and antibiotics (100 U/mL penicillin, 100 µg/mL streptomycin) were obtained from Gibco Invitrogen Corporation (Carlsbad, CA, USA). CellTiter-Glo Luminescent Cell Viability and GSH/GSSG-Glo assays were provided by Promega (Madison, MI, USA). *Bax* (N-20), *Bcl-2* (C-21), *Caspase-3* (H-277), *Caspase-9* (H-170), and *β-actin* (AC-15) antibodies were purchased from Santa Cruz Biotechnologies (Santa Cruz, CA, USA). Amersham ECL Plus Western Blotting Detection reagents were obtained from GE Healthcare (Piscataway, NJ, USA). Radioimmunoprecipitation assay (RIPA) buffer and a proteinase inhibitor cocktail were from Roche (Mannheim, Germany). Molecular weight marker BenchMark Pre-Stained Protein Ladder was from Invitrogen (Grand Island, New York, USA).

4.2. Cell Cultures

Human cancerous AGS and healthy WS-1 cells purchased from the American Type Culture Collection (ATCC, Manassas, VA, USA) were cultured in Ham's F-12 Medium which was supplemented with 10% FBS and antibiotics (100 U/mL penicillin, 100 µg/mL streptomycin). AGS and WS-1 cells were plated at a density of 15×10^3 cells/mL in 96-well plates and at 18×10^4 cells/mL in 6-well plates and incubated for 24 h at 37 °C.

4.3. Treatments

A dose range of thymol was prepared for the determination of the half-maximal inhibitory concentration (IC_{50}) value [11,15,17]. According to these literatures, different doses of thymol (0, 10, 20, 30, 50, 100, 200, and 400 µM) were prepared from a stock solution of 600 µM of thymol in DMSO. The final concentration of DMSO in the medium was 0.1%, and was used as a negative control.

4.4. Cytotoxic Activity Assay

The CellTiter-Glo Luminescent Cell Viability Assay was used for the determination of the number of viable cells in the sense of identifying the cytotoxic effect of thymol in both lines. Human AGS and WS-1 cells were seeded at a density of 15×10^3 cells mL^{-1} in each well of 96-well plates. After 24 h incubation, both cell lines were treated with different doses (0–600 µM) of thymol and incubated at 37 °C further. The CellTiter-Glo Reagent was added into each well, and then the ATP in cells was quantified using a luminometer (Varioskan Flash Multimode Reader, Thermo, Waltham, MA). The viability of cells was demonstrated as a percentage following comparison with the negative control. The IC_{50} value was calculated from the concentration response curves by non-linear regression analysis.

4.5. Prooxidant Activity Assay

Reactive oxygen species were detected and measured by oxidative-sensitive fluorescent DCFH-DA probe. Two-hundred microliters of medium and 15×10^3 mL^{-1} AGS and WS-1 cells were placed into 96-well microtiter plates for their 24 h incubation. After that, the media were replaced with a growth medium containing 5% FBS. Plates were incubated with added different concentrations of thymol (0–100 µM) for another 24 h. Both cell cultures were washed with cold PBS and incubated with 100 mM DCFH-DA for 30 min at 37 °C. The fluorescence intensity was measured using the fluorescence plate reader (Varioskan Flash Multimode Reader, Thermo, Waltham, MA) at Ex./Em. = 488/525 nm). Measurements were carried out to ensure each time that the number of cells per treatment group had the same reproducibility. The results were reported as a percentage of relative fluorescence relative to the control cells.

4.6. Antioxidant Activity Assay

The GSH/GSSG-Glo assay was used to determine and quantify the GSH level in cells which is an indicator of oxidative stress. One hundred microliters of complete medium and both cell lines were plated at a density of 15×10^3 mL^{-1} in each well of plate. Cells were treated with different doses of thymol (0–100 µM). The method was carried out according to the manufacturer's instructions. The luminescence measurements are a quantification method based on light emission existing GSH.

4.7. Apoptotic Activity Assays

AO/EB fluorescent dyes were used to investigate the apoptotic activity of thymol (0–100 µM) at the cellular level. Both cell lines were plated at a density of 18×10^4 mL^{-1} in each well of plates and were exposed to different doses of thymol for 24 h incubation. Further examinations were performed according to manufacturer instructions. Multiple photos were taken at randomly-selected areas, and a minimum of 100 cells were counted using fluorescence microscopy (Leica DM1000, Solms, Germany). Nuclear morphologies of cells were assessed according to the previously described method [14,29].

The Western blot method was used to determine the apoptotic activity of thymol (0–100 µM) at the protein expression level. After treatment with different doses of thymol (0–50 µM), AGS and WS-1 cells were lysed in a radioimmunoprecipitation assay (RIPA) buffer (50 mM Tris-HCl, pH 7.4, 150 mM NaCl, 5 mM EDTA, 1% Nonidet P-40, 1% sodium deoxycholate, 0.1% SDS, 1% aprotinin, 50 mM NaF, 0.1 mM Na_3VO_4) and a proteinase inhibitor cocktail. Lysates were centrifuged at 13.000× g for 15 min at +4 °C. The pellet was discarded, and the supernatant containing the protein was transferred into a clean tube. The cell protein was measured by the Bradford Coomassie brilliant blue dye method. Samples containing 30 µg of protein, together with the molecular weight marker were subjected to 10% SDS polyacrylamide gel electrophoresis under reducing conditions. The proteins were transferred to polyvinylidene difluoride membranes. They were blocked with 5% powdered skim milk in 0.05%, Triton X-100/Tris-buffered saline with Tween for 1 h at room temperature. Blots were incubated overnight with primary antibodies *Bax*, *Bcl-2*, *Caspase-3*, and *Caspase-9* for 1 h then incubated with peroxidase-conjugated goat anti-rabbit secondary antibody. All samples were also blotted for *β-actin* in order to normalize protein amounts. Amersham ECL Plus Western Blotting Detection Reagents (GE Healthcare, Piscataway, NJ, USA) were used to determine the protein expression levels which were captured with an imaging system (Vilber Lourmat Sté, Collégien, France).

4.8. Genotoxicity Assay

Alkaline single cell gel electrophoresis (SCGE, comet assay) was used to determine the genotoxic activity of thymol (0–50 µM) on both cell lines. Before performing the comet assay, the trypan blue exclusion test was carried out for the determination of viable cell numbers present in the cell suspensions. Human AGS and WS-1 cells were plated at a density of 2×10^5 cells/well in six-well plates and incubated at 37 °C for 24 h. Different doses of thymol (0–50 µM) were added into both cell cultures. DMSO (1%) was used as a negative control, and 50 µM H_2O_2 was applied as a positive control. The assay was performed according to the method of Singh et al. [30] with slight modifications as described earlier [14]. Additionally, a computerized image analysis system (Comet Assay IV; Perceptive Instruments) was carried out. The percentage (%) of tail DNA was determined and used as a measure for damaged DNA [31].

4.9. Statistical Analyses

The obtained data were analyzed using the Statistical Package for the Social Sciences version 23.0 (SPSS Inc, Chicago, IL, USA). All the data were expressed as the mean ± SD of the number of experiments. All performed experiments were done in triplicate, and the standard deviation was within 5%. Percentages were calculated in relation to control cells. Likewise, a non-linear regression analysis was performed for the estimation of the IC_{50} value of thymol in healthy and cancer cell lines. All the data were tested using ANOVA, and post hoc analyses of different doses of thymol were performed by Tukey's test. The means of both cell lines were compared by the Mann-Whitney-U test. Pearson's correlation coefficient test was presented to assess the associations between ROS generation and cell viability parameters. $P \leq 0.001$ was considered significant.

5. Conclusions

This study demonstrated the first in vitro comparison of a wide range of thymol concentrations in order to investigate the hormetic effect of thymol on healthy or cancer cells. The findings of the present study suggest that thymol exerts a dose-dependent hormetic impact on the different cell types. Whereas higher doses of this phenolic compound may equally harm cancerous and healthy cells, low doses seem to protect healthy cells but harm cancer cells. On the basis of the described thymol-characteristics, it seems attractive to speculate about thymol as a tentative candidate for the development of future anticancer treatment strategies. However, further studies need to provide a more detailed understanding of thymol-induced effects on cancer and healthy cells at low doses. The better understanding of hormetic mechanisms of thymol at the cellular and molecular levels can be of special value for future in vivo studies which are of utmost importance to explore whether thymol could indeed be a potential preventive and/or therapeutic option in the future.

Author Contributions: A.G.-B. and A.D. wrote the paper; A.G.-B. and A.K. conceived and designed the study; A.K. and E.M.G. performed the experiments; A.G.-B., E.M.G. and A.D. collected and analyzed the data. All authors have read and approved the final manuscript.

Funding: The authors disclosed receipt of the following financial support for the research, authorship, and/or publication of this article: this work was funded by the Bezmialem Vakif University, the Unit of Scientific Research Projects (grant numbers 12.2014/3 and 6.2016/3).

Conflicts of Interest: The authors declare no conflicts of interest.

Abbreviations

AO/EB	Acridine orange/ethidium bromide
ATP	Adenosinetriphosphate
DCFH-DA	2′,7′-dichlorofluorescein-diacetate
DMSO	Dimethyl sulfoxide
FBS	Fetal bovine serum
GC	Gastric cancer
GSH	Glutathione
Human AGS cells	Human gastric adenocarcinoma cells
Human WS-1 cells	Human fibroblast cells
IC50 level	The half-maximal growth inhibitory concentration level
Na3VO4	Sodium orthovanadate
PBS	Phosphate buffered saline
ROS	Reactive oxygen species
TBS-T	Tris-buffered saline with Tween

References

1. Calabrese, E.J. Biphasic dose responses in biology, toxicology and medicine: Accounting for their generalizability and quantitative features. *Environ. Pollut.* **2013**, *182*, 452–460. [CrossRef]
2. Calabrese, E.J. Cancer biology and hormesis: Human tumor cell lines commonly display hermetic (biphasic) dose responses. *Crit. Rev. Toxicol.* **2005**, *35*, 463–582. [CrossRef] [PubMed]
3. Nagini, S. Carcinoma of the stomach: A review of epidemiology, pathogenesis, molecular genetics and chemoprevention. *World J. Gastrointest. Oncol.* **2012**, *4*, 156–169. [CrossRef] [PubMed]
4. Ferguson, L.R. Role of plant polyphenols in genomic stability. *Mutat. Res.* **2001**, *475*, 89–111. [CrossRef]
5. Elmore, S. Apoptosis: A Review of Programmed Cell Death. *Toxicol. Pathol.* **2007**, *35*, 495–516. [CrossRef] [PubMed]
6. Circu, M.L.; Rodriguez, C.; Maloney, R.; Moyer, P.T.; Aw, T.Y. Contribution of mitochondrial GSH transport to matrix GSH status and colonic epithelial cell apoptosis. *Free Radic. Biol. Med.* **2008**, *44*, 768–778. [CrossRef]
7. Franco, R.; Schoneveld, O.J.; Pappa, A.; Panayiotidis, M.I. The central role of glutathione in the pathophysiology of human diseases. *Arch. Physiol. Biochem.* **2007**, *113*, 234–258. [CrossRef]
8. Pias, E.K.; Aw, T.Y. Apoptosis in mitotic competent undifferentiated cells is induced by cellular redox imbalance independent of reactive oxygen species production. *FASEB J.* **2002**, *16*, 781–790. [CrossRef]
9. Parsaei, P.; Bahmani, M.; Naghdi, N.; Asadi-Samani, M. A review of therapeutic and pharmacological effects of thymol. *Der Pharm. Lett.* **2016**, *8*, 150–154.
10. Aydın, S.; Basaran, A.A.; Basaran, N. Modulating effects of thyme and its major ingredients on oxidative DNA damage in human lymphocytes. *J. Agricult. Food Chem.* **2005**, *53*, 1299–1305. [CrossRef]
11. Deb, D.D.; Parimala, G.; Devi, S.S.; Chakraborty, T. Effect of thymol on peripheral blood mononuclear cell PBMC and acute promyelocytic cancer cell line HL-60. *Chem. Biol. Interact.* **2011**, *193*, 97–106. [CrossRef] [PubMed]
12. García, D.A.; Bujons, J.; Vale, C.; Suñol, C. Allosteric positive interaction of thymol with the GABA A receptor in primary cultures of mouse cortical neurons. *Neuropharmacology* **2006**, *50*, 25–35. [CrossRef] [PubMed]

13. Undeger, U.; Basaran, A.; Degen, G.H.; Başaran, N. Antioxidant activities of major thyme ingredients and lack of (oxidative) DNA damage in V79 Chinese hamster lung fibroblast cells at low levels of carvacrol and thymol. *Food Chem. Toxicol.* **2009**, *47*, 2037–2043. [CrossRef] [PubMed]
14. Günes-Bayir, A.; Kocyigit, A.; Güler, E.M. In vitro effects of two major phenolic compounds from the family *Lamiaceae* plants on the human gastric carcinoma cells. *Toxicol. Ind. Health* **2018**, *34*, 525–539.
15. Günes-Bayir, A.; Kocyigit, A.; Güler, E.M.; Kiziltan, H.S. Effects of Thymol, a Natural Phenolic Compound, on Human Gastric Adenocarcinoma Cells *in vitro*. *Altern. Ther. Health Med.* **2019**, *25*, 12–21.
16. Hsu, S.S.; Lin, K.L.; Chou, C.T.; Chiang, A.J.; Liang, W.Z.; Chang, H.T.; Tsai, J.Y.; Liao, W.C.; Huang, F.D.; Huang, J.K.; et al. Effect of thymol on Ca2+ homeostasis and viability in human glioblastoma cells. *Eur. J. Pharmacol.* **2011**, *670*, 85–91. [CrossRef]
17. Kang, S.H.; Kim, Y.S.; Kim, E.K.; Hwang, J.W.; Jeong, J.H.; Dong, X.; Lee, J.W.; Moon, S.H.; Jeon, B.T.; Park, P.J. Anticancer Effect of Thymol on AGS Human Gastric Carcinoma Cells. *J. Microbiol. Biotechnol.* **2016**, *26*, 28–37. [CrossRef]
18. Llana-Ruiz-Cabello, M.; Gutiérrez-Praena, D.; Pichardo, S.; Moreno, F.J.; Bermúdez, J.M.; Aucejo, S.; Cameán, A.M. Cytotoxicity and morphological effects induced by carvacrol and thymol on the human cell line Caco-2. *Food Chem. Toxicol.* **2014**, *64*, 281–290. [CrossRef]
19. Ozkan, A.; Erdogan, A. A comparative evaluation of antioxidant and anticancer activity of essential oil from Origanum onites (*Lamiaceae*) and its two major phenolic components. *Turkish J. Biol.* **2011**, *35*, 735–742.
20. Ozkan, A.; Erdogan, A. A comparative study of the antioxidant/prooxidant effects of thymol and thymol at various doses on membrane and DNA of parental and drug resistant H1299 cells. *Nat. Prod. Commun.* **2012**, *7*, 1557–1560.
21. Azirak, S.; Rencuzogullari, E. The in vivo genotoxic effects of carvacrol and thymol in rat bone marrow cells. *Environ. Toxicol.* **2008**, *23*, 728–735. [CrossRef] [PubMed]
22. Michiels, J.; Missotten, J.; Dierick, N.; Maene, P.; De Smet, S. In vitro degradation and in vivo passage kinetics of carvacrol, thymol, eugenol and trans-cinnamaldehyde along the gastrointestinal tract of piglets. *J. Sci. Food Agric.* **2008**, *88*, 2371–2381. [CrossRef]
23. Bao, Y.; Wang, W.; Zhou, Z.; Sun, C. Benefits and risks of the hormetic effects of dietary isothiocyanates on cancer prevention. *PLoS ONE* **2014**, *9*, e114764. [CrossRef]
24. Kuhnel, H.; Adilijiang, A.; Dadak, A.; Wieser, M.; Upur, H.; Stolze, K.; Grillari, J.; Strasser, A. Investigations into cytotoxic effects of the herbal preparation Abhealthy Savda unziq. *Chin. J. Integr. Med.* **2015**, *53*, 1–9.
25. Bakkali, F.; Averbeck, S.; Averbeck, D.; Idaomar, M. Biological effects of essential oils—A review. *Food Chem. Toxicol.* **2008**, *46*, 446–475. [CrossRef]
26. Llana-Ruiz-Cabello, M.; Gutiérrez-Praena, D.; Puerto, M.; Pichardo, S.; Jos, Á.; Cameán, A.M. In vitro pro-oxidant/antioxidant role of carvacrol, thymol and their mixture in the intestinal Caco-2 cell line. *Toxicol. In Vitro* **2015**, *29*, 647–656. [CrossRef] [PubMed]
27. Traverso, N.; Ricciarelli, R.; Nitti, M.; Marengo, B.; Furfaro, A.L.; Pronzato, M.A.; Marinari, U.M.; Domenicotti, C. Role of glutathione in cancer progression and chemoresistance. *Oxid. Med. Cell Longev.* **2013**. [CrossRef]
28. Horvathova, E.; Šramkova, M.; Labaj, J.; Slamenová, D. Study of cytotoxic, genotoxic and DNA-protective effects of selected plant essential oils on human cells cultured in vitro. *Neuro. Endocrinol. Lett.* **2006**, *27*, 44–47.
29. Kasibhatla, S.; Amarante-Mendes, G.P.; Finucane, D.; Brunner, T.; Bossy-Wetzel, E.; Green, D.R. Acridine Orange/Ethidium Bromide (AO/EB) Staining to Detect Apoptosis. *CSH Protoc.* **2006**, *2006*. [CrossRef]
30. Singh, N.P.; McCoy, M.T.; Tice, R.R.; Schneider, E.L. A simple technique for quantitation of low levels of DNA damage in individual cells. *Exp. Cell Res.* **1988**, *175*, 184–191. [PubMed]
31. Hartmann, A.; Agurell, E.; Beevers, C.; Brendler-Schwaab, S.; Burlinson, B.; Clay, P.; Collins, A.; Smith, A.; Speit, G.; Thybaud, V.; et al. Recommendations for conducting the in vivo alkaline Comet assay. *Mutagenesis* **2003**, *18*, 45–51. [CrossRef] [PubMed]

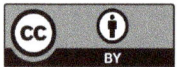

© 2020 by the authors. Licensee MDPI, Basel, Switzerland. This article is an open access article distributed under the terms and conditions of the Creative Commons Attribution (CC BY) license (http://creativecommons.org/licenses/by/4.0/).

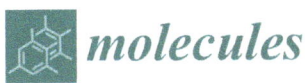

Review

Nutraceuticals and Enteric Glial Cells

Laura López-Gómez [1], Agata Szymaszkiewicz [2], Marta Zielińska [2] and Raquel Abalo [1,3,4,*]

1. High Performance Research Group in Physiopathology and Pharmacology of the Digestive System (NeuGut), Department of Basic Health Sciences, University Rey Juan Carlos, 28933 Alcorcón, Spain; laura.lopez.gomez@urjc.es
2. Department of Biochemistry, Faculty of Medicine, Medical University of Lodz, 90-419 Lodz, Poland; agata.szymaszkiewicz@stud.umed.lodz.pl (A.S.); marta.zielinska@umed.lodz.pl (M.Z.)
3. Associated Unit to Institute of Medicinal Chemistry (Unidad Asociada I+D+i del Instituto de Química Médica, IQM), Spanish National Research Council (Consejo Superior de Investigaciones Científicas, CSIC), 28006 Madrid, Spain
4. Working Group of Basic Sciences in Pain and Analgesia of the Spanish Pain Society (Grupo de Trabajo de Ciencias Básicas en Dolor y Analgesia de la Sociedad Española del Dolor), 28022 Madrid, Spain
* Correspondence: raquel.abalo@urjc.es

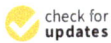

Citation: López-Gómez, L.; Szymaszkiewicz, A.; Zielińska, M.; Abalo, R. Nutraceuticals and Enteric Glial Cells. *Molecules* **2021**, *26*, 3762. https://doi.org/10.3390/molecules26123762

Academic Editors: Sokcheon Pak and Soo Liang Ooi

Received: 15 April 2021
Accepted: 15 June 2021
Published: 21 June 2021

Publisher's Note: MDPI stays neutral with regard to jurisdictional claims in published maps and institutional affiliations.

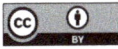

Copyright: © 2021 by the authors. Licensee MDPI, Basel, Switzerland. This article is an open access article distributed under the terms and conditions of the Creative Commons Attribution (CC BY) license (https://creativecommons.org/licenses/by/4.0/).

Abstract: Until recently, glia were considered to be a structural support for neurons, however further investigations showed that glial cells are equally as important as neurons. Among many different types of glia, enteric glial cells (EGCs) found in the gastrointestinal tract, have been significantly underestimated, but proved to play an essential role in neuroprotection, immune system modulation and many other functions. They are also said to be remarkably altered in different physiopathological conditions. A nutraceutical is defined as any food substance or part of a food that provides medical or health benefits, including prevention and treatment of the disease. Following the description of these interesting peripheral glial cells and highlighting their role in physiological and pathological changes, this article reviews all the studies on the effects of nutraceuticals as modulators of their functions. Currently there are only a few studies available concerning the effects of nutraceuticals on EGCs. Most of them evaluated molecules with antioxidant properties in systemic conditions, whereas only a few studies have been performed using models of gastrointestinal disorders. Despite the scarcity of studies on the topic, all agree that nutraceuticals have the potential to be an interesting alternative in the prevention and/or treatment of enteric gliopathies (of systemic or local etiology) and their associated gastrointestinal conditions.

Keywords: coffee; enteric glial cells; glia; inflammatory bowel disease; irritable bowel syndrome; neuropathic pain; nutraceuticals; quercetin; resveratrol

1. Introduction

The enteric nervous system (ENS) is a complex network of neurons and accompanying glial cells (enteric glial cells, EGCs) which controls the major functions of the gastrointestinal (GI) tract.

At first, glia were considered to be just a structural support for neurons, but recent findings emphasized more on their functions, and they turned out to be equally as important as neural cells, due to their involvement in all aspects of neural functions for both the central and peripheral nervous system, including the ENS.

Among the different types of glial cells (for example, astrocytes, microglia, Schwann cells), EGCs have been mostly underestimated, particularly regarding the modulation of their functions by nutraceuticals. However, EGCs are more often being recognized for their essential roles in physiology and the disease [1].

In this review, we focus on the enteric glia, their role and functions in physiology and pathology as well as the available studies on the effects of different nutraceuticals as modulators of these interesting cells.

2. Enteric Glial Cells

The ENS is a network of neurons divided into submucosal and myenteric plexuses, together with their accompanying glia, the EGCs [2]. Originally, EGCs were considered as a structural support for the enteric neurons, however recently, it was proved that they are crucial for the functioning of the GI tract under physiological (intestinal barrier support, GI motility, sensation) and pathophysiological conditions (GI motility disturbances, visceral pain).

Hanani et al. distinguished and classified EGCs into four subgroups based on their morphology (Table 1) [3].

Table 1. Division of the enteric glial cells into subtypes.

Type	Morphology		Location
Type I Protoplasmic EGCs	Star-shaped cells with short, irregularly branched processes		Intraganglionic (enteric ganglia)
Type II Fibrous EGCs	Elongated glia with branches		Within interganglionic fiber tracts
Type III Mucosal EGCs	Long branched processes		Extraganglionic: subepithelial glia
Type IV Intermuscular EGCs	Elongated glia		Extraganglionic: accompanying the nerve fibers and encircling the smooth muscles

Abbreviations: EGC, enteric glial cell. Created in biorender.com (accessed on 15 March 2021).

Besides morphology, EGCs may also be classified according to the molecular or functional differences in receptors or channels expressed on their surface or in their nuclei. The following proteins are currently used to identify EGCs, i.e., calcium-binding protein S100β [4], glial fibrillary acidic protein (GFAP) [5] and the transcription factors: SOX8, SOX9, SOX10 [6].

As shown in Table 2, EGCs share some similarities with astrocytes, the major type of glial cells of the central nervous system.

Table 2. Comparison between enteric glial cells and astrocytes [6–8].

Feature	Enteric Glial Cells	Astrocytes
Morphology	Irregularly branched processes	In vivo: numerous processes forming well-delineated bushy territories In culture: few processes, polygonal fibroblast-like shape Astrocytes show structural plasticity: their morphology differs between brain areas, and it may be changed (stellation or process growth) by different stimuli
Subtypes	Protoplasmic Fibrous Mucosal Intermuscular	Protoplasmic Fibrous
Location	Enteric nervous system (submucosal and myenteric plexus)	Central nervous system

Table 2. Cont.

Feature	Enteric Glial Cells	Astrocytes
Identification	GFAP Calcium-binding protein S100β Transcription factors (SOX8, SOX9, SOX10)	GFAP Calcium-binding protein S100β Glutamine synthase CD44 Vimentin Ran-2 Astrocytes from different brain regions can exhibit pronounced molecular differences
Adjacent cell coupling	Gap junction coupling	Gap junction coupling
Activation	Release of pro-inflammatory cytokines (i.e., IL-1β, TNF-α) Increased expression of c-fos, TrkA, ET-B, TLR-4, BR1 Enhanced expression of glial cell markers	Release of pro-inflammatory cytokines (i.e., IL-1β, IL-6, TNF-α, TGF-β) Increased expression of adhesion-related molecules (CD44) Increased expression of receptors for EGF, TNF-α Enhanced expression of glial cell markers: GFAP, vimentin, nestin
Involved in	Physiopathological modulation of GI functions	Development and plasticity of dendritic spines and synapses Elimination of dendritic spines, synapse formation Regulation of neurotransmission and plasticity

Abbreviations: BR1, bradykinin receptor 1; CD44, membrane glycoprotein; EGF, epidermal growth factor; ET-B, entothelin-1 receptor B; GFAP, glial fibrillary acidic protein; GI, gastrointestinal; IL, interleukin; Ran-2, rat neural antigen-2; TLR-4, Toll-like receptor 4; TGF-β, transforming growth factor β; TNF-α, tumor necrosis factor α; TrkA, nerve growth factor receptor.

2.1. Cellular and Tissular Roles of EGCs

Generally, EGCs are considered as non-excitable cells, as they are unable to generate an action potential. Furthermore, EGCs are interconnected and electrically coupled by gap junctions that form an extensive glial network [9], as shown in Figure 1.

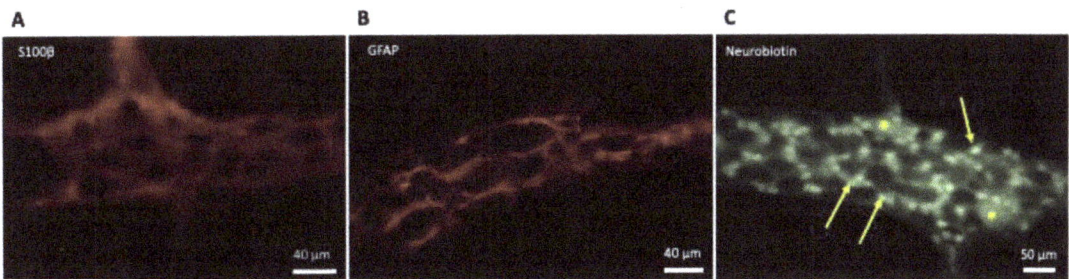

Figure 1. Appearance of enteric glial cells (EGCs). (**A,B**) Show the images obtained from the myenteric plexus of the rat distal colon; immunoreactivity to S100-β (**A**) and glial fibrillary acidic protein (GFAP) (**B**) are characteristic for EGCs. (**C**) Shows the network of electrically-coupled EGCs (arrows) in one myenteric ganglion from the guinea pig ileum; this image was taken as the result of the accidental insertion of an electrode filled with neurobiotin in one EGC while performing electrophysiological recordings of the activity of myenteric neurons (*); neurobiotin injected into one EGC diffused throughout the gap junctions connecting it with the other EGC in the myenteric ganglion, in the same way as firstly described by Hanani et al. [9] in 1989 for Lucifer yellow dye.

Enteric glial cells communicate with surrounding cells (neurons, glia, epithelial cells, immune cells) and integrate received information through calcium signaling [10]. Intercellular communication is a result of the propagation of calcium waves through connexin 43 (Cx43) hemichannels [11]. Moreover, EGCs are susceptible to the activation by neural pathways: intrinsic (from enteric neurons) or extrinsic (from autonomic or primary afferent neurons). The major neurotransmitter involved in this extracellular signaling is adenosine triphosphate (ATP) [12]. It was found that intermuscular EGCs express the purinergic receptor (P2X7) [13].

Like neurons, EGCs may release neurotransmitters and express the receptors for neurotransmitters on their surface to receive signals [13–16]. In particular, human EGCs were found to be immunoreactive to glutamate [17] and gamma amino butyric acid (GABA) transporter (GAT2) [18,19]. Furthermore, EGCs exhibit immuno-reactivity for L-arginine, a nitric oxide (NO) precursor and thus they may be involved in nitrergic neurotransmission [20,21].

Interestingly, EGCs are characterized by displaying a remarkable function: they may be activated upon stimulation (e.g., inflammation or following the injury), and switched into a reactive, pro-inflammatory phenotype [22,23]. When EGCs are activated, they have an increased ability to proliferate [24], enhance c-fos expression, and change their expression of markers and surface receptors [25]. For example, the expression of nerve growth factor (NGF) receptor, tropomyosin receptor kinase A (TrkA) [26], endothelin-1 receptor B (ET-B) [27], Toll-like receptor (TLR) 4 [28], and bradykinin receptor 1 (BR1) [29] are increased in enteric glia incubated with interleukin-1β (IL-1β), and TrkA receptor is up-regulated in response to lipopolysaccharide (LPS) stimulation [26].

Consequently, reactive glial cells are characterized by an increased expression of enteric glial markers. For instance, the expression of GFAP may be induced by the incubation with tumor necrosis factor α (TNF-α), IL-1β, LPS or LPS + interferon γ (IFN-γ) [27,30,31]. The latter also increases the expression of S100β [32]. In vivo, increased GFAP expression in the rat myenteric plexus occurred in LPS-induced intestinal inflammation [33].

Moreover, reactive EGCs are able to release neurotrophins, growth factors or cytokines and therefore enteric glia recruit immune cells (macrophages, neutrophils, mast cells) into the colonic mucosa [34–36]. This confirms an important immunomodulatory role for these cells within the GI tract.

The EGCs that are located directly underneath the epithelial layer constitute a link between the epithelium and submucosal neurons, and they participate in all steps of epithelial regeneration (cellular differentiation, migration, adhesion and proliferation) [37]. Therefore, EGCs support the epithelial barrier integrity in the intestines and have the capacity to enhance epithelial healing. Glial cell derived neurotrophic factor (GDNF) released by EGCs entails anti-inflammatory effect in the intestines through the inhibition of cellular apoptosis and decrease of pro-inflammatory cytokine level [35,38]. Furthermore, during mild inflammation, GDNF helps in the processes of epithelial reconstitution and maturation [39]. In addition, EGCs produce and release several factors involved in the processes of epithelial regeneration: pro-epithelial growth factor (pro-EGF) [40]. S-nitrosoglutathione [41] or 15-deoxy-Δ12,14-prostaglandin J2 (15d-PGJ2) [42]. EGCs support the intestinal barrier through decreasing intestinal permeability [41] or increasing the resistance to infections [43].

Enteric glial cells are also involved in the control of GI motility, as they coordinate sensory and motor signaling within the GI tract [44]. Noteworthily, according to Aubé et al. [45], a progressive loss of EGCs in transgenic mice, expressing haemagglutinin (HA), that received activated HA specific CD8+ T cells, led to the prolongation of the GI transit. In the study by Nesser et al. [46], in mice treated with fluorocitrate, a selective gliotoxin, the upper GI transit time was prolonged and the intestinal motility patterns were impaired (both the basal tone and the amplitude of contractility in response to electrical field stimulation were decreased).

Finally, ECGs are considered to be involved in visceral sensation, via directly or indirectly sensitizing or activating nociceptors. Additionally, EGCs have the potential to regulate nociceptor sensitization/activation by removing of neuromodulators [47]. Direct mechanisms of sensitization include the release of neuromodulators such as ATP, GABA, IL-1β and neurotrophins. Indirect mechanisms involve antigen presentation through major histocompatibility complex (MHC) class I and II, leading to activation of T cells followed by cytokine release, and regulation of other immune cells, leading to release of histamine and further cytokines (TNF-α, IL-1β) [47]. Moreover, pro-inflammatory signals induce glial Cx43-dependent macrophage colony-stimulating factor (M-CSF) production through protein kinase C (PKC) and TNF-α converting enzyme (TACE). This further supports the importance of EGC interaction with macrophages in the regulation of visceral hypersensitivity during chronic inflammation [48].

2.2. Physiological Changes in the Population of EGCs

The population of EGCs may be altered by many physiological factors, such as aging or diet modifications. The process of aging of the GI tract includes a progressive loss of EGCs. Philips et al. [49] compared the population of EGCs in the GI tract in young (5–6 months-old) and old (26-month-old) rats. According to their findings, there was a significant decline in the number and density of EGCs in the myenteric plexus from the duodenum up to the distal colon with age. However, there was a small, non-significant decrease of EGC number in the rectum.

Interestingly, more detailed research revealed that diet also influences the population of EGCs. A high-fat diet caused a significant loss of EGC density in duodenal submucosal plexus in mice [50]. On the contrary, the same diet increased the number of EGCs in the myenteric plexus of the antrum, while it remained unchanged in the jejunum [51]. In contrast to the alterations in the enteric glia, high-fat diet led to a substantial loss of myenteric neurons, while the population of submucosal neurons stayed within the norm [52].

On the other hand, food restrictions that slow the aging process by reducing the oxidative processes thus inhibiting of cell death, turned out to be detrimental for the EGCs. According to the study by Schoffen et al. [53], diet restriction accentuated morphologic and quantitative changes in glial cell populations in rats, whereas the 50% reduction of food supply entailed neuroprotective effects on the myenteric neurons in the colon.

Nevertheless, the mechanisms responsible for the gliopathy occurring with age or diet modifications remain unknown. It is yet to be clarified whether the changes in morphology or number of EGCs are due to a direct impact of aging/diet restrictions or rather a consequence of the concomitant degenerative processes of the neurons in the ENS.

2.3. Role of EGCs in GI Pathophysiology

As EGCs coordinate the communication between the cells in the GI tract (neurons, epithelial cells, myocytes), any alterations in their population (such as those associated with the occurrence of different diseases) may have a significant impact on the GI functions.

2.3.1. Intestinal Inflammation

Inflammatory bowel disease (IBD) is a group of chronic inflammatory conditions of the GI tract and two major types, Crohn's disease (CD) and ulcerative colitis (UC) are distinguished. The first reports regarding the importance of enteric glia in the inflammatory processes in the GI tract came from 1998. Bush et al. [54] generated transgenic mice through the ablation of GFAP-positive glial cells from the jejunum and ileum, resulting in fulminating and fatal jejuno-ileitis. The ablation of EGCs led to severe inflammations, causing degeneration of neurons in the ENS and hemorrhagic necrosis of the small intestine. The alterations within the gut were similar to the pathology in the course of IBD in both animals and humans [54]. Consequently, the concept about the involvement of EGCs in the inflammatory processes in the GI tact emerges.

Noteworthily, Pochard et al. [25] summed up the results of molecular studies on the population of EGCs in IBD: in most studies, the expression of GFAP, S100β and GDNF was elevated in inflamed colon of IBD patients (both CD and UC) in comparison to their healthy colonic tissue [55–57]. The expression of GFAP was decreased in healthy intestinal samples from CD patients [55,56], but not UC, comparing to healthy patients. The expression of S100β was downregulated in the myenteric plexus of uninflamed areas from CD patients in comparison to healthy controls [57]. Likewise, in the rectum of UC patients the submucosal expression of S100β was decreased in comparison to healthy controls [23,30]. Noteworthily, GDNF production was increased in samples collected from healthy parts of the colon of UC patients as compared to healthy controls [56]. Interestingly, GDNF ameliorated experimental colitis, inhibited mucosal inflammatory response and decreased intestinal permeability in the mouse model of colitis induced by dextran sodium sulfate (DSS) [58].

The differences in the expression of glial markers in the course of IBD do not reflect the extent of alterations in the population of EGCs in the intestines during inflammation. The decreased expression of GFAP, located in the cytoplasm of CD patients may be considered as a sign of glial loss, but GFAP immunohistochemical staining is not optimal to quantify the number of cells. The emerging approach, that could possibly be used for further assessment of the enteric glia population in the course of IBD is the utilization of proteins located in the nucleus (such as SOX 8/9/10) [59].

Besides the potential glial loss in the course of IBD, the functional differences appear to be significant. Coquenlorge et al. [60] assessed that, although EGCs isolated from controls and CD patients exhibited similar expression of glial markers (GFAP, S100β) and EGC-derived factors (IL-6, TGF-β, pro-EGF and glutathione (GSH)), they differed in their influence on the intestinal barrier. Enteric glial cells from CD patients failed in supporting the intestinal barrier and the healing process opposite to those from healthy controls. This study was further expanded on the UC patients. It assessed how EGCs isolated from UC patients affect epithelial barrier of the intestines. It was confirmed that, unlike CD patient derived EGCs, EGCs from UC patients preserve intestinal permeability. The efficiency of the intestinal barrier was similar in co-culture with EGCs derived from UC patients and healthy controls [25].

Under physiological conditions, MHC class I receptors are expressed on the enteric glia, while MHC class II remain almost undetectable [61,62]. However, after the exposure to enteroinvasive *Escherichia coli*, the expression of MHC class II on the enteroglial cells is increased [63]. Moreover, the expression of MHC class II was significantly increased in CD patients in comparison to healthy controls, in which the expression of these receptors was very low or even absent [61,62].

2.3.2. Chronic Constipation

Chronic constipation is a condition characterized by a lack of frequent bowel movements or difficulties of stool passage. Chronic constipation may be related to the organic barriers in the colon or rectum (i.e., tumor), neuronal/muscular impairment (i.e., dysmotility in Parkinson's disease), post-infection (megacolon caused by Chagas disease) or idiopathic (idiopathic constipation). The results of clinical studies on the importance of EGCs in the control of GI motility indicate that a loss of enteric glia in the ENS may be associated with dysmotility (i.e., idiopathic constipation or infectious-related dysmotility).

According to Bassotti et al. [64], who examined patients with constipation and collected samples from the ileum and colon, there was a loss of EGCs in these tissues. Notably, the decrease in the number of EGCs was accompanied by the reduction of enteric neurons density. Similar results were obtained in a group of patients with severe, intractable constipation that underwent colectomy with ileorectostomy, as they displayed a significant decrease in neurons, EGCs and interstitial cells of Cajal. Constipated patients had significantly more apoptotic enteric neurons in comparison to controls [65].

Noteworthily, the population of EGCs in the submucosal and myenteric plexus was significantly decreased in the colon of patients with severe constipation due to obstructed defecation refractory to medical treatment or biofeedback training. At the same time, the enteric neurons were reduced only in the submucosal plexus [66].

In the case of megacolon occurring in the course of Chagas disease (an infectious disease caused by *Trypanosoma cruzi*) and idiopathic megacolon, there was a remarkable reduction in the number of neurons and EGCs in the ENS in the colonic specimens collected during surgery. However, the differences in the population of EGCs were more pronounced in the group of patients with infectious megacolon [67].

2.3.3. Postoperative Ileus

Postoperative ileus (POI) is a condition that may occur after surgery of the abdominal cavity or the outer abdomen, which is associated with GI motility impairment and results in inhibition of peristalsis and distension. Although the pathophysiology of POI remains unknown, recent studies indicate that EGCs maintain an important role in this process. Stoffels et al. [68] investigated the molecular mechanism of POI in mice. They determined that the blockage of the receptor for interleukin 1 (IL-1R) attenuated the POI. These receptors were found to be expressed on the surface of EGCs in the myenteric plexus. The activation of IL-1R in cultured EGCs promoted an inflammatory response through an increase in IL-6 and monocyte chemotactic protein 1 (MCP-1) levels, which may be an important step in the development of POI.

2.3.4. Irritable Bowel Syndrome

Irritable bowel syndrome (IBS) is a chronic disease of the GI tract that manifests with recurrent abdominal pain accompanied by GI motility disturbances. This functional GI disorder may be classified as diarrhea-predominant IBS (IBS-D), constipation-predominant (IBS-C) or mixed IBS, when both diarrhea and constipation occur in an alternate manner (IBS-M).

According to Lilli et al. [69] the immunoreactivity of S100β was significantly reduced in the colonic biopsies of IBS patients, independently of the IBS subtype (IBS-C, IBS-D, and IBS-M). Furthermore, the incubation of the rodent EGCs with supernatants from the mucosal biopsies from IBS-C patients reduced the cellular proliferation. Noteworthily, exposure of rat enteric glia with IBS-D and IBS-M supernatants impaired ATP-induced Ca^{2+} response of these cells.

In some cases, one more type of IBS can be distinguished: the one followed by the bacterial, viral or parasitic infection of the GI tract (post-infectious IBS, PI-IBS) [70,71]. Notably, there were many attempts to elucidate the molecular mechanism that underlies PI-IBS, for example: hyperplasia of enterochromaffin cells, increased intestinal permeability or enhanced cytokine production [72,73]. Importantly, one of the proposed mechanisms of PI-IBS followed by *Clostridium difficile* infection involves EGCs. Toxin B produced by *C. difficile* evokes cytotoxic and pro-apoptotic effects on EGCs in vitro. This harmful impact of toxin B on enteric glia results from the disorganization of cytoskeleton, early cell rounding with Rac1 glucosylation, cell cycle inhibition and increased susceptibility to apoptosis induced by the pro-inflammatory cytokines (TNF-α and IFN-γ). Importantly, despite these direct effects of toxin B, it is important that EGCs which survive the detrimental action of toxin B, do not recover and their function is not restored (they exhibit persistent Rac1 glucosylation, disturbances in the cell cycle and low apoptosis rate) [74]. The long-term effects of *C. difficile* infection on EGCs network may be pivotal for GI homeostasis, as enteric glia coordinate cell-to-cell communication in the intestines [75].

The severity of visceral hypersensitivity in IBS patients may be associated with brain derived neurotrophic factor (BDNF), a protein described as crucial in the process of neuropathic and inflammatory pain. The level of BDNF was significantly elevated in the colonic mucosal biopsies from IBS patients and corresponded with the abdominal pain severity [76,77]. The high-affinity receptor for BDNF, tropomyosin receptor kinase B (TrkB), is expressed on the surface of EGCs [77]. Interestingly, the expression of this receptor, along with GFAP and substance P (SP), was increased in the colonic mucosa of IBS patients. It suggests that BDNF may play a key role in the occurrence of visceral hypersensitivity, i.e., in the course of IBS, through the interactions with EGCs. It was determined that the administration of fecal supernatants from IBS-D patients failed to induce visceral hypersensitivity in BDNF ± mice in contrast to wild type animals. In wild type animals, the pain threshold to colorectal distension after IBS-D fecal supernatant administration was significantly elevated when pretreated with a TrkB antagonist (TrkB/Fc). Noteworthily, the induction of visceral hypersensitivity evoked the up-regulation of the same proteins (TrkB, GFAP, SP) as in IBS patients in wild type animals, but not in the BDNF ± mice [78]. Overall, the fecal supernatant from IBS patients induced hypersensitivity that may involve a BDNF-TrkB signaling pathway. Thus, BDNF appear to act as a link between visceral hypersensitivity and EGC activation.

The first step of the non-pharmacological management of IBS is diet modification. A dietary approach may involve the consumption of a low FODMAP products (diet low in fermentable carbohydrates). It was assessed that IBS patients have a higher *Firmicutes/Bacterioidetes* ratio and bacteria from the phylum *Firmicutes* are considered as a major source of the short chain fatty acid butyrate, a small molecule metabolite arising from symbiotic bacteria fermentation from insoluble dietary fibers [79,80]. The lower supply of fermentable carbohydrates alleviates IBS symptoms [81]. Furthermore, the butyrate enemas induce visceral hypersensitivity in animals tested. It was elucidated that butyrate-induced hypersensitivity is associated with the up-regulation of NGF on messenger ribonucleic acid (mRNA) and protein level thus EGCs are one of the major sources of NGF in the GI tract. Noteworthily, NGF was co-expressed with GFAP and the co-localized immunostaining area of NGF and GFAP was increased in the colon of rats that received butyrate-enema. Furthermore, it was reported that the secretion of NGF from EGCs in the colonic lamina propria was increased after the butyrate-enema [82].

2.3.5. EGC and Pathophysiology Outer the GI Tract

Intestinal motility disfunction may also be a characteristic symptom of diseases outer the GI tract, for example neurodegenerative diseases, such as Parkinson's disease (PD) or prion diseases. PD is a long-term, multi-system disease of the CNS, which is related to degeneration of the dopaminergic neurons. Besides the motor symptoms (rigidity, tremor, dyskinesia), the intrinsic aspect of PD is a dysfunction of the GI tract. Patients experience nausea, dysphagia, abdominal distension and constipation. Studies show that, in the colon of PD patients, there was an increased expression of glial markers (GFAP, S100β, SOX10), and this was accompanied by the elevation of pro-inflammatory cytokines (TNF-α, IFN-γ, IL-1β, IL-6) at the mRNA level. However, there was no correlation found between the expression of glial markers or the inflammatory indicators and the severity of disease or GI symptoms [83]. Likewise, according to Clairembault et al. [84], in the colonic biopsies from PD patients, there was a GFAP over-expression and a reduction in GFAP phosphorylation comparing to healthy controls. These results suggest that EGCs may be involved in the GI dysfunction observed in the course of PD, nevertheless further research is needed to understand the mechanism of this process.

Prion diseases are progressive and fatal neurodegenerative conditions which are caused by spreading of pathological isoforms of cellular prion protein. This pathological process affects astrocytes in the CNS and EGCs in the GI tract [85,86]. However, it was assessed that the prion replication sites were found in the ENS prior to the replication in the CNS [87]. Thus, the enteric glia may be essential in prion neuroinvasion, as the GI system constitutes to the major exogenous prion protein entry site and acts as the starting point for the prions en route to the brain [87].

Finally, many systemic diseases may cause alterations in the GI function inducing many effects on the EGCs. For example: diabetes [88] or autoimmune diseases such as rheumatoid arthritis [89]. As shown below, some dietary components have proved beneficial in protection against EGC alterations in those diseases, thus favoring the restoration of GI altered functions.

2.4. Effects of Nutraceuticals on Enteric Glial Cells

Studies focused on the effects of nutraceuticals on EGCs are relatively scarce and include a variety of compounds with anti-inflammatory, antioxidant, or modulatory properties (Table 3).

Table 3. Effects of nutraceuticals on enteric glial cells.

Nutraceutical (Pathology)	Characteristics	Source	Effects	System	References
L-glutamine (Diabetes)	Amino acid	Protein-rich foods Available as a dietary supplement	Antioxidant	Wistar rats	[90,91]
L-glutathione (Diabetes)	Tripeptide	Supply of the raw nutritional materials used to generate GSH, such as cysteine and glycine	Antioxidant	Wistar rats	[90]
Phytotherapy (Aging, diabetes)	Procyanidin B2, epicatechin Glutamate, polyphenols Selenium, ellagic acid	*Trichilia catigua* *Agaricus blazei Murrill*, *Bertholletia excelsa* H.B., (plants/fungi extracts and foods)	Antioxidant	Wistar rats	[92–94]
15d-PGJ2	Omega-6 fatty acid metabolite	Many sources (including *B. excelsa* H.B.)	PPARγ, Nrf2 activation	Non-transformed or transformed EGCs cultures	[42,95]
Coffee compounds (Parkinson's disease)	Caffeic acid and chlorogenic acid	Coffee	Antioxidants Prevent MT-1,2 downregulation	C57BL/6 mice, EGC cultures	[96]
Quercetin (Diabetes, rheumatoid arthritis)	Flavonoid polyphenol	Fruits and vegetables Available as a dietary supplement.	Antioxidant, anti-inflammatory, Nrf 2 activation	Wistar rats, Holtzman rats	[89,97–99]
Resveratrol (Diabetes, intestinal ischemia-reperfusion)	Non-flavonoid polyphenol	Concentrated mostly in the skins and seeds of grapes and berries. Available as a dietary supplement.	Antioxidant, regulation of EGC proliferation	Wistar rats	[100–102]
PEA (IBD, HIV)	Endogenous or exogenous fatty acid amide	Soy lecithin, soybeans, egg yolk, peanuts, alfalfa. Available as a food-supplement named PeaPure.	PPARα activation, anti-inflammatory effects	Wistar rats, CD-1 mice, human intestinal biopsies.	[28,103]
Cannabidiol (UC)	Phytocannabinoid	*Cannabis sativa*	PPARγ receptor activation, anti-inflammatory effects	Mice, human biopsies	[104]
Berberine (UC)	Isoquinoline alkaloid	Plants from *Berberidaceae* family Available as a dietary supplement.	Modulation of interactions between EGCs, epithelial cells and immune cells.	C57BL/6 mice, Rat EGC cell line, CRL-2690 cultures	[105]
Probiotics (Diabetes, IBS)	*Lactobacillus plantarum* *Bifidobacterium bifidum* *Bacteroides fragilis* *Pediococcus acidilactici*	Fermented food and dairy products	Modulation of inflammation	Wistar rats, EGC cultures, pigs	[106–108]
Inulin (Diabetes)	Polysaccharide	Plants, also available in supplement form or as an ingredient	Prebiotic fiber	Wistar rats	[106]

Abbreviations: 15d-PGj2, 15-deoxy-Δ12,14-prostaglandin J2; EGC, enteric glial cell; HIV, human immunodeficiency virus; IBD, inflammatory bowel disease; IBS, irritable bowel syndrome; Nrf2, nuclear factor erythroid-derived 2-like 2; MT, Metallothionein; PEA, palmitoylethanolamide; PPARγ, peroxisome proliferator-activated receptor; UC, ulcerative colitis.

Nutraceuticals with antioxidant properties have attracted a great amount of interest motivated by their ability to counteract the damaging action of free radicals produced during pathological conditions of the GI tract affecting neurons and glial cells. Among these compounds, the usefulness of the amino acid L-glutamine [90,91] and the tripeptide glutathione (GSH) [90] has been evaluated in streptozotocin-induced (STZ) type 1 diabetic rats. In diabetes, the production of free radicals is a part of the pathological process. L-glutamine is an amino acid that acts as a substrate in the formation of GSH, an important endogenous antioxidant. The oxidative stress that occurs during diabetes is associated with an increase in cellular reactive oxygen species (ROS), which act together with proteins, nucleic acids and lipids, damaging and inducing cell death by necrosis or apoptosis. In these studies [90,91], ileal whole-mount preparations were used for immunohistochemistry to evaluate myenteric neurons and EGC, immunoreactive (IR) to HuC/D and S100β, respectively, through cell counting and morphometric analysis. Inside the GI tract, both neurons and EGCs were affected by oxidative stress and the antioxidant activity of L-glutamine and GSH prevented damaging of EGCs [90,91]. In particular, 2% L-glutamine and 1% L-GSH were shown to exert gliotrophic effects that indirectly protected the myenteric neurons in the animal model of diabetes [90,91].

Likewise, the antioxidant properties of extracts obtained from some plants such as *Trichilia catigua* [92] or fungi such as *Agaricus blazei Murril* [93] were shown to alleviate the effects of oxidative stress on EGCs in preclinical models of diabetes and aging.

The ethyl acetate fraction from *Trichilia catigua* contains two flavonoids with antioxidant properties: procyanidin B2 and epicatechin. In STZ diabetic rats, myenteric EGCs IR to S100β showed an overall reduction in the number but increase in cell body area in jejunal whole-mount preparations [92]. According to the authors, this increase in the area of EGCs could be due to development of cellular edema, provoked by the same metabolic alterations that affect neurons, or due to a specific EGC mechanism triggered to compensate for the loss of neurons and to maintain homeostasis. Furthermore, diabetes produced changes in protein expression, measured by Western blot, with an increase in S100β and a decrease in GFAP production, accompanied by a decrease in cells co-expressing S100β and GFAP in the jejunum mucosa, as observed in cryostat sections. Consistently, EGCs contribute to regulation of the barrier function in the GI tract and loosing of its integrity allows the translocation of normally excluded contents to occur through the mucosa (such as microorganisms and antigens, initializing and perpetuating inflammatory disorders and tissue damage). Thus, the reduction in EGCs could possibly contribute to diarrhea or constipation in patients with diabetes. In addition, EGCs act as a communication channel between the ENS and the local immune system, and their alteration would affect the immunity of the diabetic patients. The administration of this extract not only prevented an increase in the area of the EGC, but also caused a reduction of S100β expression, probably due to the antioxidant effects of its' flavonoids [92]. Thus, procyanidin B2 and epicatechin may be useful nutraceuticals helping to preserve GI health through their glioprotective effects.

The aging process is related to the worsening of physical and metabolic processes associated with dysfunctions of the immune system and disorders of the energy metabolism, leading to oxidative stress and, therefore, to the formation of free radicals that, if not eliminated, may damage the cells. In this context, an aqueous extract obtained from the fungus *Agaricus blazei Murril* (cogumelo du sol) containing polyphenols, flavonoids and glutamate has been investigated using rats of 7-, 12- and 23-months-old [93]. This extract was beneficial to avoid any cell damage and mitigate the reduction in the number of neurons and glial cells in the ENS, as seen in whole-mount preparations from jejunum in which myenteric S100β-IR EGCs were analyzed. Although the exact mechanism of action remains unknown, antioxidant effects of this fungus could act directly by eliminating the free radicals generated by EGC. Alternatively, the extract could have an indirect action through the conversion of glutamic acid into glutamine, which is in turn a precursor of GSH, a molecule with well-known antioxidant effects, as already mentioned.

Brazil nut (*Berthonelletis excelsa HBK*) is a natural source of selenium (whose consumption improves the action of antioxidant enzymes in the colon), unsaturated fatty acids such as omega-3 and omega-6 (which are related to neuroplasticity associated with diet and reduce oxidative stress) and polyphenols such as ellagic acid (with neuroprotective action). In healthy rats, Brazil nut supplementation decreased gastric emptying and produced changes in GFAP immunofluorescent labeling, evaluated in microtome sections of the colonic wall [94]. However, these changes were dose-dependent but not linear, since 5% supplementation produced an increase in GFAP while 10% supplementation reduced it. The effect of Brazil nut on the EGCs may be due to different factors. Firstly, selenium is involved in calcium homeostasis and EGC communication occurs through calcium waves, thus influencing enteric neurotransmission and affecting the functions of the intestine. Minerals such as selenium could condition glial behavior and responses, affecting gastric emptying and GFAP expression [94]. Secondly, Brazil nut contains unsaturated omega-3 and omega-6 fatty acids. Omega-6 fatty acid derivatives such as 15d-PGJ2 are produced by EGCs and act as glial mediators, controlling the differentiation of intestinal epithelial cells trough peroxisome proliferator-activated receptor (PPARγ) [42] and exerting neuroprotective functions in the ENS. Interestingly, in EGC cultures with the use of molecular expression analysis (Western-blot, polymerase-chain reaction, PCR) and immunofluorescence labeling, 15d-PGJ2 was shown to be capable of activating nuclear factor erythroid-derived 2-like 2 (NrF2) [95] causing an increase in GSH synthesis in neurons and protecting against oxidative stress. Thus, exogenous sources of omega-6 derivatives such as 15d-PGJ2 (such as Brazil nuts) could constitute an interesting pharmacological or nutritional intervention in pathologies where EGCs are altered [95].

Coffee is one of the most popular beverages in the world and the beneficial effects of its components have been widely studied. Among them, caffeic acid (CA) and chlorogenic acid (CGA) are compounds with major antioxidant activity. In a mouse PD model, the administration of these compounds prevented the neurodegeneration caused by rotenone (an inhibitor of the mitochondrial complex I) in the dopaminergic neurons of the *substantia nigra* and in the enteric neurons [96]. In addition, in co-cultures of enteric neurons and glial cells, CA and CGA inhibited the neurotoxic effects of rotenone, which reduced the expression of metallothionein-1,2 (MT-1,2) and caused a loss of enteric neurons. MT is a low molecular weight protein rich in cysteine that binds to metals such as zinc, copper, and cadmium. This protein participates in detoxification as well as eliminating free radicals. The MT-1 and MT-2 isoforms are considered physiologically equivalent and intervene, among other functions, in the response to oxidative stress. Thus, these coffee components could protect the enteric neurons from the action of rotenone by triggering the antioxidant properties of EGCs [96].

Polyphenols are a type of plant-derived nutraceuticals with antioxidant properties, which contribute to different plant functions such as pigmentation and resistance to environmental stress or pathogens [109]. They have one or more hydroxyl groups attached to a benzene ring in their chemical structure and two types are distinguished: flavonoids such as quercetin, and non-flavonoids such as resveratrol.

Quercetin is a flavonoid naturally found in many foods such as onions, apples, broccoli, tea and red wine. Due to its antioxidant properties, the possible beneficial effects of quercetin have been studied in the field of diabetes by several authors [97–99]. As mentioned above, diabetes causes a reduction in the number of neurons and EGCs due to the oxidative stress associated with this disease, and supplementation with quercetin results in beneficial effects in the STZ-diabetic rat model. Using immunohistochemistry in whole-mount preparations, it was demonstrated that quercetin protected, at least partially, against the diabetes-induced loss and morphometric alterations of enteric neurons and glial cells from caecum [97], duodenum [98] and jejunum [99]. As mentioned above, EGCs participate in neuroprotection by expressing the S100β protein, which has neurotrophic activity, induces the growth of neuronal extensions, dendrites and axons and participates in neuronal survival. This protein is also involved in the regulation of specific intracellular signaling pathways such as calcium homeostasis, cytoskeletal stability, and induction of apoptosis. In addition, EGCs release numerous neurotrophic and antioxidant factors, including GSH and GDNF, which activate neuropeptide Y, another antioxidant system, thus protecting against neuronal death [99]. Indeed, the authors attributed the neuroprotective effect of quercetin to its ability to increase the expression of Nrf2 in EGCs, since the increased expression of Nrf2 increases GSH synthesis and promotes neuroprotection [98]. Summing up, the antioxidant properties of quercetin include protection of EGCs and allow them to exert their neuroprotective activity in the ENS in the context of diabetes.

The antioxidant and anti-inflammatory effects of quercetin have also been shown to be beneficial in alleviating the effects of oxidative stress and the production of cytokines provoked by rheumatoid arthritis [89]. This autoimmune and inflammatory disease destroys cartilage and bone tissue, but it is considered a multisystem disease that also affects other organs. The presence of autoantibodies increases oxidative stress and production of pro-inflammatory cytokines that cause cell damage, affecting the GI tract [89]. In rats, chronic rheumatoid arthritis, induced by the intradermal injection of complete Freund's adjuvant of 5% heat-killed suspension of *Mycobacterium tuberculosis* into the right hind paw, reduced the number of neurons and EGCs in the submucosal and myenteric plexuses of the jejunum and caused mucosal inflammation. Due to the loss of EGCs, a decrease in the expression of GFAP and GNDF was observed, and there was also an increase in the expression of S100β that would activate immune and inflammatory processes. This increase in S100β corresponds to an increase of the neurons in the body area and EGCs in the myenteric plexus due to a compensatory effect to the reduction in the number of glial cells. Nevertheless, in the submucosal plexus, the EGCs reduced their area, which indicates a deleterious gliopathic effect induced by the disease, that results in a decrease of the enzymatic activity of these cells. Quercetin reversed all the effects, probably due to an elimination of free radicals that damage these cells, associated to its powerful antioxidant effects. In addition, quercetin also had anti-inflammatory effects on the mucosa, which were not found in ibuprofen [89]. However, the authors acknowledged that, in healthy animals, quercetin may result in pro-oxidant and toxic effects, depending on the dose and time of administration [110,111]. Thus, caution is needed to establish the right way of using of this nutraceutical, particularly for prophylactic purposes against inflammatory conditions.

Among the non-flavonoid polyphenols, resveratrol (3,5,4′-trihydroxy-stilbene) has been the object of great interest. It is a substance naturally present in high concentrations in the grape peel, red wine, peanuts, pistachios or chocolate and, unlike other antioxidants, high doses of resveratrol are well tolerated and not toxic [100]. This makes resveratrol a good candidate for the treatment of diseases related to oxidative stress such as diabetes or after episodes of ischemia-reperfusion, a process that usually occurs in several clinical situations (thrombosis, hernia, hemorrhagic and hypovolemic shock, infection, abdominal surgery) and in inflammatory diseases such as Crohn's disease [101,102].

In a rat model of intestinal ischemia-reperfusion (I/R) injury caused by occluding the superior mesenteric artery for 45 min, followed by 7 days of reperfusion, resveratrol reversed the proliferation of EGCs promoted by I/R (seen as an increase in cells labeled with S100β and GFAP) and was neuroprotective for the myenteric neurons. The antioxidant action of this compound seems to be key to its protective action on EGCs, through the elimination of free radicals, and the regeneration of endogenous antioxidants, mediated by the increase of GSH levels and the activity of the antioxidant enzyme glutathione peroxidase [101]. Whereas free resveratrol prevented neuronal loss, glial proliferation, and reactive gliosis in the ENS, when loaded in poly(anhydride) nanoparticulate transport systems, its effects were not improved. Moreover, empty nanoparticles caused hepatotoxicity and promoted intestinal injury [102]. Although this first attempt was not successful, it will be certainly interesting to develop nanoparticles made of more suitable materials as a means to improve the oral bioavailability of resveratrol.

Resveratrol was also tested in the STZ-diabetic rat model [100], where an increase in GFAP labeling was detected using immunohistochemistry and fluorescence analysis on whole-mount preparations of the myenteric plexus from the three segments of the small intestine (ileum, jejunum and duodenum), as a consequence of a moderate reactive gliosis. Despite its neuroprotective effect after damage, the increase in GFAP is considered detrimental to regeneration because it constitutes an obstacle to prevent the establishment of contacts and normal neural circuits. Resveratrol treatment in diabetic animals did not alter EGC density, but significantly reduced GFAP immunoreactivity, indicating a reversion of such gliosis.

It has been postulated that some nutraceuticals could modulate EGC activity through the activation of the cannabinoid system. Cannabinoids and cannabinoid-related compounds, due to their antioxidant and anti-inflammatory activity, could be interesting to modulate the inflammatory processes in which these cells intervene. EGCs do not express the typical cannabinoid CB1 and CB2 receptors [112–114]. However, EGCs express the peroxisome proliferation activation receptor α (PPARα), a nuclear hormone receptor to which transcription-related ligands bind [113,114], and whose activation may have anti-inflammatory and antinociceptive effects [28]. The presence of this receptor in EGCs has led to the study of the action of ligands of this receptor such as palmitoylethanolamide (PEA).

PEA is a cannabinoid-related molecule involved in protective mechanisms. It is an endogenous fatty acid amide naturally found in foods such as egg yolks, peanuts, and soy lecithin, and is also produced endogenously. In a mouse model of DSS-induced colitis and in colonic biopsies from UC patients PEA produced anti-inflammatory effects. These were due to its ability to activate PPARα receptors and counteract glial activation, decreasing the production of NO and the expression of pro-inflammatory proteins such as inducible isoform of nitric oxide synthase (iNOS), cyclo-oxygenase-2 (COX-2) and TNF-α [28]. Similarly, in a rat model of human immunodeficiency virus (HIV)-induced diarrhea, produced by intracolonic administration of HIV-1 trans-activator of transcription (Tat) protein, PEA was shown to decrease this symptom of HIV-1 infection. The effects of PEA were mediated through the activation of PPARα receptors, present in EGCs, the consequent reduction of S100β and iNOS overexpression in the submucosal plexus of the colon and the blockade of TLR4/nuclear factor-kappa B (NF-kB) activation [103].

CBD is a non-psychotropic cannabinoid derived from the *Cannabis sativa* plant and a key mediator of glia-mediated neuroinflammation in the GI tract. The expression of the glial protein S100β has been studied in a mouse model of intestinal inflammation induced by LPS and in cultured rectal biopsies of patients with UC, after stimulation with LPS+IFN-γ [104]. S100β is related to inflammation, as it stimulates NO production. Thus, EGCs recognize inflammatory stimuli and once activated they produce and secrete S100β, which contributes to inducing iNOS, with the consequent production of NO. Pretreatment of mice with CBD prevented glial cell hyperactivation and decreased the expression of S100β and the infiltration of immune cells in the intestine, revealing its ability to prevent the amplification of the inflammatory response and S100β-mediated immune system activation. Similar results were obtained in the cultured rectal human biopsies, which were reversed by the PPARγ antagonist GW9662, confirming the involvement of this receptor in the anti-enterogliosis effect of CBD (although, to the best of our knowledge, this receptor has not been described so far to be expressed in EGCs). Thus, CBD may be useful in IBD patients, but high-quality clinical trials that may clearly determine the efficacy and safety of this compound, used as either a nutraceutical supplement or as part of medical cannabis, are still needed [115–117].

Another interesting nutraceutical for the treatment of UC is berberine, which is able to maintain intestinal EGCs and modulate the interaction between EGCs, epithelial cells and immune cells in EGCs and epithelial cell co-cultures [105]. Berberine is an isoquinoline alkaloid with anti-inflammatory effects present in different plants such as *Hydrastis canadensis, Berberis aquifolium* and *B. vulgaris*. During UC, changes occur in the expression of the neuropeptides secreted by the EGCs of the mucosa, such as GDNF or SP, which regulate functions such as inflammation, homeostasis or intestinal barrier function. Berberine administration improved intestinal damage in the DSS-mouse model of UC through restoration of the epithelial barrier, maintenance of resident EGCs and attenuation of immune infiltration and hyperactivation of immune cells. In vitro, berberine showed direct protective effects in EGC monocultures in a simulated inflammation situation and regulated the interaction between EGCs, epithelial cells and immune cells in co-cultures, further confirming its modulatory properties of mucosal inflammation [105].

Recently, the role of the microbiota has been demonstrated in various diseases, including diabetes [106]. The alteration of the intestinal microenvironment (dysbiosis) has been related to neurological disorders and alterations in EGCs. The recovery of the healthy microbiota through feeding using probiotic compounds can help in these cases, as some studies have shown [106–108]. Probiotics are defined as live microorganisms or bacteria that, administered in the diet, have beneficial effects on the health of the host [118]. Once ingested, they are potentially capable of influencing gastrointestinal functions due to their interactions with their components [107].

The levels of GDNF, GFAP and inflammatory markers such as IL-17, IL-6 and TLR-2, measured by enzyme linked immunosorbent assay (ELISA), were increased in the colon of type 2 diabetic rats. The elevation of these markers was related to both the dysbiosis, and the inflammation caused by diabetes that would activate glial cells as a means to prevent damage and protect neurons [106]. In this study, the application for 8 weeks after diabetes induction of *Lactobacillus plantarum* combined with the prebiotic fiber inulin (but not alone) improved the composition of the microbiota and reduced the levels of inflammatory cytokines and the expression of GDNF and GFAP [106].

In piglets, the administration of the probiotic *Pediococcus acidilactici* produced modifications in the ENS, as observed immunohistochemically in microtome serial sections [107]. The glial component was affected by the diet modification, but this modification was limited to the submucosal plexus of the ileum, with a significant increase in GFAP labeling, possibly related to ensuring the functional and structural integrity of the intestinal mucosa. In the ENS, neurons modify their chemical code in response to luminal changes and this neuronal plasticity aims to allow the adaptation of GI tract to changes or damage. Indeed, neurons may react to these alterations in the intestinal environment by modifying the expression of neuropeptides. EGCs participate in this neuronal plasticity through the secretion of neurotrophic factors. Thus, this study suggests that the changes in neurons and EGCs caused by the inclusion in the diet of the probiotic would be related to neuronal plasticity [107].

Finally, in a model of intestinal inflammation established by LPS and IFNγ- administration, the possible mechanisms by which two probiotics, *Bifidobacterium bifidum* (B.b.) and *Bacteroides fragilis* (B.f.), influence EGC regulation were examined [108]. In this study, it was observed that EGCs can increase the expression of inflammatory factors if they are subjected to harmful exogenous stimuli, and *B.b* can inhibit the inflammatory process by regulating EGCs, while *B.f.* does not have similar effects. Furthermore, EGCs are involved in intestinal inflammation and *B.b.* has protective effects by regulating EGCs. Both probiotics can influence the expression of NFG, neurotrophin-3 (NT-3), inflammasomes NLRP (nod-like receptor family, pyrin domain-containing) 3 and 6, IL-18, IL-1β and caspase-1 in EGCs, promoting or inhibiting intestinal inflammation. Both probiotics have beneficial effects by facilitating the elimination of microorganisms through the upregulation of inflammasome NLRP-3, leading to the inflammatory response, through the activation of caspase-1 and the secretion of IL-1 β and IL-8. Interestingly, *B.b.* increases the regulation of NLRP-6 mRNA while *B.f.* has inhibitory effects on its expression. NLRP-6 can inhibit the inflammatory response and plays an important role in maintaining homeostasis in the intestine. Interestingly, whereas *B.b.* decreased the expression of Il-18, IL-1β and caspase-1 in EGCs to thus inhibit the inflammatory response, *B.f.* showed opposite effects (i.e., it upregulated the expression of IL-18, IL-1β and caspase-1 in EGCs and promoted the inflammatory response).

3. Conclusions

Here, we have reviewed the physiopathological roles of a relatively unstudied type of peripheral glial cells, i.e., enteric glial cells, as well as the research evaluating the effects of different nutraceuticals and food components on them.

In general, studies on the modulatory effects that nutraceuticals exert on EGCs are relatively scarce, particularly those using models of GI diseases, such as IBD, in which PEA [28], CBD [104] and berberine [105] reduced inflammation, at least partly, through modulation of EGCs. PEA was also beneficial in a model of HIV-1 induced diarrhea [103], resveratrol protected the ENS against intestinal I/R [101,102], and the probiotics *Bifidobacterium bifidum* and *Bacteroides fragilis* inhibited and promoted, respectively, intestinal inflammation after LPS+IFN-γ administration [108].

The remaining studies were focused on systemic conditions that may also affect the GI tract. Curiously enough, most of them were performed in Brazilian institutions (Universidade Estadual de Maringá; Fluminense Federal University, Niterói), particularly those using the STZ-diabetic rat model and nutraceuticals with antioxidant properties, such as L-glutamine [90,91], L-glutathione [91], extracts of *Trichilia catigua* [92], quercetin [97–99] and resveratrol [100]. These Brazilian researchers have also evaluated the effects on EGCs of quercetin in a rat model of rheumatoid arthritis [92] and performed the mentioned study of resveratrol in a rat model of intestinal I/R [101,102]. Other Brazilian studies have been performed using extracts of the fungus *Agaricus blazei Murrill* in aged rats [93] and of Brazil nut in healthy animals [94]. Apart from these studies, a Japanese group (Okayama University) found beneficial effects of the antioxidant compounds caffeic acid and chlorogenic acid, from coffee, in the rotenone-induced mouse model of PD and also in cultures of EGCs exposed to rotenone [96]. Finally, some researchers from Italian and Iranian institutions have evaluated the effect of probiotics (*Pediococcus acidilactici*, *Lactobacillus plantarum*) and prebiotics (inulin) in healthy piglets [107] and rat models of type 2 diabetes [106].

Taken together, different nutraceuticals, particularly those with antioxidant activity, seem to exert neuroprotective effects in the ENS in local and systemic conditions that may involve not only direct actions on the enteric neurons but also indirect actions through EGC modulation.

In the near future, we hope further studies will more precisely define the connections between nutraceuticals and EGCs as a possible target to treat, prevent or reduce their alterations associated with the different GI and systemic disorders in which they are involved.

Author Contributions: Conceptualization, R.A.; Writing—Original Draft Preparation, L.L.-G., A.S. and M.Z.; Writing—Review and Editing, R.A. All authors have read and agreed to the published version of the manuscript.

Funding: This research was funded by Ministerio de Ciencia, Innovación y Universidades, grant number PID2019-111510RB-I00 to RA and by National Science Center–SONATA 15 (number UMO-2019/35/D/NZ7/02830 to MZ).

Acknowledgments: The graphical abstract was created in Biorender free application.

Conflicts of Interest: The authors declare no conflict of interest. The funders had no role in the design of the study; in the collection, analyses, or interpretation of data; in the writing of the manuscript, or in the decision to publish the results.

Abbreviations

15d-PGJ2	15-deoxy-Δ12,14-prostaglandin J2
ATP	adenosin triphosphate
B.b.	Bifidobacterium bifidum
BDNF	brain derived neurotrophic factor
B.f.	Bacteroides fragilis
BR1	bradykinin receptor 1
Ca^{2+}	calcium
CA	caffeic acid
CBD	cannabidiol
CGA	chlorogenic acid
CD	Crohn's disease
CD44	membrane glycoprotein
CNS	central nervous system
COX-2	cyclo-oxygenase-2
Cx43	connexin 43
DRG	dorsal root ganglion, dorsal root ganglia
DSS	dextran sodium sulfate
EGC	enteric glial cell
ELISA	enzyme linked immunosorbent assay
ENS	enteric nervous system
ET-B	endothelin-1 receptor B
GABA	gamma amino butyric acid
GAT2	GABA transporter

GDNF	glial cell-derived neurotrophic factor
GFAP	glial fibrillary acidic protein
GI	gastrointestinal
GSH	glutathione
HA	haemagglutinin
HIV	human immunodeficiency virus
IBD	inflammatory bowel disease
IBS-C	constipation-predominant irritable bowel syndrome
IBS-D	diarrhea-irritable bowel syndrome
IBS-M	mixed irritable bowel syndrome
IBS	irritable bowel syndrome
IFN	interferon
IL	interleukin
IL-1R	receptor for interleukin 1
iNOS	inducible isoform of nitric oxide synthase
I/R	ischemia-reperfusion
IR	immunoreactive
LPS	lipopolysaccharide
M-CSF	macrophage colony-stimulating factor
MCP1	monocyte chemotactic protein 1
MHC	major histocompatibility complex
mRNA	messenger ribonucleic acid
MT	metallothionein
NF-κB	nuclear factor kappa B
NGF	nerve growth factor
NLRP	nod-like receptor family, pyrin domain-containing
NO	nitric oxide
NrF2	nuclear factor erythroid-derived 2-like 2
NT-3	neurotrophin-3
P2	purinergic receptor 2
PCR	polymerase-chain reaction
PEA	palmitoylethanolamide
PD	Parkinson's disease
PNS	peripheral nervous system
PI-IBS	post-infectious irritable bowel syndrome
PKC	protein kinase C
POI	postoperative ileus
PPAR	peroxisome proliferator-activated receptor
Pro-EGF	pro-epidermal growth factor
Ran-2	rat neural antigen-2
ROS	reactive oxygen species
SP	substance P
STZ	streptozotocin-induced
TACE	TNF-α converting enzyme
TGF	transforming growth factor
TLR	Toll-like receptor
TNF	tumor necrosis factor
Trk	tropomyosin receptor kinase
UC	ulcerative colitis

References

1. Seguella, L.; Gulbransen, B.D. Enteric glial biology, intercellular signalling and roles in gastrointestinal disease. *Nat. Rev. Gastroenterol. Hepatol.* **2021**. Available online: https://www.nature.com/articles/s41575-021-00423-7 (accessed on 15 March 2021). [CrossRef]
2. Furness, J. *The Enteric Nervous System*, 1st ed.; Blackwell Publishing: Hoboken, NJ, USA, 2007.

3. Hanani, M.; Reichenbach, A. Morphology of horseradish peroxidase (HRP)-injected glial cells in the myenteric plexus of the guinea-pig. *Cell Tissue Res.* **1994**, *278*, 153–160. [CrossRef]
4. Ferri, G.L.; Probert, L.; Cocchia, D.; Michetti, F.; Marangos, P.J.; Polak, J.M. Evidence for the presence of S-100 protein in the glial component of the human enteric nervous system. *Nature* **1982**, *297*, 409–410. [CrossRef]
5. Jessen, K.R.; Mirsky, R. Glial cells in the enteric nervous system contain glial fibrillary acidic protein. *Nature* **1980**, *286*, 736–737. [CrossRef]
6. Grundmann, D.; Loris, E.; Maas-Omlor, S.; Huang, W.; Scheller, A.; Kirchhoff, F.; Schafer, K.H. Enteric Glia: S100, GFAP, and Beyond. *Anat Rec.* **2019**, *302*, 1333–1344. [CrossRef] [PubMed]
7. Khakh, B.S.; Sofroniew, M.V. Diversity of astrocyte functions and phenotypes in neural circuits. *Nat. Neurosci.* **2017**, *18*, 942–952. [CrossRef]
8. Eddleston, M.; Mucke, L. Molecular profile of reactive astrocytes-implications for their role in neurologic disease. *Neuroscience* **1993**, *54*, 15–36. [CrossRef]
9. Hanani, M.; Zamir, O.; Baluk, P. Glial cells in the guinea pig myenteric plexus are dye coupled. *Brain Res.* **1989**, *497*, 245–249. [CrossRef]
10. Ochoa-Cortes, F.; Turco, F.; Linan-Rico, A.; Soghomonyan, S.; Whitaker, E.; Wehner, S.; Cuomo, R.; Christofi, F.L. Enteric Glial Cells: A New Frontier in Neurogastroenterology and Clinical Target for Inflammatory Bowel Diseases. *Inflamm Bowel Dis.* **2016**, *22*, 433–449. [CrossRef] [PubMed]
11. McClain, J.L.; Grubišić, V.; Fried, D.; Gomez-Suarez, R.A.; Leinninger, G.M.; Sévigny, J.; Parpura, V.; Gulbransen, B.D. Ca^{2+} responses in enteric glia are mediated by connexin-43 hemichannels and modulate colonic transit in mice. *Gastroenterology* **2014**, *146*, 497–507.e1. [CrossRef]
12. Bornstein, J.C. Purinergic mechanisms in the control of gastrointestinal motility. *Purinergic Signal.* **2008**, *4*, 197–212. [CrossRef] [PubMed]
13. Vanderwinden, J.M.; Timmermans, J.P.; Schiffmann, S.N. Glial cells, but not interstitial cells, express P2X7, an ionotropic purinergic receptor, in rat gastrointestinal musculature. *Cell Tissue Res.* **2003**, *312*, 149–154. [CrossRef]
14. Kimball, B.C.; Mulholland, M.W. Enteric Glia Exhibit P2U Receptors that Increase Cytosolic Calcium by a Phospholipase C-Dependent Mechanism. *J. Neurochem.* **2002**, *66*, 604–612. [CrossRef] [PubMed]
15. Van Nassauw, L.; Costagliola, A.; den Bosch, J.V.O.; Cecio, A.; Vanderwinden, J.M.; Burnstock, G.; Timmermans, J.P. Region-specific distribution of the P2Y4 receptor in enteric glial cells and interstitial cells of Cajal within the guinea-pig gastrointestinal tract. *Auton. Neurosci. Basic Clin.* **2006**, *126–127*, 299–306. [CrossRef] [PubMed]
16. Nasser, Y.; Keenan, C.M.; Ma, A.C.; McCafferty, D.M.; Sharkey, K.A. Expression of a functional metabotropic glutamate receptor 5 on enteric glia is altered in states of inflammation. *Glia* **2007**, *55*, 859–872. [CrossRef] [PubMed]
17. Giaroni, C.; Zanetti, E.; Chiaravalli, A.M.; Albarello, L.; Dominioni, L.; Capella, C.; Lecchini, S.; Frigo, G. Evidence for a glutamatergic modulation of the cholinergic function in the human enteric nervous system via NMDA receptors. *Eur. J. Pharmacol.* **2003**, *476*, 63–69. [CrossRef]
18. Fletcher, E.L.; Clark, M.J.; Furness, J.B. Neuronal and glial localization of GABA transporter immunoreactivity in the myenteric plexus. *Cell Tissue Res.* **2002**, *308*, 339–346. [CrossRef] [PubMed]
19. Galligan, J.J.; Lepard, K.J.; Schneider, D.A.; Zhou, X. Multiple mechanisms of fast excitatory synaptic transmission in the enteric nervous system. *J. Auton. Nerv. Syst.* **2000**, *81*, 97–103. [CrossRef]
20. Eiko, A.; Semba, R.; Kashiwamata, S. Evidence for the presence of l-arginine in the glial components of the peripheral nervous system. *Brain Res.* **1991**, *559*, 159–162. [CrossRef]
21. Nagahama, M.; Semba, R.; Tsuzuki, M.; Aoki, E. L-arginine immunoreactive enteric glial cells in the enteric nervous system of rat ileum. *Neuro Signals* **2001**, *10*, 336–340. [CrossRef]
22. Jessen, K.R.; Mirsky, R. Astrocyte-like glia in the peripheral nervous system: An immunohistochemical study of enteric glia. *J. Neurosci.* **1983**, *3*, 2206–2218. [CrossRef]
23. Cirillo, C.; Sarnelli, G.; Esposito, G.; Turco, F.; Steardo, L.; Cuomo, R. S100B protein in the gut: The evidence for enteroglial sustained intestinal inflammation. *World J. Gastroenterol.* **2011**, *17*, 1261–1266. [CrossRef]
24. Bradley, J.S.; Parr, E.J.; Sharkey, K.A. Effects of inflammation on cell proliferation in the myenteric plexus of the guinea-pig ileum. *Cell Tissue Res.* **1997**, *289*, 455–461. [CrossRef] [PubMed]
25. Pochard, C.; Coquenlorge, S.; Freyssinet, M.; Naveilhan, P.; Bourreille, A.; Neunlist, M.; Rolli-Derkinderen, M. The multiple faces of inflammatory enteric glial cells: Is Crohn's disease a gliopathy? *Am. J. Physiol. Gastrointest. Liver Physiol.* **2018**, *315*, G1–G11. [CrossRef]
26. Von Boyen, G.B.T.; Steinkamp, M.; Reinshagen, M.; Schäfer, K.-H.; Adler, G.; Kirsch, J. Nerve Growth Factor Secretion in Cultured Enteric Glia Cells is Modulated by Proinflammatory Cytokines. *J. Neuroendocrinol.* **2006**, *18*, 820–825. [CrossRef] [PubMed]
27. von Georg, B.T.; Nadine, D.; Christoph, H.; Guido Adler, M.S. The endothelin axis influences enteric glia cell functions. *Med. Sci Monit.* **2010**, *16*, 161–167.
28. Esposito, G.; Capoccia, E.; Turco, F.; Palumbo, I.; Lu, J.; Steardo, A.; Cuomo, R.; Sarnelli, G.; Steardo, L. Palmitoylethanolamide improves colon inflammation through an enteric glia/toll like receptor 4-dependent PPAR-α activation. *Gut* **2014**, *63*, 1300–1312. [CrossRef]

29. Murakami, M.; Ohta, T.; Ito, S. Interleukin-1β enhances the action of bradykinin in rat myenteric neurons through up-regulation of glial B1 receptor expression. *Neuroscience* **2008**, *151*, 222–231. [CrossRef] [PubMed]
30. Cirillo, C.; Sarnelli, G.; Esposito, G.; Grosso, M.; Petruzzelli, R.; Izzo, P.; Cali, G.; D'Armiento, F.P.; Rocco, A.; Nardone, G.; et al. Increased mucosal nitric oxide production in ulcerative colitis is mediated in part by the enteroglial-derived S100B protein. *Neurogastroenterol. Motil.* **2009**, *21*, 1209–e112. [CrossRef]
31. Von Boyen, G.B.T.; Steinkamp, M.; Reinshagen, M.; Schäfer, K.H.; Adler, G.; Kirsch, J. Proinflammatory cytokines increase glial fibrillary acidic protein expression in enteric glia. *Gut* **2004**, *53*, 222–228. [CrossRef]
32. Cirillo, C.; Sarnelli, G.; Turco, F.; Mango, A.; Grosso, M.; Aprea, G.; Masone, S.; Cuomo, R. Proinflammatory stimuli activates human-derived enteroglial cells and induces autocrine nitric oxide production. *Neurogastroenterol. Motil.* **2011**, *23*, e372–e382. [CrossRef]
33. Rosenbaum, C.; Schick, M.A.; Wollborn, J.; Heider, A.; Scholz, C.J.; Cecil, A.; Niesler, B.; Hirrlinger, J.; Walles, H.; Metzger, M. Activation of myenteric glia during acute inflammation in vitro and in vivo. *PLoS ONE* **2016**, *11*, e0151335. [CrossRef] [PubMed]
34. Burns, A.J.; Pachnis, V. Development of the enteric nervous system: Bringing together cells, signals and genes. *Neurogastroenterol. Motil.* **2009**, *21*, 100–102. [CrossRef] [PubMed]
35. Steinkamp, M.; Geerling, I.; Reinshagen, M.; Schäfer, K.; Adler, G.; Kirsch, J. Proinflammatory cytokines induce neurotrophic factor expression in enteric glia: A key to the regulation of epithelial apoptosis in Crohn's disease. *Inflamm. Bowel Dis.* **2006**, *12*, 346–354.
36. Sharkey, K.A. Emerging roles for enteric glia in gastrointestinal disorders. *J. Clin. Investig.* **2015**, *125*, 918–925. [CrossRef]
37. Liu, Y.A.; Chung, Y.C.; Pan, S.T.; Shen, M.Y.; Hou, Y.C.; Peng, S.J.; Pasricha, P.J.; Tang, S.C. 3-D imaging, illustration, and quantitation of enteric glial network in transparent human colon mucosa. *Neurogastroenterol. Motil.* **2013**, *25*, 324–338. [CrossRef]
38. Steinkamp, M.; Geerling, I.; Seufferlein, T.; von Boyen, G.; Egger, B.; Grossmann, J.; Ludwig, L.; Adler, G.; Reinshagen, M. Glial-derived neurotrophic factor regulates apoptosis in colonic epithelial cells. *Gastroenterology* **2003**, *124*, 1748–1757. [CrossRef]
39. Tanaka, F.; Tominaga, K.; Fujikawa, Y.; Nagami, Y.; Komata, N.; Yamagami, H.; Tanigawa, T.; Shiba, M.; Watanabe, T.; Fujiwara, Y.; et al. Concentration of Glial Cell Line-Derived neurotrophic Factor Positively Correlates with Symptoms in Functional Dyspepsia. *Dig. Dis. Sci.* **2016**, *61*, 3478–3485. [CrossRef]
40. Van Landeghem, L.; Chevalier, J.; Mahé, M.M.; Wedel, T.; Urvil, P.; Derkinderen, P.; Savidge, T.; Neunlist, M. Enteric glia promote intestinal mucosal healing via activation of focal adhesion kinase and release of proEGF. *Am. J. Physiol. Gastrointest. Liver Physiol.* **2011**, *300*, G976. [CrossRef]
41. Savidge, T.C.; Newman, P.; Pothoulakis, C.; Ruhl, A.; Neunlinst, M.; Bourreille, A.; Hurst, R.; Sofroniew, M.V. Enteric glia regulate intestinal barrier function and inflammation via release of S-nitrosoglutathione. *Gastroenterology* **2007**, *132*, 1344–1358. [CrossRef]
42. Bach-Ngohou, K.; Mahé, M.M.; Aubert, P.; Abdo, H.; Boni, S.; Bourreille, A.; Denis, M.G.; Lardeux, B.; Neunlist, M.; Masson, D. Enteric glia modulate epithelial cell proliferation and differentiation through 15-deoxy-Δ12,14-prostaglandin J2. *J. Physiol.* **2010**, *588*, 2533–2544. [CrossRef]
43. Flamant, M.; Aubert, P.; Rolli-Derkinderen, M.; Bourreille, A.; Neunlist, M.R.; Mahé, M.M.; Meurette, G.; Marteyn, B.; Savidge, T.; Galmiche, J.P.; et al. Enteric glia protect against Shigella flexneri invasion in intestinal epithelial cells: A role for S-nitrosoglutathione. *Gut* **2011**, *60*, 473–484. [CrossRef] [PubMed]
44. Rico, A.L.; Grants, I.; Needleman, B.J.; Williams, K.C.; Soghomonyan, S.; Turco, F.; Cuomo, R.; Grider, J.R.; Kendig, D.M.; Murthy, K.S.; et al. Gliomodulation of Neuronal and Motor Behavior in the Human GI Tract. *Gastroenterology* **2015**, *148*, S-18. [CrossRef]
45. Aubé, A.C.; Cabarrocas, J.; Bauer, J.; Philippe, D.; Aubert, P.; Doulay, F.; Liblau, R.; Galmiche, J.P.; Neunlist, M. Changes in enteric neurone phenotype and intestinal functions in a transgenic mouse model of enteric glia disruption. *Gut* **2006**, *55*, 630–637. [CrossRef]
46. Nasser, Y.; Fernandez, E.; Keenan, C.M.; Ho, W.; Oland, L.D.; Tibbles, L.A.; Schemann, M.; MacNaughton, W.K.; Ruhl, A.; Sharkey, K.A. Role of enteric glia in intestinal physiology: Effects of the gliotoxin fluorocitrate on motor and secretory function. *Am. J. Physiol. Gastrointest. Liver Physiol.* **2006**, *291*, G912–G927. [CrossRef]
47. Morales-Soto, W.; Gulbransen, B.D. Enteric Glia: A New Player in Abdominal Pain. *Cell Mol. Gastroenterol. Hepatol.* **2019**, *7*, 433–445. [CrossRef] [PubMed]
48. Grubišić, V.; McClain, J.L.; Fried, D.E.; Grants, I.; Rajasekhar, P.; Csizmadia, E.; Ajijola, O.; Watson, R.E.; Poole, D.P.; Robson, S.C.; et al. Enteric Glia Modulate Macrophage Phenotype and Visceral Sensitivity following Inflammation. *Cell Rep.* **2020**, *32*, 108100. [CrossRef] [PubMed]
49. Phillips, R.J.; Kieffer, E.J.; Powley, T.L. Loss of glia and neurons in the myenteric plexus of the aged Fischer 344 rat. *Anat Embryol.* **2004**, *209*, 19–30. [CrossRef]
50. Stenkamp-Strahm, C.; Patterson, S.; Boren, J.; Gericke, M.; Balemba, O. High-fat diet and age-dependent effects on enteric glial cell populations of mouse small intestine. *Auton. Neurosci. Basic Clin.* **2013**, *177*, 199–210. [CrossRef]
51. Baudry, C.; Reichardt, F.; Marchix, J.; Bado, A.; Schemann, M.; des Varannes, S.B.; Neunlist, M.; Moriez, R. Diet-induced obesity has neuroprotective effects in murine gastric enteric nervous system: Involvement of leptin and glial cell line-derived neurotrophic factor. *J. Physiol.* **2012**, *590*, 533–544. [CrossRef]
52. Voss, U.; Sand, E.; Olde, B.; Ekblad, E. Enteric neuropathy can be induced by high fat diet in vivo and palmitic acid exposure in vitro. *PLoS ONE* **2013**, *8*, e81413. [CrossRef]

53. Schoffen, J.P.F.; Santi Rampazzo, A.P.; Cirilo, C.P.; Zapater, M.C.U.; Vicentini, F.A.; Comar, J.F.; Bracht, A.; Marcal Natali, M.R. Food restriction enhances oxidative status in aging rats with neuroprotective effects on myenteric neuron populations in the proximal colon. *Exp. Gerontol.* **2014**, *51*, 54–64. [CrossRef] [PubMed]
54. Bush, T.G.; Savidge, T.C.; Freeman, T.C.; Cox, H.J.; Campbell, E.A.; Mucke, L.; Johnson, M.H.; Sofroniew, M.V. Fulminant jejuno-ileitis following ablation of enteric gila in adult transgenic mice. *Cell* **1998**, *93*, 189–201. [CrossRef]
55. Cornet, A.; Savidge, T.C.; Cabarrocas, J.; Deng, W.L.; Colombel, J.F.; Lassmann, H.; Desreumaux, P.; Liblau, R.S. Enterocolitis induced by autoimmune targeting of enteric glial cells: A possible mechanism in Crohn's disease? *Proc. Natl. Acad. Sci. USA* **2001**, *98*, 13306–13311. [CrossRef]
56. Von Boyen, G.B.T.; Schulte, N.; Pflüger, C.; Spaniol, U.; Hartmann, C.; Steinkamp, M. Distribution of enteric glia and GDNF during gut inflammation. *BMC Gastroenterol.* **2011**, *11*, 3. [CrossRef] [PubMed]
57. Villanacci, V.; Bassotti, G.; Nascimbeni, R.; Antonelli, E.; Cadei, M.; Fisogni, S.; Salerni, B.; Geboes, K. Enteric nervous system abnormalities in inflammatory bowel diseases. *Neurogastroenterol. Motil.* **2008**, *20*, 1009–1016. [CrossRef]
58. Zhang, D.K.; He, F.Q.; Li, T.K.; Pang, X.H.; Cui, D.J.; Xie, Q.; Huang, L.H.; Gan, H.T. Glial-derived neurotrophic factor regulates intestinal epithelial barrier function and inflammation and is therapeutic for murine colitis. *J. Pathol.* **2010**, *222*, 213–222. [CrossRef]
59. Hoff, S.; Zeller, F.; von Weyhern, C.W.H.; Wegner, M.; Schemann, M.; Klaus, M.; Ruhl, A. Quantitative assessment of glial cells in the human and guinea pig enteric nervous system with an anti-Sox8/9/10 antibody. *J. Comp. Neurol.* **2008**, *509*, 356–371. [CrossRef]
60. Coquenlorge, S.; Van Landeghem, L.; Jaulin, J.; Cenac, N.; Vergnolle, N.; Duchalais, E.; Neunlist, M.; Rolli-Derkinderen, M. The arachidonic acid metabolite 11β-ProstaglandinF2α controls intestinal epithelial healing: Deficiency in patients with Crohn's disease. *Sci. Rep.* **2016**, *6*, 25203. [CrossRef] [PubMed]
61. Geboes, K.; Rutgeerts, P.; Ectors, N.; Mebis, J.; Penninckx, F.; Vantrappen, G.; Desmet, V.J. Major histocompatibility class II expression on the small intestinal nervous system in Crohn's disease. *Gastroenterology* **1992**, *103*, 439–447. [CrossRef]
62. Koretz, K.; Momburg, F.; Otto, H.F.; Möller, P. Sequential induction of MHC antigens on autochthonous cells of ileum affected by Crohn's disease. *Am. J. Pathol.* **1987**, *129*, 493–502.
63. Turco, F.; Sarnelli, G.; Cirillo, C.; Palumbo, I.; De Giorgi, F.; D'Alessandro, A.; Cammarota, M.; Giuliano, M.; Cuomo, R. Enteroglial-derived S100B protein integrates bacteria-induced Toll-like receptor signalling in human enteric glial cells. *Gut* **2014**, *63*, 105–115. [CrossRef] [PubMed]
64. Bassotti, G.; Villanacci, V.; Cathomas, G.; Maurer, C.A.; Fisogni, S.; Cadei, M.; Baron, L.; Morelli, A.; Valloncini, E.; Salerni, B. Enteric neuropathology of the terminal ileum in patients with intractable slow-transit constipation. *Hum. Pathol.* **2006**, *37*, 1252–1258. [CrossRef] [PubMed]
65. Bassotti, G.; Villanacci, V.; Maurer, C.A.; Fisogni, S.; Di Fabio, F.; Cadei, M.; Morelli, A.; Panagiotis, T.; Cathomas, G.; Salerni, B. The role of glial cells and apoptosis of enteric neurones in the neuropathology of intractable slow transit constipation. *Gut* **2006**, *55*, 41–46. [CrossRef] [PubMed]
66. Bassotti, G.; Villanacci, V.; Nascimbeni, R.; Asteria, C.R.; Fisogni, S.; Nesi, G.; Legrenzi, L.; Mariano, M.; Tonelli, F.; Morelli, A.; et al. Colonic neuropathological aspects in patients with intractable constipation due to obstructed defecation. *Mod. Pathol.* **2007**, *20*, 367–374. [CrossRef] [PubMed]
67. Iantorno, G.; Bassotti, G.; Kogan, Z.; Lumi, C.M.; Cabanne, A.M.; Fisogni, S.; Varrica, L.M.; Bilder, C.R.; Munoz, J.P.; Liserre, B.; et al. The Enteric Nervous System in Chagasic and Idiopathic Megacolon. *Am. J. Surg. Pathol.* **2007**, *31*, 460–468. [CrossRef] [PubMed]
68. Stoffels, B.; Hupa, K.J.; Snoek, S.A.; Van Bree, S.; Stein, K.; Schwandt, T.; Vilz, T.O.; Lysson, M.; Van't Veer, C.; Kummer, M.P.; et al. Postoperative ileus involves interleukin-1 receptor signaling in enteric glia. *Gastroenterology* **2014**, *146*, 176–187.e1. [CrossRef]
69. Lilli, N.L.; Quénéhervé, L.; Haddara, S.; Brochard, C.; Aubert, P.; Rolli-Derkinderen, M.; Durand, T.; Naveilhan, P.; Hardouin, J.B.; De Giorgio, R.; et al. Glioplasticity in irritable bowel syndrome. *Neurogastroenterol. Motil.* **2018**, *30*, e13232. [CrossRef]
70. Jackson, M.; Olefson, S.; MacHan, J.T.; Kelly, C.R. A high rate of alternative diagnoses in patients referred for presumed clostridium difficile infection. *J. Clin. Gastroenterol.* **2016**, *50*, 742–746. [CrossRef]
71. Klem, F.; Wadhwa, A.; Prokop, L.J.; Sundt, W.J.; Farrugia, G.; Camilleri, M.; Singh, S.; Grover, M. Prevalence, Risk Factors, and Outcomes of Irritable Bowel Syndrome After Infectious Enteritis: A Systematic Review and Meta-analysis. *Gastroenterology* **2017**, *152*, 1042–1054.e1. [CrossRef] [PubMed]
72. Swan, C.; Duroudier, N.P.; Campbell, E.; Zaitoun, A.; Hastings, M.; Dukes, G.E.; Cox, J.; Kelly, F.M.; Wilde, J.; Lennon, M.G.; et al. Identifying and testing candidate genetic polymorphisms in the irritable bowel syndrome (IBS): Association with TNFSF15 and TNFα. *Gut* **2013**, *62*, 985–994. [CrossRef] [PubMed]
73. Spiller, R.C.; Jenkins, D.; Thornley, J.P.; Hebden, J.M.; Wright, T.; Skinner, M.; Neal, K. Increased rectal mucosal enteroendocrine cells, T lymphocytes, and increased gut permeability following acute Campylobacter enteritis and in post-dysenteric irritable bowel syndrome. *Gut* **2000**, *47*, 804–811. [CrossRef]
74. Fettucciari, K.; Ponsini, P.; Gioè, D.; Macchioni, L.; Palumbo, C.; Antonelli, E.; Coaccioli, S.; Villanacci, V.; Corazzi, L.; Marconi, P.; et al. Enteric glial cells are susceptible to Clostridium difficile toxin B. *Cell Mol. Life Sci.* **2017**, *74*, 1527–1551. [CrossRef] [PubMed]
75. Bassotti, G.; Macchioni, L.; Corazzi, L.; Marconi, P.; Fettucciari, K. Clostridium difficile-related postinfective IBS: A case of enteroglial microbiological stalking and/or the solution of a conundrum? *Cell Mol. Life Sci.* **2018**, *75*, 1145–1149. [CrossRef] [PubMed]

76. Yu, Y.B.; Zuo, X.L.; Zhao, Q.J.; Chen, F.X.; Yang, J.; Dong, Y.Y.; Wang, P.; Li, Y.Q. Brain-derived neurotrophic factor contributes to abdominal pain in irritable bowel syndrome. *Gut* **2012**, *61*, 685–694. [CrossRef]
77. Hoehner, J.C.; Wester, T.; Pahlman, S.; Olsen, L. Localization of neurotrophins and their high-affinity receptors during human enteric nervous system development. *Gastroenterology* **1996**, *110*, 756–767. [CrossRef]
78. Wang, P.; Du, C.; Chen, F.X.; Li, C.Q.; Yu, Y.B.; Han, T.; Akhtar, S.; Zuo, Z.L.; Di Tan, X.; Li, Y.-Q. BDNF contributes to IBS-like colonic hypersensitivity via activating the enteroglia-nerve unit. *Sci. Rep.* **2016**, *6*, 20320. [CrossRef] [PubMed]
79. Rajilić-Stojanović, M.; Biagi, E.; Heilig, H.G.H.J.; Kajander, K.; Kekkonen, R.A.; Tims, S.; de Vos, V.M. Global and deep molecular analysis of microbiota signatures in fecal samples from patients with irritable bowel syndrome. *Gastroenterology* **2011**, *141*, 1792–1801. [CrossRef]
80. Jeffery, I.B.; O'Toole, P.W.; Ohman, L.; Claesson, M.J.; Deane, J.; Quigley, E.M.M.; Simren, M. An irritable bowel syndrome subtype defined by species-specific alterations in faecal microbiota. *Gut* **2012**, *61*, 997–1006. [CrossRef]
81. Staudacher, H.M.; Lomer, M.C.E.; Anderson, J.L.; Barrett, J.S.; Muir, J.G.; Irving, P.M.; Whelan, K. Fermentable Carbohydrate Restriction Reduces Luminal Bifidobacteria and Gastrointestinal Symptoms in Patients with Irritable Bowel Syndrome. *J. Nutr.* **2012**, *142*, 1510–1518. [CrossRef]
82. Long, X.; Li, M.; Li, L.-X.; Sun, Y.-Y.; Zhang, W.-X.; Zhao, D.-Y.; Li, Y.Q. Butyrate promotes visceral hypersensitivity in an IBS-like model via enteric glial cell-derived nerve growth factor. *Neurogastroenterol. Motil.* **2018**, *30*, e13227. [CrossRef] [PubMed]
83. Devos, D.; Lebouvier, T.; Lardeux, B.; Biraud, M.; Rouaud, T.; Pouclet, H.; Coron, E.; des Varannes, S.B.; Naveilhan, P.; Nguyen, J.-M.; et al. Colonic inflammation in Parkinson's disease. *Neurobiol Dis.* **2013**, *50*, 42–48. [CrossRef] [PubMed]
84. Clairembault, T.; Kamphuis, W.; Leclair-Visonneau, L.; Rolli-Derkinderen, M.; Coron, E.; Neunlist, M.; Hol, E.M.; Derkinderen, P. Enteric GFAP expression and phosphorylation in Parkinson's disease. *J. Neurochem.* **2014**, *130*, 805–815. [CrossRef] [PubMed]
85. Lima, F.R.S.; Arantes, C.P.; Muras, A.G.; Nomizo, R.; Brentani, R.R.; Martins, V.R. Cellular prion protein expression in astrocytes modulates neuronal survival and differentiation. *J. Neurochem.* **2007**, *103*, 2164–2176. [CrossRef] [PubMed]
86. Natale, G.; Ferrucci, M.; Lazzeri, G.; Paparelli, A.; Fornai, F. Transmission of prions within the gut and toward the central nervous system. *Prion* **2011**, *5*, 142–149. [CrossRef]
87. Kujala, P.; Raymond, C.R.; Romeijn, M.; Godsave, S.F.; van Kasteren, S.I.; Wille, H.; Prusiner, S.B.; Mabbott, N.A.; Peters, P.J. Prion uptake in the gut: Identification of the first uptake and replication sites. *PLoS Pathog.* **2011**, *7*, 1002449. [CrossRef] [PubMed]
88. Luo, P.; Liu, D.; Li, C.; He, W.-X.; Zhang, C.-L.; Chang, M.-J. Enteric glial cell activation protects enteric neurons from damage due to diabetes in part via the promotion of neurotrophic factor release. *Neurogastroenterol. Motil.* **2018**, *30*, e13368. [CrossRef]
89. Piovezana Bossolani, G.D.; Silva, B.T.; Colombo Martins Perles, J.V.; Lima, M.M.; Vieira Frez, F.C.; Garcia de Souza, S.R.; Sehaber-Sierakowski, C.C.; Bersani-Amado, C.A.; Zanoni, J.N. Rheumatoid arthritis induces enteric neurodegeneration and jejunal inflammation, and quercetin promotes neuroprotective and anti-inflammatory actions. *Life Sci.* **2019**, *238*, 116956. [CrossRef]
90. Panizzon, C.P. do N.B.; Zanoni, J.N.; Hermes-Uliana, C.; Trevizan, A.R.; Sehaber, C.C.; Pereira, R.V.F.; Linden, D.R.; Hubner, M.; Neto, M. Desired and side effects of the supplementation with L-glutamine and L-glutathione in enteric glia of diabetic rats. *Acta Histochem.* **2016**, *118*, 625–631. [CrossRef]
91. Pereira, R.V.F.; Tronchini, E.A.; Tashima, C.M.; Alves, E.P.B.; Lima, M.M.H.; Zanoni, J.N. L-glutamine supplementation prevents myenteric neuron loss and has gliatrophic effects in the ileum of diabetic rats. *Dig. Dis Sci.* **2011**, *56*, 3507–3516. [CrossRef]
92. Do Nascimento Bonato Panizzon, C.P.; De Miranda Neto, M.H.; Ramalho, F.V.; Longhini, R.; De Mello, J.C.P.; Zanoni, J.N. Ethyl acetate fraction from Trichilia catigua confers partial neuroprotection in components of the enteric innervation of the jejunum in diabetic rats. *Cell Physiol. Biochem.* **2019**, *53*, 76–86.
93. De Santi-Rampazzo, A.P.; Schoffen, J.P.F.; Cirilo, C.P.; Zapater, M.C.V.U.; Vicentini, F.A.; Soares, A.A.; Peralta, R.M.; Bracht, A.; Buttow, N.C.; Natali, M.R.M. Aqueous extract of Agaricus blazei Murrill prevents age-related changes in the myenteric plexus of the jejunum in rats. *Evid. Based Complement. Alternat Med.* **2015**, *2015*, 287153.
94. Almeida, P.P.D.; Thomasi, B.B.D.M.; Costa, N.D.S.; Valdetaro, L.; Pereira, A.D.A.; Gomes, A.L.T.; Stockler-Pinto, M.B. Brazil Nut (Bertholletia excelsa H.B.K) Retards Gastric Emptying and Modulates Enteric Glial Cells in a Dose-Dependent Manner. *J. Am. Coll Nutr.* **2020**, 1–9. [CrossRef]
95. Abdo, H.; Mahé, M.M.; Derkinderen, P.; Bach-Ngohou, K.; Neunlist, M.; Lardeux, B. The omega-6 fatty acid derivative 15-deoxy-$\Delta^{12,14}$-prostaglandin J2 is involved in neuroprotection by enteric glial cells against oxidative stress. *J. Physiol.* **2012**, *590*, 2739–2750. [CrossRef] [PubMed]
96. Miyazaki, I.; Isooka, N.; Wada, K.; Kikuoka, R.; Kitamura, Y.; Asanuma, M. Effects of Enteric Environmental Modification by Coffee Components on Neurodegeneration in Rotenone-Treated Mice. *Cells* **2019**, *8*, 221. [CrossRef] [PubMed]
97. Ferreira, P.E.B.; Lopes, C.R.P.; Alves, A.M.P.; Alves, É.P.B.; Linden, D.R.; Zanoni, J.N.; Buttow, N.C. Diabetic neuropathy: An evaluation of the use of quercetin in the cecum of rats. *World J. Gastroenterol.* **2013**, *19*, 6416–6426. [CrossRef] [PubMed]
98. Lopes, C.R.P.; Ferreira, P.E.B.; Zanoni, J.N.; Alves, A.M.P.; Alves, É.P.B.; Buttow, N.C. Neuroprotective effect of quercetin on the duodenum enteric nervous system of streptozotocin-induced diabetic rats. *Dig. Dis. Sci.* **2012**, *57*, 3106–3115. [CrossRef]
99. De Souza, S.R.G.; de Neto, M.H.; Perles, J.V.C.M.; Frez, F.C.V.; Zignani, I.; Ramalho, F.V.; Hermes-Uliana, C.; Piovezana Bossolani, G.D.; Zanoni, J.N. Antioxidant effects of the quercetin in the jejunal myenteric innervation of diabetic rats. *Front. Med.* **2017**, *4*, 8. [CrossRef] [PubMed]
100. Ferreira, P.E.B.; Beraldi, E.J.; Borges, S.C.; Natali, M.R.M.; Buttow, N.C. Resveratrol promotes neuroprotection and attenuates oxidative and nitrosative stress in the small intestine in diabetic rats. *Biomed. Pharmacother.* **2018**, *105*, 724–733. [CrossRef]

101. Borges, S.C.; da Silva de Souza, A.C.; Beraldi, E.J.; Schneider, L.C.L.; Buttow, N.C. Resveratrol promotes myenteric neuroprotection in the ileum of rats after ischemia-reperfusion injury. *Life Sci.* **2016**, *166*, 54–59. [CrossRef]
102. Borges, S.C.; Ferreira, P.E.B.; da Silva, L.M.; de Paula Werner, M.F.; Irache, J.M.; Cavalcanti, O.A.; Buttow, N.C. Evaluation of the treatment with resveratrol-loaded nanoparticles in intestinal injury model caused by ischemia and reperfusion. *Toxicology* **2018**, *396–397*, 13–22. [CrossRef]
103. Sarnelli, G.; Seguella, L.; Pesce, M.; Lu, J.; Gigli, S.; Bruzzese, E.; Lattanzi, R.; D'Alessandro, A.; Cuomo, R.; Steardo, L.; et al. HIV-1 Tat-induced diarrhea is improved by the PPARalpha agonist, palmitoylethanolamide, by suppressing the activation of enteric glia. *J. Neuroinflammation.* **2018**, *15*, 94. [CrossRef]
104. De Filippis, D.; Esposito, G.; Cirillo, C.; Cipriano, M.; De Winter, B.Y.; Scuderi, C.; Sarnelli, G.; Cuomo, R.; Steardo, L.; De Man, J.G.; et al. Cannabidiol Reduces Intestinal Inflammation through the Control of Neuroimmune Axis. Gaetani S, editor. *PLoS ONE* **2011**, *6*, e28159. [CrossRef]
105. Li, H.; Fan, C.; Lu, H.; Feng, C.; He, P.; Yang, X.; Xiang, C.; Zuo, J.; Tang, W. Protective role of berberine on ulcerative colitis through modulating enteric glial cells–intestinal epithelial cells–immune cells interactions. *Acta Pharm Sin. B* **2020**, *10*, 447–461. [CrossRef]
106. Hosseinifard, E.S.; Morshedi, M.; Bavafa-Valenlia, K.; Saghafi-Asl, M. The novel insight into anti-inflammatory and anxiolytic effects of psychobiotics in diabetic rats: Possible link between gut microbiota and brain regions. *Eur J. Nutr.* **2019**, *58*, 3361–3375. [CrossRef] [PubMed]
107. Di Giancamillo, A.; Vitari, F.; Bosi, G.; Savoini, G.; Domeneghini, C. The chemical code of porcine enteric neurons and the number of enteric glial cells are altered by dietary probiotics. *Neurogastroenterol. Motil.* **2010**, *22*, e271-8. [CrossRef]
108. Yang, P.C.; Li, X.J.; Yang, Y.H.; Qian, W.; Li, S.Y.; Yan, C.H.; Wang, J.; Wang, Q.; Hou, X.H.; Dai, C.B. The Influence of Bifidobacterium bifidum and Bacteroides fragilis on Enteric Glial Cell–Derived Neurotrophic Factors and Inflammasome. *Inflammation* **2020**, *43*, 2166–2177. [CrossRef] [PubMed]
109. Serra, D.; Almeida, L.M.; Dinis, T.C.P. Dietary polyphenols: A novel strategy to modulate microbiota-gut-brain axis. *Trends Food Sci. Technol.* **2018**, *78*, 224–233. [CrossRef]
110. Kessler, M.; Ubeaud, G.; Jung, L. Anti- and pro-oxidant activity of rutin and quercetin derivatives. *J. Pharm Pharmacol.* **2003**, *55*, 131–142. [CrossRef] [PubMed]
111. Choi, E.J.; Kim, G.H. Quercetin accumulation by chronic administration causes the caspase-3 activation in liver and brain of mice. *Biofactors* **2010**, *36*, 216–221. [CrossRef] [PubMed]
112. Sibaev, A.; Yüce, B.; Kemmer, M.; Van Nassauw, L.; Broedl, U.; Allescher, H.D.; Goke, B.; Timmermans, J.P.; Storr, M. Cannabinoid-1 (CB1) receptors regulate colonic propulsion by acting at motor neurons within the ascending motor pathways in mouse colon. *Am. J. Physiol. Gastrointest Liver Physiol.* **2009**, *296*, G119–G128. [CrossRef]
113. Stanzani, A.; Galiazzo, G.; Giancola, F.; Tagliavia, C.; De Silva, M.; Pietra, M.; Fracassi, F.; Chiocchetti, R. Localization of cannabinoid and cannabinoid related receptors in the cat gastrointestinal tract. *Histochem Cell Biol.* **2020**, *153*, 339–356. [CrossRef]
114. Galiazzo, G.; Giancola, F.; Stanzani, A.; Fracassi, F.; Bernardini, C.; Forni, M.; Pietra, M.; Chiocchetti, R. Localization of cannabinoid receptors CB1, CB2, GPR55, and PPARα in the canine gastrointestinal tract. *Histochem Cell Biol.* **2018**, *150*, 187–205. [CrossRef]
115. Maselli, D.B.; Camilleri, M. Pharmacology, Clinical Effects, and Therapeutic Potential of Cannabinoids for Gastrointestinal and Liver Diseases. *Clin. Gastroenterol. Hepatol.* **2020**, S1542–S3565, 30504–30508. [CrossRef] [PubMed]
116. Inglet, S.; Winter, B.; Yost, S.E.; Entringer, S.; Lian, A.; Biksacky, M.; Pitt, R.D.; Mortensen, W. Clinical Data for the Use of Cannabis-Based Treatments: A Comprehensive Review of the Literature. *Ann. Pharmacother.* **2020**, *54*, 1109–1143. [CrossRef] [PubMed]
117. Martínez, V.; Iriondo De-Hond, A.; Borrelli, F.; Capasso, R.; Del Castillo, M.D.; Abalo, R. Cannabidiol and Other Non-Psychoactive Cannabinoids for Prevention and Treatment of Gastrointestinal Disorders: Useful Nutraceuticals? *Int. J. Mol. Sci.* **2020**, *21*, 3067. [CrossRef] [PubMed]
118. Hill, C.; Guarner, F.; Reid, G.; Gibson, G.R.; Merenstein, D.J.; Pot, B.; Morelli, L.; Canani, R.B.; Flint, H.J.; Salminen, S.; et al. The International Scientific Association for Probiotics and Prebiotics consensus statement on the scope and appropriate use of the term probiotic. *Nat. Rev. Gastroenterol. Hepatol.* **2014**, *11*, 506–514. [CrossRef]

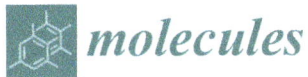

Review

Nutraceuticals: Transformation of Conventional Foods into Health Promoters/Disease Preventers and Safety Considerations

Mudhi AlAli [1], Maream Alqubaisy [1], Mariam Nasser Aljaafari [1], Asma Obaid AlAli [1], Laila Baqais [1], Aidin Molouki [2], Aisha Abushelaibi [3], Kok-Song Lai [1] and Swee-Hua Erin Lim [1,*]

1. Health Sciences Division, Abu Dhabi Women's College, Higher Colleges of Technology, Abu Dhabi 41012, United Arab Emirates; H00349412@hct.ac.ae (M.A.); H00349801@hct.ac.ae (M.A.); H00349760@hct.ac.ae (M.N.A.); H00323776@hct.ac.ae (A.O.A.); H00307981@hct.ac.ae (L.B.); lkoksong@hct.ac.ae (K.-S.L.)
2. Department of Avian Disease Research and Diagnostic, Razi Vaccine and Serum Research Institute, Agricultural Research Education and Extension Organization (AREEO), Karaj 31585-854, Iran; aidinmolouki@gmail.com
3. Dubai Colleges, Higher Colleges of Technology, Dubai 16062, United Arab Emirates; aabushelaibi@hct.ac.ae
* Correspondence: erinlimsh@gmail.com or lerin@hct.ac.ae; Tel.: +971-56-389-3757

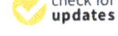

Citation: AlAli, M.; Alqubaisy, M.; Aljaafari, M.N.; AlAli, A.O.; Baqais, L.; Molouki, A.; Abushelaibi, A.; Lai, K.-S.; Lim, S.-H.E. Nutraceuticals: Transformation of Conventional Foods into Health Promoters/Disease Preventers and Safety Considerations. *Molecules* **2021**, *26*, 2540. https://doi.org/10.3390/molecules26092540

Academic Editors: Luisa Tesoriere and Sokcheon Pak

Received: 30 December 2020
Accepted: 27 March 2021
Published: 27 April 2021

Publisher's Note: MDPI stays neutral with regard to jurisdictional claims in published maps and institutional affiliations.

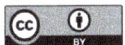

Copyright: © 2021 by the authors. Licensee MDPI, Basel, Switzerland. This article is an open access article distributed under the terms and conditions of the Creative Commons Attribution (CC BY) license (https://creativecommons.org/licenses/by/4.0/).

Abstract: Nutraceuticals are essential food constituents that provide nutritional benefits as well as medicinal effects. The benefits of these foods are due to the presence of active compounds such as carotenoids, collagen hydrolysate, and dietary fibers. Nutraceuticals have been found to positively affect cardiovascular and immune system health and have a role in infection and cancer prevention. Nutraceuticals can be categorized into different classes based on their nature and mode of action. In this review, different classifications of nutraceuticals and their potential therapeutic activity, such as anti-cancer, antioxidant, anti-inflammatory and anti-lipid activity in disease will be reviewed. Moreover, the different mechanisms of action of these products, applications, and safety upon consumers including current trends and future prospect of nutraceuticals will be included.

Keywords: functional foods; anti-cancer; anti-inflammation; antioxidant activity; anti-lipid activity; nutraceuticals safety and toxicity

1. Introduction

Since ancient times, conventional food and herbal extracts have been recognized as a fundamental part of the holistic approach to achieve complete wellness and health, especially in the ancient ayurvedic system in India, in addition to traditional Chinese, Roman, and Greek medicine [1]. The Greek physician Hippocrates adopted the philosophy of food as medicine, with his renowned quote "Let food be the medicine and medicine be the food" [2]. Throughout human history, many natural sources were utilized for their healing and strength restoring effects upon consumption, such as cinnamon, saffron, honey, garlic, ginger, pomegranate, mint, and many more [3].

Nutraceuticals are known as bioactive substances that are present in common food or botanical-based sources that can be delivered in the form of dietary supplements or functional food, supplying beneficial effects in addition to the nutritional essential components [4]. Nutraceuticals comprise a wide range of bioactive derivatives accumulated in edible sources including antioxidants, phytochemicals, fatty acids, amino acids, and probiotics. With either established previously or potential effects, nutraceuticals are well-known for their role of being involved in disease treatment and prevention, anti-aging properties, and malignancy prevention. Consuming probiotics is encouraged due to its significant role in the treatment and prevention of gastroenterological diseases [5]. Garlic, for example, has been suggested as a complementary therapy for high blood pressure and cholesterol [6].

With the presence of side effects induced by some pharmaceutical drugs and the emergence of antimicrobial resistance, nutraceutical compounds have gained attention as an alternative therapeutic and preventive approach alongside the advantages of being more affordable and available. Several studies have significantly shown the beneficial effects of nutraceutical ingredients on immune system functions. Such functions include enhancing the infection response mechanism, boosting immunomodulatory activity, and contributing to reducing the impacts of autoimmune disorders and hypersensitivity. Nutraceuticals have also been shown to exert lipid-lowering, anti-inflammatory, anti-cancer and antioxidant activity [7–10].

The immune system is a sophisticated host defense system, composed of different specialized cells and protein components acting as a unit in the defensive mechanism against diseases. The immune system is divided into two subsystems, commonly known as the innate and the adaptive immune systems. Both subsystems involve humoral and cellular responses. The innate immune system is based on unspecific defense strategies and components that are present from birth, starting with the first line defense (skin and mucous) and the second line, which comprises cellular mediated (granulocytes, macrophages, and dendritic cells), as well as humoral components including cytokines and complements. On the other hand, the adaptive immune system attains the immunological memory throughout previous exposure to several antigens. Therefore, this will induce a corresponding response regulated by a series of cell-mediated responses which consists of T lymphocytes responsible for recognizing pathogens and destroying them. In addition to B lymphocytes that produce specific antibodies corresponding to antigens or pathogens, it will also provide a neutralizing effect and protection against any harm that the body might encounter [11].

When it comes to boosting external immunity, vitamin C is the one of most popularly consumed compounds. Many studies have suggested the beneficial effects of vitamin C in improving the immune system by supporting the innate and adaptive systems, augmenting defense mechanisms such as phagocytosis and chemotaxis, as well as possessing antioxidant properties [12].

The acknowledgment of the science of nutraceuticals has been growing, with increased interest in finding novel therapeutic options by utilizing new technologies and scientific methods. Although many nutraceuticals have been reported for their effective properties in the immune system, there is a necessity of conducting more high-level, clearly evidenced clinical trials for further investigation regarding the long-term effects and public safety. We have observed that it is necessary to broadly exploit the medicinal properties and nutritional values of those compounds separately, because nutraceuticals still lie in the grey zone; being confused by many whether they should be administered as medicine, or if they are a basic nutrient need. The advanced exploration of their safety, bioactivity, and bioavailability perspective is crucial because it will contribute to translate these hypothetically potential natural nutraceutical compounds into implementable, validated, regulated, and approved effective medicinal products.

The main aim of this review is to highlight recent studies' outcomes of the immune-boosting properties of nutraceutical compounds and the potential therapeutic activities, including an overview on several types of nutraceuticals and different mechanisms of action on the immune system. Additionally, the safety of nutraceuticals, possible applications, and future prospects will be discussed.

2. Types of Nutraceuticals Based on Source, Nature and Application

Nutraceuticals have been classified based on their application into traditional, non-traditional, fortified, recombinant, phytochemical, herbal, functional foods, dietary supplements, probiotics and prebiotics [13,14]. Nutraceuticals with their different classes have a variety of applications and uses depending on their nature. The following subsections will discuss different nutraceutical classes. Table 1 also summarizes the classes of nutraceuticals with their beneficial effects to health.

The classification of nutraceuticals and their definitions tend to overlap due to the similarity among their chemical constituents and functions in delivering health benefits. The Institute of Food Technologists (IFT) defines functional foods as "foods and food components that provide a health benefit beyond basic nutrition". Examples may include conventional foods; fortified, enriched, or enhanced foods; and dietary supplements [15]. Traditional nutraceuticals are defined as natural foods with their potential health attributes: this may include, but is not limited to, fruits, vegetables, grains, fish, dairy and meat products [16]. Traditional foods or nutraceuticals can positively affect health by stimulating the immune system, and lowering the risk of heart diseases and cancers [17–19]. Looking at these definitions, the conclusion we have drawn is that nutraceuticals can be classified into traditional and non-traditional groups. Further subclassification of each will be discussed below, although some may overlap.

2.1. Traditional Nutraceuticals and Products

2.1.1. Functional Foods

Functional foods are foods with benefits in health improvement and disease prevention other than only providing nutrients [13,20]. These foods have ingredients that enhance antioxidant and anti-inflammatory activities, which are functional to prevent diseases such as type-2 diabetes [21]. These foods are made available for daily consumption for a specific population with a similar quality of other traditional foods in the market [22,23]. Examples of these functional foods are rice, wheat, kidney beans, soybeans, lentils, chocolate, citrus fruits, nuts, and fermented milk [13,24]. Rice is the first staple food consumed by the majority of populations; its nutritional value is as a source of carbohydrates, containing low levels of fat, salt and sugar, because all types of rice are gluten free and contain resistant starch that helps in the growth of healthy bowel bacteria [25]. Traditional rice varieties in India represent a great origin of minerals and vitamins such as niacin, thiamine, iron, riboflavin, vitamin D, and calcium; in addition, they hold higher fiber and lower amounts of sugar [26]. Wheat is the second staple food consumed across the world: wholegrain wheat is made up of three layers which are the bran, the endosperm, and the germ; wholegrain wheat can be processed to produce wheat bran and wheat germ [27]. Wheat brans represent the most beneficial part of wholegrain wheat due it their fiber content which is believed to play a role in improving gastrointestinal health [28].

Additionally, carrots and broccoli are examples of functional foods due to their active components such as sulforaphane, and lycopene [29]. Although functional foods have various health benefits due to several active ingredients, more studies with scientific evidence are needed to provide these products with health claims in their labels [22,30–32]. Some of the active ingredients in functional foods are carotenoids, collagen hydrolysate, dietary fibers, and fatty acids that possess various health benefits such as anti-inflammatory activity and enhance body immunity. In the following subsections, the nature and various health benefits of these functional ingredients will be discussed.

2.1.2. Carotenoids

Carotenoids are natural compounds and sources of pigmentation that accumulate abundantly in plants, fruits and vegetables, and algae. A wide range of carotenoid derivatives are found in the human diet, including α-carotene, β-carotene, β-cryptoxanthin, lutein, lycopene, zeaxanthin, crocetin, fucoxanthin and astaxanthin [33,34]. They are renowned for their wide spectrum of beneficial effects to health, including antioxidant and anti-inflammatory properties [35]. In addition, carotenoids exert health benefits over human vision, cognitive functions, heart functions, cancer prevention, and immune functions [36–38]. A study revealed the anti-inflammatory activity of two forms of carotenoids, astaxanthin and β-carotene, where both were found to be able to suppress the inflammation induced by *Helicobacter pylori* by inhibiting the production of reactive oxygen species and diminishing the level of inflammatory mediators being expressed [39].

Carotenoids are also known for their antioxidant activity, which is credited to their chemical structure consisting of a series of conjugated C=C bonds. This structure provides carotenoids with the ability to interact with free radicals and act as effective antioxidants [40]. Although carotenoids exhibit radical scavenging activity, which aids in diseases associated with increased oxidative stress, they also exhibit cyto-genotoxic activity.

2.1.3. Collagen Hydrolysate

Collagen is a primary protein in mammals that can be extracted from bovine connective tissues such as skin, bone, cartilage, and tendons. Collagen extraction is obtained by subjecting it to sources of hot water; this provides a partially hydrolyzed product called gelatin. In order to completely hydrolyze gelatin, a process of enzymatic hydrolysis takes place to produce collagen hydrolysates. Collagen hydrolysates provide various beneficial effects such as antioxidant, anti-aging, antitumor, anti-inflammatory and anti-obesity effects [41,42]. A study has shown the immune-boosting effects of collagen hydrolysates that have been extracted from domestic yak (*Bos grunniens*) bone and its potential in improving the adaptive and innate immunity in mice [43]. Furthermore, a study conducted to investigate the health benefits of collagen hydrolysate in females diagnosed with photoaged skin showed a remarkable improvement in skin hydration, wrinkling, and elasticity [44].

2.1.4. Dietary Fibers

Fibers are plant-based non-starch carbohydrates that are poorly digestible and provide various health benefits, as mentioned in many studies, and can be found naturally in a wide variety of foods including vegetables, fruits, wheat bran, oats and ispaghula husk [45–47]. Dietary fibers can be classified into more than two categories on the basis of their solubility in hot water, water-retaining capacity, and viscosity into soluble and insoluble fibers. Soluble fibers comprise viscous components such as β-glucans, fructans, and non-viscous fibers such as hemicellulose. Insoluble fibers tend to lose the characteristic of viscosity and they are insoluble in water; insoluble fibers tend to accelerate gastric emptying time which helps in relieving constipation, while soluble fibers tend to delay gastric emptying time [48]. High fiber diets are found to have a positive impact on inflammatory bowel diseases, because they can lessen the risk of Crohn's disease and ulcerative colitis [49].

2.1.5. Fatty Acids

Fatty acids are the component of oils and fats that are present in animal fats, fish oil supplements, seeds, olive oil, and coconuts. Aside from their role in energy storage, they have been documented for their ability to act as an anti-inflammatory and immunomodulatory component in various studies. In one study, the omega-3 polyunsaturated fatty acids (PUFAs) administered at a dose of >2.7 g/day for at least three months to patients with rheumatoid arthritis (RA) showed reductions in the severity of rheumatoid arthritis (RA) symptoms [50].

2.1.6. Phytochemicals

Phytochemicals are beneficial, concentrated or purified chemicals from plants that have active components for biochemical and metabolic reactions in humans, such as lutein and lycopene [13]. Phytochemicals can help in maintaining chemical balance of the brain, thus providing neuroprotective activity [51]. Additionally, high consumption of vegetables and fruits that contain phytochemicals can reduce the risk of cancers, and cardiac and neurodegenerative disorders [29,51].

2.1.7. Herbs

Herbs are plants that have no woody tissue and can be processed in many ways depending on each individual preference. Herbs can be dried; however, the drying process leads to a reduction in the effectiveness of herbal properties [52]. Herbs that are rich in antioxidant have been used in flavoring and aroma for more than two thousand years [53]. Garlic extracts, ginger root, and aloe gel are herbs that have health benefits such as reducing cholesterol, wound healing, and anti-ulcer and antioxidant activities [13,54].

2.1.8. Probiotics

Probiotics are microbes that are beneficial to health and used in food, especially in milk products, which are important to promote health by providing immunologic and digestive properties [55]. In addition, these live microbes can improve microbial intestinal balance. *Lactobacillus* with its different species is the most common probiotic used that will survive in the human gut. Currently, *Bifidobacterium* spp., and *Streptococcus* are also used as probiotic strains [56].

2.1.9. Prebiotics

Prebiotics are ingredients consisting of short chain carbohydrates that improve the probiotics' activity [57]. These prebiotics are literally fertilizing agents for probiotics that are not affected by gastric pH and stomach acids [13]. Prebiotics are non-digestible ingredients that promote the growth of productive microorganism and affect the composition and activity of gut microbiota. Fructo-oligosaccharides and inulin are examples of prebiotics used in functional foods to improve gastric health [57,58].

2.1.10. Dietary Supplements

Although not entirely a traditional approach, dietary supplements are products that can be taken as a dietary ingredient by individuals to maintain and improve health and not to cure diseases [13,59]. These supplements are found in various forms, such as tablets, liquid-based, capsules, powder, and concentrated with specific doses [2,60]. Omega-3, vitamins A, B, C, D, and E, iron, folic acid, minerals, calcium, magnesium, etc., are some examples of dietary supplements that can either be taken by an individual with or without prescription [2,59]. Moreover, these supplements can be consumed to ensure that a diet meets the sufficient nutrient requirements for the body and to prevent any deficiencies [61]. At the beginning of the 20th century, food extracts that contain important nutrients such as vitamin C, and B were shown to be helpful to prevent some serious conditions such as scurvy, pellagra, and beriberi [61,62].

2.2. Non-Conventional Approach

Non-traditional nutraceuticals, as a non-conventional approach, are artificially synthesized foods or food products. The application of biotechnology or agriculture breeding is used to add nutrient ingredients for the enhancement of food properties and human health. Based on the processing method, non-traditional nutraceuticals may be differentiated into fortified and recombinant nutraceuticals [14,60,63]. Rice enriched with β-carotene, and cereals infused with vitamins and minerals are some examples of this class of nutraceuticals which contain provitamin A that can boost antioxidant activity [13,64,65].

2.2.1. Fortified Nutraceuticals

Fortified nutraceuticals such as orange juice with calcium added, or milk with cholecalciferol vitamin are foods that contain additional micronutrients or vitamins added to them to improve their value [13,14,60]. These foods supply the body with important nutrients that can prevent anemia and improve health [2,66]. For example, if calcium is added to specific food such as orange juice, the orange juice can enhance glycemic control [67,68].

2.2.2. Recombinant Nutraceuticals

Recombinant nutraceuticals are foods that are produced by both genetic recombination and biotechnology [14]. This type of foods and crops are genetically modified to develop products that contain recombinant compounds and proteins that would be make them more beneficial to health [69]. Iron rice, golden rice, maize, golden mustard, multivitamin corn, and gold kiwifruit are examples of these nutraceuticals. Gold kiwifruit contains a recombinant gene that increases ascorbic acid levels, carotenoid, and lutein to enhance immune function. Additionally, it is considered a source of vitamins, potassium and fiber [70–72].

Table 1. Summary of types of nutraceuticals and their potential effects on health.

Class/Type of Nutraceutical	Examples	Active Ingredient	Advantages	References
Traditional approaches				
Functional foods	Tomatoes	Lycopene	Anticancer activities, e.g., lung and prostate, reduce blood pressure	[17]
	Salmon	Omega 3	Lower cardiovascular, diabetes disease risk	[19]
	Soy	Saponins	Antioxidant, detoxification of enzymes, stimulate immune response, hormonal metabolism	[18]
	Fermented milk and milk products	*L. acidophilus*, *Bifidobacterium* spp.	Prevent gastrointestinal infections, lower the level of cholesterol	[73]
	Marine algae	Fucoidans	Antioxidant, anticancer, anticoagulant activity	[74]
	Broccoli	Sulforaphane, glucosinolates	Decrease risk of several cancers, antioxidant	[29,75]
	Carrots	β-carotene	Reduce cancer risk, improve immune system	[29,76]
	Aloe	Aloins	Wound healing, antiulcer, anti-inflammatory, immunostimulant, antimicrobial activity, hematopoietic stimulation	[77,78]
	Turmeric	Curcumin	Anti-inflammatory, anticarcinogenic	[77,79]
Dietary supplements	Folic acid		Prevent defect in neural tubes, Red blood cells formation	[77,80]
	Vitamin A		Antioxidant, growth, treat some skin diseases	[60]
	Calcium		Bone, muscles, teeth nerve health, prevent osteoporosis	[81,82]
	Iron		Carry oxygen, produce energy	[60]
	Vitamin D		Bone and teeth health, help in calcium absorption, musculoskeletal health	[83]
Probiotics	*Lactobacillus acidophilus*, *Bifidobacterium* spp., *Streptococci*, *Enterococci*		Gut health, replace diarrhea-causing bacteria, anticancer	[60,84,85]

Table 1. Cont.

Class/Type of Nutraceutical	Examples	Active Ingredient	Advantages	References
Prebiotics	Fructo-oligosaccharides		Enhance probiotics growth, *bifidobacteria* growth enhancement	[58]
	Inulin		Enhance immune system, minerals absorption, protect bones	[57,84,86]
Non-conventional approach				
Fortified	Orange juice with calcium	Calcium, ascorbic acid	Glycemic control enhancement, sensitivity to insulin	[67]
	Anthocyanin-fortified bread	Anthocyanin	Reduce digestion rate	[68]
Recombinant	Gold kiwifruit	Ascorbic acid, carotenoids	Immune system enhancement	[13,71]

3. Classification of Nutraceuticals Based on Modes of Action

It is believed that nutraceuticals enhance human health and increase life expectancy along with many other processes that delay aging and prevent chronic diseases [87]. Many nutraceutical supplements have shown a positive impact on cardiovascular disease, cancer, diabetes, obesity, osteoporosis and immune functions [88–90]. Generally, nutraceutical modes of action take place to increase functional components which will lead to health enhancement [91]. This section will discuss various biological activities in nutraceuticals.

3.1. Anti-Cancer Activity

The use of nutraceuticals as chemo-preventative agents has been studied, and promising results were obtained as per their ability to prevent and treat cancer. Nutraceuticals of different origins have been shown to exhibit anti-cancer activity. Plants such as garlic, ginseng, curcumin, ginger, and green tea extract express several mechanisms of action against oncogenesis. Such mechanisms include the inhibition of DNA alkylation, tumor initiation, proliferation, and metastasis, in addition to the promotion of autophagy and intrinsic apoptosis [92]. Furthermore, nutraceuticals have been found to attenuate cancer signaling pathways that are believed to play a role in carcinogenesis [93]. Many studies have been conducted to evaluate nutraceuticals' modes of action against various types of cancer, and a wide range of nutraceuticals have been found to express anti-cancer properties against oral cancer, prostate cancer, breast cancer, lung cancer and colon cancer cells [94,95].

Activation of vitamin D receptor (VDR) results in cell cycle arrest, apoptosis, and anti-angiogenesis [96,97]. This receptor is an intracellular nuclear receptor found in organs and tissues. The active form of vitamin D binds to VDR, leading to activation of the growth arrest gene and *DNA-damage-inducible* gene [96,97]. This concludes that vitamin D deficiency would give rise to many diseases, while sufficient intake of vitamin D aids in disease prevention. In addition, the potentials of vitamins such as vitamin A, C and D have been studied for their mechanisms as anti-cancer agents. On the other hand, complementary therapy incorporating the nutraceutical herb *Clinacanthus nutans* and gemcitabine has been investigated. It has been found that application of *C. nutans* alone or combined with gemcitabine exhibited anti-proliferative effects on pancreatic cancer cells. The summary of this combinatory therapy is the upregulation of Bax and downregulation of Bcl-2, cIAP-2, and XIAP in human pancreatic cancer cells [98].

The role of prebiotics and probiotics has been investigated widely in colorectal cancer (CRC). Both prebiotics and probiotics are believed to be of benefit in promoting human health, specifically in the gastrointestinal tract. A study investigating the effect of prebiotics' anti-cancer activity showed that high fiber intake elevates the number of short chain fatty acids (SCFAs), thus producing bacteria and resulting in reduced number of colon tumors [99]. Similarly, a study aiming to investigate the prophylactic activity of *Lactobacillus rhamnosus* on the carcinogenesis of CRC showed that oral administration of this probiotic inhibited inflammation associated with tumor development by observing an increase in the expression of inflammatory proteins such as NFκB-p65, TNFα and iNOS [100]. Moreover, tumor incidence, tumor multiplicity, and tumor size are all reduced via consumption of probiotics *Lactobacilus acidophilus*, *Bifidobacteria* spp., and a combination of fructo-oligosaccharide and maltodextrin [101]. Additionally, the synbiotic mechanism lies in facilitating apoptotic responses to carcinogenesis-induced DNA damage in the colon, SCFA production, and downregulation of carcinogenic enzymes [102]. This concludes that the consumption of prebiotics and probiotics exerts immunomodulatory and anti-inflammatory activity and increases lactic acid-producing bacteria, which in return express their anti-cancer activity in colorectal cancer.

Prostate, breast, skin, lung, and liver cancer have been shown to be targeted by polyphenols particularly in green tea as chemo-preventive agents. Green tea is abundant with catechins that possess antioxidant, anti-inflammatory, antiproliferative, and antiangiogenic activity against cancer [103]. A study investigating habitual green tea consumption among human subjects revealed that Epigallocatechin gallate (EGCG) reduced the risk of prostate cancer [104]. Furthermore, the treatment of prostatic carcinoma cell line PC-3 with green tea polyphenol E induced cell death by prompting intracellular oxidative stress that subsequently inhibits the pro-survival pathway Akt [105]. Additionally, the administration of EGCG demonstrated an inhibitory effect on lung cancer cells by activating reactive oxygen species (ROS) that lead to oxidative DNA damage, causing cancerous growth inhibition [106]. Apart from this, a practical study evaluating the effect of EGCG on mammary tumors showed that the administration of poly E resulted in slowing tumor progression, reductions in metastasis, inhibiting mammary ductal growth, and affecting angiogenesis by reducing vascular endothelial growth factor (VEGF) levels. VEGF is an influential angiogenic factor that allows for tumor proliferation and metastatic growth [107]. Additionally, EGCG has shown its potential in inhibiting hepatocellular carcinoma growth by inhibiting the proliferation of HepG2 and PC12, as well as inducing tumor cell apoptosis [108].

Chemopreventive, chemosensitization, and radiosensitization effects have been indicated by curcumin. The curcumin mode of action refers to its ability in inhibiting multiple cell signaling pathways such as AP-1 signaling, NF-κB signaling, and the Wnt/beta-catenin signaling pathway [109]. The inhibition of NF-κB signaling increases cancer cells' vulnerability to radiotherapy; thus, curcumins' ability in inhibiting signaling pathways serves as one of its radiosensitizing activity. The administration of curcumin demonstrated the effects on T cell lymphoma, and the results indicate a decline in VEGF proteins resulting in angiogenesis inhibition [110]. In addition, the same study found that curcumin inhibits Glut1, thus resulting in decreased glucose uptake leading to induced apoptosis [110]. An in vitro study on breast cancer cells showed that curcumin decreased cell viability and induced apoptosis by targeting the PI3K signaling pathway [111]. Additionally, it has been found that curcumin up-regulates the expression of miR-99a, which consequently lead to deactivation of the JAK/STAT signaling pathway. The previous processes exerted antitumor results such as inhibited proliferation, migration, invasion, and induced apoptosis in retinoblastoma cells [112]. These examples explain curcumin's activity against tumor progression factors, which justify its chemopreventive effect.

Cell signaling modulation activity has been shown by resveratrol, a polyphenol acting as a chemosensitizer by inhibiting NF-κB and STAT3 pathways [113]. Furthermore, due to resveratrol's ability in reducing oxidative stress and upregulating the expression of survival proteins, it is used to reduce the cellular damage of chemotherapeutic agents [114].

A study conducted to assess the anti-cancer activity of resveratrol in melanoma determined that resveratrol downregulates NF-κB expression, which in return inhibits the expression of miR-221. The subsequent inhibition process leads to reductions in metastasis and cancer cell proliferation [115]. Additionally, a study revealed that the administration of resveratrol at high concentrations together with long-term treatment led to the promotion of apoptosis and suppression of cancerous cell growth in human non-small cell lung cancer [116]. Overall, nutraceuticals and functional foods participate in cancer treatment as either chemopreventive or chemosensitizing agents. Table 2 summarizes anti-cancer modes of action.

Table 2. Selected anti-cancer modes of action classified based on cancer type and nutraceutical.

Type of Cancer	Mode of Action	Nutraceutical	References
Prostate cancer	Antiproliferation, cell cycle inhibition, angiogenesis inhibition and promotion of apoptosis	Vitamin D	[117]
	Antioxidation, antiproliferation, and promotion of apoptosis	Catechins in green tea	[118,119]
Colon cancer	Tumor marker suppression, promotion of apoptosis, metastasis inhibition, and antiproliferation	Polyphenols	[120,121]
	Antioxidant, antiproliferation, promotion of apoptosis, inflammatory protein inhibition	Terpenoids	[122,123]
	Autophagy induction and promotion of apoptosis	Alkaloids	[124–126]
	Induction of DNA hypomethylation, promotion of apoptosis, and antiproliferation	Micronutrients	[127,128]
Breast cancer	Antiproliferation, angiogenesis inhibition, and promotion of apoptosis	Allicin in garlic	[129–131]
	Antiproliferation and promotion of apoptosis	Curcumin	[132]
	Cell cycle inhibition, promotion of apoptosis, and inhibition of metastasis	Vitamin D	[133,134]
Oral cancer	Prevent tumor initiation	Strawberry	[127]
	Antioxidation	Rosemary	[128]
	Antiproliferation, promotion of apoptosis, and angiogenesis inhibition	Geraniol	[135]

3.2. Anti-Inflammatory Activity

Nutraceuticals exert anti-inflammatory activities which help in the prevention and treatment of chronic inflammation-associated diseases [136]. Another benefit of nutraceuticals as anti-inflammatory agents is that they can be used as a complementary alternative to anti-inflammatory therapeutic drugs, which leads to a reduction in drug dosage, and therefore reducing side effects [137]. Chronic inflammation is the major cause of chronic diseases such as cardiovascular diseases, pulmonary diseases, diabetes, and cancer [136].

Suppression of inflammatory cytokines such as interleukins, TNF-α and cyclooxygenase-2 (COX-2) can occur upon the administration of a potent anti-inflammatory such as curcumin [138]. Curcumin can act as an anti-inflammatory agent which can help in the prevention and treatment of periodontitis [139]. Curcumin can reduce inflammation in patients suffering from chronic cutaneous complications and improve patient's condition suffered from chronic pruritis caused by a chemical sulfur mustard by reducing IL-8 and high-sensitivity c-reactive protein (hs-CRP) [140].

PUFAs are an example of nutraceuticals that have been shown to control inflammatory disorders [141]. Treatment with PUFA reduced the expression of NF-κB. In addition, a reduction in proinflammatory markers and an increase in IL-10 anti-inflammatory marker was observed in patients suffering from Duchenne muscular dystrophy [142]. Another example of a nutraceutical component is lycopene, which is an anti-inflammatory molecule found in tomatoes that can protect the heart and prevent cardiovascular diseases such as atherosclerosis and myocarditis [143,144]. A meta-analysis conducted to evaluate the association between lycopene and cardiovascular disease (CVD) showed a reduction in CVD risk by 17% [145].

Probiotics with anti-inflammatory activity, exert its anti-inflammatory effect through modulation of the NF-κB signaling pathway, inflammatory cytokines, and the regulatory T cell response [146]. For instance, the mixture of probiotics *L. rhamnosus*, *Bifidobacterium lactis*, and *Bifidobacterium longum* exhibited anti-inflammatory activity by inducing IL-10 and reducing proinflammatory cytokine production [147]. Additionally, prebiotics have also been suggested to express anti-inflammatory and immunomodulatory functions [148]. Pretreatment with β-(1,3)-glucan prevented clinical manifestations of dextran sulfate sodium-induced inflammatory bowel disease and inhibited the expression of inflammatory cytokines and reactive oxygen species (ROS) in mice [149].

Anti-inflammatory activities have also been exhibited by ginger, cinnamon, peppermint, and lycopene. Ginger and its compounds exert anti-inflammation activity which can reduce the inflammation [150]. In a study, orally administered ginger to newborn rats with necrotizing enterocolitis showed a reduction in TNF-α, IL-1β, and IL-6, which indicated a significant reduction in the inflammation [150], as well as inhibiting the acute inflammatory response in ulcerative colitis [151]. Furthermore, cinnamon extracts were able to inhibit more than 90% of the expression of IL-1 at the concentration of 50 μg/mL, and peppermint extracts were capable of reducing 90% of the expression of IL-6 at the concentration of 50 μg/mL; both indicated potent levels of anti-inflammatory activity [152]. Table 3 summarizes anti-inflammatory modes of action.

Table 3. Selected anti-inflammatory modes of action classified based on nutraceutical and benefits.

Mode of Action	Nutraceutical	Benefits	Reference
Reduce nitric oxide synthase (iNOS), tumor necrosis factor-α (TNF-α), production of nitric oxide (NO), interleukin-1β (IL-1β), nuclear factor kappa B (NF-κB)	Resveratrol	Neuroprotective	[153]
Inhibit the activation of NF-κB and limits the inflammatory response, such as ICAM-1, MCP-1, Cox-2, TNF-α, IL-1β, and IL-6	Baicalin	Improvement of trinitrobenzene sulphonic acid (TNBS) induced colitis	[154]
Reduce the expression of TNF-α, COX-2, 5-LOX, and IL-6 and increase IL-10 levels	Flavocoxid	Protects from sepsis	[155]

Table 3. Cont.

Mode of Action	Nutraceutical	Benefits	Reference
Reduces the expression of TNFα, IL-1β and reduces myeloperoxidase (MPO) activity	Curcumin	Improve dextran sulfate sodium (DSS)-induced colitis	[156]
Decreases the expression of iNOS and COX-2	6-Gingerol	Protects from carbon tetrachloride (CCl4)-induced liver fibrosis	[157]
Inhibits the expression of TLR4 and NF-κB and suppress iNOS, COX-2, TNF-α, IL-6, and IL-1β	Apigenin	Protects against blood-brain barrier disruption	[158]
Reduced the expression of TNF-α, IL-1β, and IL-6 and increases IL-10 expression. Decreases TLR-2 and TLR-4 expression Inhibits phosphorylation of I-κB, p65, p38, ERK, and JNK	Piperine	Reduces inflammatory injury in *Staphylococcus aureus* endometritis.	[159]
Suppresses the activity of renal MPO	Naringin	Decreases neutrophil infiltration in the kidneys.	[160]
Reduces NF-kappa B p65 subunit activation which decreases inflammatory cells and reduces cytokine secretion	Eucalyptol	Potential agent in the treatment of cigarette smoke-induced acute lung inflammation.	[161]
Suppresses NF-kB and p38 and reduces the level of TNF-α and IL-1β levels	Ortho-eugenol	Treatment of pain and inflammation.	[162]

3.3. Antioxidant Activity

Oxidative stress is a result of the accumulation of free radicals in the body which can subsequently lead to the development of various chronic diseases such as cancer, cardiovascular and autoimmune disease, ischemic disease, atherosclerosis, diabetes mellitus, and hypertension [163,164]. Normally, redox (reduction and oxidation) balance of the cell maintains the generation and the removal of reactive oxygen species (ROS) [165]. However, an imbalance in redox will result in the accumulation of ROS and reducing antioxidant ability to neutralize ROS effects, which subsequently induces oxidative stress [166,167].

Exogenous antioxidants such as vitamin C, vitamin E, and phenolic antioxidants are capable of removing free radicals [168]. Free radicals such as hydroxyl radicals and superoxide anion radicals can be scavenged by vitamin C [168]. Vitamin C is a potent antioxidant that protects cells and DNA from oxidative stress by scavenging free radicals [169]. Vitamin E and vitamin C are capable of protecting cells from lipid peroxidation [170].

Ginger extract and quercetin are also antioxidants; however, the ability of ginger extract to inhibit hydroxyl radicals is greater than quercetin [171]. Ginger extract showed an increase in the antioxidant enzyme and a reduction in the oxidative stress in blood [172].

The main sources of antioxidants are food, vitamins, and supplements. Foods such as fruits and vegetables are considered a great source of antioxidants due to their high levels of vitamins and phytochemicals [173]. Beetroot contains betalain and phenolic compounds which cause an increase in the resistance of low-density lipoproteins (LDLs) to oxidation [174], protect the liver from damage [175], and decrease blood pressure [176]. Dried fruits are a good source of antioxidants and have health benefits to humans. They can reduce glucose levels in the blood in addition to reducing risk factors associated with heart disease [177].

Dates are an example of dried fruit which contains two compounds, isoflavones and lignans; these two compounds can act as antioxidants which have a role in diabetes and are capable of modulating the secretion of pancreatic insulin [178]. Nuts such as pistachios are a rich source of antioxidants [179] which can reduce oxidative stress and prevent or lower the risk of chronic diseases [180]. Pistachios and other nuts such as walnuts and pecans contain polyphenolic compounds which act as antioxidants [181] that might protect against diseases associated with the accumulation of free radicals [180].

3.4. Anti-Lipid Activity

Nutraceuticals such as vitamins, minerals, and antioxidants are considered useful in the management of hypercholesterolemia in many conditions such as hypertension, diabetes, and cardiovascular disease [88,182,183]. Hypercholesterolemia is a term used to describe the presence of excessive low-density lipoproteins in blood [184]. The effects of nutraceuticals on lowering lipid profiles in hypercholesterolemic patients have been investigated; therefore, this section will discuss nutraceuticals' activity on multiple conditions associated with elevated lipid levels. The application of nutraceuticals as hypolipidemic agents has shown great potential in lowering total cholesterol (TC) and low-density lipoprotein (LDL) concentrations. Lipid-lowering nutraceuticals can be classified into three groups based on their mechanism of action. Such mechanisms include the inhibition of cholesterol absorption, inhibition of cholesterol synthesis, and excretion of LDL [185].

Plant sterol foods or supplements have displayed effectiveness in lowering lipid profiles. It has been established that plant sterols modify lipid profiles by decreasing the intestinal absorption of cholesterol [186]. It has been found that the intake of plant sterols demonstrated an effect on lipid profiles by lowering the concentrations of triglycerides and LDL in individuals at risk or suffering from type-2 diabetes mellitus [187]. A study examining the effectiveness of plant sterol-enriched yogurt has demonstrated a modified lipid profile resulting in reduced TC and LDL concentrations [188]. Moreover, the additive effect of plant sterols with lipid-lowering therapies have been investigated, and it has been determined that the addition of plant sterols to atorvastatin or ezetimibe resulted in further reductions in total and low density cholesterol [189].

Red yeast rice (RYR) exhibited potent effects on lowering lipid profiles in patients suffering from cardiovascular disease and dyslipidemia [190–192]. A study was conducted to assess a group of nutraceuticals on their lipid modifying ability; the nutraceuticals of choice were berberine, RYR and monacolin K, policosanol, and folic acid. The results demonstrated that RYR significantly lowered TC and LDL [183]. The combination of fermented red rice, liposomal berberine, and curcumin showed great results in improving lipid profiles and reducing inflammatory markers in individuals suffering from hypercholesterolemia [193]. RYR possess many functional components, although monacolin K may be a major contributor to its effectiveness. Monacolin K mechanism of action lies in decreasing hepatic cholesterol synthesis and inhibiting cholesterol absorption [194].

The consumption of dietary fibers is considered an effective approach in modulating lipid profiles. Dietary fibers are divided into soluble and insoluble fibers. Soluble fibers are more beneficial because they are fermented by the microbiota of the large intestine [195].

Cholesterol-lowering activity has been demonstrated by berberine, a plant alkaloid known for its cholesterol-lowering activity [196]. Similarly, curcumin is also considered a hypolipidemic agent that reduces TC, LDL and triglycerides, which is explained by increased cholesterol excretion [197].

In summary, many nutraceuticals and functional foods have been proven for their ability in regulating lipid profiles. Owing to their mechanism of action, nutraceuticals can either inhibit cholesterol synthesis, inhibit cholesterol absorption, or enhance cholesterol excretion. Each nutraceutical mentioned above may display a single or combined mechanism of action, resulting in lowered TC and LDL.

4. Nutraceuticals' Safety on Consumers

The majority of nutraceuticals on the market are safe for human consumption and only in some instances may cause harm because some nutraceuticals have toxic effects on human health. Studies have shown that some widely consumed nutraceuticals possess many health benefits with very minimal toxicity when used in correct controllable amounts. Nutraceuticals such as anthocyanins, polyphenols, and catechins are widely used and are safe for human consumption on controlled use. There have been very few studies that have indicated how these substances are harmful to human health.

Nevertheless, studies on nutraceuticals have shown that benefits of use outweigh the risk, and they are widely approved for human use within the correct amounts and dosages [185]. However, misuse and overuse of these products may pose health risks to humans. The safety of these nutraceuticals on consumers basically depends on the type, time, and the quantity used. Use of some nutraceuticals, especially when one is under medication, can result in interactions between the drug and the nutraceutical compounds causing very harmful effects on the body [198]. Thus, for safe usage, they should be used only when prescribed by qualified personnel at the right quantity, the correct quality, and timing.

Among the most important features of nutraceuticals are their cost effectiveness, broad safety profiles both in humans and animals, tolerability, and easy availability [199]. Despite a broad safety profile, few of them are reported to have been compromised due to contamination with heavy metals, toxic pesticides, drugs having potentials for abuse, potentially toxic plants, fertilizers, and mycotoxins [200,201]. Unfortunately, the safety profile of a large number of nutraceuticals is yet to be explored, and thus insufficient safety data are available for these agents. Understanding of the pharmacokinetic behavior of every drug is extremely important for the understanding of safety profile (toxico-kinetics), onset of action, required dose, and dose frequency. Furthermore, interactions with other drugs as well as nutrients/foods are another vital aspect of safety evaluations of nutraceuticals that assess the effect of interactions on safety, efficacy, half-life and subsequent therapeutic response [198].

In a majority of countries, including the United States, nutraceuticals are included in the dietary supplements list and may not be subject to the laws and regulations for safety standards of allopathic drugs. In 1994, the U.S. Congress established a regulation called the "Dietary Supplements Health & Education Act" which included nutraceuticals in a dietary list. These are not considered drugs; therefore, their sale without any safety and efficacy evaluation is permitted. However, as per regulations of the European Union, these herbal agents must prove scientific evidence of safety, efficacy, and quality before being licensed for use in the public. Toxicity and therapeutic evaluations of nutraceuticals are difficult as compared to pure synthetic compound-based products because they have multiple compounds and usually are a complex mixture of several compounds. Furthermore, their chemical composition varies based on the area of plant collection, variable effects of fertilizers/pesticides, and effect of stress [202]. All of the above factors, in addition to the unavailability of well-established techniques for extraction, identification, chemical composition, purity, potency, and safety of active pharmaceutical ingredients are the limiting factors of nutraceuticals, responsible for batch to batch variation and the un-reproducibility of therapeutic responses [203]. Furthermore, nutraceuticals comprise numerous compounds which can act synergistically as well as mediate an antagonistic response. Both of these effects may range from high therapeutic outcomes to toxicity and possibly a sub-therapeutic response [204].

In short, the use of nutraceuticals is tremendously increased both in humans as well as in veterinary products. Consequently, toxicity risks associated with their use are also increased due to the unavailability of large-scale evaluations of their safety and efficacy in clinical trials. Furthermore, controlling variations and the presence of adulterants such as heavy metals, agricultural chemicals, and mycotoxins, as well as proper pharmacokinetic and dynamic evaluations are extremely necessary for more effective utilization of these important alternative agents.

4.1. Nutraceuticals Associated with Genotoxicity and Carcinogenicity

Nutraceutical-associated genotoxicity is the potential of a nutraceutical product or its component to cause DNA lesion resulting in cellular death or genetic mutations, which may lead to various types of cancers. However, *Aloe vera* is recommended as a remedy for many diseases; studies involving oral therapy with *Aloe vera* whole leaf extract for two years in F344/N rats evidenced some carcinogenic effects [205–208]. *Aloe vera* gel has been generally found to be less genotoxic and less mutagenic as compared to whole leaf extracts [209], and in agreement, it was unable to induce significant mutagenic effects in *S. typhimurium* TA100 strain [210]. However, a positive mutagenic response was observed when an *E. coli* repair-deficient mutant was treated with *A. vera* pulp extract [211]. Danthron, an aloe constituent, is reported to initiate DNA damage and cause caspase-induced apoptosis via Bax-elicited and mitochondrial permeability transition pore pathways in human gastric cancer cells [212].

In a different study, mutagenic effects were observed via the development of hepatocellular carcinoma and hepa-blastoma in B6C3F1 mice in the presence and absence of external S9 (liver extract from hamsters and rats) metabolic activation after chronic administration of *Ginkgo biloba*. Mutagenic effects in *S. typhimurium* strains TA98 and TA, and *E. coli* WP2 *uvrA* pKM101 strain were also observed [213]. Several in-vitro studies using cell lines demonstrated *G. biloba* as well as its isolated components including quercetin, kaempferol-induced cytotoxicity, and mutagenicity [214]. However, no genotoxicity was experienced in androstane receptor knockout and *gpt* delta mice following oral administration of 2000 mg/kg *G. biloba* extract [215,216]. Therefore, testing against *S. typhimurium* (TA98, TA100 strains) and *E. coli* (WP2 *uvrA*/pKM101 strain) revealed that 1–10 mg/plate of goldenseal root powder was not mutagenic, while hepatocellular carcinoma/adenoma were observed in F344/N rats and B6C3F1 mice orally supplemented with the same nutraceutical for two years. However, when supplementation was performed only for three months, increases in micro-nucleated erythrocyte frequencies were not significant [217]. In vitro studies on HepG2 cells using commercial goldenseal products suggested that it damages DNA, indicated by the induction of gamma-H2AX, which is a biomarker of DNA damage and breaks [218].

Consumption of herbal products has been tremendously increased worldwide despite inconsistencies in scientific evidence, although their health promoting benefits are reported by numerous studies. Results of these studies suggest that despite dietary supplements, herbs, and nutraceuticals are generally considered safe, however there is still a need for rigorous toxicological testing. The currently available data regarding genotoxic and mutagenic effects of these products are insufficient to provide conclusive outcomes of the safe use of all nutraceuticals.

4.2. Models to Evaluate Safety, Efficacy, and Potential Toxicities of Nutraceuticals

Several models have been developed to evaluate the safety, efficacy, and toxicity of nutraceutical products and their active ingredients. Bioactive ingredients present in nutraceuticals have exhibited diverse pharmacological properties such as antioxidant, sedative, hypnotic, anti-inflammatory, immuno-modulatory and adaptogenic attributes [219–223]. Subsequently, these products were applied and their efficiency appraised using in vitro, in vivo, in silico, high-throughput in vitro, and omics technology-reliant assays [224]. Furthermore, various animal models have been used for in vivo, invasive, and non-invasive studies depending upon study design [225]. Some invertebrate models have been developed for safety and efficacy evaluations of nutraceuticals [226,227]. Currently, some alternative safety evaluation models are more preferred [228]. Novel and mechanism-based predictive kinetic models have also been developed, which provide very useful information regarding pathways involved in toxicity and efficacy [229,230].

4.3. Toxicities Based on Interactions of Nutraceuticals with Other Drugs

Interaction of a drug with any herbal or dietary supplement may lead to severe undesirable health consequences [231]. Several factors including age, simultaneously administered drugs, and multiple co-morbidities such as hypertension, diabetes, cancer, and infectious diseases contribute to these unwanted interactions and pre-dispose patients to the side effects of nutraceuticals. Of particular importance are drugs with a low therapeutic index such as digitalis glycosides, anticoagulant drugs, chemotherapeutics, psychoactive agents, and immune-modulators which can lead to life threatening reactions if their concentrations rise beyond the safety range due to interactions [231]. Some nutraceuticals are inducers and inhibitors of cytochrome P450 (CYTP450) iso-enzymes, and thus induce or inhibit liver enzymes responsible for the metabolism of these drugs [232–234]. For instance, several phytochemicals present in *G. biloba* are inducers as well as inhibitors of CYP450 [235,236]. Ginseng is an inducer of CYP450, whereas grapefruit juice is an inhibitor of it. Likewise, peppermint oil is a well-studied inducer of several CYP450 isoforms including CYP1A2, CYP2C9, CYP2C19 and CYP3A4 [237]. Furthermore, St. John's wort and its constituents inhibit CYP3A4-induced metabolism of testosterone and midazolam. Studies revealed that several fold increases in the metabolic activity of hepatic CYP3A2 were observed fourteen days subsequently of St. John's wort administration [238,239]. Moreover, ginseng, an inhibitor of P-glycoproteins type efflux pumps, causes a 3–4-fold increase in the activity of several drugs [238]. St. John's wort administration has major effects on the kinetics and dynamics of several drugs, especially when poly-pharmacy is involved [240,241]. Most types of drug may affect nutriture, directly or indirectly, whereas nutriture affects drug disposition and subsequent therapeutic responses.

4.4. Contaminants Compromising the Quality of Nutraceuticals

Several toxic adulterants or contaminants such as heavy metals, pesticides, mycotoxins, phytotoxicants, and abused drugs can significantly compromise the quality as well as use of nutraceuticals. Mixing of these adulterants in high amounts can lead to severe health consequences and even death [242]. For instance, pyrrolizidine alkaloids are among the most toxic alkaloids present in several plant species. These alkaloids contaminate several foods and nutraceuticals and react with proteins causing abnormal mitosis, tissue necrosis, and cellular dysfunctions [243–245]. These are hepatotoxic and have carcinogenic and cytotoxic potentials [242].

On the other hand, microbial contamination may contribute to a deterioration in the quality and stability of dietary foods and supplements [246]. For example, a Polish study showed that from 152 products and samples tested, 92.1% and 86.8% exhibited different degrees of bacterial and fungal contamination, respectively [246].

Mycotoxins are fungal secondary metabolites which significantly affect food and nutraceutical quality. These are usually unintentionally added to the foods/products during cultivation, storage, and transportation. Some common mycotoxins include citrinin, aflatoxins, ochratoxins and other molds and their spores [247,248]. Likewise, heavy metals including mercury, arsenic, cadmium and lead are contaminates added during harvesting or storage; therefore, the World Health Organization (WHO) strongly recommends to evaluate all herbal products for heavy metal contents due to their severe side effects [249]. Similarly, widespread use of pesticides causes accumulation in the products and causes toxicity [250].

4.5. Regulatory Status of Nutraceuticals

Several organizations including government agencies have promoted nutraceuticals and functional foods, and the public awareness regarding the use of these products has been increased. In several countries, no specific standard guidelines are available regarding the production and use of nutraceuticals. In the United States, some guidelines are provided in the Dietary Supplement Health and Education Act (DSHEA), adopted by congress for implementation in 1994. Likewise, in Poland, the Food and Nutrition Safety Act was adopted in 2006, whereas Canada has framed specific guidelines in their Food and Drugs Act [16,251]. Proper regulatory recognition of these products will excel the pharmaceutical industry with many new products and subsequent expansion of its market. A majority of countries have not adopted specific regulatory guidelines for nutraceuticals, which could possibly cause flooding of the healthcare sector with low-quality products, especially in developing countries. Thus, there is a dire need for the global health community to prepare regulatory guidelines for nutraceuticals to protect the market from the entry of spurious and low-quality drugs. Furthermore, rigorous scientific research is necessary both in the field of functional foods and nutraceuticals to uncover their exact mechanisms of action as well as potential adverse effects.

4.6. Effects of Processing on Nutraceuticals

Previous work considering some post-harvest abiotic elicitors proposed nonthermal processing technologies (i.e., ultrasound, high pressure processing (HPP), and pulsed electric fields (PEF)) to enhance the production of secondary metabolites. Interestingly, however, the outcome of these effects have been shown to be highly similar to conditions of plants under duress [252]. These treatments activate the biosynthesis of nutraceuticals in crops by a similar mechanism exerted by wound stress. Another study has shown that ultrasound treatment increases the levels of carotenoids in carrots [253]. Furthermore, the same treatment enhanced phenylalanine ammonia-lyase activity (PAL) and phenolic compounds in Panax ginseng [254], while phenolic compounds were increased in romaine lettuce [255]. A different study has shown that HHP increased ascorbic acid, phenolic compounds, and carotenoids in ataulfo mango [256]. Additionally, potato metabolism showed PEF-specific responses characterized by changes in the hexose pool, which may result in starch and ascorbic acid degradation [257]. The inadvertent production of metabolites may further enhance the exerted health benefits of such foods compared to foods which are consumed directly post-harvest. However, this is an area that is still under research, and the perceived benefits in the long term to human health are very much unexplored.

5. Current Trends and Future Prospects of Nutraceuticals

Over the last 20 years, there has been a rapid increase in the use of nutraceuticals due to mass information available on internet sources coupled with increased public awareness of health issues [258]. The marked side effects and ineffectiveness of modern pharmaceuticals have compelled people to look for nutraceuticals as alternative therapy [259]. Nutraceuticals for a medicinal use have been justified on the basis that they treat disease caused by the deficiency of nutrients. Clear evidence has been reported that nutraceutical supplementation improves health and prevents diseases [260]. The treatment through nutraceutical supplementation does not involve diagnosis by a trained practitioner, and nutraceuticals with antioxidant activity are expected to have beneficial effects on the whole body rather than to treat symptoms of a disease state. Consumers of nutraceuticals control their health comfortably without needing consultation with their physicians.

Self-medications with nutraceutical for the long term may result in cost implications to the consumers and may be more expensive as compared to other medications, despite their benefits [261]. This is due to glorification of the benefits of nutraceuticals via advertising and media coverage. Health professionals such as general physicians, nurses, pharmacists, and nutritionist are well aware of nutraceuticals, and educate their patients or consumers about the appropriate use of such products. Self-medication of nutraceuticals for serious diseases is inappropriate, while their long-term use is safe and beneficial for the prevention of chronic diseases. Nutraceuticals for serious diseases involve carnitine and flaxseed oil mostly used for cardiovascular disease, and antioxidants mostly for the prevention of cancer. Currently, many nutraceutical consumers believe that dietary supplements may be safer than other synthetic substances, but their presumption could be wrong and medical diagnosis is required for serious disease to prescribe effective conventional medicines. It has been reported that self-medication with complementary medicine has increased in diabetic patients [262,263].

Manufacturers of nutraceuticals are well informed about the production cost and profit. Manufacturers of nutraceuticals are also frequently launching new products into the market to expand the nutraceutical industry. The use of nutraceuticals has been encouraged for the prevention and treatment of chronic diseases. For example, green tea and soy products are used to prevent cancer [264].

The developments of new medicines are more expensive and riskier than the already available drugs in the market; therefore, most pharmaceutical companies are turning to marketing nutraceuticals. The drug company "Novartis" has also launched functional food for the health of consumer in the market and pharmacies [265]. In October 1998, Dean Farms, Tring and Hertfordshire introduced "Columbus healthier eggs" which were rich in fatty acid and available in all major supermarkets [266]. Similarly, burgeon bread is another example of function food, which was introduced by Allied Bakeries in September 1997. This bread contains soya and flaxseed and is rich in natural plant estrogen and is used to treat menopausal symptoms [266–268].

Meanwhile, government sponsorship for clinical trial has grown, and funding for nutraceutical research has increased. The supply of nutraceuticals and writing of analytical monographs of nutraceuticals for routine quality assurance is controlled by the regulatory authorities. Analytical profiles of products published by consumer organizations enables the consumer to pick out the best quality products. Available data showing the use of nutraceuticals against certain life-threatening diseases are still insufficient to prove the use of nutraceuticals for which they are sold in the market. Therefore, government support is mandatory to improve or strengthen the research in these areas.

The identification of single nucleotide polymorphisms among the human population has enabled us to predict variations in individual responses to drugs and materialize the new concept of personalized medicines. Subsequently nutritional genomics has emerged, which includes dietary component interactions with genomes and results in proteomic and metabolic changes called "nutrigenomics". Additionally, understanding of genetic differences among individuals has developed; people respond differently to the same nutraceutical, which is called nutrigenetics. The availability of genomic information accelerates the progress of disease treatment, and genotyping is used by the pharmaceutical companies to predict the efficacy, safety, and toxicity of drugs during clinical trials. In pharmacogenomics, the patient's response to medication is studied, whereas to study the effect of nutraceuticals and dietary components on the health of particular individual, "nutrigenomics" has been developed. Nutrigenomics uses genetic information of a particular individual to predict nutraceutical supplementation for to maintain health or prevent diseases.

6. Conclusions

Nutraceuticals embody a novel and exhilarating research field for the discovery of innovative health products with tremendous potentials of health benefits including safety, efficacy, and economy. Globally, researchers have realized the fact that proper nutrition and dietary supplements can prevent and cure chronic diseases. Several types of nutraceuticals have been isolated from foods, and massive quantities are produced using biotechnology and genetic engineering tools which provide pharmaco-economic benefits. These products, beside their nutritional aspects, provide tremendous health benefits via the prevention of several diseases. Nutraceuticals have proven efficacy in numerous diseases, including cancer, rheumatism, diabetes, and other chronic diseases. The use of scientifically and medically approved nutraceuticals can definitely improve health and prevent certain diseases, and some have exhibited the same efficacy as that of conventional pharmaceuticals. Generally, nutraceuticals have lower incidences of side effects, adverse effects, and drug interactions as compared to both complementary medicines and conventional pharmaceuticals. However, risk-benefit uses of nutraceuticals have not yet been documented as well as for other conventional pharmaceuticals, and the absence of side effects, adverse effects, and drug interactions does not indicate that nutraceuticals lack these properties.

This research area has major attractions both for academia and pharmaceutical/food industries. A few pharma-industries including Ranbaxy and Abbot have taken the initiative of synthesizing a range of nutraceutical products for different age consumers. The preventive role of these products is uncovered by researchers to a great extent; therefore, further extensive research both from academia as well as the pharmaceutical sector is necessary regarding their safety and efficacy. Furthermore, use of advanced and high-throughput technologies can help us understand the underlying mechanisms of action and develop this exciting area of research to new horizons for the betterment of humanity, both in terms of economic benefits as well as health outcomes.

Author Contributions: Conceptualization, S.-H.E.L.; writing—original draft preparation, M.A. (Mudhi AlAli), M.A. (Maream Alqubaisy), M.N.A., A.O.A., L.B., A.M.; writing—review and editing, all authors; visualization and supervision, S.-H.E.L. and K.-S.L.; project administration and funding acquisition, A.A. All authors have read and agreed to the published version of the manuscript.

Funding: This research was funded by a Higher Colleges of Technology Interdisciplinary Research Grant (1340).

Institutional Review Board Statement: Not applicant.

Informed Consent Statement: Not applicant.

Data Availability Statement: Not applicant.

Acknowledgments: The authors gratefully thank the Higher Colleges of Technology (HCT) for funding this research via the HCT Interdisciplinary Research Grant (Interdisciplinary_1340).

Conflicts of Interest: The authors declare no conflict of interest.

References

1. Misra, L. Traditional Phytomedicinal Systems, Scientific Validations and Current Popularity as Nutraceuticals. 2013. Available online: https://www.semanticscholar.org/paper/Traditional-Phytomedicinal-Systems%2C-Scientific-and-Misra/7df8a6c6cc432a4cd711b8b6a96702f1908353d4 (accessed on 23 April 2020).
2. Helal, N.A.; Eassa, H.A.; Amer, A.M.; Eltokhy, M.A.; Edafiogho, I.; Nounou, M.I. Nutraceuticals' Novel Formulations: The Good, the Bad, the Unknown and Patents Involved. *Recent Pat. Drug Deliv. Formul.* **2019**, *13*, 105–156. [CrossRef]
3. Petrovska, B.B. Historical review of medicinal plants' usage. *Pharmacogn. Rev.* **2012**, *6*, 1–5. [CrossRef]
4. Nasri, H.; Baradaran, A.; Shirzad, H.; Rafieian-Kopaei, M. New Concepts in Nutraceuticals as Alternative for Pharmaceuticals. *Int. J. Prev. Med.* **2014**, *5*, 1487–1499. [PubMed]
5. Caramia, G.; Silvi, S. Probiotics: From the Ancient Wisdom to the Actual Therapeutical and Nutraceutical Perspective. In *Probiotic Bacteria and Enteric Infections: Cytoprotection by Probiotic Bacteria*; Malago, J.J., Koninkx, J.F.J.G., Marinsek-Logar, R., Eds.; Springer: Dordrecht, The Netherlands, 2011; pp. 3–37.
6. Ried, K. Garlic Lowers Blood Pressure in Hypertensive Individuals, Regulates Serum Cholesterol, and Stimulates Immunity: An Updated Meta-analysis and Review. *J. Nutr.* **2016**, *146*, 389S–396S. [CrossRef] [PubMed]
7. Affuso, F.; Ruvolo, A.; Micillo, F.; Saccà, L.; Fazio, S. Effects of a nutraceutical combination (berberine, red yeast rice and policosanols) on lipid levels and endothelial function randomized, double-blind, placebo-controlled study. *Nutr. Metab. Cardiovasc. Dis.* **2010**, *20*, 656–661. [CrossRef] [PubMed]
8. Chen, G.-L.; Chen, S.-G.; Chen, F.; Xie, Y.-Q.; Han, M.-D.; Luo, C.-X.; Zhao, Y.-Y.; Gaob, Y.-Q. Nutraceutical potential and antioxidant benefits of selected fruit seeds subjected to an in vitro digestion. *J. Funct. Foods* **2016**, *20*, 317–331. [CrossRef]
9. Pitchaiah, G.; Akula, A.; Chandi, V. Anticancer Potential of Nutraceutical Formulations in MNU-induced Mammary Cancer in Sprague Dawley Rats. *Pharmacogn. Mag.* **2017**, *13*, 46–50.
10. Singla, V.; Pratap Mouli, V.; Garg, S.K.; Rai, T.; Choudhury, B.N.; Verma, P.; Deb, R.; Tiwari, V.; Rohatgi, S.; Dhingra, R.; et al. Induction with NCB-02 (curcumin) enema for mild-to-moderate distal ulcerative colitis—A randomized, placebo-controlled, pilot study. *J. Crohn's Colitis* **2014**, *8*, 208–214. [CrossRef] [PubMed]
11. Chaplin, D.D. Overview of the Immune Response. *J. Allergy Clin. Immunol.* **2010**, *125*, S3–S23. [CrossRef]
12. Carr, A.C.; Maggini, S. Vitamin C and Immune Function. *Nutrients* **2017**, *9*, 1211. [CrossRef]
13. Ruchi, S. Role of nutraceuticals in health care: A review. *Int. J. Green Pharm.* **2017**, *11*. [CrossRef]
14. Singh, J.; Sinha, S. Classification, regulatory acts and applications of nutraceuticals for health. *Int. J. Pharm. Bio Sci.* **2012**, *2*, 177–187.

15. Scrinis, G. Functional foods or functionally marketed foods? A critique of, and alternatives to, the category of "functional foods". *Public Health Nutr.* **2008**, *11*, 541–545. [CrossRef] [PubMed]
16. Prabu, S.L.; SuriyaPrakash, T.N.K.; Kumar, C.D.; SureshKuma, S.; Ragavendran, T. Nutraceuticals: A review. *Elixir Int. J.* **2012**, *46*, 8372–8377.
17. Bhowmik, D.; Kumar, K.P.S.; Paswan, S.; Srivastava, S. Tomato-A Natural Medicine and Its Health Benefits. *J. Pharmacogn. Phytochem.* **2012**, *1*, 33–43.
18. Singh, B.; Singh, J.P.; Kaur, A. Saponins in pulses and their health promoting activities: A review. *Food Chem.* **2017**, *233*, 540–549. [CrossRef]
19. Smith, L.K.; Guentzel, L.J. Mercury concentrations and omega-3 fatty acids in fish and shrimp: Preferential consumption for maximum health benefits. *Mar. Pollut. Bull.* **2010**, *60*, 1615–1618. [CrossRef] [PubMed]
20. Heldman, D.R. Food Science Text Series. 1994. Available online: http://www.springer.com/series/5999 (accessed on 22 April 2020).
21. Alkhatib, A.; Tsang, C.; Tiss, A.; Bahorun, T.; Arefanian, H.; Barake, R.; Khadir, A.; Tuomilehto, J. Functional Foods and Lifestyle Approaches for Diabetes Prevention and Management. *Nutrients* **2017**, *9*, 1310. [CrossRef] [PubMed]
22. Lau, T.-C.; Chan, M.-W.; Tan, H.-P.; Kwek, C.-L. Functional Food: A Growing Trend among the Health Conscious. *Asian Soc. Sci.* **2012**, *9*, 198. [CrossRef]
23. Smith, J.; Charter, E. *Functional Food Product Development*; John Wiley & Sons: Hoboken, NJ, USA, 2011; p. 673.
24. Sikand, G.; Kris-Etherton, P.; Boulos, N.M. Impact of functional foods on prevention of cardiovascular disease and diabetes. *Curr. Cardiol. Rep.* **2015**, *17*, 39. [CrossRef]
25. Umadevi, M.; Pushpa, R.; Sampathkumar, K.; Bhowmik, D. Rice-Traditional Medicinal Plant in India. *J. Pharmacogn. Phytochem.* **2012**, *1*, 6–12.
26. Bhat, F.M.; Riar, C.S. Health Benefits of Traditional Rice Varieties of Temperate Regions. *Med. Aromat. Plants* **2015**, *4*, 1000198.
27. Stevenson, L.; Phillips, F.; O'Sullivan, K.; Walton, J. Wheat bran: Its composition and benefits to health, a European perspective. *Int. J. Food Sci. Nutr.* **2012**, *63*, 1001–1013. [CrossRef]
28. Prückler, M.; Siebenhandl-Ehn, S.; Apprich, S.; Höltinger, S.; Haas, C.; Schmid, E.; Kneifel, W. Wheat bran-based biorefinery 1: Composition of wheat bran and strategies of functionalization. *LWT Food Sci. Technol.* **2014**, *56*, 211–221. [CrossRef]
29. Lobo, V.; Patil, A.; Phatak, A.; Chandra, N. Free radicals, antioxidants and functional foods: Impact on human health. *Pharmacogn. Rev.* **2010**, *4*, 118–126. [CrossRef] [PubMed]
30. El Sohaimy, S.A. Functional foods and nutraceuticals-modern approach to food science. *World Appl. Sci. J.* **2012**, *20*, 691–708.
31. Hasler, C.M. Functional foods: Benefits, concerns and challenges-a position paper from the american council on science and health. *J Nutr.* **2002**, *132*, 3772–3781. [CrossRef]
32. Wildman, R.E.C.; Bruno, R.S. *Handbook of Nutraceuticals and Functional Foods*, 3rd ed.; CRC Press: Boca Raton, FL, USA, 2019; p. 412.
33. Lee, Y.; Hu, S.; Park, Y.-K.; Lee, J.-Y. Health Benefits of Carotenoids: A Role of Carotenoids in the Prevention of Non-Alcoholic Fatty Liver Disease. *Prev. Nutr. Food Sci.* **2019**, *24*, 103–113. [CrossRef]
34. Shardell, M.D.; Alley, D.E.; Hicks, G.E.; El-Kamary, S.S.; Miller, R.R.; Semba, R.D.; Ferrucci, L. Low-serum carotenoid concentrations and carotenoid interactions predict mortality in US adults: The Third National Health and Nutrition Examination Survey. *Nutr Res.* **2011**, *31*, 178–189. [CrossRef] [PubMed]
35. Eggersdorfer, M.; Wyss, A. Carotenoids in human nutrition and health. *Arch. Biochem. Biophys.* **2018**, *652*, 18–26. [CrossRef]
36. Cheng, H.M.; Koutsidis, G.; Lodge, J.K.; Ashor, A.W.; Siervo, M.; Lara, J. Lycopene and tomato and risk of cardiovascular diseases: A systematic review and meta-analysis of epidemiological evidence. *Crit. Rev. Food Sci. Nutr.* **2019**, *59*, 141–158. [CrossRef]
37. Chew, E.; Clemons, T.; SanGiovanni, J.P.; Denis, R.; Ferris, I.I.I.F.; Elman, M.; Antoszyk, A.N.; Ruby, A.J.; Orth, D.; Bressler, S.B.; et al. Secondary Analyses of the Effects of Lutein/Zeaxanthin on Age-Related Macular Degeneration Progression. *JAMA Ophthalmol.* **2014**, *132*, 142–149. [CrossRef]
38. Walk, A.M.; Khan, N.A.; Barnett, S.M.; Raine, L.B.; Kramer, A.F.; Cohen, N.J.; Moulton, C.J.; Renzi-Hammond, L.M.; Hammond, B.R.; Hillman, C.H. From neuro-pigments to neural efficiency: The relationship between retinal carotenoids and behavioral and neuroelectric indices of cognitive control in childhood. *Int. J. Psychophysiol.* **2017**, *118*, 1–8. [CrossRef]
39. Kang, H.; Kim, H. Astaxanthin and β-carotene in Helicobacter pylori-induced Gastric Inflammation: A Mini-review on Action Mechanisms. *J. Cancer Prev.* **2017**, *22*, 57–61. [CrossRef] [PubMed]
40. Young, A.J.; Lowe, G.L. Carotenoids-Antioxidant Properties. *Antioxidants* **2018**, *7*, 28. [CrossRef] [PubMed]
41. Gómez-Guillén, M.C.; Giménez, B.; López-Caballero, M.E.; Montero, M.P. Functional and bioactive properties of collagen and gelatin from alternative sources: A review. *Food Hydrocoll.* **2011**, *25*, 1813–1827. [CrossRef]
42. Song, H.; Li, B. Beneficial Effects of Collagen Hydrolysate: A Review on Recent Developments. *J. Sci. Tech. Res.* **2017**, *1*. [CrossRef]
43. Fan, J.; Zhuang, Y.; Li, B. Effects of Collagen and Collagen Hydrolysate from Jellyfish Umbrella on Histological and Immunity Changes of Mice Photoaging. *Nutrients* **2013**, *5*, 223–233. [CrossRef]
44. Do-Un, K.; Chung, H.-C.; Choi, J.; Sakai, Y.; Boo-Yong, L. Oral Intake of Low-Molecular-Weight Collagen Peptide Improves Hydration, Elasticity, and Wrinkling in Human Skin: A Randomized, Double-Blind, Placebo-Controlled Study. *Nutrients* **2018**, *10*, 826.
45. Gidley, M.J.; Yakubov, G.E. Functional categorisation of dietary fibre in foods: Beyond 'soluble' vs. 'insoluble'. *Trends Food Sci. Technol.* **2019**, *86*, 563–568. [CrossRef]

46. McRorie, J.W.; McKeown, N.M. Understanding the Physics of Functional Fibers in the Gastrointestinal Tract: An Evidence-Based Approach to Resolving Enduring Misconceptions about Insoluble and Soluble Fiber. *J. Acad. Nutr. Diet.* **2017**, *117*, 251–264. [CrossRef]
47. Turner, N.D.; Lupton, J.R. Dietary Fiber. *Adv. Nutr.* **2011**, *2*, 151–152. [CrossRef] [PubMed]
48. Soliman, G.A. Dietary Fiber, Atherosclerosis, and Cardiovascular Disease. *Nutrients* **2019**, *11*, 1155. [CrossRef]
49. Hou, J.K.; Abraham, B.; El-Serag, H. Dietary intake and risk of developing inflammatory bowel disease: A systematic review of the literature. *Am. J. Gastroenterol.* **2011**, *106*, 563–573. [CrossRef] [PubMed]
50. Lee, Y.-H.; Bae, S.-C.; Song, G.-G. Omega-3 Polyunsaturated Fatty Acids and the Treatment of Rheumatoid Arthritis: A Meta-analysis. *Arch. Med. Res.* **2012**, *43*, 356–362. [CrossRef] [PubMed]
51. Kumar, G.P.; Khanum, F. Neuroprotective potential of phytochemicals. *Pharmacogn. Rev.* **2012**, *6*, 81–90. [CrossRef] [PubMed]
52. Lust, J. *The Herb Book: The Most Complete Catalog of Herbs Ever Published*; Courier Corporation: North Chelmsford, MA, USA, 2014; p. 642.
53. Embuscado, M.E. Spices and herbs: Natural sources of antioxidants—A mini review. *J. Funct. Foods* **2015**, *18*, 811–819. [CrossRef]
54. Borkar, N.; Saurabh, S.; Rathore, K.; Pandit, A.; Khandelwal, K. An Insight on Nutraceuticals. *PharmaTutor* **2015**, *3*, 13–23.
55. Kechagia, M.; Basoulis, D.; Konstantopoulou, S.; Dimitriadi, D.; Gyftopoulou, K.; Skarmoutsou, N.; Fakiri, E.M. Health Benefits of Probiotics: A Review. *ISRN Nutr.* **2013**, *2013*, 7. [CrossRef] [PubMed]
56. Fuller, R. *Probiotics: The Scientific Basis*; Springer Science & Business Media: Berlin/Heidelberg, Germany, 2012; p. 405.
57. Al-Sheraji, S.H.; Ismail, A.; Manap, M.Y.; Mustafa, S.; Yusof, R.M.; Hassan, F.A. Prebiotics as Functional Foods: A review. *J. Funct. Foods* **2013**, *5*, 1542–1553. [CrossRef]
58. Caetano, B.F.R.; De Moura, N.A.; Almeida, A.P.S.; Dias, M.C.; Sivieri, K.; Barbisan, L.F. Yacon (*Smallanthus sonchifolius*) as a Food Supplement: Health-Promoting Benefits of Fructooligosaccharides. *Nutrients* **2016**, *8*, 436. [CrossRef] [PubMed]
59. Bailey, R.L.; Gahche, J.J.; Miller, P.E.; Thomas, P.R.; Dwyer, J.T. Why US adults use dietary supplements. *JAMA Intern. Med.* **2013**, *173*, 355–361. [CrossRef]
60. Gupta, S.; Chauhan, D.; Mehla, K.; Sood, P.; Nair, A. An Overview of Nutraceuticals: Current Scenario. *J. Basic Clin. Pharm.* **2010**, *1*, 55–62.
61. Webb, G.P. *Dietary Supplements and Functional Foods*; John Wiley & Sons: Hoboken, NJ, USA, 2011; p. 297.
62. Nabarro, L.; Morris-Jones, S.; Moore, D.A.J. 7—Nutrition. In *Peter's Atlas of Tropical Medicine and Parasitology*, 7th ed.; Nabarro, L., Morris-Jones, S., Moore, D.A.J., Eds.; Elsevier: London, UK, 2020; pp. 322–332.
63. Anjali Garg, V.; Dhiman, A.; Dutt, R.; Ranga, S. Health benefits of nutraceuticals. *Pharm. Innov. J.* **2018**, *7*, 178–181.
64. Roadjanakamolson, M.; Suntornsuk, W. Production of beta-carotene-enriched rice bran using solid-state fermentation of Rhodotorula glutinis. *J. Microbiol. Biotechnol.* **2010**, *20*, 525–531. [PubMed]
65. Shekhar, V.; Jha, A.K.; Dangi, J.S. Nutraceuticals: A Re-emerging Health Aid. In Proceedings of the International Conference on Food, Biological and Medical Sciences (FBMS-2014), Bangkok, Thailand, 28–29 January 2014.
66. Kalra, E.K. Nutraceutical-definition and introduction. *AAPS Pharmsci.* **2003**, *5*, 27–28. [CrossRef] [PubMed]
67. Swaroopa, G.; Srinath, D. Nutraceuticals and their Health Benefits. *Int. J. Pure Appl. Biosci.* **2017**, *5*, 1151–1155.
68. Sui, X.; Zhang, Y.; Zhou, W. Bread fortified with anthocyanin-rich extract from black rice as nutraceutical sources: Its quality attributes and in vitro digestibility. *Food Chem.* **2016**, *196*, 910–916. [CrossRef]
69. Drake, P.M.W.; Szeto, T.H.; Paul, M.J.; Teh, A.Y.-H.; Ma, J.K. Recombinant biologic products versus nutraceuticals from plants—A regulatory choice? *Br. J. Clin. Pharmacol.* **2017**, *83*, 82–87. [CrossRef]
70. Alamgir, A.N.M. Therapeutic Use of Medicinal Plants and Their Extracts. In *Pharmacognosy*; Springer: Berlin/Heidelberg, Germany, 2017; Volume 1, p. 554.
71. Skinner, M.A.; Loh, J.M.S.; Hunter, D.C.; Zhang, J. Gold kiwifruit (*Actinidia chinensis* 'Hort16A') for immune support. *Proc. Nutr. Soc.* **2011**, *70*, 276–280. [CrossRef]
72. Stonehouse, W.; Gammon, C.S.; Beck, K.L.; Conlon, C.A.; von Hurst, P.R.; Kruger, R. Kiwifruit: Our daily prescription for health. *Can. J. Physiol. Pharmacol.* **2012**, *91*, 442–447. [CrossRef]
73. Shiby, V.K.; Mishra, H.N. Fermented Milks and Milk Products as Functional Foods—A Review. *Crit. Rev. Food Sci. Nutr.* **2013**, *53*, 482–496. [CrossRef] [PubMed]
74. Vo, T.-S.; Kim, S.-K. Fucoidans as a natural bioactive ingredient for functional foods. *J. Funct. Foods* **2013**, *5*, 16–27. [CrossRef]
75. Latté, K.P.; Appel, K.-E.; Lampen, A. Health benefits and possible risks of broccoli—An overview. *Food Chem. Toxicol.* **2011**, *49*, 3287–3309. [CrossRef]
76. Irw Jaswir, I.; Noviendri, D.; Hasrini, R.F.; Octavianti, F. Carotenoids: Sources, medicinal properties and their application in food and nutraceutical industry. *JMPR* **2011**, *5*, 7119–7131. [CrossRef]
77. Chauhan, B.; Kumar, G.; Kalam, N.; Ansari, S.H. Current concepts and prospects of herbal nutraceutical: A review. *J. Adv. Pharm. Technol. Res.* **2013**, *4*, 4–8. [PubMed]
78. Kispotta, A.; Srivastava, M.K.; Dutta, M. Free radical scavenging activity of ethanolic extracts and determination of aloin from *Aloe vera* L. leaf extract. *Int. J. Med. Aromat. Plants* **2012**, *2*, 612–618.
79. Souyoul, S.A.; Saussy, K.P.; Lupo, M.P. Nutraceuticals: A Review. *Dermatol. Ther.* **2018**, *8*, 5–16. [CrossRef] [PubMed]

80. Bailey, R.L.; Dodd, K.W.; Gahche, J.J.; Dwyer, J.T.; McDowell, M.A.; Yetley, E.A.; Sempos, C.A.; Burt, V.L.; Radimer, K.L.; Picciano, M.F. Total folate and folic acid intake from foods and dietary supplements in the United States: 2003–2006. *Am. J. Clin. Nutr.* **2010**, *91*, 231–237. [CrossRef] [PubMed]
81. Areco, V.; Rivoira, M.A.; Rodriguez, V.; Marchionatti, A.M.; Carpentieri, A.; de Talamoni, N.T. Dietary and pharmacological compounds altering intestinal calcium absorption in humans and animals. *Nutr. Res. Rev.* **2015**, *28*, 83–99. [CrossRef] [PubMed]
82. Martini, M.; Altomonte, I.; Licitra, R.; Salari, F. Nutritional and Nutraceutical Quality of Donkey Milk. *J. Equine Vet. Sci.* **2018**, *65*, 33–37. [CrossRef]
83. Hossein-nezhad, A.; Holick, M.F. Vitamin D for Health: A Global Perspective. *Mayo Clin. Proc.* **2013**, *88*, 720–755. [CrossRef]
84. Keservani, R.K.; Kesharwani, R.K.; Vyas, N.; Jain, S.; Sharma, A.K. Nutraceutical and Functional Food as Future Food: A Review. *Der Pharm. Lett.* **2010**, *2*, 106–116.
85. Prasanna, P.H.P.; Grandison, A.S.; Charalampopoulos, D. Bifidobacteria in milk products: An overview of physiological and biochemical properties, exopolysaccharide production, selection criteria of milk products and health benefits. *Food Res. Int.* **2014**, *55*, 247–262. [CrossRef]
86. Shoaib, M.; Shehzad, A.; Omar, M.; Rakha, A.; Raza, H.; Sharif, H.R.; Shakeel, A.; Ansari, A.; Niazi, S. Inulin: Properties, health benefits and food applications. *Carbohydr. Polym.* **2016**, *147*, 444–454. [CrossRef] [PubMed]
87. Golla, U. Emergence of nutraceuticals as the alternative medications for pharmaceuticals. *IJCAM* **2018**, *11*, 155–158. [CrossRef]
88. Dav, G.; Santilli, F.; Patrono, C. Nutraceuticals in Diabetes and Metabolic Syndrome. *Cardiovasc. Ther.* **2010**, *28*, 216–226. [CrossRef]
89. Johnston, T.P.; Korolenko, T.A.; Pirro, M.; Sahebkar, A. Preventing cardiovascular heart disease: Promising nutraceutical and non-nutraceutical treatments for cholesterol management. *Pharmacol. Res.* **2017**, *120*, 219–225. [CrossRef]
90. Kramer, K.; Hoppe, P.-P.; Packer, L. *Nutraceuticals in Health and Disease Prevention*; CRC Press: Boca Raton, FL, USA, 2001; p. 340.
91. Bele, A.A.; Khale, A. An approach to a Nutraceutical. *Asian J. Res. Chem.* **2013**, *6*, 1161–1164.
92. Gupta, S.V.; Pathak, Y.V. *Advances in Nutraceutical Applications in Cancer: Recent Research Trends and Clinical Applications*; CRC Press LLC: Milton, UK, 2019.
93. Sarkar, F.H.; Li, Y.; Wang, Z.; Kong, D. The role of nutraceuticals in the regulation of Wnt and Hedgehog signaling in cancer. *Cancer Metastasis Rev.* **2010**, *29*, 383–394. [CrossRef] [PubMed]
94. De Mejia, E.G.; Dia, V.P. The role of nutraceutical proteins and peptides in apoptosis, angiogenesis, and metastasis of cancer cells. *Cancer Metastasis Rev.* **2010**, *29*, 511–528. [CrossRef]
95. Shukla, Y.; George, J. Combinatorial strategies employing nutraceuticals for cancer development. *Ann. N. Y. Acad. Sci.* **2011**, *1229*, 162–175. [CrossRef]
96. Fathi, N.; Ahmadian, E.; Shahi, S.; Roshangar, L.; Khan, H.; Kouhsoltani, M.; Dizaj, S.M.; Sharifi, S. Role of vitamin D and vitamin D receptor (VDR) in oral cancer. *Biomed. Pharmacother.* **2019**, *109*, 391–401. [CrossRef] [PubMed]
97. Vuolo, L.; Faggiano, A.; Colao, A. Vitamin D and Cancer. *Front. Endocrinol.* **2012**, *3*. [CrossRef] [PubMed]
98. Hii, L.-W.; Swee-Hua, E.L.; Leong, C.-O.; Swee-Yee, C.; Tan, N.-P.; Kok-Song, L.; Mai, C.-W. The synergism of Clinacanthus nutans Lindau extracts with gemcitabine: Downregulation of anti-apoptotic markers in squamous pancreatic ductal adenocarcinoma. *BMC Complement. Altern. Med.* **2019**, *19*. [CrossRef] [PubMed]
99. Bishehsari, F.; Engen, P.A.; Preite, N.Z.; Tuncil, Y.E.; Naqib, A.; Shaikh, M.; Rossi, M.; Wilber, S.; Green, S.J.; Hamaker, B.R.; et al. Dietary Fiber Treatment Corrects the Composition of Gut Microbiota, Promotes SCFA Production, and Suppresses Colon Carcinogenesis. *Genes* **2018**, *9*, 102. [CrossRef] [PubMed]
100. Gamallat, Y.; Meyiah, A.; Kuugbee, E.D.; Hago, A.M.; Chiwala, G.; Awadasseid, A.; Bamba, D.; Zhang, X.; Shang, X.; Luo, F.; et al. Lactobacillus rhamnosus induced epithelial cell apoptosis, ameliorates inflammation and prevents colon cancer development in an animal model. *Biomed. Pharmacother.* **2016**, *83*, 536–541. [CrossRef]
101. Kuugbee, E.D.; Shang, X.; Gamallat, Y.; Bamba, D.; Awadasseid, A.; Suliman, M.A.; Zang, S.; Ma, Y.; Chiwala, G.; Xin, Y.; et al. Structural Change in Microbiota by a Probiotic Cocktail Enhances the Gut Barrier and Reduces Cancer via TLR2 Signaling in a Rat Model of Colon Cancer. *Dig. Dis. Sci.* **2016**, *61*, 2908–2920. [CrossRef]
102. Raman, M.; Ambalam, P.; Kondepudi, K.K.; Pithva, S.; Kothari, C.; Patel, A.T.; Purama, R.K.; Dave, J.M.; Vyas, B.R.M. Potential of probiotics, prebiotics and synbiotics for management of colorectal cancer. *Gut Microbes* **2013**, *4*, 181–192. [CrossRef]
103. Juneja, L.R.; Kapoor, M.P.; Okubo, T.; Rao, T. *Green Tea Polyphenols: Nutraceuticals of Modern Life*; CRC Press LLC: Boca Raton, FA, USA, 2013.
104. Lee, P.M.Y.; Ng, C.F.; Liu, Z.M.; Ho, W.M.; Lee, M.K.; Wang, F.; Kan, H.D.; He, Y.H.; Ng, S.S.M.; Wong, S.Y.S.; et al. Reduced prostate cancer risk with green tea and epigallocatechin 3-gallate intake among Hong Kong Chinese men. *Prostate Cancer Prostatic Dis.* **2017**, *20*, 318–322. [CrossRef]
105. Posadino, A.M.; Phu, H.T.; Cossu, A.; Giordo, R.; Fois, M.; Thuan, D.T.B.; Piga, A.; Sotgia, S.; Zinellu, A.; Carru, C.; et al. Oxidative stress-induced Akt downregulation mediates green tea toxicity towards prostate cancer cells. *Toxicol. Vitr.* **2017**, *42*, 255–262. [CrossRef] [PubMed]
106. Huang, J.; Li, F.; Chen, S.; Shi, Y.; Wang, X.; Wang, C.; Meng, Q.-h.; Jiang, C.; Zhu, Z.-y.; Li, C.-H. Green tea polyphenol induces significant cell death in human lung cancer cells. *Trop. J. Pharm. Res.* **2017**, *16*, 1021–1028. [CrossRef]
107. Leong, H.; Mathur, P.S.; Greene, G.L. Inhibition of mammary tumorigenesis in the C3(1)/SV40 mouse model by green tea. *Breast Cancer Res. Treat.* **2008**, *107*, 359–369. [CrossRef] [PubMed]

108. Jian, W.; Fang, S.; Chen, T.; Fang, J.; Mo, Y.; Li, D.; Xiong, S.; Liu, W.; Song, L.; Shen, J.; et al. A novel role of HuR in -Epigallocatechin-3-gallate (EGCG) induces tumour cells apoptosis. *J. Cell Mol. Med.* **2019**, *23*, 3767–3771. [CrossRef]
109. Kunnumakkara, A.B.; Anand, P.; Aggarwal, B.B. Curcumin inhibits proliferation, invasion, angiogenesis and metastasis of different cancers through interaction with multiple cell signaling proteins. *Cancer Lett.* **2008**, *269*, 199–225. [CrossRef]
110. Vishvakarma, N.K.; Kumar, A.; Singh, S.M. Role of curcumin-dependent modulation of tumor microenvironment of a murine T cell lymphoma in altered regulation of tumor cell survival. *Toxicol. Appl. Pharmacol.* **2011**, *252*, 298–306. [CrossRef]
111. Akkoç, Y.; Berrak, Ö.; Arısan, E.D.; Obakan, P.; Çoker-Gürkan, A.; Palavan-Ünsal, N. Inhibition of PI3K signaling triggered apoptotic potential of curcumin which is hindered by Bcl-2 through activation of autophagy in MCF-7 cells. *Biomed. Pharmacother.* **2015**, *71*, 161–171. [CrossRef]
112. Li, Y.; Sun, W.; Han, N.; Zou, Y.; Yin, D. Curcumin inhibits proliferation, migration, invasion and promotes apoptosis of retinoblastoma cell lines through modulation of miR-99a and JAK/STAT pathway. *BMC Cancer* **2018**, *18*, 1230. [CrossRef]
113. Gupta, S.C.; Kannappan, R.; Reuter, S.; Kim, J.H.; Aggarwal, B.B. Chemosensitization of tumors by resveratrol. *Ann. N. Y. Acad. Sci.* **2011**, *1215*, 150–160. [CrossRef]
114. Jiang, Z.; Chen, K.; Cheng, L.; Yan, B.; Qian, W.; Cao, J.; Li, J.; Wu, E.; Ma, Q.; Yang, W. Resveratrol and cancer treatment: Updates. *Ann. N. Y. Acad. Sci.* **2017**, *1403*, 59–69. [CrossRef]
115. Wu, F.; Cui, L. Resveratrol suppresses melanoma by inhibiting NF-κB/miR-221 and inducing TFG expression. *Arch. Dermatol. Res.* **2017**, *309*, 823–831. [CrossRef]
116. Li, W.; Ma, X.; Li, N.; Liu, H.; Dong, Q.; Zhang, J.; Yang, C.; Liu, Y.; Liang, Q.; Zhang, S.; et al. Resveratrol inhibits Hexokinases II mediated glycolysis in non-small cell lung cancer via targeting Akt signaling pathway. *Exp. Cell Res.* **2016**, *349*, 320–327. [CrossRef] [PubMed]
117. Karlsson, S.; Olausson, J.; Lundh, D.; Sögård, P.; Mandal, A.; Holmström, K.-O.; Stahel, A.; Bengtsson, J.; Larsson, D. Vitamin D and prostate cancer: The role of membrane initiated signaling pathways in prostate cancer progression. *J. Steroid Biochem. Mol. Biol.* **2010**, *121*, 413–416. [CrossRef]
118. Lassed, S.; Deus, C.M.; Djebbari, R.; Zama, D.; Oliveira, P.J.; Rizvanov, A.A.; Dahdouh, A.; Benayache, F.; Benayache, S. Protective Effect of Green Tea (*Camellia sinensis* (L.) Kuntze) against Prostate Cancer: From In Vitro Data to Algerian Patients. *Evid. Based Complement Altern. Med.* **2017**, *2017*. [CrossRef]
119. Yang, K.; Gao, Z.-Y.; Li, T.-Q.; Song, W.; Xiao, W.; Zheng, J.; Chen, H.; Chen, G.-H.; Zou, H.-Y. Anti-tumor activity and the mechanism of a green tea (*Camellia sinensis*) polysaccharide on prostate cancer. *Int. J. Biol. Macromol.* **2019**, *122*, 95–103. [CrossRef]
120. Johnson, J.J.; Mukhtar, H. Curcumin for chemoprevention of colon cancer. *Cancer Lett.* **2007**, *255*, 170–181. [CrossRef] [PubMed]
121. Umesalma, S.; Sudhandiran, G. Differential Inhibitory Effects of the Polyphenol Ellagic Acid on Inflammatory Mediators NF-κB, iNOS, COX-2, TNF-α, and IL-6 in 1,2-Dimethylhydrazine-Induced Rat Colon Carcinogenesis. *Basic Clin. Pharmacol. Toxicol.* **2010**, *107*, 650–655. [CrossRef]
122. Akrout, A.; Gonzalez, L.A.; El Jani, H.; Madrid, P.C. Antioxidant and antitumor activities of Artemisia campestris and Thymelaea hirsuta from southern Tunisia. *Food Chem. Toxicol.* **2011**, *49*, 342–347. [CrossRef]
123. Jayaprakasha, G.K.; Murthy, K.N.C.; Uckoo, R.M.; Patil, B.S. Chemical composition of volatile oil from Citrus limettioides and their inhibition of colon cancer cell proliferation. *Ind. Crops Prod.* **2013**, *45*, 200–207. [CrossRef]
124. Mondal, A.; Gandhi, A.; Fimognari, C.; Atanasov, A.G.; Bishayee, A. Alkaloids for cancer prevention and therapy: Current progress and future perspectives. *Eur. J. Pharmacol.* **2019**, *858*, 172472. [CrossRef] [PubMed]
125. Shoeb, M.; MacManus, S.M.; Jaspars, M.; Trevidu, J.; Nahar, L.; Kong-Thoo-Lin, P.; Sarkere, S.D. Montamine, a unique dimeric indole alkaloid, from the seeds of *Centaurea montana* (Asteraceae), and its in vitro cytotoxic activity against the CaCo2 colon cancer cells. *Tetrahedron* **2006**, *62*, 11172–11177. [CrossRef]
126. Zhou, J.; Feng, J.-H.; Fang, L. A novel monoterpenoid indole alkaloid with anticancer activity from Melodinus khasianus. *Bioorg. Med. Chem. Lett.* **2017**, *27*, 893–896. [CrossRef]
127. Chang, H.-F.; Yang, L.-L. Gamma-Mangostin, a Micronutrient of Mangosteen Fruit, Induces Apoptosis in Human Colon Cancer Cells. *Molecules* **2012**, *17*, 8010–8021. [CrossRef] [PubMed]
128. Prinz-langenohl, R.; Fohr, I.; Pietrzik, K. Beneficial role for folate in the prevention of colorectal and breast cancer. *Eur. J. Nutr.* **2001**, *40*, 98–105. [CrossRef] [PubMed]
129. Modem, S.; DiCarlo, S.E.; Reddy, T.R. Fresh Garlic Extract Induces Growth Arrest and Morphological Differentiation of MCF7 Breast Cancer Cells. *Genes Cancer* **2012**, *3*, 177–186. [CrossRef] [PubMed]
130. Talib, W.H. Consumption of garlic and lemon aqueous extracts combination reduces tumor burden by angiogenesis inhibition, apoptosis induction, and immune system modulation. *Nutrition* **2017**, *43*, 89–97. [CrossRef] [PubMed]
131. Vijayakumar, S.; Malaikozhundan, B.; Saravanakumar, K.; Durán-Lara, E.F.; Wang, M.-H.; Vaseeharan, B. Garlic clove extract assisted silver nanoparticle—Antibacterial, antibiofilm, antihelminthic, anti-inflammatory, anticancer and ecotoxicity assessment. *J. Photochem. Photobiol. B* **2019**, *198*, 111558. [CrossRef]
132. Kronski, E.; Fiori, M.E.; Barbieri, O.; Astigiano, S.; Mirisola, V.; Killian, P.H.; Bruno, A.; Pagani, A.; Rovera, F.; Pfeffer, U.; et al. miR181b is induced by the chemopreventive polyphenol curcumin and inhibits breast cancer metastasis via down-regulation of the inflammatory cytokines CXCL1 and -2. *Mol. Oncol.* **2014**, *8*, 581–595. [CrossRef]
133. Simboli-campbell, M.; Narvaez, C.J.; Vanweelden, K.; Tenniswood, M.; Welsh, J. Comparative effects of 1,25(OH)$_2$D$_3$ and EB1089 on cell cycle kinetics and apoptosis in MCF-7 breast cancer cells. *Breast Cancer Res. Treat.* **1997**, *42*, 31–41. [CrossRef]

134. Wang, Q.; Lee, D.; Sysounthone, V.; Chandraratna, R.A.S.; Christakos, S.; Korah, R.; Wieder, R. 1,25-dihydroxyvitamin D_3 and retonic acid analogues induce differentiation in breast cancer cells with function- and cell-specific additive effects. *Breast Cancer Res. Treat.* **2001**, *67*, 157–168. [CrossRef]
135. Zhu, X.; Xiong, L.; Zhang, X.; Shi, N.; Zhang, Y.; Ke, J.; Sun, Z.; Chen, T. Lyophilized strawberries prevent 7,12-dimethylbenz[α]anthracene (DMBA)-induced oral squamous cell carcinogenesis in hamsters. *J. Funct. Foods* **2015**, *15*, 476–486. [CrossRef]
136. Petiwala, S.M.; Johnson, J.J. Diterpenes from rosemary (*Rosmarinus officinalis*): Defining their potential for anti-cancer activity. *Cancer Lett.* **2015**, *367*, 93–102. [CrossRef]
137. Vinothkumar, V.; Manoharan, S.; Sindhu, G.; Nirmal, M.R.; Vetrichelvi, V. Geraniol modulates cell proliferation, apoptosis, inflammation, and angiogenesis during 7,12-dimethylbenz[a]anthracene-induced hamster buccal pouch carcinogenesis. *Mol. Cell Biochem.* **2012**, *369*, 17–25. [CrossRef]
138. Nair, H.B.; Sung, B.; Yadav, V.R.; Kannappan, R.; Chaturvedi, M.M.; Aggarwal, B.B. Delivery of antiinflammatory nutraceuticals by nanoparticles for the prevention and treatment of cancer. *Biochem. Pharmacol.* **2010**, *80*, 1833–1843. [CrossRef] [PubMed]
139. Al-Okbi, S.Y. Nutraceuticals of anti-inflammatory activity as complementary therapy for rheumatoid arthritis. *Toxicol. Ind. Health* **2014**, *30*, 738–749. [CrossRef] [PubMed]
140. Vecchione, R.; Quagliariello, V.; Calabria, D.; Calcagno, V.; De Luca, E.; Iaffaioli, R.V.; Netti, P.A. Curcumin bioavailability from oil in water nano-emulsions: In vitro and in vivo study on the dimensional, compositional and interactional dependence. *J. Control. Release.* **2016**, *233*, 88–100. [CrossRef] [PubMed]
141. Kunnumakkara, A.B.; Bordoloi, D.; Padmavathi, G.; Monisha, J.; Roy, N.K.; Prasad, S.; Aggarwal, B.B. Curcumin, the golden nutraceutical: Multitargeting for multiple chronic diseases. *Br. J. Pharmacol.* **2017**, *174*, 1325–1348. [CrossRef]
142. Panahi, Y.; Sahebkar, A.; Amiri, M.; Davoudi, S.M.; Beiraghdar, F.; Hoseininejad, S.L.; Kolivand, M. Improvement of sulphur mustard-induced chronic pruritus, quality of life and antioxidant status by curcumin: Results of a randomised, double-blind, placebo-controlled trial. *Br. J. Nutr.* **2012**, *108*, 1272–1279. [CrossRef] [PubMed]
143. Mijan, M.A.; Lim, B.O. Diets, functional foods, and nutraceuticals as alternative therapies for inflammatory bowel disease: Present status and future trends. *World J. Gastroenterol.* **2018**, *24*, 2673–2685. [CrossRef] [PubMed]
144. Rodríguez-Cruz, M.; del Cruz-Guzmán, O.R.; Almeida-Becerril, T.; Solís-Serna, A.D.; Atilano-Miguel, S.; Sánchez-González, J.R.; Barbosa-Cortés, L.; Ruíz-Cruz, E.D.; Huicochea, J.C.; Cárdenas-Conejo, A.; et al. Potential therapeutic impact of omega-3 long chain-polyunsaturated fatty acids on inflammation markers in Duchenne muscular dystrophy: A double-blind, controlled randomized trial. *Clin. Nutr.* **2018**, *37*, 1840–1851. [CrossRef]
145. Bansal, P.; Gupta, S.K.; Ojha, S.K.; Nandave, M.; Mittal, R.; Kumari, S.; Arya, D.S. Cardioprotective effect of lycopene in the experimental model of myocardial ischemia-reperfusion injury. *Mol. Cell. Biochem.* **2006**, *289*, 1–9. [CrossRef] [PubMed]
146. Ojha, S.; Goyal, S.; Sharma, C.; Arora, S.; Kumari, S.; Arya, D.S. Cardioprotective effect of lycopene against isoproterenol-induced myocardial infarction in rats. *Hum. Exp. Toxicol.* **2013**, *32*, 492–503. [CrossRef] [PubMed]
147. Song, B.; Liu, K.; Gao, Y.; Zhao, L.; Fang, H.; Li, Y.; Pei, L.; Xu, Y. Lycopene and risk of cardiovascular diseases: A meta-analysis of observational studies. *Mol. Nutr. Food Res.* **2017**, *61*. [CrossRef]
148. Srutkova, D.; Schwarzer, M.; Hudcovic, T.; Zakostelska, Z.; Drab, V.; Spanova, A.; Rittich, B.; Kozakova, H.; Schabussova, I. Bifidobacterium longum CCM 7952 Promotes Epithelial Barrier Function and Prevents Acute DSS-Induced Colitis in Strictly Strain-Specific Manner. *PLoS ONE* **2015**, *10*, e0134050.
149. Sichetti, M.; De Marco, S.; Pagiotti, R.; Traina, G.; Pietrella, D. Anti-inflammatory effect of multistrain probiotic formulation (*L. rhamnosus*, *B. lactis*, and *B. longum*). *Nutrition* **2018**, *53*, 95–102. [CrossRef]
150. Liu, X.; Wu, Y.; Li, F.; Zhang, D. Dietary fiber intake reduces risk of inflammatory bowel disease: Result from a meta-analysis. *Nutr. Res.* **2015**, *35*, 753–758. [CrossRef] [PubMed]
151. Lee, K.-H.; Park, M.; Ji, K.-Y.; Lee, H.-Y.; Jang, J.-H.; Yoon, I.-J.; Oh, S.-S.; Kim, S.-M.; Jeong, Y.-H.; Yun, C.-H.; et al. Bacterial β-(1,3)-glucan prevents DSS-induced IBD by restoring the reduced population of regulatory T cells. *Immunobiology* **2014**, *219*, 802–812. [CrossRef]
152. Cakir, U.; Tayman, C.; Serkant, U.; Yakut, H.I.; Cakir, E.; Ates, U.; Koyuncu, I.; Karaogul, E. Ginger (*Zingiber officinale* Roscoe) for the treatment and prevention of necrotizing enterocolitis. *J. Ethnopharmacol.* **2018**, *225*, 297–308. [CrossRef]
153. El-Abhar, H.S.; Hammad, L.N.A.; Gawad, H.S.A. Modulating effect of ginger extract on rats with ulcerative colitis. *J. Ethnopharmacol.* **2008**, *118*, 367–372. [CrossRef] [PubMed]
154. Lv, J.; Huang, H.; Yu, L.; Whent, M.; Niu, Y.; Shi, H.; Wang, T.T.Y.; Luthria, D.; Charles, D.; Yu, L.L. Phenolic composition and nutraceutical properties of organic and conventional cinnamon and peppermint. *Food Chem.* **2012**, *132*, 1442–1450. [CrossRef]
155. Hassanzadeh, P.; Arbabi, E.; Atyabi, F.; Dinarvand, R. The endocannabinoid system and NGF are involved in the mechanism of action of resveratrol: A multi-target nutraceutical with therapeutic potential in neuropsychiatric disorders. *Psychopharmacology* **2016**, *233*, 1087–1096. [CrossRef] [PubMed]
156. Cui, L.; Feng, L.; Zhang, Z.H.; Jia, X.B. The anti-inflammation effect of baicalin on experimental colitis through inhibiting TLR4/NF-κB pathway activation. *Int. Immunopharmacol.* **2014**, *23*, 294–303. [CrossRef] [PubMed]
157. Bitto, A.; Minutoli, L.; David, A.; Irrera, N.; Rinaldi, M.; Venuti, F.S.; Squadrito, F.; Altavilla, D. Flavocoxid, a dual inhibitor of COX-2 and 5-LOX of natural origin, attenuates the inflammatory response and protects mice from sepsis. *Crit. Care* **2012**, *16*, R32. [CrossRef] [PubMed]

158. Liu, L.; Shang, Y.; Li, M.; Han, X.; Wang, J.; Wang, J. Curcumin ameliorates asthmatic airway inflammation by activating nuclear factor-E2-related factor 2/haem oxygenase (HO)-1 signalling pathway. *Clin. Exp. Pharmacol. Physiol.* **2015**, *42*, 520–529. [CrossRef] [PubMed]
159. Algandaby, M.M.; El-halawany, A.M.; Abdallah, H.M.; Alahdal, A.M.; Nagy, A.A.; Ashour, O.M.; Abdel-Naim, A.B. Gingerol protects against experimental liver fibrosis in rats via suppression of pro-inflammatory and profibrogenic mediators. *Naunyn Schmiedeberg Arch. Pharmacol.* **2016**, *389*, 419–428. [CrossRef]
160. Zhang, T.; Su, J.; Guo, B.; Wang, K.; Li, X.; Liang, G. Apigenin protects blood–brain barrier and ameliorates early brain injury by inhibiting TLR4-mediated inflammatory pathway in subarachnoid hemorrhage rats. *Int. Immunopharmacol.* **2015**, *28*, 79–87. [CrossRef]
161. Zhai, W.; Zhang, Z.; Xu, N.; Guo, Y.; Qiu, C.; Li, C.; Deng, G.Z.; Guo, M.Y. Piperine Plays an Anti-Inflammatory Role in Staphylococcus aureus Endometritis by Inhibiting Activation of NF-κB and MAPK Pathways in Mice. *Evid. Based Complement Altern. Med.* **2016**, *2016*. [CrossRef]
162. Sahu, B.D.; Tatireddy, S.; Koneru, M.; Borkar, R.M.; Kumar, J.M.; Kuncha, M.; Srinivas, R.; Sunder R, S.; Sistla, R. Naringin ameliorates gentamicin-induced nephrotoxicity and associated mitochondrial dysfunction, apoptosis and inflammation in rats: Possible mechanism of nephroprotection. *Toxicol. Appl. Pharmacol.* **2014**, *277*, 8–20. [CrossRef] [PubMed]
163. Kennedy-Feitosa, E.; Okuro, R.T.; Pinho Ribeiro, V.; Lanzetti, M.; Barroso, M.V.; Zin, W.A.; Porto, L.C.; Brito-Gitirana, L.; Valenca, S.S. Eucalyptol attenuates cigarette smoke-induced acute lung inflammation and oxidative stress in the mouse. *Pulm. Pharmacol. Ther.* **2016**, *41*, 11–18. [CrossRef]
164. Fonsêca, D.; Salgado, P.; de Aragão Neto, H.; Golzio, A.; Caldas Filho, M.; Melo, C.; Leite, F.; Piuvezam, M.; Pordeus, L.; Barbosa Filho, J.; et al. Ortho-eugenol exhibits anti-nociceptive and anti-inflammatory activities. *Int. Immunopharmacol.* **2016**, *38*, 402–408. [CrossRef] [PubMed]
165. Simioni, C.; Zauli, G.; Martelli, A.M.; Vitale, M.; Sacchetti, G.; Gonelli, A.; Neri, L.M. Oxidative stress: Role of physical exercise and antioxidant nutraceuticals in adulthood and aging. *Oncotarget* **2018**, *9*, 17181–17198. [CrossRef]
166. Wu, Q.; Liu, L.; Miron, A.; Klímová, B.; Wan, D.; Kuca, K. The antioxidant, immunomodulatory, and anti-inflammatory activities of Spirulina: An overview. *Arch. Toxicol. Arch. Toxikol.* **2016**, *90*, 1817–1840. [CrossRef]
167. Trachootham, D.; Lu, W.; Ogasawara, M.A.; Valle, N.R.-D.; Huang, P. Redox Regulation of Cell Survival. *Antioxid. Redox Signal.* **2008**, *10*, 1343–1374. [CrossRef]
168. Lushchak, V.I. Free radicals, reactive oxygen species, oxidative stress and its classification. *Chem. Biol. Interact.* **2014**, *224*, 164–175. [CrossRef]
169. McCubrey, J.A.; Lertpiriyapong, K.; Steelman, L.S.; Abrams, S.L.; Yang, L.V.; Murata, R.M.; Rosalen, P.L.; Scalisi, A.; Neri, L.M.; Cocco, L.; et al. Effects of resveratrol, curcumin, berberine and other nutraceuticals on aging, cancer development, cancer stem cells and microRNAs. *Aging* **2017**, *9*, 1477–1536. [CrossRef]
170. Liguori, I.; Russo, G.; Curcio, F.; Bulli, G.; Aran, L.; Della-Morte, D.; Gargiulo, G.; Testa, G.; Cacciatore, F.; Bonaduce, D.; et al. Oxidative stress, aging, and diseases. *Clin. Interv. Aging.* **2018**, *13*, 757–772. [CrossRef]
171. Naveen, J.; Baskaran, V. Antidiabetic plant-derived nutraceuticals: A critical review. *Eur. J. Nutr.* **2018**, *57*, 1275–1299. [CrossRef] [PubMed]
172. Neha, K.; Haider, M.R.; Pathak, A.; Yar, M.S. Medicinal prospects of antioxidants: A review. *Eur. J. Med. Chem.* **2019**, *178*, 687–704. [CrossRef] [PubMed]
173. Srinivasan, K. Antioxidant Potential of Spices and Their Active Constituents. *Crit. Rev. Food Sci. Nutr.* **2014**, *54*, 352–372. [CrossRef] [PubMed]
174. Danwilai, K.; Konmun, J.; Sripanidkulchai, B.; Subongkot, S. Antioxidant activity of ginger extract as a daily supplement in cancer patients receiving adjuvant chemotherapy: A pilot study. *Cancer Manag. Res.* **2017**, *9*, 11–18. [CrossRef]
175. Cao, C.; Pathak, S.; Patil, K. *Antioxidant Nutraceuticals: Preventive and Healthcare Applications*, 1st ed.; Taylor & Francis Group: Milton, UK, 2018; p. 428.
176. Tesoriere, L.; Allegra, M.; Butera, D.; Livrea, M.A. Absorption, excretion, and distribution of dietary antioxidant betalains in LDLs: Potential health effects of betalains in humans. *Am. J. Clin. Nutr.* **2004**, *80*, 941–945. [CrossRef]
177. Krajka-Kuźniak, V.; Szaefer, H.; Ignatowicz, E.; Adamska, T.; Baer-Dubowska, W. Beetroot juice protects against N-nitrosodiethylamine-induced liver injury in rats. *Food Chem. Toxicol.* **2012**, *50*, 2027–2033. [CrossRef]
178. Coles, L.T.; Clifton, P.M. Effect of beetroot juice on lowering blood pressure in free-living, disease-free adults: A randomized, placebo-controlled trial. *Nutr. J.* **2012**, *11*, 106. [CrossRef]
179. Jeszka-Skowron, M.; Zgoła-Grześkowiak, A.; Stanisz, E.; Waśkiewicz, A. Potential health benefits and quality of dried fruits: Goji fruits, cranberries and raisins. *Food Chem.* **2017**, *221*, 228–236. [CrossRef] [PubMed]
180. Chang, S.K.; Alasalvar, C.; Shahidi, F. Review of dried fruits: Phytochemicals, antioxidant efficacies, and health benefits. *J. Funct. Foods* **2016**, *21*, 113–132. [CrossRef]
181. Hernández-Alonso, P.; Bulló, M.; Salas-Salvadó, J. Pistachios for Health. *Nutr. Today* **2016**, *51*, 133–138. [CrossRef]
182. Bulló, M.; Juanola-Falgarona, M.; Hernández-Alonso, P.; Salas-Salvadó, J. Nutrition attributes and health effects of pistachio nuts. *Br. J. Nutr.* **2015**, *113*, S79–S93. [CrossRef] [PubMed]

183. Bolling, B.W.; Chen, C.-Y.O.; McKay, D.L.; Blumberg, J.B. Tree nut phytochemicals: Composition, antioxidant capacity, bioactivity, impact factors. A systematic review of almonds, Brazils, cashews, hazelnuts, macadamias, pecans, pine nuts, pistachios and walnuts. *Nutr. Res. Rev.* **2011**, *24*, 244–275. [CrossRef]
184. Houston, M.C. Treatment of hypertension with nutraceuticals, vitamins, antioxidants and minerals. *Expert Rev. Cardiovasc. Ther.* **2007**, *5*, 681–691. [CrossRef] [PubMed]
185. Riccioni, G.; Gammone, M.A.; Currenti, W.; D'Orazio, N. Effectiveness and Safety of Dietetic Supplementation of a New Nutraceutical on Lipid Profile and Serum Inflammation Biomarkers in Hypercholesterolemic Patients. *Molecules* **2018**, *23*, 1168. [CrossRef]
186. Lyseng-Williamson, K.A. Ezetimibe/Simvastatin: A Guide to its Clinical Use in Hypercholesterolemia. *Am. J. Cardiovasc. Drugs* **2012**, *12*, 49–56. [CrossRef]
187. Cicero, A.F.G.; Colletti, A.; Bajraktari, G.; Descamps, O.; Djuric, D.M.; Ezhov, M.; Fras, Z.; Katsiki, N.; Langlois, M.; Latkovskis, G.; et al. Lipid lowering nutraceuticals in clinical practice: Position paper from an International Lipid Expert Panel. *Arch. Med. Sci.* **2017**, *13*, 965–1005. [CrossRef] [PubMed]
188. Brown, A.W.; Hang, J.; Dussault, P.H.; Carr, T.P. Phytosterol Ester Constituents Affect Micellar Cholesterol Solubility in Model Bile. *Lipids* **2010**, *45*, 855–862. [CrossRef] [PubMed]
189. Trautwein, E.A.; Koppenol, W.P.; Jong, A.; de Hiemstra, H.; Vermeer, M.A.; Noakes, M.; Luscombe-Marsh, N.D. Plant sterols lower LDL-cholesterol and triglycerides in dyslipidemic individuals with or at risk of developing type 2 diabetes; a randomized, double-blind, placebo-controlled study. *Nutr. Diabetes* **2018**, *8*, 1–13. [CrossRef] [PubMed]
190. Amir Shaghaghi, M.; Harding, S.V.; Jones, P.J.H. Water dispersible plant sterol formulation shows improved effect on lipid profile compared to plant sterol esters. *J. Funct. Foods* **2014**, *6*, 280–289. [CrossRef]
191. Malina, D.M.T.; Fonseca, F.A.; Barbosa, S.A.; Kasmas, S.H.; Machado, V.A.; França, C.N.; Borges, N.C.; Moreno, R.A.; Izar, M.C. Additive effects of plant sterols supplementation in addition to different lipid-lowering regimens. *J. Clin. Lipidol.* **2015**, *9*, 542–552. [CrossRef]
192. Becker, D.J.; Gordon, R.Y.; Halbert, S.C.; French, B.; Morris, P.B.; Rader, D.J. Red yeast rice for dyslipidemia in statin-intolerant patients: A randomized trial. *Ann. Intern. Med.* **2009**, *150*, 830. [CrossRef]
193. Verhoeven, V.; Van der Auwera, A.; Van Gaal, L.; Remmen, R.; Apers, S.; Stalpaert, M.; Wens, J.; Hermans, N. Can red yeast rice and olive extract improve lipid profile and cardiovascular risk in metabolic syndrome? A double blind, placebo controlled randomized trial. *BMC Complement Altern. Med.* **2015**, *15*, 52. [CrossRef] [PubMed]
194. Yang, C.W.; Mousa, S.A. The effect of red yeast rice (*Monascus purpureus*) in dyslipidemia and other disorders. *Complement Ther. Med.* **2012**, *20*, 466–474. [CrossRef]
195. Biagi, M.; Minoretti, P.; Bertona, M.; Emanuele, E. Effects of a nutraceutical combination of fermented red rice, liposomal berberine, and curcumin on lipid and inflammatory parameters in patients with mild-to-moderate hypercholesterolemia: An 8-week, open-label, single-arm pilot study. *Arch. Med. Sci. Atheroscler. Dis.* **2018**, *3*, e137–e141. [CrossRef] [PubMed]
196. Xiong, Z.; Cao, X.; Wen, Q.; Chen, Z.; Cheng, Z.; Huang, X.; Zhang, Y.; Long, C.; Zhang, Y.; Huang, Z. An overview of the bioactivity of monacolin K/lovastatin. *Food Chem. Toxicol.* **2019**, *131*, 110585. [CrossRef] [PubMed]
197. Surampudi, P.; Enkhmaa, B.; Anuurad, E.; Berglund, L. Lipid Lowering with Soluble Dietary Fiber. *Curr. Atheroscler. Rep.* **2016**, *18*, 75. [CrossRef] [PubMed]
198. Pirillo, A.; Catapano, A.L. Berberine, a plant alkaloid with lipid- and glucose-lowering properties: From in vitro evidence to clinical studies. *Atherosclerosis* **2015**, *243*, 449–461. [CrossRef]
199. Kim, M.; Kim, Y. Hypocholesterolemic effects of curcumin via up-regulation of cholesterol 7a-hydroxylase in rats fed a high fat diet. *Nutr. Res. Pract.* **2010**, *4*, 191–195. [CrossRef]
200. Anadón, A.; Martínez-Larrañaga, M.R.; Ares, I.; Martínez, M.A. Interactions between Nutraceuticals/Nutrients and Therapeutic Drugs. In *Nutraceuticals*, 1st ed.; Gupta, R.C., Ed.; Academic Press: Cambridge, MA, USA, 2016.
201. Gul, K.; Singh, A.K.; Jabeen, R. Nutraceuticals and Functional Foods: The Foods for the Future World. *Crit. Rev. Food Sci. Nutr.* **2016**, *56*, 2617–2627. [CrossRef]
202. Gil, F.; Hernández, A.F.; Martín-Domingo, M.C. Toxic Contamination of Nutraceuticals and Food Ingredients. In *Nutraceuticals*; Gupta, R.C., Ed.; Academic Press: Cambridge, MA, USA, 2016.
203. Gupta, R.C.; Srivastava, A.; Lall, R. Toxicity Potential of Nutraceuticals. In *Computational Toxicology: Methods and Protocols (Methods in Molecular Biology)*; Nicolotti, O., Ed.; Springer: New York, NY, USA, 2018; pp. 367–394. [CrossRef]
204. Gupta, R.C. *Nutraceuticals: Efficacy, Safety and Toxicity*; Academic Press: Cambridge, MA, USA, 2016; p. 1042.
205. Girdhar, S.; Pandita, D.; Girdhar, A.; Lather, V. Safety, Quality and Regulatory Aspects of Nutraceuticals. *Appl. Clin. Res. Clin. Trials Regul. Aff.* **2017**, *4*, 36–42. [CrossRef]
206. Ayaz, M.; Ullah, F.; Sadiq, A.; Ullah, F.; Ovais, M.; Ahmed, J.; Devkota, H.P. Synergistic interactions of phytochemicals with antimicrobial agents: Potential strategy to counteract drug resistance. *Chem. Biol. Interact.* **2019**, *308*, 294–303. [CrossRef]
207. Guo, X.; Mei, N. *Aloe vera*: A review of toxicity and adverse clinical effects. *J. Environ. Sci. Health C* **2016**, *34*, 77–96. [CrossRef]
208. Boudreau, M.D.; Mellick, P.W.; Olson, G.R.; Felton, R.P.; Thorn, B.T.; Beland, F.A. Toxicology and carcinogenesis studies of a nondecolorized [corrected] whole leaf extract of Aloe barbadensis Miller (*Aloe vera*) in F344/N rats and B6C3F1 mice (drinking water study). *Natl. Toxicol. Program. Tech. Rep. Ser.* **2013**, *577*, 1–266.

209. Pandiri, A.R.; Sills, R.C.; Hoenerhoff, M.J.; Peddada, S.D.; Ton, T.-V.T.; Hong, H.-H.L.; Flake, G.P.; Malarkey, D.E.; Olson, G.R.; Pogribny, I.P.; et al. *Aloe vera* Non-Decolorized Whole Leaf Extract-Induced Large Intestinal Tumors in F344 Rats Share Similar Molecular Pathways with Human Sporadic Colorectal Tumors. *Toxicol. Pathol.* **2011**, *39*, 1065–1074. [CrossRef]
210. Shao, A.; Broadmeadow, A.; Goddard, G.; Bejar, E.; Frankos, V. Safety of purified decolorized (low anthraquinone) whole leaf *Aloe vera* (L) Burm. f. juice in a 3-month drinking water toxicity study in F344 rats. *Food Chem. Toxicol.* **2013**, *57*, 21–31. [CrossRef]
211. Williams, L.D.; Burdock, G.A.; Shin, E.; Kim, S.; Jo, T.H.; Jones, K.N.; Matulka, R.A. Safety studies conducted on a proprietary high-purity *Aloe vera* inner leaf fillet preparation, Qmatrix®. *Reg. Toxicol. Pharmacol.* **2010**, *57*, 90–98. [CrossRef] [PubMed]
212. Sehgal, I.; Winters, W.D.; Scott, M.; Kousoulas, K. An in vitro and in vivo toxicologic evaluation of a stabilized *Aloe vera* gel supplement drink in mice. *Food Chem. Toxicol.* **2013**, *55*, 363–370. [CrossRef]
213. Paes-Leme, A.A.; Motta, E.S.; De Mattos, J.C.P.; Dantas, F.J.S.; Bezerra, R.J.A.C.; Caldeira-de-Araujo, A. Assessment of *Aloe vera* (L.) genotoxic potential on Escherichia coli and plasmid DNA. *J. Ethnopharmacol.* **2005**, *102*, 197–201. [CrossRef]
214. Chiang, J.-H.; Yang, J.-S.; Ma, C.-Y.; Yang, M.-D.; Huang, H.-Y.; Hsia, T.-C.; Kuo, H.-M.; Wu, P.-P.; Lee, T.-H.; Chung, J.-G. Danthron, an Anthraquinone Derivative, Induces DNA Damage and Caspase Cascades-Mediated Apoptosis in SNU-1 Human Gastric Cancer Cells through Mitochondrial Permeability Transition Pores and Bax-Triggered Pathways. *Chem. Res. Toxicol.* **2011**, *24*, 20–29. [CrossRef] [PubMed]
215. National Toxicology Program. *Ntp Technical Report on the Toxicology and Carcinogenesis Studies of Ginkgo Biloba Extract (cas No. 90045-36-6) in F344/N Rats and B6c3f1/N Mice (Gavage Studies)*; Technical Report Series; U.S. Public Health Service; National Toxicology Program: Research Triangle Park, NC, USA, 2013; pp. 1–183.
216. Lin, H.; Guo, X.; Zhang, S.; Dial, S.L.; Guo, L.; Manjanatha, M.G.; Moore, M.M.; Mei, N. Mechanistic Evaluation of Ginkgo biloba Leaf Extract-Induced Genotoxicity in L5178Y Cells. *Toxicol. Sci.* **2014**, *139*, 338–349. [CrossRef] [PubMed]
217. Maeda, J.; Kijima, A.; Inoue, K.; Ishii, Y.; Ichimura, R.; Takasu, S.; Kuroda, K.; Matsushita, K.; Kodama, Y.; Saito, N.; et al. In Vivo Genotoxicity of Ginkgo Biloba Extract in gpt Delta Mice and Constitutive Androstane Receptor Knockout Mice. *Toxicol. Sci.* **2014**, *140*, 298–306. [CrossRef] [PubMed]
218. Resende, F.A.; Vilegas, W.; Dos Santos, L.C.; Varanda, E.A. Mutagenicity of Flavonoids Assayed by Bacterial Reverse Mutation (Ames) Test. *Molecules* **2012**, *17*, 5255–5268. [CrossRef] [PubMed]
219. National Toxicology Program. *Toxicology and Carcinogenesis Studies of Goldenseal Root Powder (Hydrastis canadensis) in F344/N Rats and B6c3f1 Mice (Feed Studies)*; Technical Report Series; National Toxicology Program; U.S. Public Health Service; National Toxicology Program: Research Triangle Park, NC, USA, 2010; pp. 1–188.
220. Chen, S.; Wan, L.; Couch, L.; Lin, H.; Li, Y.; Dobrovolsky, V.N.; Mei, N.; Guo, L. Mechanism study of goldenseal-associated DNA damage. *Toxicol. Lett.* **2013**, *221*, 64–72. [CrossRef]
221. Ajayi, A.M.; Umukoro, S.; Ben-Azu, B.; Adzu, B.; Ademowo, O.G. Toxicity and Protective Effect of Phenolic-Enriched Ethylacetate Fraction of *Ocimum gratissimum* (Linn.) Leaf against Acute Inflammation and Oxidative Stress in Rats. *Drug Dev. Res.* **2017**, *78*, 135–145. [CrossRef] [PubMed]
222. Arslan Burnaz, N.; Küçük, M.; Akar, Z. An on-line HPLC system for detection of antioxidant compounds in some plant extracts by comparing three different methods. *J. Chromatogr. B* **2017**, *1052*, 66–72. [CrossRef]
223. Gulati, K.; Anand, R.; Ray, A. Nutraceuticals as Adaptogens: Their Role in Health and Disease. In *Nutraceuticals*; Gupta, R.C., Ed.; Academic Press: Cambridge, MA, USA, 2016.
224. Sobrinho, A.P.; Minho, A.S.; Ferreira, L.L.C.; Martins, G.R.; Boylan, F.; Fernandes, P.D. Characterization of anti-inflammatory effect and possible mechanism of action of Tibouchina granulosa. *J. Pharm. Phramacol.* **2017**, *69*, 706–713. [CrossRef]
225. Wang, K. Adverse Reaction Prediction and Pharmacovigilance of Nutraceuticals: Examples of Computational and Statistical Analysis on Big Data. In *Nutraceuticals*; Gupta, R.C., Ed.; Academic Press: Cambridge, MA, USA, 2016.
226. Gonçalves, R.F.S.; Martins, J.T.; Duarte, C.M.M.; Vicente, A.A.; Pinheiro, A.C. Advances in nutraceutical delivery systems: From formulation design for bioavailability enhancement to efficacy and safety evaluation. *Trends Food Sci. Technol.* **2018**, *78*, 270–291. [CrossRef]
227. Peterson, J.D. Noninvasive In Vivo Optical Imaging Models for Safety and Toxicity Testing. In *Nutraceuticals*; Gupta, R.C., Ed.; Academic Press: Cambridge, MA, USA, 2016.
228. Barnett, R.E.; Bailey, D.C.; Hatfield, H.E.; Fitsanakis, V.A. Caenorhabditis elegans: A Model Organism for Nutraceutical Safety and Toxicity Evaluation. In *Nutraceuticals*; Gupta, R.C., Ed.; Academic Press: Cambridge, MA, USA, 2016.
229. Bian, W.-P.; Pei, D.-S. Zebrafish Model for Safety and Toxicity Testing of Nutraceuticals. In *Nutraceuticals*; Gupta, R.C., Ed.; Academic Press: Cambridge, MA, USA, 2016.
230. Krishna, G.; Gopalakrishnan, G. Alternative In Vitro Models for Safety and Toxicity Evaluation of Nutraceuticals. In *Nutraceuticals*; Gupta, R.C., Ed.; Academic Press: Cambridge, MA, USA, 2016.
231. Gonzalez-Suarez, I.; Martin, F.; Hoeng, J.; Peitsch, M.C. Mechanistic Network Models in Safety and Toxicity Evaluation of Nutraceuticals. In *Nutraceuticals*; Gupta, R.C., Ed.; Academic Press: Cambridge, MA, USA, 2016.
232. Kadakkuzha, B.M.; Liu, X.; Swarnkar, S.; Chen, Y. Genomic and Proteomic Mechanisms and Models in Toxicity and Safety Evaluation of Nutraceuticals. In *Nutraceuticals*; Gupta, R.C., Ed.; Academic Press: Cambridge, MA, USA, 2016.
233. Mouly, S.; Lloret-Linares, C.; Sellier, P.-O.; Sene, D.; Bergmann, J.-F. Is the clinical relevance of drug-food and drug-herb interactions limited to grapefruit juice and Saint-John's Wort? *Pharmacol. Res.* **2017**, *118*, 82–92. [CrossRef]

234. Mooiman, K.D.; Maas-Bakker, R.F.; Hendrikx, J.J.M.A.; Bank, P.C.D.; Rosing, H.; Beijnen, J.H.; Schellens, J.H.M.; Meijerman, I. The effect of complementary and alternative medicines on CYP3A4-mediated metabolism of three different substrates: 7-benzyloxy-4-trifluoromethyl-coumarin, midazolam and docetaxel. *J. Pharm. Phramacol.* **2014**, *66*, 865–874. [CrossRef] [PubMed]
235. Oh, H.-A.; Lee, H.; Kim, D.; Jung, B.H. Development of GC-MS based cytochrome P450 assay for the investigation of multi-herb interaction. *Anal. Biochem.* **2017**, *519*, 71–83. [CrossRef] [PubMed]
236. Zhang, L.; Sparreboom, A. Predicting transporter-mediated drug interactions: Commentary on: "Pharmacokinetic evaluation of a drug transporter cocktail consisting of digoxin, furosemide, metformin and rosuvastatin" and "Validation of a microdose probe drug cocktail for clinical drug interaction assessments for drug transporters and CYP3A". *Clin. Pharmacol. Ther.* **2017**, *101*, 447–449.
237. Gaudineau, C.; Beckerman, R.; Welbourn, S.; Auclair, K. Inhibition of human P450 enzymes by multiple constituents of the Ginkgo biloba extract. *Biochem. Biophys. Res. Commun.* **2004**, *318*, 1072–1078. [CrossRef] [PubMed]
238. Shao, F.; Zhang, H.; Xie, L.; Chen, J.; Zhou, S.; Zhang, J.; Lv, J.; Hao, W.; Ma, Y.; Liu, Y.; et al. Pharmacokinetics of ginkgolides A, B and K after single and multiple intravenous infusions and their interactions with midazolam in healthy Chinese male subjects. *Eur. J. Clin. Pharmacol.* **2017**, *73*, 537–546. [CrossRef]
239. Unger, M.; Frank, A. Simultaneous determination of the inhibitory potency of herbal extracts on the activity of six major cytochrome P450 enzymes using liquid chromatography/mass spectrometry and automated online extraction. *Rapid Commun. Mass Spetrom.* **2004**, *18*, 2273–2281. [CrossRef]
240. Dürr, D.; Stieger, B.; Kullak-Ublick, G.A.; Rentsch, K.M.; Steinert, H.C.; Meier, P.J.; Fattinger, K. St John's Wort induces intestinal P-glycoprotein/MDR1 and intestinal and hepatic CYP3A4. *Clin. Pharmacol. Ther.* **2000**, *68*, 598–604. [CrossRef] [PubMed]
241. Goey, A.K.L.; Mooiman, K.D.; Beijnen, J.H.; Schellens, J.H.M.; Meijerman, I. Relevance of in vitro and clinical data for predicting CYP3A4-mediated herb–drug interactions in cancer patients. *Cancer Treat. Rev.* **2013**, *39*, 773–783. [CrossRef] [PubMed]
242. Dormán, G.; Flachner, B.; Hajdú, I.; András, C.D. Target Identification and Polypharmacology of Nutraceuticals. In *Nutraceuticals*; Gupta, R.C., Ed.; Academic Press: Cambridge, MA, USA, 2016.
243. Herr, M.; Grondin, H.; Sanchez, S.; Armaingaud, D.; Blochet, C.; Vial, A.; Denormandie, P.; Ankri, J. Polypharmacy and potentially inappropriate medications: A cross-sectional analysis among 451 nursing homes in France. *Eur. J. Clin. Pharmacol.* **2017**, *73*, 601–608. [CrossRef]
244. Yang, X.; Li, W.; Sun, Y.; Guo, X.; Huang, W.; Peng, Y.; Zheng, J. Comparative Study of Hepatotoxicity of Pyrrolizidine Alkaloids Retrosine and Monocrotaline. *Chem. Res. Toxicol.* **2017**, *30*, 532–539. [CrossRef]
245. Merz, K.-H.; Schrenk, D. Interim relative potency factors for the toxicological risk assessment of pyrrolizidine alkaloids in food and herbal medicines. *Toxicol. Lett.* **2016**, *263*, 44–57. [CrossRef]
246. Panter, K.E.; Welch, K.D.; Gardner, D.R. Poisonous Plants: Biomarkers for Diagnosis. In *Nutraceuticals*; Gupta, R.C., Ed.; Academic Press: Cambridge, MA, USA, 2019.
247. Preliasco, M.; Gardner, D.; Moraes, J.; González, A.C.; Uriarte, G.; Rivero, R. Senecio grisebachii Baker: Pyrrolizidine alkaloids and experimental poisoning in calves. *Toxicon* **2017**, *133*, 68–73. [CrossRef]
248. Dlugaszewska, J.; Ratajczak, M.; Kamińska, D.; Gajecka, M. Are dietary supplements containing plant-derived ingredients safe microbiologically? *Saudi Pharm. J.* **2019**, *27*, 240–245. [CrossRef]
249. Bugno, A.; Almodovar, A.A.B.; Pereira, T.C.; Pinto, T. de, J.A.; Sabino, M. Occurrence of toxigenic fungi in herbal drugs. *Braz. J. Microbiol.* **2006**, *37*, 47–51. [CrossRef]
250. Prado, G.; Altoé, A.F.; Gomes, T.C.B.; Leal, A.S.; Morais, V.A.D.; Oliveira, M.S.; Ferreira, M.B.; Gomes, M.B.; Paschoal, F.N.; Souza, R.V.S.; et al. Occurrence of aflatoxin B1 in natural products. *Braz. J. Microbiol.* **2012**, *43*, 1428–1435. [CrossRef]
251. Sarma, H.; Deka, S.; Deka, H.; Saikia, R.R. Accumulation of Heavy Metals in Selected Medicinal Plants. In *Reviews of Environmental Contamination and Toxicology*; Whitacre, D.M., Ed.; Springer: New York, NY, USA, 2011; pp. 63–86. [CrossRef]
252. Tong, M.; Gao, W.; Jiao, W.; Zhou, J.; Li, Y.; He, L.; Hou, R. Uptake, Translocation, Metabolism, and Distribution of Glyphosate in Nontarget Tea Plant (*Camellia sinensis* L.). *J. Agric. Food Chem.* **2017**, *65*, 7638–7646. [CrossRef]
253. Hasler, C.M. *Regulation of Functional Foods and Nutraceuticals: A Global Perspective*; John Wiley & Sons: Hoboken, NJ, USA, 2005; p. 425.
254. Jacobo-Velázquez, D.A.; del Rosario Cuéllar-Villarreal, M.; Welti-Chanes, J.; Cisneros-Zevallos, L.; Ramos-Parra, P.A.; Hernández-Brenes, C. Nonthermal processing technologies as elicitors to induce the biosynthesis and, accumulation of nutraceuticals in plant foods. *Trends Food Sci. Technol.* **2017**, *60*, 80–87. [CrossRef]
255. Del Cuéllar-Villarreal, M.R.; Ortega-Hernández, E.; Becerra-Moreno, A.; Welti-Chanes, J.; Cisneros-Zevallos, L.; Jacobo-Velázquez, D.A. Effects of ultrasound treatment and storage time on the extractability and biosynthesis of nutraceuticals in carrot (*Daucus carota*). *Postharvest Biol. Technol.* **2016**, *119*, 18–26. [CrossRef]
256. Wu, J.; Lin, L. Ultrasound-Induced Stress Responses of Panax ginsengCells: Enzymatic Browning and Phenolics Production. *Biotechnol. Prog.* **2002**, *18*, 862–866. [CrossRef] [PubMed]
257. Yu, J.; Engeseth, N.J.; Feng, H. High Intensity Ultrasound as an Abiotic Elicitor—Effects on Antioxidant Capacity and Overall Quality of Romaine Lettuce. *Food Bioprocess Technol.* **2016**, *9*, 262–273. [CrossRef]
258. Ortega, V.G.; Ramírez, J.A.; Velázquez, G.; Tovar, B.; Mata, M.; Montalvo, E. Effect of high hydrostatic pressure on antioxidant content of "Ataulfo" mango during postharvest maturation. *Food Sci. Technol.* **2013**, *33*, 561–568. [CrossRef]
259. Galindo, F.G.; Dejmek, P.; Lundgren, K.; Rasmusson, A.G.; Vicente, A.; Moritz, T. Metabolomic evaluation of pulsed electric field-induced stress on potato tissue. *Planta* **2009**, *230*, 469–479. [CrossRef]

260. Anita, S.; Mangesh, T.; Prasad, V.S.; SinghMeera, C. Nutraceuticals-Global Status and Applications: A Review. 2013. Available online: https://www.semanticscholar.org/paper/Nutraceuticals-Global-status-and-applications-%3A-a-Anita-Mangesh/a1e4ce0f21e585b554e86b203f3bd8166b1cb112 (accessed on 21 May 2020).
261. Santini, A.; Tenore, G.C.; Novellino, E. Nutraceuticals: A paradigm of proactive medicine. *Eur. J. Pharm. Sci.* **2017**, *96*, 53–61. [CrossRef]
262. Brower, V. A nutraceutical a day may keep the doctor away. *EMBO Rep.* **2005**, *6*, 708–711. [CrossRef]
263. Mechanick, J.I.; Brett, E.M. Nutrition and the chronically critically ill patient. *Curr. Opin. Clin. Nutr. Metab. Care* **2005**, *8*, 33–39. [CrossRef]
264. Blades, M. Functional foods or nutraceuticals. *Nutr. Food Sci.* **2000**, *30*, 73–76. [CrossRef]
265. Pandey, M.; Verma, R.K.; Saraf, S.A. Nutraceuticals: New era of medicine and health. *Asian J. Pharm. Clin. Res.* **2010**, *3*, 6.
266. Rudra, S.G.; Nishad, J.; Jakhar, N.; Kaur, C. Food Industry Waste: Mine of Nutraceuticals. *Int. J. Sci.* **2015**, *4*, 205–229.
267. Camacho, F.; Macedo, A.; Malcata, F. Potential Industrial Applications and Commercialization of Microalgae in the Functional Food and Feed Industries: A Short Review. *Mar. Drugs* **2019**, *17*, 312. [CrossRef] [PubMed]
268. Schröder, M.J.A. (Ed.) Food Additives, Functional Food Ingredients and Food Contaminants. In *Food Quality and Consumer Value: Delivering Food That Satisfies*; Springer: Berlin/Heidelberg, Germany, 2003; pp. 167–196. [CrossRef]

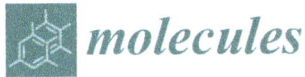

Review

The Health-Promoting Properties and Clinical Applications of Rice Bran Arabinoxylan Modified with Shiitake Mushroom Enzyme—A Narrative Review

Soo Liang Ooi [1], Sok Cheon Pak [1,*], Peter S. Micalos [1], Emily Schupfer [1], Catherine Lockley [1], Mi Houn Park [2] and Sung-Joo Hwang [2,3]

1. School of Biomedical Sciences, Charles Sturt University, Bathurst, NSW 2795, Australia; sooi@csu.edu.au (S.L.O.); pmicalos@csu.edu.au (P.S.M.); eschupfer@csu.edu.au (E.S.); clockley@csu.edu.au (C.L.)
2. EROM R&D Center, EROM Co., Ltd., Chuncheon-si 24427, Gangwon-do, Korea; mhpark@eromplus.com (M.H.P.); mcity007@gmail.com (S.-J.H.)
3. Love Care Clinic, Bundang-gu, Seongnam-si 13724, Gyeonggi-do, Korea
* Correspondence: spak@csu.edu.au; Tel.: +61-2-6338-4952; Fax: +61-2-6338-4993

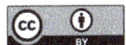

Abstract: Rice bran arabinoxylan compound (RBAC) is derived from defatted rice bran hydrolyzed with *Lentinus edodes* mycelial enzyme. It has been marketed as a functional food and a nutraceutical with health-promoting properties. Some research has demonstrated this rice bran derivative to be a potent immunomodulator, which also possesses anti-inflammatory, antioxidant, and anti-angiogenic properties. To date, research on RBAC has predominantly focused on its immunomodulatory action and application as a complementary therapy for cancer. Nonetheless, the clinical applications of RBAC can extend beyond cancer therapy. This article is a narrative review of the research on the potential benefits of RBAC for cancer and other health conditions based on the available literature. RBAC research has shown it to be useful as a complementary treatment for cancer and human immunodeficiency virus infection. It can positively modulate serum glucose, lipid and protein metabolism in diabetic patients. Additionally, RBAC has been shown to ameliorate irritable bowel syndrome and protect against liver injury caused by hepatitis or nonalcoholic fatty liver disease. It can potentially ease symptoms in chronic fatigue syndrome and prevent the common cold. RBAC is safe to consume and has no known side effects at the typical dosage of 2–3 g/day. Nevertheless, further research in both basic studies and human clinical trials are required to investigate the clinical applications, mechanisms, and effects of RBAC.

Keywords: complementary therapy; BioBran; MGN-3; rice bran exo-biopolymer; functional food; nutraceuticals

1. Introduction

Rice bran is the rough brown layer sandwiched between the outer husk of paddy and its endosperm (kernel), as shown in Figure 1. The bran constitutes roughly 8% of a rice grain before milling and is a source of many nutrients, such as lipids (20–29%), carbohydrates (20–27%, including fibers), proteins (10–15%), B-complex vitamins, minerals, as well as a variety of phytochemicals and antioxidants [1,2]. Many of the bioactive compounds within rice bran possess cancer-preventing properties, including γ-oryzanol, ferulic acid, caffeic acid, tricin, coumaric acid, phytic acid, tocopherols, phytosterols, and carotenoids [3]. As such, this by-product of rice production is now gaining increasing attention for its nutritional, functional, and commercial potentials beyond its traditional use as animal feed [4]. For instance, there is a growing use of defatted rice bran as a functional ingredient in food production, such as baking, to increase the protein, dietary fiber, and antioxidant contents [5].

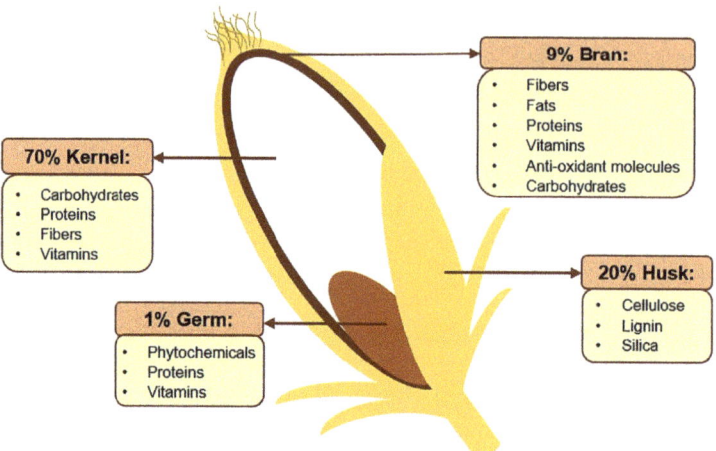

Figure 1. Schematic representation of rice before the milling process with the percentage of all its components and the main constituents. Reprinted under CC-BY 4.0 license from Fraterrigo Garofalo S., Tommasi T., & Fino, D. (2021). A short review of green extraction technologies for rice bran oil. *Biomass Conv. Bioref., 11*, 569–587.

A primary component of the dietary fibers found in rice bran is arabinoxylan, a hemicellulose type belonging to the non-starch polysaccharide group. The structure of arabinoxylan consists of backbone chains of β-(1-4)-linked D-xylopyranosyl (xylan) with α-L-arabinofuranose units linked as side chains via the second and third carbon positions [6]. Along with arabinose, some galactose, xylose, and glucuronic acid residues can also exist as side branches. With a molecular weight ranging between 10 to 10,000 kDa, the cross-links of many side chains make arabinoxylan mostly resistant to extraction by water [7]. Additional treatments using enzymes, alkali solutions or mechanical methods are needed to remove arabinoxylans from the stable cross-link networks to produce soluble hemicellulose and arabinoxylan compounds with low molecular weights [7,8].

One approach to facilitate the extraction of arabinoxylan from rice bran is via the use of mycelium enzymes. In one study, rice bran was treated with enzymes cultured from nine different fungi types and tested for their macrophage stimulating activities [9]. Treatment with the enzyme from *L. edodes* (shiitake mushroom) exhibited the highest macrophage stimulating activity. Further research has shown that this rice bran arabinoxylan compound (RBAC) possesses immunomodulating, anti-inflammatory, antioxidant, and anti-angiogenesis properties. From this, RBAC has shown significant potential for clinical applications as a nutraceutical [8].

This article reviews available in vivo, in vitro, and human studies from the literature to uncover the health-promoting properties of RBAC. Potential clinical applications of RBAC in cancer, human immunodeficiency viruses (HIV) infection, diabetes, irritable bowel syndrome (IBS), liver diseases, chronic fatigue syndrome (CFS), and the common cold, which are supported by research evidence, will also be presented.

2. The Production and Composition of RBAC

RBAC is currently available as dietary supplements or nutraceuticals for immune system improvement and disease prevention. Most prominently, a functional food called Biobran MGN-3 is developed in Japan by Daiwa Pharmaceutical Co., Ltd. This product is marketed worldwide under many different brand names, such as Biobran, Ribraxx (in Australia), Lentin Plus (in Asia), or BRM4 (in the United States) [10]. Rice bran exo-biopolymer is another variant of RBAC independently developed in Korea by Erom Co., Ltd. [8,11,12]. It is the main ingredient of Erom's immune-related products distributed not only in Korea but also in the United States and other countries. This review adopts RBAC as the generic name for any hydrolyzed extract of defatted rice bran modified with the *L. edodes* mycelial enzyme.

The production of RBAC is depicted in the following Figure 2.

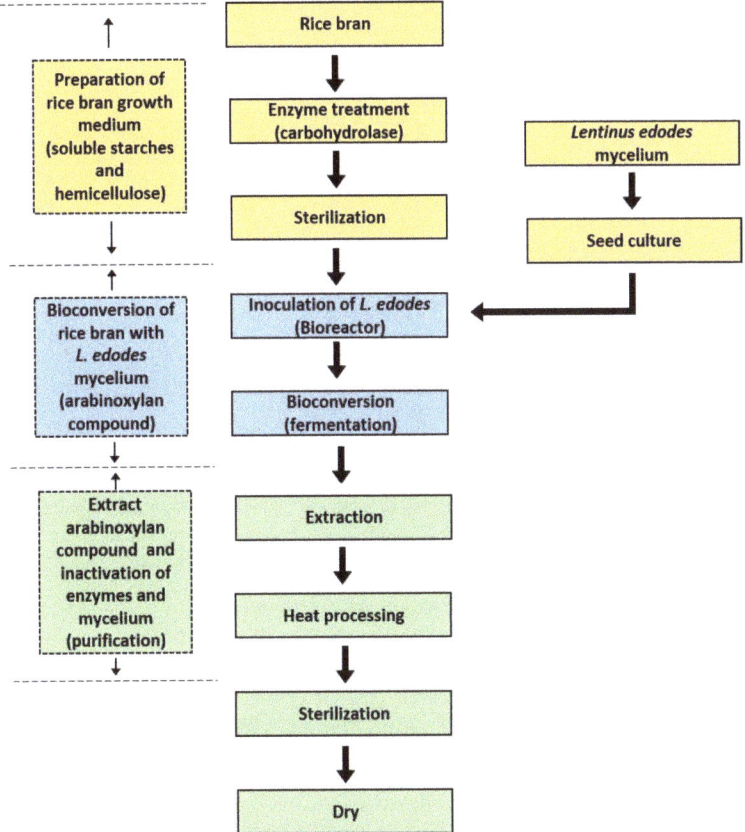

Figure 2. The steps to produce rice bran arabinoxylan compound: (1) Preparation: Defatted rice bran is enzymatically treated and *Lentinus edodes* is prepared as a seed culture. (2) Bioconversion: Inoculation of *L. edodes* as a bioreactor to instigate fermentation. (3) Extraction: The arabinoxylan compound is extracted through heat processing, sterilization and drying.

Biobran Research Foundation [10] described the steps to produce RBAC as follows:

Preparation: Defatted rice bran is thoroughly mixed with hot water at the ratio of 1:5. The insoluble polysaccharide is removed from the mixture leaving only soluble starch. Glucoamylase is then added to hydrolyze the starch by cleaving the 1,4-α-glycosidic bonds of the nonreducing end of the glycosidic chains resulting in the release of d-glucose. This process increases the content of fermentable carbohydrates [13]. *L. edodes* is cultured in a liquid medium. The mycelia of *L. edodes* and any insoluble residues are then removed to obtain the carbohydrase complexes, including xylanase, glucosidase, monosidase, and hemicellulose [10].

Bioconversion: This step involves mixing and heating the hemicellulose extract (from rice bran) with the carbohydrase complexes (from *L. edodes*), resulting in the bioconversion or fermentation of the raw materials.

Extraction: The bioconversion produces partially hydrolyzed rice bran hemicellulose, which has a high arabinoxylan content. The extract is then heated, sterilized, condensed, and added with excipient resulting in the final product as a powder [10].

This powdered product is 98.4% soluble in purified water consisting of heteropolysaccharide structures with molecular weights between 30–100 kDa [14,15]. The active ingredient responsible for its immunomodulatory property is likely to be a modified arabinoxylan with a xylose in its main chain and an arabinose polymer side chain [14], as shown in Figure 3.

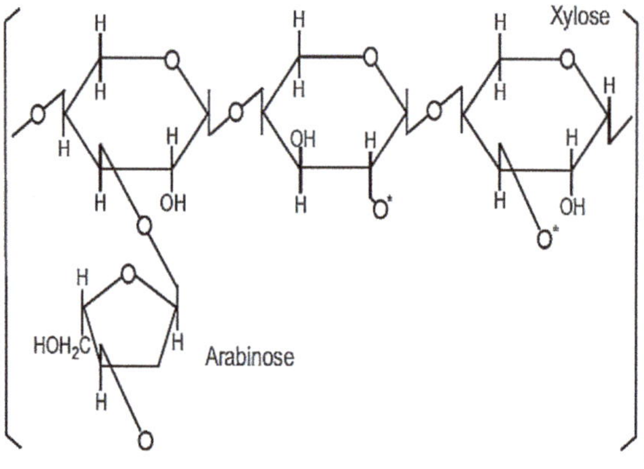

Figure 3. Chemical structure of MGN-3/Biobran. Reprinted from Wheat and Rice in Disease Prevention and Health, 1st ed., M. H. Ghoneum, Chapter 31—Apoptosis and arabinoxylan rice bran, pp. 401–408, Copyright 2014, with permission from Elsevier.

3. Health-Promoting Properties

3.1. Immunomodulatory Action

RBAC has been promoted as a plant-based biological response modifier that acts to modify the body's immune response [16]. RBAC can enhance both innate and adaptive immune systems in eliminating pathogens and malignant cells.

The innate immunity is enhanced via up-regulating the cytotoxic activity of natural killer (NK) cells with increased granularity [17]. RBAC's effects on NK cell activity were demonstrated in vivo in different mouse models [18–22], in vitro with different cell lines [11,19,23], and in human trials [17,23–29]. RBAC can also enhance the phagocytic cellular functions of macrophages, neutrophils, and monocytes. Macrophages cultured with RBAC demonstrated better efficacy in phagocytosis, enhanced spreading ability, and increased production of cytokines (tumor necrosis factor-alpha [TNF-α] and interleukin [IL]-6) to regulate B-cell function [9,12,30,31]. Similarly, neutrophils and monocytes treated with RBAC have also shown enhanced anti-bacterial activity characterized by increased oxidative burst and cytokine production in the presence of bacteria [32].

RBAC influences the adaptive immune response via the dendritic cells (DCs). Immature DCs derived from peripheral monocytes showed increased expression of maturation markers after treatment with RBAC [33,34] The effect of RBAC as a potent inducer of DC maturation and activation has also been confirmed in a placebo randomized control trial (RCT) with 48 multiple myeloma patients [28,29]. Activation of DCs also triggers T lymphocyte responses with the increased proliferation of T and B lymphocytes, as revealed in several studies [17,23,33,35,36]. In patients with underactive immune systems, RBAC may also enhance immune function by inhibiting the immunosuppression effects of Treg lymphocytes [36].

3.2. Anti-Inflammatory Effect

The mechanism of how RBAC can trigger the immune-inflammatory response remains unclear. Experiments by Endo and Kanbayashi [37] have confirmed that molecules of immunoreactive polysaccharides can be detected in blood after oral administration of

RBAC. Due to the similarity in structure and molecular weight with lipopolysaccharide from Gram-negative bacteria, it has been suggested that enzyme-treated arabinoxylan may mimic pathogen-associated molecular patterns [6]. As lipopolysaccharide binds to the toll-like receptor 4 on phagocytes' surface, low-molecular-weight arabinoxylan may also activate phagocytes through the same receptor [6]. RBAC administration was shown to exert transient activation of inflammatory cytokines in healthy individuals [25]. However, in the presence of infection or inflammation, it could down-regulate the overall inflammatory response through competing with pathogens at the immune-stimulating ligands [6]. Many pre-clinical [20,22,24,31–33,35] and clinical studies [25,28,38] demonstrated RBAC affecting the production of both pro-inflammatory (tumor necrosis factor [TNF]-α, interferon [INF]-γ, IL-1β, IL-2, IL-6, IL-7, and IL-12) and anti-inflammatory (IL-1RA and IL-10) cytokines. Hence, RBAC plays a role in regulating the immuno-inflammatory mechanism by modulating these signaling proteins in a complex multifactorial manner.

The dysfunction of localized inflammatory regulation can lead to chronic and systemic inflammation, which is the underlying cause of many chronic conditions, including asthma, autoimmune conditions, cardiovascular diseases, obesity, diabetes, depression, osteoarthritis, and cancer [39]. Ichihashi [40] reported the potential beneficial effect of RBAC on chronic inflammation in a case series. Eight patients with chronic rheumatism on steroids were given RBAC as a food supplement for 6 to 12 months. Three of them responded to RBAC, showing a reduction in rheumatoid factor and C-reactive protein (CRP) post-treatment. Ghoneum and El Sayed [41] further demonstrated that RBAC has a protective effect against neuroinflammation in a mouse model of sporadic Alzheimer's disease by lowering IL-6 and intercellular adhesion molecule-1 in brain tissues.

RBAC was also shown in clinical trials to exert effects on lowering the biomarkers for systemic inflammation. A small study (n = 10) that combined RBAC and curcumin reported a potential effect in reducing the raising erythrocyte sedimentation rate in 44% of the participants with early B-cell lymphoid malignancies [42]. In another study involving patients with mixed-type IBS, supplementation of four weeks with RBAC was shown to have an anti-inflammatory effect by lowering CRP value and the neutrophil-to-lymphocyte ratio [43].

3.3. Antioxidant Action

RBAC has been shown to augment the function of the antioxidant defense system. Solutions of RBAC in ethanol were assessed by Tazawa et al. [44] as having a high scavenging rate on hypoxanthine-xanthine oxidase generated superoxide anion radicals, ferrous sulphate-hydrogen peroxide and ultra-violet light reaction system-generated hydroxyl radicals. In an animal study with Ehrlich carcinoma-bearing mice, Noaman et al. [45] reported that RBAC efficiently suppressed tumor growth with an associated normalization of lipid peroxidation and glutathione contents.

RBAC was also shown to enhance the activity of the endogenous antioxidant scavenging enzymes, which include superoxide dismutase (SOD), glutathione peroxidase (GPx), catalase (CAT) and glutathione-S-transferase (GST), in blood, liver, and tumor tissue [45]. Similarly, the messenger ribonucleic acid (mRNA) expressions of GPx, SOD1 and CAT in the liver were up-regulated, demonstrating RBAC's protective properties against oxidative stress [45].

In another murine model, sporadic Alzheimer's disease was induced via intracerebroventricular injection of streptozotocin [41]. After administering RBAC for 21 days, the streptozotocin-treated mouse showed improvement in oxidative stress biomarkers with the significant increase of malondialdehyde and glutathione levels in the hippocampus ($p < 0.0001$). Oxidative stress was further studied via the expression of nuclear factor erythroid 2-related factor 2 (Nrf2) and antioxidant response element (ARE). RBAC was shown to increase the hippocampal Nrf2 and ARE levels significantly ($p < 0.0001$) in a dose-dependent manner where a high level of RBAC (200 mg/kg) approximately returned the Nrf2 and ARE levels to that of control [41].

This protective effect against oxidative stress was also shown in another murine study examining gamma radiation's effects [46]. Exposure to ionizing radiation is known to induce oxidative stress that can damage cellular macromolecules leading to the demise of hematopoietic tissues [47]. Mice exposed to gamma radiation showed significant depression in their full blood count, hypocellularity of their bone marrow, and a remarkable decrease in splenic weight. In contrast, pre-treatment with RBAC resulted in protection against such irradiation-induced damages [46]. RBAC's ability to augment the antioxidant defense system to counteract the severe adverse effects and toxicity of radiation therapy is confirmed in a double-blind, placebo RCT with head-and-neck cancer patients (n = 65) undergoing radiotherapy by Tan and Flores [48].

3.4. Angiogenesis Inhibition

RBAC can affect new blood vessel growth through the vascular endothelial growth factor (VEGF) pathway. An in vitro study by Zhu et al. [49] demonstrated that RBAC significantly inhibited VEGF-induced tube formation in human umbilical vein endothelial cells co-cultured with human dermal fibroblasts. Furthermore, RBAC also suppressed the VEGF-induced proliferation and migration of human umbilical vein endothelial cells in a dose-dependent manner [49]. The anti-angiogenic mechanism of RBAC operates through the reduction of not only the VEGF-induced activation of VEGF receptor 2, but also the downstream proteins of protein kinase B, extracellular signal-regulated protein kinase 1/2, and p38 mitogen-activated protein kinase [49]. Therefore, RBAC can potentially mediate angiogenesis, implicated in the pathological progression of conditions such as cancer, cardiac and limb ischemia, diabetic retinopathy, rheumatoid arthritis, and neoplasms [50]. Figure 4 summarizes the medicinal actions and effects of rice bran arabinoxylan compound discussed in this section.

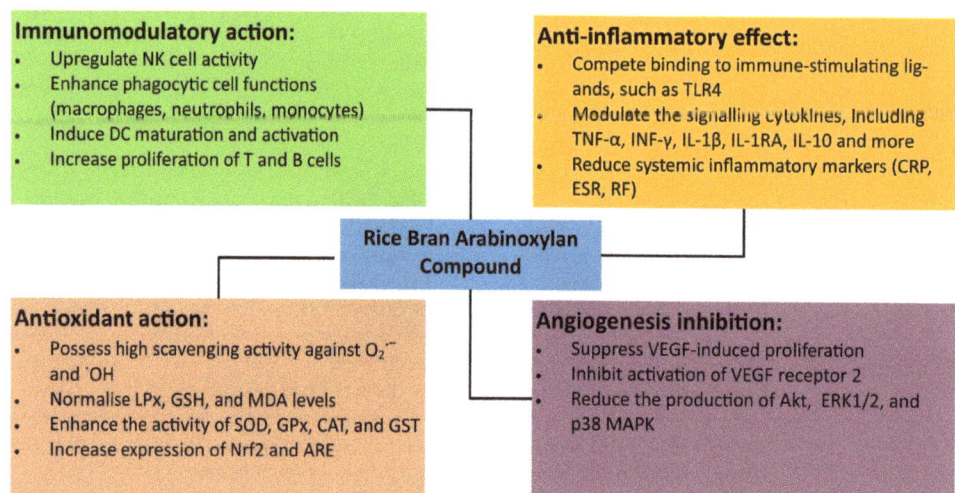

Abbreviations: Akt, protein kinase B; ARE, antioxidant response element; CRP, C-reactive protein; CAT, catalase; DC, dendritic cell; ERK, extracellular signal-regulated protein kinase; ESR, erythrocyte sedimentation rate; GPx, glutathione peroxidase; GSH, glutathione; GST, glutathione-S-transferase; INF, interferon; IL, interleukin; LPx, lipid peroxidation; MAPK, mitogen-activated protein kinase; MDA, malondialdehyde; NK, natural killer; Nrf2, nuclear factor erythroid 2-related factor 2; $O_2^{·-}$, superoxide anion radical; ·OH, hydroxyl radical; RF, rheumatoid factor; SOD, superoxide dismutase; TLR, toll-like receptor; TNF, tumour necrosis factor; VEGF, vascular endothelial growth factor.

Figure 4. A summary of the key health-promoting attributes of rice bran arabinoxylan compound.

4. Clinical Applications

4.1. Cancer

The immunomodulatory effects of RBAC make it a potential anti-cancer lead compound [16]. The antiproliferative actions on cancer cells were demonstrated in several in vitro studies that cultured human and murine cancer cell lines with RBAC [19,51–53]. In models of animals implanted with malignancies, including gastric cancer [21], neuroblastoma [19], melanoma [11], and Ehrlich carcinoma [20,45], RBAC demonstrated its ability to inhibit cancer growth. RBAC was also shown to work synergistically with other natural anti-cancer substances, such as Baker's yeast [51] and curcumin [53]. It also enhanced the effectiveness of chemotherapeutic agents, including cisplatin [37,54], daunorubicin [54,55] and paclitaxel [56,57] as well as radiotherapy [48,58].

Many successful RBAC-treated clinical cases have been reported in current literature with primary cancers, including leukemia, prostate, breast, colorectal, pancreatic, liver, lung, skin, and ovarian [59]. Favorable outcomes reported in these cases include improvements in tumor markers, immunocompetence profile, and initial symptoms after taking RBAC [60,61]. Some patients' conditions stabilized and showed no indication of recurrence at follow-up [17]. Improvement in cancer patient's quality of life (QoL) in terms of subjective sleep quality, appetite, digestion, physical activity and decrease in anxiety and pain, as well as reduced adverse events during chemotherapy, were also reported [62,63]. One case reported remission of metastatic lung tumor after 34 months of self-treatment with RBAC [64]. Complete or near-complete remission of hepatic metastases was also reported by Hajto and Kirsch [65] in seven cases of patients treated with a combination of RBAC, mistletoe lectins and wheat germ extract. In three case reports, patients with terminal cancer exceeded their initially clinically projected lifespans and reported significantly improved QoL [60,66,67].

A recent systematic review conducted by the lead authors found evidence supporting RBAC as a complementary therapy alongside conventional cancer treatment [59]. The review identified 11 RBAC clinical trials with cancer patients, including six RCTs. As an adjunct therapy during conventional chemo- and radiotherapy, the reported effects of RBAC include improvement of the immune profile, reduction of side effects, and improvement of treatment outcomes [29,68–71]. Investigating the efficacy of administering RBAC as a follow-up therapy after conventional treatment, three clinical studies [17,27,36] reported favorable results in the restoration of the immune system profiles, improvement in QoL, and enhancing the long-term survival rate of late-stage cancer patients. The review also found RBAC as safe with no related adverse events reported in the clinical trials and recommended RBAC as an adjunct or follow-up therapy to complement conventional cancer treatment [59]. A more recent trial by Tan and Flores [48] further confirmed the benefits of RBAC for head-and-neck cancer patients during radiation treatment. Patients who took RBAC before, during and after treatment had better clinical outcomes compared to the placebo group. A new study is currently underway to confirm the effects of RBAC on patients' QoL during active cancer treatment [72]. Table 1 shows a summary of the systematic review and recent clinical trials evaluating the effects of RBAC on cancer patients.

Table 1. Summary of systematic reviews and recent clinical trials evaluating the effects of RBAC on cancer patients.

Study	Design	Condition	Objectives	N	Dosage	Findings
Ooi et al. (2018), Australia	Systematic review (includes studies until May 2017)	Various malignancies	To comprehensively review the available evidence on the effects and efficacies of MGN-3 as a complementary therapy for conventional cancer treatment.	11 studies (NRT = 5, RCT = 6). N = 566 (RBAC = 351, control = 215)	1–3 g/day with duration ranging from 2 weeks to 4 years.	Available evidence suggests RBAC as an effective immunomodulator that can complement conventional cancer treatment. More well-designed RCT is needed to strengthen the evidence base.
Tan & Flores (2020), Philippines	Double-blind placebo RCT	Head-and-neck carcinoma	To investigate the effects of RBAC on hematologic profile, nutritional status, and QoL of head-and-neck cancer patients undergoing radiation therapy or concurrent chemotherapy.	N = 65 (RBAC = 33, placebo = 32)	3 g/day. 2 weeks before the start of treatment, during treatment and 2 months after treatment.	The results showed better clinical outcomes for the RBAC group with fewer blood transfusions, treatment delays and hospital admissions, avoidance of treatment mortalities and morbidities, and improved QoL.
Ooi et al. (2020), Australia	Double-blind placebo RCT	Solid organ cancers stage II and above	To evaluate the effects of RBAC on cancer patients' QoL, inflammatory and nutritional status, cytokine profile, and gut microbiota during active treatment, compared to placebo.	N = 50 (RBAC = 25, placebo = 25)	3 g/day for 6 months during active treatment.	This trial is ongoing. Trial Reg No: ACTRN12619000562178p. Targeted completion date: May 2022.

Abbreviation: NRT, non-randomized trial; QoL, quality of life; RBAC, rice bran arabinoxylan compound; RCT, randomized control trial.

4.2. HIV Infection

The anti-HIV activity of RBAC was first reported by Ghoneum [73]. In an in vitro study, the peripheral blood mononuclear cells from three healthy donors were incubated with HIV-1 SF strains (HIV-1 p24 of 3000 pg/106 cells) at 37 °C for one hour. The infected cells were then kept in complete media for seven days at 37 °C with or without RBAC at a range of concentrations (0, 12.5, 25, 50, 100 µg/mL). The mean production of HIV-1 p24 antigen, compared to control, was reduced by 18.3%, 42.8%, 59% and 75%, at concentrations of 12.5, 25, 50, and 100 µg/mL of RBAC, respectively [73]. Thus, RBAC inhibited HIV-1 replication in a dose-dependent manner. RBAC was also shown to inhibit HIV-induced syncytia formation. A syncytium is a fusion of an infected cell with neighboring cells forming a multinucleated product. Syncytia formation is known to contribute to virus dissemination [74]. Ghoneum investigated syncytia formation with the mononuclear cell fusion array from five patients with acquired immunodeficiency syndrome (AIDS) [73]. The mononuclear cells were cultured for seven days at 37 °C with or without RBAC at different concentrations (0, 12.5, 25, 50, 100 µg/mL). RBAC was shown to significantly inhibit the syncytia formation in a dose-dependent manner, with the maximum inhibition of 75% observed at a concentration of 100 µg/mL [73].

The effects of RBAC on the immune, hepatic, and renal functions of HIV-positive individuals were examined by Lewis et al. [75]. in a double-blind, placebo RCT. Forty-seven HIV+ participants on stable antiretroviral therapy (ART) were randomly assigned to consume either 3 g/day of RBAC (n = 22) or placebo (n = 25) supplement for six months. Participants were assessed at the third and sixth month for cluster differentiation (CD)4+ T cells and CD8+ T cells, liver enzymes, and kidney function for comparison with baseline. Both groups' liver and kidney markers remained within normal limits throughout the study, with no significant difference between groups. However, there was a statistically significant difference in the percentage change in CD8+ T cells between the groups ($F[1,32] = 4.8$, $p = 0.04$), with the placebo group showing rising CD8+. Furthermore, the RBAC group showed a clinically significant increase in the CD4+/CD8+ ratio (+8.6%) compared to a decrease (−12.2%) in the placebo group, even though the change was only statistically marginal ($F[1, 31] = 3.2$, $p = 0.085$). Elevated CD8+ T cell count under ART is recognized as an early warning indicator for future treatment failure [76]. With its ability to attenuate the CD8+ overstimulation, RBAC can potentially prevent the resultant complications of ART in HIV+ patients [75].

Another double-blind, placebo RCT for HIV+ patients using RBAC was conducted by Cadden et al. [77]. The study aimed to investigate RBAC's anti-inflammatory effects in ART-suppressed HIV infection for its potential use in preventing end-organ disease in AIDS patients. Analysis of the biomarkers from 24 participants (RBAC = 12, placebo = 12) consisting of hsCRP, CD14, sCD163, lipoprotein binding protein, and IL-6 did not reveal any statistically significant difference between the RBAC and placebo groups after 12 weeks of supplementation. Hence, the clinical application of RBAC for the HIV+ population requires further investigation.

4.3. Common Cold

The common cold is an acute self-limiting viral infection of the upper respiratory tract. The preventive effect of RBAC against common cold in older adults was examined in a double-blind, cross-over RCT [78]. The study recruited 50 elderly aged 70 to 95 years from a residential care facility. Each participant consumed RBAC in one period and water-soluble fractions of rice bran as a control in another period. Each administration period was six weeks with a two-week washout interval. Participants were randomly assigned to receive either RBAC or control substance as their starting treatment in the first period. Common cold symptoms were assessed and scored by care personnel daily. Data from 36 participants who completed both periods were analyzed. Withdrawal reasons were due to healthy participants leaving the care facility and were unrelated to the treatment protocols. The control group's total symptom score was significantly higher ($p < 0.05$), three times more than the RBAC group. Furthermore, the mean duration of common cold symptoms was shorter in the RBAC group (1.2 days) than the control (2.6 days), albeit not statistically significant. The results demonstrated that RBAC could prevent the upper respiratory tract viral infection and reduce common cold symptoms in older adults [78].

4.4. Liver Diseases

RBAC can potentially protect against liver injury caused by viral hepatitis. In an in vivo study by Zheng et al. [79], male Wistar rats were injected with D-galactosamine to induce liver injury similar to human hepatitis B. Rats were pre-treated with RBAC at 20 mg/kg body weight or 60 mg/kg body weight, intraperitoneally. Compared to control, pre-treated rats had significantly ($p < 0.05$) lower serum transaminase levels. The study also found that the low-molecular-weight ($\leqslant 0.4$ kDa) fractions of RBAC were more effective than both medium (0.4 − 2000 kDa) and high (>2000 kDa) molecular-weight fractions in lowering serum transaminase levels. The hepatoprotective mechanisms were partly mediated by the down-regulation of both the IL-18 mRNA expression in the liver and serum IL-18 concentration in RBAC-administered rats [79]. Further experiments also show that the suppressive effects of RBAC on hepatitis induced by D-galactosamine are related to the inhibition of nuclear factor-κB, mitogen-activated protein kinase, and CD14 expression [80].

In a non-inferiority clinical trial, two groups of hepatitis C patients were randomized to receive either RBAC (n = 16, 1 g/day) or the standard treatment (pegylated interferon plus ribavirin, n = 21) for three months [81]. Post-treatment viral load in both groups reduced similarly and significantly relative to baseline ($p < 0.05$). Treatment with RBAC was shown to significantly increase the level of IFN-γ after three months ($p < 0.001$). The standard treatment group reported adverse events, including fever, anemia, thrombocytopenia, and fatigue, whereas no adverse effects were reported in the RBAC group. Hence, RBAC could be a viable alternative to pegylated interferon plus ribavirin treatment for hepatitis C with fewer side effects [81].

RBAC supplementation also benefits patients with nonalcoholic fatty liver disease (NAFLD). In a 90-day double-blind, placebo RCT [82], 23 NAFLD patients were randomly assigned to consume 1 g/day of either RBAC or placebo. Serum biomarkers were assessed at baseline, 45, and 90 days. Alkaline phosphatase, a hallmark of liver damage, significantly decreased ($p = 0.03$) in the RBAC group compared to placebo. Significant increases in the eosinophils ($p = 0.02$), monocytes ($p < 0.001$), and IL-18 ($p = 0.03$) in the RBAC group compared to placebo were also detected at the 90-day follow-up, suggestive of the immunomodulatory effects of RBAC [82]. Decreases in both neutrophils and neutrophil-to-lymphocyte ratio in RBAC group compared to placebo were also observed, even though not statistically significant, may be clinically relevant. No adverse events caused by RBAC was reported in this study [82]. Overall, the evidence on the beneficial effects of RBAC for managing NAFLD is promising.

4.5. Chronic Fatigue Syndrome

The potential beneficial effects of RBAC on CFS was first reported in a small observational study with patients diagnosed with CFS (n = 10) consuming 3 g/day of RBAC for two months [83]. Symptom severity was assessed with Chalder fatigue score and the visual analogue scale at baseline and after two months. This study observed symptom improvement in patients with clear viral etiology (4 out of 10 patients). The author postulated a potential link between the increased NK cell activity during RBAC supplementation and fatigue symptoms [83].

To validate the effectiveness of RBAC in reducing fatigue in CFS patients, McDermott et al. [84] conducted a placebo RCT with 71 participants. Participants were given oral RBAC supplement (n = 37) or matching placebo (n = 34) for eight weeks at a dosage of 6 g/day (2 g × 3 times daily). The primary outcome measure was the Chalder physical fatigue score. Additional outcome measures included self-reported fatigue, self-assessment of improvement, change in key symptoms, QoL, anxiety and depression. Both groups of participants experienced marked improvement over the study duration but without significant differences between groups. As such, the study did not find RBAC to be superior to placebo for reducing fatigue in CFS patients [84]. However, this study did not differentiate patients based on their CFS aetiology, a potential factor influencing the treatment efficacy of RBAC observed by Kenyon [83].

RBAC was combined with oncothermia therapy to treat patients with CFS due to cancer treatment in an RCT [71]. Fifty patients completed the study, with 25 of them taking RBAC (1 g × 3 per day) plus receiving 15 weekly oncothermia treatment, in addition to their standard cancer treatment (chemotherapy or radiotherapy) over six months. Another 25 control patients received only standard cancer treatment. The severity of CFS was assessed with Chalder fatigue score, patient global impression of change, and QoL questionnaire (EORTC QLQ-C30). The study found a significant reduction in the mean fatigue score in the RBAC+ oncothermia group after treatment compared to baseline ($p < 0.01$), whereas no significant change in fatigue score was detected in the control group. In terms of the mean patient global impression of change, the RBAC+ oncothermia group indicated 'much improved' after treatment compared to 'no change' in the control group. Therefore, the study found the combined therapy (RBAC+ oncothermia) effectively reduced fatigue in cancer patients suffering from CFS [71].

Overall, the effects of RBAC on CFS remain unclear, with mixed results from the low number of studies conducted. Further research is needed to investigate the applicability of RBAC for CFS patients with the disease aetiology being a potential determinant factor for fatigue reduction.

4.6. Irritable Bowel Syndrome

In a pilot study by Kamiya et al. [43], 40 patients with diarrhea-predominant or mixed-type IBS were randomly assigned to receive an oral supplement of either 1g of RBAC or placebo powder twice a day for four weeks. Global symptom assessments were conducted at baseline and weekly intervals using a five-point Likert scale. Other outcome measures, including gastrointestinal-specific QoL and anxiety, were evaluated using self-reported questionnaires before and at the end of supplementation. The participants also had blood tests at baseline and week four [43].

The results showed that RBAC supplementation was effective for 63.2% of the patients RBAC group compared to only 30% in the placebo group ($p < 0.05$) at the end of the study [43]. Significant between-group differences in serum neutrophil ($p = 0.0184$) and lymphocyte ($p = 0.0384$) were also reported. A lower neutrophil-to-lymphocyte ratio in the RBAC group suggests reduced subclinical inflammation. The RBAC group also reported significant improvement in the symptoms of reflux ($p = 0.013$), diarrhea ($p < 0.001$), and constipation ($p < 0.024$) compared to baseline. No significant changes in the placebo group's symptom ratings were detected at the end of the study, compared to baseline. However, comparisons of all symptom changes between-group were not significant due to the small sample size [43]. A full-scale trial validating the effects of RBAC on mixed-type IBS is warranted.

4.7. Diabetes

Ohara et al. [85,86] explored the effects of RBAC in streptozotocin-induced diabetic rats. In one study [85], the diabetic rats were administered with 0.5 g/kg body mass of RBAC via stomach tube for two months. Compared to controlled diabetic rats administered with inert substance (0.5% sodium alginate), RBAC-fed rats showed significantly reduced water intake ($p \leq 0.05$), suggested as an improvement in polyuria. The RBAC-fed rats also had significantly ($p \leq 0.05$) lower triglycerides, total cholesterol, total protein, and zinc levels in serum at the end of the study. However, no significant difference in body mass, serum glucose and insulin were detected between the two groups [85].

In another study [86], adult rats with diabetes induced with streptozotocin as neonates were fed with experimental diets consisting of only 1.7% cellulose or 1.7% cellulose plus 1% RBAC for 60 days. Oral glucose tolerance tests were performed after 20 h of fasting on day 58. Diabetic rats fed with RBAC, compared to control, had significantly lower glucose level ($p < 0.05$) at 30 min after being fed with glucose (2 g/kg body mass) via stomach tubes. Like the previous study, serum biochemistry analysis also revealed a significantly lower total cholesterol level ($p < 0.05$) in RBAC-fed diabetic rats than those on the control diet [86]. Supplementation with RBAC potentially improves blood glucose spike as well as lipid and protein metabolism in diabetic rats. To date, there is no published human study on the potential beneficial effects of RBAC for diabetes.

Table 2 is a summary of all clinical trials evaluating the effects of RBAC on health conditions other than cancer.

Table 2. Summary of clinical trials evaluating the effects of RBAC on health conditions other than cancer.

Study	Design	Condition	Objectives	N	Dosage	Findings
Kenyon et al. (2001), UK	Single-arm prospective study	CFS	To assess the effect of RBAC on the fatigue symptoms in patients with CFS.	N = 10	3 g/day for 2 months	In those patients with a clear viral aetiology of CFS, RBAC produced significant improvement.
Maeda et al. (2004), Japan	Double-blind cross-over, active-control RCT	Common cold	To examine the preventive effect of RBAC against the common cold symptoms in older adults (age 70–95) compared to a water-soluble rice bran supplement.	N = 36	0.5 g/day for 6 weeks	The rice bran group's total symptom score was three times higher than that for the RBAC group. The average duration of symptoms was 2.6 days for the rice bran group, whereas it was only 1.2 days for the RBAC group.
McDermott et al. (2006), UK	Double-blind placebo RCT	CFS	To evaluate the effectiveness of RBAC as a putative natural killer cell stimulant in reducing fatigue in CFS patients.	N = 67 (RBAC = 35, placebo = 32)	2 g/day for 8 weeks	Both groups showed marked improvement over the study duration but without significant differences. The findings do not support a specific therapeutic effect for RBAC in CFS.
Kamiya et al. (2014), Japan	Double-blind placebo RCT	IBS	To investigate the immune modulation effect of RBAC in patients with diarrhea-predominant IBS or mixed IBS.	N = 39 (RBAC = 19, placebo = 20)	2 g/day for 4 weeks	RBAC group showed a significant decrease ($p < 0.05$) in the score of reflux, diarrhea, and constipation. The placebo group showed no significant difference in symptom scores.
Petrovics et al. (2016), Hungary	Double-blind, active-control RCT	CFS	To evaluate the efficacy of a combined oncothermia and RBAC therapy to treat cancer patients suffering from CFS.	N = 50 (RBAC = 25, control = 25)	1 g/day for 24 weeks	The mean fatigue score was significantly reduced ($p < 0.01$) after treatment in the intervention group but not in the control group.
Salama et al. (2016), Egypt	Double-blind RCT	HCV	To examine the anti-HCV effects of RBAC in restricting viremia in chronic HCV patients compared to the standard PEG IFN therapy.	N = 37 (RBAC = 16, control = 21)	1 g/day for 3 months	RBAC showed a similar effect in reducing HCV load compared to PEG IFN without any side effects.
Lewis et al. (2018), USA	Double-blind placebo RCT	NAFLD	To evaluate the effect of RBAC on biomarkers in adults with NAFLD.	N = 23 (RBAC = 12, placebo = 11)	1 g/day for 90 days	RBAC had beneficial effects on several biomarkers (monocytes, eosinophils, IFN-γ. IL-18), demonstrating immunomodulatory activities in patients with NAFLD.
Lewis et al. (2020), USA	Double-blind placebo RCT	HIV	To evaluate the effects of RBAC on immune, hepatic, and renal function in HIV+ individuals on stable antiretroviral therapy.	N = 47 (RBAC = 22, placebo = 25)	3 g/day for 6 months	The results showed promising immunomodulatory and anti-senescent activities of RBAC with a statistically significant decrease in CD8+ count and a clinically significant increase in CD4+/CD8+ ratio.
Cadden et al. (2020), USA	Double-blind placebo RCT	HIV	To evaluate the anti-inflammatory effects of RBAC in virologically suppressed HIV patients who had incomplete immune reconstitution.	N = 24 (RBAC = 12, placebo = 12)	3 g/day for 12 weeks	The study found no evidence of a beneficial effect of 12 weeks of RBAC supplementation compared to placebo.

Abbreviation: CD, cluster differentiation; CFS, chronic fatigue syndrome; HCV, hepatitis C virus; HIV, human immunodeficiency virus; IBS, irritable bowel syndrome; IFN, interferon; IL, interleukin; NAFLD, nonalcoholic fatty liver disease; PEG IFN, pegylated interferon; RBAC, rice bran arabinoxylan compound; RCT, randomized control trial; UK, United Kingdom; USA, United States of America.

5. Safety and Adverse Events

The safety of RBAC has been well established in both human and animal studies. The resultant product's median lethal dose (LD50) is above 36 g/kg, and the No-Observed-Adverse-Effect-Level is 200 mg/kg/day or above [87]. The compound also tested negative in a reverse mutagenicity array and low antigenicity in a controlled test with guinea pigs with no positive allergic responses observed [87]. Twenty-four healthy volunteers were given RBAC at different concentrations of 15, 30, and 45 mg/kg body weight daily. Blood chemistry analysis using Panel 20, which includes liver enzymes, was conducted to assess toxicity. After one month of treatment, no abnormalities were detected in these parameters, as compared to baseline [16]. RBAC also has an excellent safety record. In the systematic review of RBAC conducted by the authors summarized earlier, no adverse events at the typical dosage of 2–3 g/day, was reported in any of the included clinical trials (total 11) or clinical case reports (total 14) [59]. Hence, RBAC is considered safe to consume with no known side-effect at the typical dosages used in research and clinical settings.

6. Conclusions

Research evidence supports the use of hydrolyzed rice bran enzymatically modified with shiitake mushroom as a functional food and nutraceutical with health-promoting properties. RBAC is a plant-based immunomodulator that can affect both innate and adaptive responses. It balances the inflammatory cytokines, protects against oxidative stress, and inhibits the uncontrolled proliferation of new blood vessels. RBAC has been successfully applied to restore the immune profiles, improve QoL, and enhance cancer patients' long-term survival. The available research literature also suggests that RBAC supplement can be beneficial for HIV infection, diabetes, IBS, hepatitis, NAFLD, CFS, and the common cold. Therefore, the potential clinical applications of RBAC are wide-ranging.

However, the understanding of the health-promoting properties and clinical applications of RBAC is still limited. The bulk of the available basic research was on the compound's immunomodulatory properties, with only a small number of studies on its anti-inflammatory and antioxidant properties. More research is needed to explore the physiological pathways of RBAC exerting these effects. The anti-angiogenic property of RBAC is a new discovery from a recent study and the findings need validation.

Although there is good evidence supporting the use of RBAC as a complementary therapy in cancer, evidence for RBAC beyond cancer remains insufficient. Further research in both basic and human clinical studies are needed to establish the potential mechanisms by which RBAC may affect the pathophysiology of different disease conditions.

Author Contributions: Conceptualization, writing, S.L.O.; review and editing, S.C.P., P.S.M., E.S., C.L., M.H.P., and S.-J.H. All authors have read and agreed to the published version of the manuscript.

Funding: This research received no external funding.

Institutional Review Board Statement: Not applicable.

Informed Consent Statement: Not applicable.

Data Availability Statement: Not applicable.

Conflicts of Interest: S.J.H. is a founder and director of Erom Co., Ltd. which develops and markets RBAC products commercially. All other authors declare no conflict of interest.

Abbreviations

The following abbreviations are used in this manuscript:

AIDS	Acquired immunodeficiency syndrome
ARE	Antioxidant response element
ART	Antiretroviral therapy
CAT	Catalase
CD	Cluster differentiation
CFS	Chronic fatigue syndrome
CRP	C-reactive protein
DC	Dendritic cells
GPx	Glutathione peroxidase
GST	Glutathione-S-transferase
HIV	Human immunodeficiency viruses

IBS	Irritable bowel syndrome
IL	Interleukin
INF	Interferon
mRNA	Messenger ribonucleic acid
NAFLD	Nonalcoholic fatty liver disease
Nrf2	nuclear factor erythroid 2-related factor 2
QoL	Quality of life
RBAC	Rice bran arabinoxylan compound
RCT	Randomized control trial
SOD	Superoxide dismutase
TNF	Tumor necrosis factor
VEGF	Vascular endothelial growth factor

References

1. Park, H.Y.; Lee, K.W.; Choi, H.D. Rice bran constituents: Immunomodulatory and therapeutic activities. *Food Funct.* **2017**, *8*, 935–943. [CrossRef]
2. Fraterrigo Garofalo, S.; Tommasi, T.; Fino, D. A short review of green extraction technologies for rice bran oil. *Biomass Convers. Biorefin.* **2021**, *11*, 569–587. [CrossRef]
3. Henderson, A.J.; Ollila, C.A.; Kumar, A.; Borresen, E.C.; Raina, R.; Agarwal, R.; Ryan, E.P. Chemopreventive properties of dietary rice bran: Current status and future prospects. *Adv. Nutr.* **2012**, *3*, 643–653. [CrossRef]
4. Sharif, M.K.; Butt, M.S.; Anjum, F.M.; Khan, S.H. Rice bran: A novel functional ingredient. *Crit. Rev. Food Sci. Nutr.* **2014**, *54*, 807–816. [CrossRef] [PubMed]
5. Sairam, S.; Gopala Krishna, A.G.; Urooj, A. Physico-chemical characteristics of defatted rice bran and its utilization in a bakery product. *J. Food Sci. Technol.* **2011**, *48*, 478–483. [CrossRef]
6. Fadel, A.; Plunkett, A.; Nyaranga, R.R.; Ashworth, J. Arabinoxylans from rice bran and wheat immunomodulatory potentials: A review article. *Nutr. Food Sci.* **2018**, *48*, 97–110. [CrossRef]
7. Mendez-Encinas, M.A.; Carvajal-Millan, E.; Rascon-Chu, A.; Astiazaran-Garcia, H.F.; Valencia-Rivera, D.E. Ferulated Arabinoxylans and Their Gels: Functional Properties and Potential Application as Antioxidant and Anticancer Agent. *Oxid. Med. Cell. Longev.* **2018**, *2018*, 22. [CrossRef] [PubMed]
8. Hong, S. Development of immunostimulation materials from rice bran. *Food Ind. Nutr.* **2005**, *10*, 42–47.
9. Yu, K.W.; Shin, K.S.; Choi, Y.M.; Suh, H.J. Macrophage stimulating activity of exo-biopolymer from submerged culture of Lentinus edodes with rice bran. *J. Microbiol. Biotechnol.* **2004**, *14*, 658–664.
10. BioBran Research Foundation. The summary of Biobran/MGM-3. In *BioBran/MGN-3 (Rice Bran Arabinoxylan Compound): Basic and Clinical Application to Integrative Medicine*, 2nd ed.; BioBran Research Foundation: Tokyo, Japan, 2013; Chapter I-1, pp. 3–8.
11. Kim, H.Y.; Kim, J.H.; Yang, S.B.; Hong, S.G.; Lee, S.A.; Hwang, S.J.; Shin, K.S.; Suh, H.J.; Park, M.H. A Polysaccharide Extracted from Rice Bran Fermented with Lentinus edodes Enhances Natural Killer Cell Activity and Exhibits Anticancer Effects. *J. Med. Food* **2007**, *10*, 25–31. [CrossRef] [PubMed]
12. Kim, H.Y.; Han, J.T.; Hong, S.G.; Yang, S.B.; Hwang, S.J.; Shin, K.S.; Suh, H.J.; Park, M.H. Enhancement of immunological activity in exo-biopolymer from submerged culture of Lentinus edodes with rice bran. *Nat. Prod. Sci.* **2005**, *11*, 183–187.
13. Trono, D. Recombinant enzymes in the food and pharmaceutical industries. In *Biomass, Biofuels, Biochem*; Singh, R.S., Singhania, R.R., Pandey, A., Larroche, C., Eds.; Elsevier: Amsterdam, The Netherlands, 2019; Chapter 13, pp. 349–387. [CrossRef]
14. Ghoneum, M. Apoptosis and arabinoxylan rice bran. In *Wheat and Rice in Disease Prevention and Health*; Watson, R.R., Preedy, V.R., Zibadi, S., Eds.; Elsevier: San Diego, CA, USA, 2014; Chapter 31, pp. 399–404. [CrossRef]
15. Miura, T.; Chiba, M.; Miyazaki, Y.; Kato, Y.; Maeda, H. Chemical structure of the component involved in immunoregulation. In *BioBran/MGN-3 (Rice Bran Arabinoxylan Coumpound): Basic and Clinical Application to Integrative Medicine*, 2nd ed.; BioBran Research Foundation: Tokyo, Japan, 2013; Chapter I-3, pp. 14–22.
16. Ghoneum, M. From bench to bedside: The growing use of arabinoxylan rice bran (MGN-3/Biobran) in cancer immunotherapy. *Austin Immunol.* **2016**, *1*, 1006.
17. Ghoneum, M.; Brown, J. NK Immunorestoration and cancer patients by BioBran/MGN-3, a modified aracbynoxylan rice bran (Study of 32 patients followed for up to 4 years). In *Anti-Aging Medical Therapeutics Vol III*; Klatz, R.M., Goldman, R., Eds.; Health Quest Publications: Marina del Rey, CA, USA, 1999; Chapter 30, pp. 217–226.
18. Ghoneum, M.; Abedi, S. Enhancement of natural killer cell activity of aged mice by modified arabinoxylan rice bran (MGN-3/Biobran). *J. Pharm. Pharmacol.* **2004**, *56*, 1581–1588. [CrossRef] [PubMed]
19. Pérez-Martínez, A.; Valentín, J.; Fernández, L.; Hernández-Jiménez, E.; López-Collazo, E.; Zerbes, P.; Schwörer, E.; Nuñéz, F.; Martín, I.G.; Sallis, H.; et al. Arabinoxylan rice bran (MGN-3/Biobran) enhances natural killer cell-mediated cytotoxicity against neuroblastoma in vitro and in vivo. *Cytotherapy* **2015**, *17*, 601–612. [CrossRef]
20. Badr El-Din, N.K.; Noaman, E.; Ghoneum, M. In vivo tumor inhibitory effects of nutritional rice bran supplement MGN-3/Biobran on ehrlich carcinoma-bearing mice. *Nutr. Cancer* **2008**, *60*, 235–244. [CrossRef] [PubMed]

21. Badr El-Din, N.K.; Abdel Fattah, S.M.; Pan, D.; Tolentino, L.; Ghoneum, M. Chemopreventive activity of MGN-3/Biobran against chemical induction of glandular stomach carcinogenesis in rats and its apoptotic effect in gastric cancer cells. *Integr. Cancer Ther.* **2016**. [CrossRef]
22. Giese, S.; Sabell, G.R.; Coussons-Read, M. Impact of ingestion of rice bran and shitake mushroom extract on lymphocyte function and cytokine production in healthy rats. *J. Diet. Suppl.* **2008**, *5*, 47–61. [CrossRef]
23. Ghoneum, M. Enhancement of human natural killer cell activity by modified arabinoxylane from rice bran (MGN-3). *Int. J. Immunother.* **1998**, *14*, 89–99.
24. Ghoneum, M.; Jewett, A. Production of tumor necrosis factor-alpha and interferon-gamma from human peripheral blood lymphocytes by MGN-3, a modified arabinoxylan from rice bran, and its synergy with interleukin-2 in vitro. *Cancer Detect. Prev.* **2000**, *24*, 314–324.
25. Ali, K.H.; Melillo, A.B.; Leonard, S.M.; Asthana, D.; Woolger, J.M.; Wolfson, A.H.; Mcdaniel, H.R.; Lewis, J.E. An open-label, randomized clinical trial to assess the immunomodulatory activity of a novel oligosaccharide compound in healthy adults. *Funct. Foods Health Dis.* **2012**, *2*, 265–279. [CrossRef]
26. Elsaid, A.F.; Shaheen, M.; Ghoneum, M. Biobran/MGN-3, an arabinoxylan rice bran, enhances NK cell activity in geriatric subjects: A randomized, double-blind, placebo-controlled clinical trial. *Exp. Ther. Med.* **2018**, *15*, 2313–2320. [CrossRef]
27. Tsunekawa, H. Effect of long-term administration of immunomodulatory food on cancer patients completing conventional treatments. *Clin. Pharmacol. Ther.* **2004**, *14*, 295–302.
28. Cholujova, D.; Jakubikova, J.; Sulikova, M.; Chovancova, J.; Czako, B.; Martisova, M.; Mistrik, M.; Pastorek, M.; Gronesova, P.; Hunakova, L.; et al. The effect of MGN-3 arabinoxylan on natural killer and dendritic cells in multiple myeloma patients. *Haematologica* **2011**, *96*, S117–S118.
29. Cholujova, D.; Jakubikova, J.; Czako, B.; Martisova, M.; Hunakova, L.; Duraj, J.; Mistrik, M.; Sedlak, J. MGN-3 arabinoxylan rice bran modulates innate immunity in multiple myeloma patients. *Cancer Immunol. Immunother.* **2013**, *62*, 437–445. [CrossRef] [PubMed]
30. Ghoneum, M.; Matsuura, M. Augmentation of macrophage phagocytosis by modified arabinoxylan rice bran (MGN-3/Biobran). *Int. J. Immunopathol. Pharmacol.* **2004**, *17*, 283–292. [CrossRef]
31. Chae, S.; Shin, S.; Bae, M.; Park, M.; Song, M.; Hwang, S.; Yee, S. Effect of arabinoxylane and PSP on activation of immune cells. *J. Korean Soc. Food Sci. Nutr.* **2004**, *33*, 278–286.
32. Ghoneum, M.; Matsuura, M.; Gollapudi, S. Modified arabinoxylan rice bran (Mgn-3/Biobran) enhances intracellular killing of microbes by human phagocytic cells in vitro. *Int. J. Immunopathol. Pharmacol.* **2008**, *21*, 87–95. [CrossRef]
33. Ghoneum, M.; Agrawal, S. Activation of human monocyte-derived dendritic cells in vitro by the biological response modifier arabinoxylan rice bran (MGN-3/Biobran). *Int. J. Immunopathol. Pharmacol.* **2011**, *24*, 941–948. [CrossRef] [PubMed]
34. Cholujova, D.; Jakubikova, J.; Sedlak, J. BioBran-augmented maturation of human monocyte-derived dendritic cells. *Neoplasma* **2009**, *56*, 89–95. [CrossRef]
35. Ghoneum, M.; Agrawal, S. MGN-3/Biobran enhances generation of cytotoxic CD8+ T cells via upregulation of DEC-205 expression on dendritic cells. *Int. J. Immunopathol. Pharmacol.* **2014**, *27*, 523–530. [CrossRef]
36. Lissoni, P.; Messina, G.; Brivio, F.; Fumagalli, L.; Rovelli, F.; Maruelli, L.; Miceli, M.; Marchiori, P.; Porro, G.; Held, M.; et al. Modulation of the anticancer immunity by natural agents: Inhibition of T regulatory lymphocyte generation by arabinoxylan in patients with locally limited or metastatic solid tumors. *Cancer Ther.* **2008**, *6*, 1011–1016.
37. Endo, Y.; Kanbayashi, H. Modified rice bran beneficial for weight loss of mice as a major and acute adverse effect of cisplatin. *Pharmacol. Toxicol.* **2003**, *92*, 300–303. [CrossRef]
38. Choi, J.Y.; Paik, D.J.; Kwon, D.Y.; Park, Y. Dietary supplementation with rice bran fermented with Lentinus edodes increases interferon-γ activity without causing adverse effects: A randomized, double-blind, placebo-controlled, parallel-group study. *Nutr. J.* **2014**, *13*, 35. [CrossRef]
39. Bennett, J.M.; Reeves, G.; Billman, G.E.; Sturmberg, J.P. Inflammation-nature's way to efficiently respond to all types of challenges: Implications for understanding and managing "the epidemic" of chronic diseases. *Front. Med.* **2018**, *5*, 316. [CrossRef]
40. Ichihashi, K. Experience with administration of BioBran in patients with chronic rheumatism. *Clin. Pharmacol. Ther.* **2004**, *14*, 459–463.
41. Ghoneum, M.H.; El Sayed, N.S. Protective effect of Biobran/MGN-3 against sporadic Alzheimer's disease mouse model: Possible role of oxidative stress and apoptotic pathways. *Oxid. Med. Cell. Longev.* **2021**, *2021*, 8845064. [CrossRef]
42. Golombick, T.; Diamond, T.H.; Manoharan, A.; Ramakrishna, R. Addition of rice bran arabinoxylan to curcumin therapy may be of benefit to patients with early-stage B-cell lymphoid malignancies (monoclonal gammopathy of undetermined significance, smoldering multiple myeloma, or stage 0/1 chronic lymphocytic leukemia). *Integr. Cancer Ther.* **2016**, *15*, 183–189. [CrossRef] [PubMed]
43. Kamiya, T.; Shikano, M.; Tanaka, M.; Ozeki, K.; Ebi, M.; Katano, T.; Hamano, S.; Nishiwaki, H.; Tsukamoto, H.; Mizoshita, T.; et al. Therapeutic effects of biobran, modified arabinoxylan rice bran, in improving symptoms of diarrhea predominant or mixed type irritable bowel syndrome: A pilot, randomized controlled study. *Evid.-Based Complement. Altern. Med.* **2014**, *2014*, 828137. [CrossRef] [PubMed]
44. Tazawa, K.; Namikawa, H.; Oida, N.; Itoh, K.; Yatsuzuka, M.; Koike, J.; Masada, M.; Maeda, H. Scavenging activity of MGN-3 (arabinoxylane from rice bran) with natural killer cell activity on free radicals. *Biotherapy* **2000**, *14*, 493–495.

45. Noaman, E.; Badr El-Din, N.K.; Bibars, M.A.; Abou Mossallam, A.A.; Ghoneum, M. Antioxidant potential by arabinoxylan rice bran, MGN-3/biobran, represents a mechanism for its oncostatic effect against murine solid Ehrlich carcinoma. *Cancer Lett.* **2008**, *268*, 348–359. [CrossRef]
46. Ghoneum, M.; Badr El-Din, N.K.; Fattah, S.M.A.; Tolentino, L. Arabinoxylan rice bran (MGN-3/Biobran) provides protection against whole-body γ-irradiation in mice via restoration of hematopoietic tissues. *J. Radiat. Res.* **2013**, *54*, 419. [CrossRef] [PubMed]
47. Shao, L.; Luo, Y.; Zhou, D. Hematopoietic stem cell injury induced by ionizing radiation. *Antioxid. Redox Signal.* **2014**, *20*, 1447–1462. [CrossRef] [PubMed]
48. Tan, D.F.S.; Flores, J.A.S. The immunomodulating effects of arabinoxylan rice bran (Lentin) on hematologic profile, nutritional status and quality of life among head and neck carcinoma patients undergoing radiation therapy: A double blind randomized control trial. *Radiol. J. Off. Publ. Philipp. Coll. Radiol.* **2020**, *12*, 11–16.
49. Zhu, X.; Okubo, A.; Igari, N.; Ninomiya, K.; Egashira, Y. Modified rice bran hemicellulose inhibits vascular endothelial growth factor-induced angiogenesis in vitro via VEGFR2 and its downstream signaling pathways. *Biosci. Microbiota Food Health* **2017**, *36*, 45–53. [CrossRef]
50. Pang, R.W.C.; Poon, R.T.P. Clinical implications of angiogenesis in cancers. *Vasc. Health Risk Manag.* **2006**, *2*, 97–108. [CrossRef]
51. Ghoneum, M.; Gollapudi, S. Modified arabinoxylan rice bran (MGN-3/Biobran) enhances yeast-induced apoptosis in human breast cancer cells in vitro. *Anticancer Res.* **2005**, *25*, 859–870.
52. Ghoneum, M.; Gollapudi, S. Synergistic role of arabinoxylan rice bran (MGN-3/Biobran) in S. cerevisiae-induced apoptosis of monolayer breast cancer MCF-7 cells. *Anticancer Res.* **2005**, *25*, 4187–4196. [PubMed]
53. Ghoneum, M.; Gollapudi, S. Synergistic apoptotic effect of arabinoxylan rice bran (MGN-3/Biobran) and curcumin (turmeric) on human multiple myeloma cell line U266 in vitro. *Neoplasma* **2011**, *58*, 118–123. [CrossRef]
54. Jacoby, H.I.; Wnorowski, G.; Sakata, K.; Maeda, H. The effect of MGN-3 on cisplatin and doxorubicin induced toxicity in the rat. *J. Nutraceuticals Funct. Med. Foods* **2001**, *3*, 3–12. [CrossRef]
55. Gollapudi, S.; Ghoneum, M. MGN-3/Biobran, modified arabinoxylan from rice bran, sensitizes human breast cancer cells to chemotherapeutic agent, daunorubicin. *Cancer Detect. Prev.* **2008**, *32*, 1–6. [CrossRef]
56. Ghoneum, M.; Badr El-Din, N.K.; Ali, D.A.; El-Dein, M.A. Modified arabinoxylan from rice bran, MGN-3/Biobran, sensitizes metastatic breast cancer cells to paclitaxel in vitro. *Anticancer Res.* **2014**, *34*, 81–87.
57. Badr El-Din, N.K.; Ali, D.A.; Alaa El-Dein, M.; Ghoneum, M. Enhancing the apoptotic effect of a low dose of paclitaxel on tumor cells in mice by arabinoxylan rice bran (MGN-3/Biobran). *Nutr. Cancer* **2016**, *68*, 1010–1020. [CrossRef] [PubMed]
58. Badr El-Din, N.K.; Areida, S.K.; Ahmed, K.O.; Ghoneum, M. Arabinoxylan rice bran (MGN-3/Biobran) enhances radiotherapy in animals bearing Ehrlich ascites carcinoma. *J. Radiat. Res.* **2019**, *60*, 747–758. [CrossRef]
59. Ooi, S.L.; McMullen, D.; Golombick, T.; Pak, S.C. Evidence-based review of BioBran/MGN-3 arabinoxylan compound as a complementary therapy for conventional cancer treatment. *Integr. Cancer Ther.* **2018**, *17*, 165–178. [CrossRef]
60. Okamura, Y. The clinical significance of modified arabinoxylan from rice bran (BioBran/MGN-3) in immunotherapy for cancer. *Clin. Pharmacol. Ther.* **2004**, *14*, 289–294.
61. Meshitsuka, K. A case of stage IV hepatocellular carcinoma treated by KM900, Biobran, and psychotherapy has presented significant good results. *Pers. Med. Univ. (Jpn. Ed.)* **2013**, *1*, 46–48.
62. Hajto, T.; Baranyai, L.; Kirsch, A.; Kuzma, M.; Perjési, P. Can a synergistic activation of pattern recognition receptors by plant immunomodulators enhance the effect of oncologic therapy? Case Report of a patient with uterus and ovary sarcoma. *Clin. Case Rep. Rev.* **2015**, *1*, 235–238. [CrossRef]
63. Hajtó, T.; Horvath, A.; Papp, S. Improvement of quality of life in tumor patients after an immunomodulatory treatment with standardized mistletoe lectin and arabinoxylan plant extracts. *Int. J. Neurorehabilit.* **2016**, *3*, 2–4. [CrossRef]
64. Markus, J.; Miller, A.; Smith, M.; Orengo, I. Metastatic hemangiopericytoma of the skin treated with wide local excision and MGN-3. *Dermatol. Surg.* **2006**, *32*, 145–147. [CrossRef]
65. Hajto, T.; Kirsch, A. Case reports of cancer patients with hepatic metastases treated by standardized plant immunomodulatory preparations. *J. Can. Res. Updat.* **2013**, 1–9. [CrossRef]
66. Kawai, T. One case of a patient with umbilical metastasis of recurrent cancer (Sister Mary Joseph's Nodule, SMJN) who has survived for a long time under immunomodulatory supplement therapy. *Clin. Pharmacol. Ther.* **2004**, *14*, 281–288.
67. Kaketani, K. A case where an immunomodulatory food was effective in conservative therapy for progressive terminal pancreatic cancer. *Clin. Pharmacol. Ther.* **2004**, *14*, 273–279.
68. Bang, M.H.; Riep, T.V.; Thinh, N.T.; Song, L.H.; Dung, T.T.; Troung, L.V.; Don, L.V.; Ky, T.D.; Pan, D.; Shaheen, M.; et al. Arabinoxylan rice bran (MGN-3) enhances the effects of interventional therapies for the treatment of hepatocellular carcinoma: A three-year randomized clinical trial. *Anticancer Res.* **2010**, *30*, 5145–5151. [PubMed]
69. Masood, A.I.; Sheikh, R.; Anwer, R.A. "BIOBRAN MGN-3"; Effect of reducing side effects of chemotherapy in breast cancer patients. *Prof. Med. J.* **2013**, *20*, 13–16.
70. Itoh, Y.; Mizuno, M.; Ikeda, M.; Nakahara, R.; Kubota, S.; Ito, J.; Okada, T.; Kawamura, M.; Kikkawa, F.; Naganawa, S. A randomized, double-blind pilot trial of hydrolyzed rice bran versus placebo for radioprotective effect on acute gastroenteritis secondary to chemoradiotherapy in patients with cervical cancer. *Evid. Based. Complement. Alternat. Med.* **2015**, *2015*, 974390. [CrossRef]

71. Petrovics, G.; Szigeti, G.; Hamvas, S.; Máté, Á.; Betlehem, J.; Hegyi, G. Controlled pilot study for cancer patients suffering from chronic fatigue syndrome due to chemotherapy treated with BioBran (MGN-3-Arabinoxylane) and targeted radiofrequency heat therapy. *Eur. J. Integr. Med.* **2016**, *8*, 29–35. [CrossRef]
72. Ooi, S.L.; Pak, S.C.; Micalos, P.S.; Schupfer, E.; Zielinski, R.; Jeffries, T.; Harris, G.; Golombick, T.; McKinnon, D. Rice bran arabinoxylan compound and quality of life of cancer patients (RBAC-QoL): Study protocol for a randomized pilot feasibility trial. *Contemp. Clin. Trials Commun.* **2020**, *19*, 100580. [CrossRef] [PubMed]
73. Ghoneum, M. Anti-HIV activity in vitro of MGN-3, an activated arabinoxylane from rice bran. *Biochem. Biophys. Res. Commun.* **1998**, *243*, 25–29. [CrossRef] [PubMed]
74. Symeonides, M.; Murooka, T.T.; Bellfy, L.N.; Roy, N.H.; Mempel, T.R.; Thali, M. HIV-1-Induced Small T Cell Syncytia Can Transfer Virus Particles to Target Cells through Transient Contacts. *Viruses* **2015**, *7*, 6590–6603. [CrossRef]
75. Lewis, J.E.; Atlas, S.E.; Abbas, M.H.; Rasul, A.; Farooqi, A.; Lantigua, L.A.; Michaud, F.; Goldberg, S.; Lages, L.C.; Higuera, O.L.; et al. The Novel Effects of a Hydrolyzed Polysaccharide Dietary Supplement on Immune, Hepatic, and Renal Function in Adults with HIV in a Randomized, Double-Blind, Placebo-Control Trial. *J. Diet. Suppl.* **2020**, *17*, 429–441. [CrossRef]
76. Ku, N.S.; Jiamsakul, A.; Ng, O.T.; Yunihastuti, E.; Cuong, D.D.; Lee, M.P.; Sim, B.L.H.; Phanuphak, P.; Wong, W.W.; Kamarulzaman, A.; et al. Elevated CD8 T-cell counts and virological failure in HIV-infected patients after combination antiretroviral therapy. *Medicine* **2016**, *95*, e4570. [CrossRef] [PubMed]
77. Cadden, J.; Loomis, K.; Kallia, R.; Louie, S.; Dubé, M. Anti-inflammatory effects of arabinoxylan rice bran supplementation in participants with treated, suppressed HIV infection and inadequate immune reconstitution: A randomized, doubleblind trial. *Antivir. Ther.* **2020**, *25*, A26.
78. Maeda, H.; Ichihashi, K.; Fujii, T.; Omura, K.; Zhu, X.; Anazawa, M.; Tazawa, K. Oral administration of hydrolyzed rice bran prevents the common cold syndrome in the elderly based on its immunomodulatory action. *BioFactors* **2004**, *21*, 185–187. [CrossRef] [PubMed]
79. Zheng, S.; Sanada, H.; Dohi, H.; Hirai, S.; Egashira, Y. Suppressive effect of modified arabinoxylan from rice bran (MGN-3) on D-galactosamine-induced IL-18 expression and hepatitis in rats. *Biosci. Biotechnol. Biochem.* **2012**, *76*, 942–946. [CrossRef] [PubMed]
80. Zheng, S.; Sugita, S.; Hirai, S.; Egashira, Y. Protective effect of low molecular fraction of MGN-3, a modified arabinoxylan from rice bran, on acute liver injury by inhibition of NF-κB and JNK/MAPK expression. *Int. Immunopharmacol.* **2012**, *14*, 764–769. [CrossRef] [PubMed]
81. Salama, H.; Medhat, E.; Shaheen, M.; Zekri, A.R.N.; Darwish, T.; Ghoneum, M. Arabinoxylan rice bran (Biobran) suppresses the viremia level in patients with chronic HCV infection: A randomized trial. *Int. J. Immunopathol. Pharmacol.* **2016**, *29*, 647–653. [CrossRef]
82. Lewis, J.E.; Atlas, S.E.; Higuera, O.L.; Fiallo, A.; Rasul, A.; Farooqi, A.; Kromo, O.; Lantigua, L.A.; Tiozzo, E.; Woolger, J.M.; et al. The effect of a hydrolyzed polysaccharide dietary supplement on biomarkers in adults with nonalcoholic fatty liver disease. *Evid.-Based Complement. Altern. Med.* **2018**, *2018*, 1751583. [CrossRef]
83. Kenyon, J. A descriptive questionnaire-based study on the use of Biobran (MGN3), in chronic fatigue syndrome. *Townsend Lett. Dr. Patients* **2001**, *220*, 48–50.
84. McDermott, C.; Richards, S.C.M.; Thomas, P.W.; Montgomery, J.; Lewith, G. A placebo-controlled, double-blind, randomized controlled trial of a natural killer cell stimulant (BioBran MGN-3) in chronic fatigue syndrome. *QJM Int. J. Med.* **2006**, *99*, 461–468. [CrossRef]
85. Ohara, I.; Tabuchi, R.; Onai, K.; Econ, M.H. Effects of modified rice bran on serum lipids and taste preference in streptozotocin-induced diabetic rats. *Nutr. Res.* **2000**, *20*, 59–68. [CrossRef]
86. Ohara, I.; Onai, K.; Maeda, H. Modified rice bran improves glucose tolerance in NIDDM adult rats given streptozotocin as neonates. *Stud. Aichi Gakusen Univ.* **2002**, *37*, 17–23.
87. BioBran Research Foundation. The safety of Biobran/MGN-3. In *BioBran/MGN-3 (Rice Bran Arabinoxylan Compound): Basic and Clinical Application to Integrative Medicine*, 2nd ed.; BioBran Research Foundation: Tokyo, Japan, 2013; Chapter I-2, pp. 9–13.

Review
Anti-Inflammatory Action and Mechanisms of Resveratrol

Tiantian Meng [1], Dingfu Xiao [1,*], Arowolo Muhammed [1], Juying Deng [1], Liang Chen [2] and Jianhua He [1,*]

1. College of Animal Science and Technology, Hunan Agricultural University, Changsha 410128, China; meng-tiantian@foxmail.com (T.M.); mbayor88@gmail.com (A.M.); djuyingyx@foxmail.com (J.D.)
2. Huaihua Institute of Agricultural Sciences, No.140 Yingfeng East Road, Hecheng District, Huaihua 418000, China; chenliang890709@163.com
* Correspondence: xiaodingfu2001@163.com (D.X.); jianhuahy@hunau.net (J.H.)

Abstract: Resveratrol (3,4′,5-trihy- droxystilbene), a natural phytoalexin polyphenol, exhibits antioxidant, anti-inflammatory, and anti-carcinogenic properties. This phytoalexin is well-absorbed and rapidly and extensively metabolized in the body. Inflammation is an adaptive response, which could be triggered by various danger signals, such as invasion by microorganisms or tissue injury. In this review, the anti-inflammatory activity and the mechanism of resveratrol modulates the inflammatory response are examined. Multiple experimental studies that illustrate regulatory mechanisms and the immunomodulatory function of resveratrol both in vivo and in vitro. The data acquired from those studies are discussed.

Keywords: resveratrol; absorption and metabolism; anti-inflammation; antioxidant; mechanism

1. Introduction

In 1976, resveratrol (3,4′,5-trihy- droxystilbene) was thought to be just a phytoalexin [1], one of the polyphenolic compounds produced by plants in response to environmental stress [2]. Subsequently, resveratrol was found to exhibit multiple bioactivities, including anti-oxidative [3], anti-inflammatory [4], cardiovascular protective [5], and anti-aging [6] properties, in animals. This phytoalexin has been found in at least 72 plant species, such as mulberries, peanuts, and grapes (Table 1). As a nonflavonoid polyphenol, resveratrol exists as two geometric isomers, trans- and cis- (Figure 1), and their glucosides, trans- and cis- piceids [7].

Table 1. The content of resveratrol in some food products.

Plants	Content
Mulberries	5 mg of resveratrol per 100 g
Lingonberries	3 mg per 100 g
Cranberries	1.92 mg of resveratrol per 100 g
Red currants	1.57 mg of resveratrol per 100 g
Bilberries	0.67 mg of resveratrol per 100 g
Blueberries	0.383 mg per 100 g
Peanuts	1.12 mg of resveratrol per 100 g
Pistachios	0.11 mg of resveratrol per 100 g
Fresh grapes	0.24 to 1.25 mg per cup (160 g)
Red grape juice	0.5 mg per liter

Since there may be important clinical implications for the positive roles of resveratrol on inflammatory response control, the aim of this article is to examine its strong anti-inflammatory action and the potential molecular mechanisms of such effects.

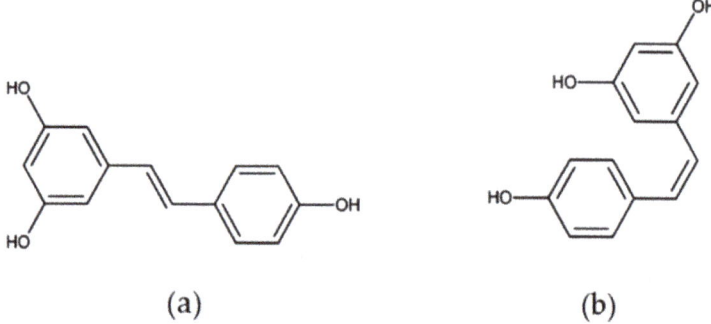

Figure 1. Structure of trans-resveratrol (a) and cis-resveratrol (b).

2. Absorption and Metabolism of Resveratrol

Previous studies have characterized in vitro and in vivo resveratrol absorption rates [8,9]. Resveratrol is absorbed in large quantities by enterocytes after oral administration [10], but only a small part of this compound ingested from the diet reaches the bloodstream and body tissues [9]. Additionally, owing to the complex structure and high molecular weight, the well-operating metabolism of resveratrol in the liver and intestine leads to oral bioavailability of about 12% of trans-resveratrol [8].

Resveratrol is absorbed by passive diffusion or carrier-mediated transport across the enterocyte apical membrane, and then rapidly and extensively metabolized to resveratrol glucuronides or sulfates [11]. Meanwhile, a significant portion (about 90%) of ingested resveratrol reaches the colon in their intact form and is subsequently subjected to gut fermentation. Once absorbed through the portal vein, the produced polyphenolic metabolites enter the liver where they are further methylated, glucuronidated or sulfated. Then, the metabolites will penetrate into the systematic circulation and reach the target tissues and cells where physiological significance can be demonstrated. Resveratrol and unused metabolites can be recycled back to the small intestine through the bile or excreted through urine [9].

Rapid absorption, poor bioavailability, and low aqueous solubility are some of the crucial limitations and challenges of the in vivo use of resveratrol [12,13]. Therefore, different methodological approaches, such as solid lipid nanoparticles (SLNs) and nanostructured lipid carriers (NLCs), have been used to improve the poor aqueous solubility and the low bioavailability of resveratrol [14].

3. The Anti-Inflammatory Activity of Resveratrol

Inflammatory response is a multi-stage process involving multiple cell types as well as mediator signals [15]. Inflammation is an adaptive response, which can be triggered by various danger signals, such as invasion by microorganisms or tissue injury [16]. The exogenous and endogenous signaling molecules are known as pathogen-associated molecular patterns (PAMPs) and damage-associated molecular patterns (DAMPs), respectively [15–17].

Both PAMPs and DAMPs are recognized by various pattern recognition receptors (PRRs), such as Toll-like receptors (TLRs) [18–20]. The activation of PRR induces intracellular signaling cascades, such as kinases and transcription factors [19,21]. The signaling pathways mentioned above can promote the production of a variety of inflammatory mediators (such as cytokines) for inflammation development.

Multiple lines of evidence from laboratory studies, both in vivo and in vitro, have shown that the anti-inflammatory properties of resveratrol may be explained though inhibiting the production of anti-inflammatory factors. For example, resveratrol has been stated to suppress the proliferation of spleen cells induced by concanavalin A (ConA), interleukin (IL)-2, or allo-antigens, and to more effectively prevent lymphocytes from producing

IL-2 and interferon-gamma (IFN-γ) and macrophages from producing tumor necrosis factor alpha (TNF-α) or IL-12 [22]. Resveratrol has been found to induce a dose-dependent suppression of the production of IL-1α, IL-6, and TNF-α and down-regulate both mRNA expression and protein secretion of IL-17 in vitro [23]. Dietary resveratrol supplementation is capable of improving tight junction protein zonula occludens-1, Occludin, and claudin-1 expression to reduce intestinal permeability in vivo [24,25]. Resveratrol treatment also reduced the expression of the inflammatory factors, glycation end product receptor (RAGE), NF-B (P65) and nicotinamide adenine dinucleotide phosphate (NADPH) oxidase 4 (NOX4) and improved the renal pathological structure [26]. In addition, as the natural precursor of resveratrol, polydatin (a resveratrol glycoside isolated from Polygonum cuspidatum) significantly downregulated IL-6, IL-1β, and TNF-α expression induced by Mycoplasma gallisepticum both in vivo and in vitro, suggested that polydatin also has anti-inflammatory effect [27].

The anti-inflammatory activity of this compound was also demonstrated in a rat model of carrageenan-induced paw edema [28]. Additionally, it has been reported that resveratrol preconditioning modulates inflammatory response of hippocampus after global cerebral ischemia in rat [29]. In addition, resveratrol has been documented to be able to suppress neuro-inflammation mediated by microglia, protect neurons from inflammatory damage, and relieve inflammation of the airway caused by asthma and airway remodeling [30,31].

Heat stress may induce reactive oxygen species (ROS) production, cause antioxidant system disorders, and cause damage to the immune organs in vivo [32]. In a recent report, our research group observed that dietary resveratrol supplementation in broilers was successful in partially alleviating the detrimental effects of heat stress on the function of the intestinal barrier, by restoring the damaged villus-crypt structure, altering the mRNA expression of intestinal heat-shock proteins, secreted immunoglobulin A, and close junction-related genes and inhibiting pro-inflammation secretion [33]. Zhang et al. [34] reported that dietary supplementation with resveratrol in broilers could partly reverse the adverse effects of heat stress on the growth of immune organ by reestablishing redox status and inhibiting apoptosis. Importantly, our recent study demonstrated that resveratrol could alleviate heat stress-induced innate immunity and inflammatory response by inhibiting the activation of PRRs signaling in the spleen of broilers [35].

Lipopolysaccharides (LPS) is an essential glycolipid component of Gram-negative bacterial endotoxin which can trigger inflammatory responses to the host [36]. The addition of resveratrol has also led to decreases in inflammatory mediator expression, including prostaglandin (PG)E2, COX-2, IL-1β, IL-8, TNF-α, and monocyte chemoattractant protein-1 in BV-2 or monocyte LPS stimulation cells [37,38]. Additionally, Toll-like receptor-4 (TLR-4) expression in LPS-stimulated cells was attenuated after resveratrol pre-treatment [39]. Long-term treatment with this compound is able to increase brain defenses in aged animals against acute LPS pro-inflammatory stimuli [40]. Moreover, palmitate-induced IL-6 and TNF-α at mRNA and protein levels in C2C12 cells can also be substantially prevented by resveratrol pretreatment [41].

On the other hand, resveratrol can induce anti-inflammatory properties by suppressing the production of ROS and nitric oxide (NO). Oxidative stress caused by the accumulation of ROS plays a role in promoting inflammation in a wide spectrum of diseases, such as chronic inflammation and cancer [42]. It was found that resveratrol was able to suppress strongly the generation of NO in activated macrophages, as well as decrease strongly the amount of cytosolic inducible nitric oxide synthase (iNOS) protein and steady state mRNA levels [43]. Dietary resveratrol supplementation also can effectively eliminate free radicals, enhance the activities of SOD, CAT, and GPX [32,44]. Babu et al. [45] showed that the cytoprotective effect of resveratrol is predominantly due to mitigation of mitochondrial ROS. A recent study conducted by Kortam et al. [46] showed that resveratrol increased the liver's antioxidant and anti-inflammatory activity against chronic unpredictable mild stress induced depression in the animal model, as explained by the normalization of total antioxidant ability, glutathione, malondialdehyde (MDA), NF-B, TNF-α, and myeloperoxidase. Additionally, resveratrol down-regulated the expression of iNOS mRNA and protein expression in the LPS-stimulated intestinal cells in a dose-dependent manner, resulting in a decreased production of NO [39]. Similarly, resveratrol dose-dependently inhibited the expression of iNOS and IL-6 in LPS-treated RAW264.7 cells, therefore, suppressed the production of NO and the secretion of IL-6 [47].

4. Potential Anti-Inflammatory Pathways of Resveratrol

Many studies have reported that resveratrol regulates inflammatory response through a variety of signaling pathways, such as AA pathway [48], nuclear factor kappa B (NF-κb) [49], Mitogen-activated protein kinase (MAPK) [50], and activator protein-1 (AP-1) [51].

4.1. Arachidonic Acid (AA) Pathway

Inhibition of the AA pathway plays a major role, among other anti-inflammatory pathways facilitated by polyphenols [48,52]. AA is released by membrane phospholipids with the cleavage of phospholipase A2, and then metabolized by COX with generation of PGs (such as PGD2, PGE2, PGI2) and thromboxane (TX) A2 [53] (Figure 2). There is evidence that both COX forms (include COX-1 and COX-2) are significant sources of PGs [54,55]. Prostanoids produced via COX-1 exert renal homeostasis, cytoprotective, immunomodulatory, and platelet function [56], while those derived from COX-2 participates in the inflammatory response [57]. COX-2 expression is affected by many inflammatory factors, such as ultraviolet B (UVB)-radiation, TPA (12-O-tetradecanoylphorbol-13-acetate) or PMA (Phorbol 12-myristate 13-acetate) (a tumor promoter), and tobacco [58,59].

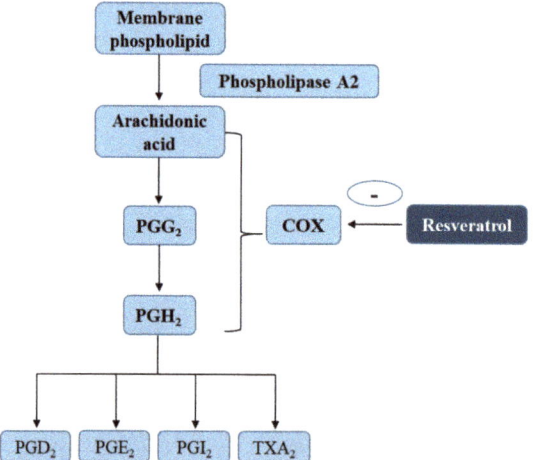

Figure 2. Inhibition of arachidonic acid metabolic pathway by resveratrol. Key abbreviations: COX, cyclooxygenase; PGD2, prostaglandin D2; PGE2, prostaglandin E2; PGI2, prostaglandin I2; TXA2, thromboxane A2.

Resveratrol has been stated to exhibit anti-inflammatory responses and inhibit the functions of COX and hydroperoxidase, although the results have been inconsistent in various previous studies. Jang et al. [28] found that this polyphenol was able to selectively suppress the COX activity of COX-1 and this isoenzyme's hydroperoxidase activity, thus inhibiting PG synthesis. It has also been shown that resveratrol was able to discriminate between two COX isoforms, suggesting it is a potent inhibitor of COX-1 catalytic activity, but only a poor inhibitor of COX-2 peroxidase activity, the isoform target for non-steroidal anti-inflammatory drugs [60].

In comparison, it has been demonstrated that resveratrol inhibits PGE2 synthesis by directly blocking the activity of COX-2, and suppresses the transcription of COX-2 gene without changing the amount of COX-1 in PMA-treated human mammary epithelial cells [61]. A subsequent study reported that resveratrol induced a decrease of PGs as well as COX-2 expression by reducing AA release, as well as COX-2 induction by an antioxidant action, because this phytoalexin is able to decrease O29- as well as hydrogen peroxide (H_2O_2) produced by PMA- or LPS-treated murine peritoneal macrophages [62]. Murias et al. [63] evaluated some methoxylated and hydroxylated resveratrol derivatives for their ability to inhibit COX isoenzymes and the results showed that hydroxylated resveratrol analogs are selective inhibitors of COX-2. Resveratrol was stated to be able to reduce the degree of colonic injury by decreasing the production of PGD2 and PGE2, as well as lowering COX-2 expression in the colon of resveratrol-treated rats compared with inflamed colon [64,65].

Resveratrol in a certain concentration can suppress human colorectal cancer and pulmonary epithelial cell (A549 cells) proliferation by inhibiting COX-2 expression [48,66]. A recent study found that this phytoalexin inhibited microphthalmia-associated transcription factor and tyrosinase activity via extracellular signal-regulated kinase (ERK) 1/2 and PI-3K/Akt pathway-mediated suppression of COX-2 [67]. Additionally, resveratrol is able to improve neuroimmune dysregulation by inhibiting of neuronal TLRs and COX-2 signaling pathways in vivo [68]. Transient transfections using deletion constructs of the COX-2 promoter as well as COX-2 promoter constructs in which unique enhancer elements are mutagenized has shown that resveratrol's effects are mediated by a cyclic AMP response element [61].

Moreover, the literature shows that resveratrol decreases PMA-dependent PGE2 production through the down-regulation of gene transcription of COX-2 in rats indirectly by inhibiting the protein kinase C (PKC), ERK1, c-Juns, and AP-1 activities, which provides an additional mechanism for resveratrol inactivation of COX-2 [61]. A subsequent study showed that this polyphenol was able to suppress COX-2 promoter-induced transcriptional activity (include NF-κB and AP-1) and PKC activation [69,70]. Kundu et al. [71] also reported that this compound was able to inhibit oxidative stress, expression and activity of COX-2 by inhibiting NF-κB, AP-1, and Janus kinase/signal transducers and transcript activators (JAK/STAT) activation pathways in mouse skin induced by TPA. TPA/PMA is known to induce expression of COX-2 via transcriptional activation of NF-κB and AP-1 [59]. The anti-inflammatory action of resveratrol is dependent on activation of AMP-activated kinase (AMPK) and is related to inhibition of the LPS stimulation NF-κB-induced COX-2 signaling pathway in RAW 264.7 macrophages [72].

In fact, the overexpression of COX-2 isoenzymes in cancer is due to abnormal transcription and post-transcriptional control [70]. Hence, the suppression of COX-2 activity exerted by resveratrol provides a mechanistic basis for this compound's the chemo-preventive properties [61]. Again, both COX-1 and COX-2 are potently suppressed by resveratrol [73]. Therefore, resveratrol exerts an anti-inflammatory action partly due to the suppression of COX-1, COX-2, and its antioxidant effect.

4.2. NF-κB Pathway

As a ubiquitous nuclear transcription factor, NF-κB modulates a wide variety of genes expression regulating inflammatory responses. The family of NF-κB/Rel transcription factor includes NF-κB1 (p50/p105), NF-κB2 (p52/p100), p65 (RelA), RelB, and c-Rel [74]. NF-κB normally exists in the cytoplasm in an inactive form, and interacts with inhibitors of κB (IκB), including IκBα and IκBβ. IKK-mediated phosphorylation of IκB is a significant step in NF-κB activation [75]. Recently, it has become very clear that there are two separate NF-κB activation pathways: the classical pathway and the alternative pathway [76,77]. The activation of NF-κB can lead to the expression of inflammatory cytokines such as IL-1, IL-6, IL-10, and TNF in LPS-stimulation cells [78]. The abilities of resveratrol inhibition of NO synthase (NOS) and the down-regulation of NF-κB activation in macrophages is higher than naringenin and naringin [43]. Furthermore, the inhibition of NF-κB activation and

NF-κB-regulated gene expression by resveratrol are related to the suppression of the IκB kinase activation [79].

Resveratrol can block PMA-induced NF-κB activation [51], LPS [43], H_2O_2, okadaic acid, TNF-α-, IL-1β [80,81], and UVB [49]. Actually, resveratrol suppresses TNF-induced NF-κB activation in a dose- and time-dependent fashion, as demonstrated in myeloid cells, lymphoid, and epithelial cells [51]. In the same study, resveratrol was also reported to suppress phosphorylation and nuclear translocation of the p65 subunit induced by TNF-α, as well as transcription of NF-κB-dependent reporter gene. A previous study demonstrated that cells treated with LPS in addition to resveratrol exhibited suppression of NF-κB activation and phosphorylation, as well as IκBα degradation, and NF-κB subunits' nuclear content was reduced [43]. In addition, it has been shown that resveratrol decreases the TLR-4 expression and induces the development of IL-6, NO, and iNOS induced by LPS, inhibits IκBα phosphorylation, subsequently preventing NF-κB p65 translocation from the cytoplasm to the nucleus [39,47].

Resveratrol decreases IL-1β production and also inhibits the NF-κB activation dependent by IL-1β in vitro, which regulates several signals controlling cellular survival, proliferation, and inflammatory cytokine production [22,80]. In the normal human epidermal keratinocytes, this compound has been reported to block the activation of NF-κB in a dose- and time-dependent manner caused by UVB (40 mJ/cm^2), via inhibition of phosphorylation and degradation of IκBα as well as IKKα activation [49]. Zhang et al. [82] demonstrated that resveratrol was able to attenuate anoxia/reoxygenation injury-reduced expression of TLR4, inhibit NF-κB activation and downregulate the expression of inflammatory factors genes including TNF-α and IL-1β in vitro. Furthermore, Ren et al. [83] found that resveratrol suppressed endogenous and TNF-α-induced NF-κB activation in a dose-dependent manner. Further investigation revealed that resveratrol blocked the ubiquitination of NEMO and inhibited IκBβ-mediated NF-κB activation. Yi et al. [81] also reported that resveratrol was able to dramatically suppress the IL-1β-induced inflammation (including the COX-2, matrix metalloproteinase-1 (MMP-1), MMP-3, MMP-13, and iNOs expression) by inhibiting IL-1β-induced the degradation of IκB-α and the activation of NF-κB.

Uchida et al. [84] reported that resveratrol markedly and dose-dependently enhanced NF-κB activation triggered by pro-inflammatory cytokinesinglomerular mesangial cells. This compound was also able to suppress the ERK1/2/NF-κB pathway to inhibit oxidative stress and inflammation, and then inhibit neointimal hyperplasia after balloon injury [85]. Resveratrol can also attenuate liver fibrosis though the inhibition of the Akt/NF-κB pathways [86]. Liver fibrosis is a significant pathological change in chronic liver injury in which multiple inflammatory cytokines and signaling pathways are involved [87]. Qi et al. [88] demonstrated that resveratrol might play an important role in protection of the ethanol-induced neuro inflammatory responses by blocking TLR2-MyD88-NF-κB signal pathway. Rasheduzzaman et al. [89] pointed out that resveratrol could also be the effective TRAIL-based cancer therapy regimen by attenuating TNF-included apoptosis-inducing ligand (TRAIL) resistance, as well as inducing TRAIL-mediated apoptosis via the NF-κB p65 pathway.

In addition, resveratrol treatment improved neuroimmune dysregulation via inhibiting pro-inflammatory mediators and TLRs/NF-κB pathway [68]. In a recent study conducted by Lopes Pinheiro et al. [38], resveratrol treatment initiated substantial changes in protein acetylation and methylation patterns, indicating deacetylase induction and demethylase reduction activities that primarily affect regulatory cascades NF-B- and JAK/STAT- mediated pathway. In summary, NF-κB is a molecular target for the treatment of inflammatory diseases. These studies suggested that NF-κB transcriptional activity suppression leads to resveratrol's anti-inflammatory properties.

Further study of the NF-κB mechanism of resveratrol found that resveratrol can act on the corresponding cellular kinases. As a Ca_2/CaM-dependent Ser/Thr protein kinase, Death-associated protein kinase 1 (DAPK1) has many functions to participate in several pathological and physiological processes, such as cell necrosis, apoptosis, autophagy, and innate immunity [90,91]. It has been found that DAPK can suppress NF-κB activation and expression of pro-inflammatory cytokine induced by TNF-α or LPS [92,93]. DAPK1 knockdown using siRNA abolished resveratrol-induced autophagy, while it almost did not affect the phosphorylation level of AMPK, a target of resveratrol. Resveratrol-induced autophagy in human dermal fibroblasts can be DAPK1-mediated, raising the possibility that its anti-inflammatory effects are related to its regulation of DAPK1 [94].

Resveratrol exhibits anti-inflammatory effects and immunomodulating functions via sirtuin-1 (Sirt-1) activation [95]. As a deacetylase, Sirt-1 plays a vital role in immune tolerance [96,97], and it operates by blocking the TLR-4/NF-κB/STAT pathway with decreased inflammatory factors production [6,98]. For example, it was demonstrated that Sirt1 exhibited anti-inflammatory effects by regulating NLRP3 expression in mesenchymal stem cells partially via the NF-κB signaling [99], and it suppressed Porphyromonas endodontalis LPS-induced MMP-13 expression in osteoblasts via the inhibition of NF-κB signaling [100]. Resveratrol binding to Sirt-1 enhanced its attachment to RelA/p65 substrate [101], which activated leukocytes and the pro-inflammatory cytokine pathway [102]. Resveratrol inhibited RelA acetylation via Sirt1 activation, and in turn lowered expression of genes including TNF-α, IL-1β, IL-6, MMPs, and Cox-2 induced by NF-κB [96,103]. Resveratrol has been shown to be a double inhibitor of NF-κB signaling, for the reason that treated cells are less responsive to NF-κB signaling and apoptosis initiation induced by TNF-α [51]. Moreover, resveratrol could suppress p300 expression and promote IκBα degradation, while it remains unclear whether this process occurs through the activation of Sirt1 [104]. The activation of SIRT1 by resveratrol, leading to the inhibition of phospho-p38 MAPK as well as the reduced NF-κB p65 activity [105].

4.3. MAPK Pathway

MAPK is activated by translocation to the nucleus, where they phosphorylate various target transcription factors, including Nrf2, NF-κb, and AP-1 [106,107]. MAPK signal transduction pathways are pivotal in many biological processes, including proliferation, differentiation, apoptosis, inflammation, and responses to environmental stresses [108]. MAPKs are a family of stress-inducible kinases, including the c-jun Nterminal kinase (JNK), extracellular-signal regulated kinase (ERK), Big MAP kinase (BMK), and p38 (Figure 3) [109,110]. Among these, the p38 MAPK is activated by several pro-inflammatory stimuli such as oxidative stress, UBV, and inflammatory cytokines [111,112].

It has been reported that resveratrol suppresses COX-2 expression in mouse skin ex vivo by suppressing the activation of ERKs and p38 MAPK pathways induced by PMA [64]. The inhibitory effects of this compound probably involve suppression of the p38 MAPK-cytosolic phospholipase A2-AA-TxA2-$[Ca^{2+}]_i$ cascade and NO/cyclic GMP activation, then lead to suppression of phospholipase C and/or PKC activation [113]. Resveratrol in combination with pemetrexed shows a synergistic cytotoxic effect, accompanied with the reduction of protein levels of phospho-p38 MAPK and ERCC1, as well as a DNA repair capacity [114]. Resveratrol has also been reported to suppress invasion and migration of pancreatic cancer cells by blocking the ERKs and p38 MAPK induced by hyperglycemia-driven ROS [115]. In vivo studies reported that maternal dietary resveratrol addition decreased the levels of T cell receptor genes, MAPK signal transduction pathways in weaning piglets, and it alleviated weaning-associated diarrhea and intestinal inflammatory disorders in porcine offspring [116]. Moreover, many studies have shown that this compound could potentially induce apoptosis and in vitro ROS accumulation through p38 MAPK signaling pathways [117–119]. Yang et al. [120] also reported that resveratrol was able to reduce ROS accumulation, inflammation, and angiogenesis both in vivo and in vitro, then displaying preventive effects for rheumatoid arthritis (RA). Additionally, it can alleviate the nervous inflammatory responses after injury via decreasing the extracellular levels of gliotransmitter, as well as blocking p38 MAPK activation [121,122]. Moreover, the inhibition of MAPK signaling pathways probably contributes to the anti-inflammatory effects of resveratrol.

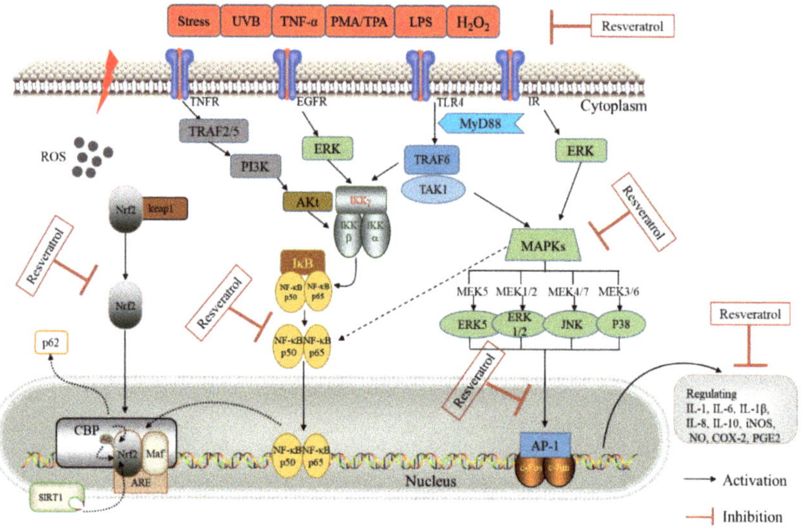

Figure 3. Schematic presentation of possible signaling cascades of resveratrol in suppression inflammatory response. Key abbreviations: UVB, ultraviolet B; TNF-α, tumor necrosis factor alpha; TPA, 12-O-tetradecanoylphorbol-13-acetate; PMA, Phorbol 12-myristate 13-acetate; H_2O_2, hydrogen peroxide; LPS, lipopolysaccharide; TLR4, Toll-like receptor 4; MyD88, myeloid differentiation factor 88; TRAF6, tumor necrosis factor receptor associated factor 6; MAPKs, mitogen-activated protein kinases; IκB, inhibitor kappa B; IKK, inhibitor-κB kinase; NF-κBp65, nuclear factor kappa B 3; IL, interleukin; NO, nitric oxide; iNOS, inducible nitric oxide synthase; COX-2, cyclooxygenase-2; PGE2, prostaglandin E2.

Resveratrol is able to suppress the inflammatory response though blocking the phosphorylation protein expression of p65 and IκB from the NF-κB signaling as well as phosphorylation of p38 and ERK from MAPK signaling under mastitis conditions [123]. Our recently study also demonstrated that dietary resveratrol supplementation in broilers could inhibit inflammatory response by inhibiting NF-κB, MAPK, and PI3K/AKT signaling under heat stress condition [35]. Wang et al. [124] pointed out that this phytoalexins could block the signaling cascades of NF-κB p65 and MAPKs in vivo by downregulating the mRNA expression of genes involved in NF-κB and MAPKs in LPS-induced liver and lung in rats, and inhibiting the dynamic changes of proteins and phosphorylated proteins which include IκBα, NF-κB p65, JNK, ERK1/2, ERK5, and p38 MAPK from tissue cytoplasm to nucleus.

4.4. AP-1 Pathway

AP-1 is another transcription factor typically comprised of one member each from the Jun (c-Jun, JunB and JunD) and Fos (c-Fos, FosB, Fra1 and Fra2) families [125]. AP-1 regulates an array of cell processes, including proliferation, differentiation, inflammation, and apoptosis [126]. AP-1 can be activated by various extracellular stimuli [125], and resveratrol can block PMA- or TNF- induced activation of AP-1-mediated gene expression (Figure 3) [51,61]. Resveratrol can suppress IL-8 production in U937 cells induced by PMA at both mRNA and protein levels [127], suggesting that the block on IL-8 gene transcription by this compound is due partly to suppression of AP-1 activation. The downregulation of AP-1 activity may contribute to resveratrol's anti-proliferative activity in A431 cells [128]. Although studies have shown that resveratrol can easily inhibit COX-2 activity directly, the indirect inhibitory effect of reducing COX-2 expression appears to be more significant after inhibiting AP-1 [129].

In addition, suppression of NF-κB correlated with inhibition of AP-1, and the anti-carcinogenic and anti-inflammatory effects of resveratrol can therefore be partly due to blocking both NF-κB and AP-1 activation as well as related kinases [51]. Resveratrol provides chemical protection against cancer through the NF-κB and AP-1 pathways [129]. This has been shown in mouse skin models in which abnormal NF-κB and AP-1 activities lead to skin tumors [130]. Furthermore, in vitro study conducted by Donnelly et al. [131] found that the inhibitory effects of this phytoalexin are greater than those of the glucocorticosteroid dexamethasone, due to the suppression of transcription of NF-κB- and AP-1-, as well as the protein-dependent cyclic adenosine monophosphate response element binding.

4.5. Antioxidant Defense Pathways

Resveratrol exhibits strong antioxidant activity, mainly via the control of major antioxidant enzymes and block on DNA damage by free radicals. The anti-inflammatory activity of this compound may be due to the antioxidant properties by inhibiting pro-inflammatory signaling pathways (Figure 3). Many studies have demonstrated that resveratrol can reduce H_2O_2-dependent oxidative damage in calf thymus DNA [117,132], as well as in several cancer cell lines [133,134]. As a known marker of oxidative DNA damage, the levels of 8-oxo-7,8-dihydroxy-29-deoxyguanosine decrease with the addition of resveratrol in vivo [135]. Moreover, resveratrol is able to alleviate intestinal injury and dysfunctions though improving oxidative status and inhibiting inflammatory responses in rats under heat stress [136].

High levels of NO are produced by iNOS in inflammation, and the inhibition of iNOS expression, might play a major role in anti-inflammatory responses [137]. It has been shown that resveratrol can protect IPEC-J2 cells from oxidative damage by stimulating the Nrf2 pathway [138]. Additionally, resveratrol upregulates the protein expression of Nrf2 and HO-1 signaling pathway, thus attenuating oxidative stress and inflammatory response by hypoxic-ichemically induced in neonatal rats [139]. In addition, resveratrol also inhibits the activation of MAPKs and reduces the production of inflammatory mediators by activating SIRT1/AMPK and Nrf2 antioxidant defense pathways [140]. Therefore, one of the anti-inflammatory effects of resveratrol may be explained by the suppression of the antioxidant properties.

5. Summary and Perspectives

Multiple lines of compelling evidence indicate that resveratrol has a promising role in the prevention and treatment of many autoimmune and inflammatory chronic diseases, such as inflammatory, neurological, and multiple cancers. This phytoalexin was demonstrated to modulate many cellular and molecular mediators of inflammation, but the molecular mechanisms of polyphenol are complex and involve multiple signal transduction pathways, and have not been fully elucidated.

Therefore, future research should focus on: (1) further evaluating the compound during clinical trials and improving oral absorption efficiency; and (2) elucidating the underlying mechanisms of resveratrol action in several physiological conditions, in order to make this compound a cutting-edge therapeutic strategy for the prevention and treatment of a wide variety of chronic diseases.

Author Contributions: Conceptualization, T.M., D.X. and J.H.; writing—original draft preparation, T.M.; writing—review and editing, D.X., J.H., A.M., J.D. and L.C. All authors have read and agreed to the published version of the manuscript.

Funding: This research was funded by the National Natural Science Foundation of China, grant number NO.31972600, 31872991; Natural Science Foundation of Hunan Province-China, grant number 2020JJ4364; "Double first class" Construction Project of Hunan Agricultural University, grant number kxk201801004; Project of science and Technology Department of Hunan Province, grant number 2020NK4247.

Conflicts of Interest: The authors have declared no conflict of interest.

References

1. Langcake, P.; Pryce, R.J. The production of resveratrol by Vitis vinifera and other members of the Vitaceae as a response to infection or injury. *Physiol. Plant Pathol.* **1976**, *9*, 77–86. [CrossRef]
2. Lastra, C.A.; Villegas, I. Resveratrol as an antioxidant and pro-oxidant agent: Mechanisms and clinical implications. *Biochem. Soc. Trans.* **2007**, *35*, 1156–1160. [PubMed]
3. Meng, Q.; Guo, T.; Li, G.; Sun, S.; He, S.; Cheng, B.; Shi, B.; Shan, A. Dietary resveratrol improves antioxidant status of sows and piglets and regulates antioxidant gene expression in placenta by Keap1-Nrf2 pathway and Sirt1. *J. Anim. Sci. Biotechnol.* **2018**, *9*, 34. [CrossRef] [PubMed]
4. Nunes, S.; Danesi, F.; Del Rio, D.; Silva, P. Resveratrol and inflammatory bowel disease: The evidence so far. *Nutr. Res. Rev.* **2018**, *31*, 85–97. [CrossRef] [PubMed]
5. Duthie, G.G.; Duthie, S.J.; Kyle, J.A.M. Plant polyphenols in cancer and heart disease: Implications as nutritional antioxidants. *Nutr. Res. Rev.* **2000**, *13*, 79–106. [CrossRef]
6. Lastra, C.A.; Villegas, I. Resveratrol as an anti-inflammatory and anti-aging agent: Mechanisms and clinical implications. *Mol. Nutr. Food Res.* **2005**, *49*, 405–430. [CrossRef]
7. Signorelli, P.; Ghidoni, R. Resveratrol as an anticancer nutrient: Molecular basis, open questions and promises. *J. Nutr. Biochem.* **2005**, *16*, 449–466. [CrossRef]
8. Walle, T. Bioavailability of resveratrol. *Ann. N. Y. Acad. Sci.* **2011**, *1215*, 9–15. [CrossRef]
9. Gowda, V.; Karima, N.; Rezaul Islam Shishira, M.; Xie, L.; Chen, W. Dietary polyphenols to combat the metabolic diseases via altering gut microbiota. *Trends Food Sci. Technol.* **2019**, *93*, 81–93. [CrossRef]
10. Bhat, K.P.L.; Kosmeder, J.W.; Pezzuto, J.M. Biological effects of resveratrol. *Antioxid. Redox. Signal.* **2001**, *3*, 1041–1064. [CrossRef]
11. Lancon, A.; Delmas, D.; Osman, H.; Thenot, J.P.; Jannin, B.; Latruffe, N. Human hepatic cell uptake of resveratrol: Involvement of both passive diffusion and carrier-mediated process. *Biochem. Biophys. Res. Commun.* **2004**, *316*, 1132–1137. [CrossRef] [PubMed]
12. Walle, T.; Hsieh, F.; DeLegge, M.H.; Oatis, J.E., Jr.; Walle, U.K. High absorption but very low bioavailability of oral resveratrol in humans. *Drug Metab. Dispos.* **2004**, *32*, 1377–1382. [CrossRef] [PubMed]
13. Ferraz da Costa, D.C.; Pereira Rangel, L.; Quarti, J.; Santos, R.A.; Silva, J.L.; Fialho, E. Bioactive Compounds and Metabolites from Grapes and Red Wine in Breast Cancer Chemoprevention and Therapy. *Molecules* **2020**, *25*, 3531. [CrossRef] [PubMed]
14. Chimento, A.; De Amicis, F.; Sirianni, R.; Sinicropi, M.S.; Puoci, F.; Casaburi, I.; Saturnino, C.; Pezzi, V. Progress to Improve Oral Bioavailability and Beneficial Effects of Resveratrol. *Int. J. Mol. Sci.* **2019**, *20*, 1381. [CrossRef] [PubMed]
15. Lugrin, J.; Rosenblatt-Velin, N.; Parapanov, R.; Liaudet, L. The role of oxidative stress during inflammatory processes. *Biol. Chem.* **2014**, *395*, 203–230. [CrossRef] [PubMed]
16. Medzhitov, R. Origin and physiological roles of inflammation. *Nature* **2008**, *454*, 428–435. [CrossRef]
17. Iwasaki, A.; Medzhitov, R. Control of adaptive immunity by the innate immune system. *Nat. Immunol.* **2015**, *16*, 343–353. [CrossRef]
18. Nathan, C. Points of control in inflammation. *Nature* **2002**, *420*, 846–852. [CrossRef]
19. Liu, J.; Cao, X. Cellular and molecular regulation of innate inflammatory responses. *Cell Mol. Immunol.* **2016**, *13*, 711–721. [CrossRef]
20. Fitzgerald, K.A.; Kagan, J.C. Toll-like Receptors and the Control of Immunity. *Cell* **2020**, *180*, 1044–1066. [CrossRef]
21. Singh, A.; Yau, Y.F.; Leung, K.S.; El-Nezami, H.; Lee, J.C.-Y. Interaction of Polyphenols as Antioxidant and Anti-Inflammatory Compounds in Brain–Liver–Gut Axis. *Antioxidants* **2020**, *9*, 669. [CrossRef] [PubMed]
22. Gao, X.; Xu, Y.X.; Janakiraman, N.; Chapman, R.A.; Gautam, S.C. Immunomodulatory activity of resveratrol: Suppression of lymphocyte proliferation, development of cell-mediated cytotoxicity, and cytokine production. *Biochem. Pharmacol.* **2001**, *62*, 1299–1308. [CrossRef]
23. Fuggetta, M.P.; Bordignon, V.; Cottarelli, A.; Macchi, B.; Frezza, C.; Cordiali-Fei, P.; Ensoli, F.; Ciafre, S.; Marino-Merlo, F.; Mastino, A.; et al. Downregulation of proinflammatory cytokines in HTLV-1-infected T cells by Resveratrol. *J. Exp. Clin. Cancer Res.* **2016**, *35*, 118. [CrossRef] [PubMed]
24. Zhang, C.; Zhao, X.H.; Yang, L.; Chen, X.Y.; Jiang, R.S.; Jin, S.H.; Geng, Z.Y. Resveratrol alleviates heat stress-induced impairment of intestinal morphology, microflora, and barrier integrity in broilers. *Poult. Sci.* **2017**, *96*, 4325–4332. [CrossRef] [PubMed]
25. Zhang, H.; Chen, Y.; Chen, Y.; Ji, S.; Jia, P.; Li, Y.; Wang, T. Comparison of the protective effects of resveratrol and pterostilbene against intestinal damage and redox imbalance in weanling piglets. *J. Anim. Sci. Biotechnol.* **2020**, *11*, 52. [CrossRef]
26. Xian, Y.; Gao, Y.; Lv, W.; Ma, X.; Hu, J.; Chi, J.; Wang, W.; Wang, Y. Resveratrol prevents diabetic nephropathy by reducing chronic inflammation and improving the blood glucose memory effect in non-obese diabetic mice. *Naunyn Schmiedebergs Arch. Pharmacol.* **2020**, *393*, 2009–2017. [CrossRef] [PubMed]
27. Zou, M.; Yang, W.; Niu, L.; Sun, Y.; Luo, R.; Wang, Y.; Peng, X. Polydatin attenuates Mycoplasma gallisepticum (HS strain)-induced inflammation injury via inhibiting the TLR6/ MyD88/NF-kappaB pathway. *Microb. Pathog.* **2020**, *149*, 104552. [CrossRef]

28. Jang, M.; Cai, L.; Udeani, G.O.; Slowing, K.V.; Thomas, C.F.; Beecher, C.W.; Fong, H.H.; Farnsworth, N.R.; Kinghorn, A.D.; Mehta, R.G.; et al. Cancer chemopreventive activity of resveratrol, a natural product derived from grapes. *Science* **1997**, *275*, 218–220. [CrossRef]
29. Simao, F.; Matte, A.; Pagnussat, A.S.; Netto, C.A.; Salbego, C.G. Resveratrol preconditioning modulates inflammatory response in the rat hippocampus following global cerebral ischemia. *Neurochem. Inter.* **2012**, *61*, 659–665. [CrossRef]
30. Hou, Y.; Zhang, Y.; Mi, Y.; Wang, J.; Zhang, H.; Xu, J.; Yang, Y.; Liu, J.; Ding, L.; Yang, J.; et al. A Novel Quinolyl-Substituted Analogue of Resveratrol Inhibits LPS-Induced Inflammatory Responses in Microglial Cells by Blocking the NF-κB/MAPK Signaling Pathways. *Mol. Nutr. Food. Res.* **2019**, *63*, e1801380. [CrossRef]
31. Jiang, H.; Duan, J.; Xu, K.; Zhang, W. Resveratrol protects against asthma-induced airway inflammation and remodeling by inhibiting the HMGB1/TLR4/NF-kappa B pathway. *Exp. Ther. Med.* **2019**, *18*, 459–466. [PubMed]
32. Liu, L.L.; He, J.H.; Xie, H.B.; Yang, Y.S.; Li, J.C.; Zou, Y. Resveratrol induces antioxidant and heat shock protein mRNA expression in response to heat stress in black-boned chickens. *Poult. Sci.* **2014**, *93*, 54–62. [CrossRef]
33. He, S.; Chen, L.; He, Y.; Chen, F.; Ma, Y.; Xiao, D.; He, J. Resveratrol alleviates heat stress-induced impairment of intestinal morphology, barrier integrity and inflammation in yellow-feather broilers. *Anim. Prod. Sci.* **2020**, *60*, 1547. [CrossRef]
34. Zhang, C.; Chen, K.; Zhao, X.; Geng, Z. Protective effects of resveratrol against high ambient temperature-induced spleen dysplasia in broilers through modulating splenic redox status and apoptosis. *J. Sci. Food Agric.* **2018**, *98*, 5409–5417. [CrossRef] [PubMed]
35. He, S.; Yu, Q.; He, Y.; Hu, R.; Xia, S.; He, J. Dietary resveratrol supplementation inhibits heat stress-induced high-activated innate immunity and inflammatory response in spleen of yellow-feather broilers. *Poult. Sci.* **2019**, *98*, 6378–6387. [CrossRef]
36. Rietschel, E.T.; Kirikae, T.; Schade, F.U.; Mamat, U.; Schmidt, G.; Loppnow, H.; Ulmer, A.J.; Zahringer, U.; Seydel, U.; Di Padova, F.; et al. Bacterial endotoxin: Molecular relationships of structure to activity and function. *FASEB J.* **1994**, *8*, 217–225. [CrossRef]
37. Zhong, L.M.; Zong, Y.; Sun, L.; Guo, J.Z.; Zhang, W.; He, Y.; Song, R.; Wang, W.M.; Xiao, C.J.; Lu, D. Resveratrol inhibits inflammatory responses via the mammalian target of rapamycin signaling pathway in cultured LPS-stimulated microglial cells. *PLoS ONE* **2012**, *7*, e32195. [CrossRef]
38. Lopes Pinheiro, D.M.; Sales de Oliveira, A.H.; Coutinho, L.G.; Fontes, F.L.; de Medeiros Oliveira, R.K.; Oliveira, T.T.; Fonseca Faustino, A.L.; da Silva, V.L.; Araujo de Melo Campos, J.T.; Petta Lajus, T.B.; et al. Resveratrol decreases the expression of genes involved in inflammation through transcriptional regulation. *Free Radic. Biol. Med.* **2019**, *130*, 8–22. [CrossRef]
39. Panaro, M.A.; Carofiglio, V.; Acquafredda, A.; Cavallo, P.; Cianciulli, A. Anti-inflammatory effects of resveratrol occur via inhibition of lipopolysaccharide-induced NF-κB activation in Caco-2 and SW480 human colon cancer cells. *Br. J. Nutr.* **2012**, *108*, 1623–1632. [CrossRef]
40. Palomera-Avalos, V.; Grinan-Ferre, C.; Izquierdo, V.; Camins, A.; Sanfeliu, C.; Canudas, A.M.; Pallas, M. Resveratrol modulates response against acute inflammatory stimuli in aged mouse brain. *Exp. Gerontol.* **2018**, *102*, 3–11. [CrossRef]
41. Sadeghi, A.; Ebrahimi, S.S.S.; Golestani, A.; Meshkani, R. Resveratrol Ameliorates Palmitate-Induced Inflammation in Skeletal Muscle Cells by Attenuating Oxidative Stress and JNK/NF-kappa B Pathway in a SIRT1-Independent Mechanism. *J. Cell. Biochem.* **2017**, *118*, 2654–2663. [CrossRef] [PubMed]
42. Reuter, S.; Gupta, S.C.; Chaturvedi, M.M.; Aggarwal, B.B. Oxidative stress, inflammation, and cancer: How are they linked? *Free Radic. Biol. Med.* **2010**, *49*, 1603–1616. [CrossRef] [PubMed]
43. Tsai, S.H.; Lin-Shiau, S.Y.; Lin, J.K. Suppression of nitric oxide synthase and the down- regulation of the activation of NF-kappa B in macrophages by resveratrol. *Br. J. Pharmacol.* **1999**, *126*, 673–680. [CrossRef] [PubMed]
44. Das, A. Heat stress-induced hepatotoxicity and its prevention by resveratrol in rats. *Toxicol. Mech. Methods* **2011**, *21*, 393–399. [CrossRef]
45. Babu, D.; Leclercq, G.; Goossens, V.; Remijsen, Q.; Vandenabeele, P.; Motterlini, R.; Lefebvre, R.A. Antioxidant potential of CORM-A1 and resveratrol during TNF-alpha/cycloheximide-induced oxidative stress and apoptosis in murine intestinal epithelial MODE-K cells. *Toxicol. Appl. Pharmacol.* **2015**, *288*, 161–178. [CrossRef]
46. Kortam, M.A.; Ali, B.M.; Fathy, N. The deleterious effect of stress-induced depression on rat liver: Protective role of resveratrol and dimethyl fumarate via inhibiting the MAPK/ERK/JNK pathway. *J. Biochem. Mol. Toxicol.* **2020**, 1–11. [CrossRef]
47. Ma, C.; Wang, Y.; Dong, L.; Li, M.; Cai, W. Anti-inflammatory effect of resveratrol through the suppression of NF-kappa B and JAK/STAT signaling pathways. *Acta Biochim. Biophys. Sin.* **2015**, *47*, 207–213. [CrossRef]
48. Li, X.; Li, F.; Wang, F.; Li, J.; Lin, C.; Du, J. Resveratrol inhibits the proliferation of A549 cells by inhibiting the expression of COX-2. *Oncotargets Ther.* **2018**, *11*, 2981–2989. [CrossRef]
49. Adhami, V.M.; Afaq, F.; Ahmad, N. Suppression of Ultraviolet B Exposure-Mediated Activation of NF-κB in Normal Human Keratinocytes by Resveratrol. *Neoplasia* **2003**, *5*, 74–82. [CrossRef]
50. Pirola, L.; Frojdo, S. Resveratrol: One molecule, many targets. *IUBMB Life* **2008**, *60*, 323–332. [CrossRef]
51. Manna, S.K.; Mukhopadhyay, A.; Aggarwal, B.B. Resveratrol suppresses TNF-induced activation of nuclear transcription factors NF-kappa B, activator protein-1, and apoptosis: Potential role of reactive oxygen intermediates and lipid peroxidation. *J. Immunol.* **2000**, *164*, 6509–6519. [CrossRef] [PubMed]
52. Magrone, T.; Magrone, M.; Russo, M.A.; Jirillo, E. Recent Advances on the Anti-Inflammatory and Antioxidant Properties of Red Grape Polyphenols: In Vitro and In Vivo Studies. *Antioxidants* **2019**, *9*, 35. [CrossRef] [PubMed]

53. Chandrasekharan, N.V.; Dai, H.; Roos, K.L.; Evanson, N.K.; Tomsik, J.; Elton, T.S.; Simmons, D.L. COX-3, a cyclooxygenase-1 variant inhibited by acetaminophen and other analgesic/antipyretic drugs: Cloning, structure, and expression. *Proc. Natl. Acad. Sci. USA* **2002**, *99*, 13926–13931. [CrossRef] [PubMed]
54. Dinchuk, J.E.; Liu, R.Q.; Trzaskos, J.M. COX-3: In the wrong frame in mind. *Immunol. Lett.* **2003**, *86*, 121. [CrossRef]
55. Schmassmann, A.; Peskar, B.M.; Stettler, C.; Netzer, P. Effects of inhibition of prostaglandin endoperoxide synthase-2 in chronic gastrointestinal ulcer models in rats. *Br. J. Pharmacol.* **1998**, *123*, 795–804. [CrossRef]
56. Vane, J.R.; Botting, R.M. Mechanism of action of nonsteroidal anti-inflammatory drugs. *Am. J. Med.* **1998**, *104*, 2S–8S. [CrossRef]
57. Greenhough, A.; Smartt, H.J.; Moore, A.E.; Roberts, H.R.; Williams, A.C.; Paraskeva, C.; Kaidi, A. The COX-2/PGE2 pathway: Key roles in the hallmarks of cancer and adaptation to the tumour microenvironment. *Carcinogenesis* **2009**, *30*, 377–386. [CrossRef]
58. Rundhaug, J.E.; Fischer, S.M. Cyclo-oxygenase-2 plays a critical role in UV-induced skin carcinogenesis. *Photochem. Photobiol.* **2008**, *84*, 322–329. [CrossRef]
59. Kundu, J.K.; Shin, Y.K.; Kim, S.H.; Surh, Y.-J. Resveratrol inhibits phorbol ester-induced expression of COX-2 and activation of NF-kappaB in mouse skin by blocking IkappaB kinase activity. *Carcinogenesis* **2006**, *27*, 1465–1474. [CrossRef]
60. Szewczuk, L.M.; Forti, L.; Stivala, L.A.; Penning, T.M. Resveratrol is a peroxidase-mediated inactivator of COX-1 but not COX-2: A mechanistic approach to the design of COX-1 selective agents. *J. Biol. Chem.* **2004**, *279*, 22727–22737. [CrossRef]
61. Subbaramaiah, K.; Chung, W.J.; Michaluart, P.; Telang, N.; Tanabe, T.; Inoue, H.; Jang, M.; Pezzuto, J.M.; Dannenberg, A.J. Resveratrol inhibits cyclooxygenase-2 transcription and activity in phorbol ester-treated human mammary epithelial cells. *J. Biol. Chem.* **1998**, *273*, 21875–21882. [CrossRef] [PubMed]
62. Martinez, J.; Moreno, J.J. Effect of resveratrol, a natural polyphenolic compound, on reactive oxygen species and prostaglandin production. *Biochem. Pharmacol.* **2000**, *59*, 865–870. [CrossRef]
63. Murias, M.; Handler, N.; Erker, T.; Pleban, K.; Ecker, G.; Saiko, P.; Szekeres, T.; Jäger, W. Resveratrol analogues as selective cyclooxygenase-2 inhibitors: Synthesis and structure–activity relationship. *Bioorg. Med. Chem.* **2004**, *12*, 5571–5578. [CrossRef]
64. Martín, A.R.; Villegas, I.; La Casa, C.; de la Lastra, C.A. Resveratrol, a polyphenol found in grapes, suppresses oxidative damage and stimulates apoptosis during early colonic inflammation in rats. *Biochem. Pharmacol.* **2004**, *67*, 1399–1410. [PubMed]
65. Zykova, T.A.; Zhu, F.; Zhai, X.; Ma, W.Y.; Ermakova, S.P.; Lee, K.W.; Bode, A.M.; Dong, Z. Resveratrol directly targets COX-2 to inhibit carcinogenesis. *Mol. Carcinog.* **2008**, *47*, 797–805. [CrossRef] [PubMed]
66. Gong, W.H.; Zhao, N.; Zhang, Z.M.; Zhang, Y.X.; Yan, L; Li, J.B. The inhibitory effect of resveratrol on COX-2 expression in human colorectal cancer: A promising therapeutic strategy. *Eur. Rev. Med. Pharmacol. Sci.* **2017**, *21*, 1136–1143.
67. Eo, S.-H.; Kim, S.J. Resveratrol-mediated inhibition of cyclooxygenase-2 in melanocytes suppresses melanogenesis through extracellular signal-regulated kinase 1/2 and phosphoinositide 3-kinase/Akt signalling. *Eur. J. Pharmacol.* **2019**, *860*, 172586. [CrossRef]
68. Ahmad, S.F.; Ansari, M.A.; Nadeem, A.; Alzahrani, M.Z.; Bakheet, S.A.; Attia, S.M. Resveratrol Improves Neuroimmune Dysregulation Through the Inhibition of Neuronal Toll-Like Receptors and COX-2 Signaling in BTBR T(+) Itpr3(tf)/J Mice. *Neuromol. Med.* **2018**, *20*, 133–146. [CrossRef]
69. Garcia-Garcia, J.; Micol, V.; de Godos, A.; Gomez-Fernandez, J.C. The cancer chemopreventive agent resveratrol is incorporated into model membranes and inhibits protein kinase C alpha activity. *Arch. Biochem. Biophys.* **1999**, *372*, 382–388. [CrossRef]
70. Dorai, T.; Aggarwal, B.B. Role of chemopreventive agents in cancer therapy. *Cancer Lett.* **2004**, *215*, 129–140. [CrossRef]
71. Kundu, J.K.; Chun, K.S.; Kim, S.O.; Surh, Y.J. Resveratrol inhibits phorbol ester-induced cyclooxygenase-2 expression in mouse skin: MAPKs and AP-1 as potential molecular targets. *BioFactors* **2004**, *21*, 33–39. [CrossRef] [PubMed]
72. Yi, C.-O.; Jeon, B.T.; Shin, H.J.; Jeong, E.A.; Chang, K.C.; Lee, J.E.; Lee, D.H.; Kim, H.J.; Kang, S.S.; Cho, G.J.; et al. Resveratrol activates AMPK and suppresses LPS-induced NF-kappaB-dependent COX-2 activation in RAW 264.7 macrophage cells. *Anat. Cell Boil.* **2011**, *44*, 194–203. [CrossRef] [PubMed]
73. Calamini, B.; Ratia, K.; Malkowski, M.G.; Cuendet, M.; Pezzuto, J.M.; Santarsiero, B.D.; Mesecar, A.D. Pleiotropic mechanisms facilitated by resveratrol and its metabolites. *Biochem. J.* **2010**, *429*, 273–282. [CrossRef] [PubMed]
74. Chen, F.; Castranova, V.; Shi, X. New Insights into the Role of Nuclear Factor-κB in Cell Growth Regulation. *Am. J. Pathol.* **2001**, *159*, 387–397. [CrossRef]
75. Tak, P.P.; Firestein, G.S. NF-κB: A key role in inflammatory diseases. *Clin. Investig.* **2001**, *107*, 7–11. [CrossRef]
76. Hoesel, B.; Schmid, J.A. The complexity of NF-κB signaling in inflammation and cancer. *Mol. Cancer* **2013**, *12*, 1–15. [CrossRef]
77. Lawrence, T. The nuclear factor NF-kappaB pathway in inflammation. *Cold Spring Harb. Perspect.* **2009**, *1*, a001651.
78. Wang, T.; Wu, F.; Jin, Z.; Zhai, Z.; Wang, Y.; Tu, B.; Yan, W.; Tang, T. Plumbagin inhibits LPS-induced inflammation through the inactivation of the nuclear factor-kappa B and mitogen activated protein kinase signaling pathways in RAW 264.7 cells. *Food Chem. Toxicol.* **2014**, *64*, 177–183. [CrossRef]
79. Holmes-McNary, M.; Baldwin, A.S., Jr. Chemopreventive Properties of trans-Resveratrol Are Associated with Inhibition of Activation of the IB Kinase. *Cancer Res.* **2000**, *60*, 3477–3483.
80. Estrov, Z.; Shishodia, S.; Faderl, S.; Harris, D.; Van, Q.; Kantarjian, H.M.; Talpaz, M.; Aggarwal, B.B. Resveratrol blocks interleukin-1beta-induced activation of the nuclear transcription factor NF-kappaB, inhibits proliferation, causes S-phase arrest, and induces apoptosis of acute myeloid leukemia cells. *Blood* **2003**, *102*, 987–995. [CrossRef]
81. Yi, H.; Zhang, W.; Cui, Z.-M.; Cui, S.-Y.; Fan, J.-B.; Zhu, X.-H.; Liu, W. Resveratrol alleviates the interleukin-1beta-induced chondrocytes injury through the NF-kappaB signaling pathway. *J. Orthop. Surg. Res.* **2020**, *15*, 424. [CrossRef] [PubMed]

82. Zhang, C.; Lin, G.; Wan, W.; Li, X.; Zeng, B.; Yang, B.; Huang, C. Resveratrol, a polyphenol phytoalexin, protects cardiomyocytes against anoxia/reoxygenation injury via the TLR4/NF-kappa B signaling pathway. *Int. J. Mol. Med.* **2012**, *29*, 557–563. [CrossRef] [PubMed]
83. Ren, Z.; Wang, L.; Cui, J.; Huoc, Z.; Xue, J.; Cui, H.; Mao, Q.; Yang, R. Resveratrol inhibits NF-kB signaling through suppression of p65 and IkappaB kinase activities. *Pharmazie* **2013**, *68*, 689–694.
84. Uchida, Y.; Yamazaki, H.; Watanabe, S.; Hayakawa, K.; Meng, Y.; Hiramatsu, N.; Kasai, A.; Yamauchi, K.; Yao, J.; Kitamura, M. Enhancement of NF-kappaB activity by resveratrol in cytokine-exposed mesangial cells. *Clin. Exp. Immunol.* **2005**, *142*, 76–83. [CrossRef] [PubMed]
85. Zhang, J.; Chen, J.; Yang, J.; Xu, C.-W.; Pu, P.; Ding, J.-W.; Jiang, H. Resveratrol Attenuates Oxidative Stress Induced by Balloon Injury in the Rat Carotid Artery Through Actions on the ERK1/2 and NF-Kappa B Pathway. *Cell. Physiol. Biochem.* **2013**, *31*, 230–241. [CrossRef]
86. Zhang, H.; Sun, Q.; Xu, T.; Hong, L.; Fu, R.; Wu, J.; Ding, J. Resveratrol attenuates the progress of liver fibrosis via the Akt/nuclear factor-kappa B pathways. *Mol. Med. Rep.* **2016**, *13*, 224–230. [CrossRef]
87. Friedman, S.L. Evolving challenges in hepatic fibrosis. *Nat. Rev. Gastroenterol. Hepatol.* **2010**, *7*, 425–436. [CrossRef]
88. Qi, B.; Shi, C.; Meng, J.; Xu, S.; Liu, J. Resveratrol alleviates ethanol-induced neuroinflammation in vivo and in vitro: Involvement of TLR2-MyD88-NF-kappa B pathway. *Int. J. Biochem. Cell Biol.* **2018**, *103*, 56–64. [CrossRef]
89. Rasheduzzaman, M.; Jeong, J.K.; Park, S.Y. Resveratrol sensitizes lung cancer cell to TRAIL by p53 independent and suppression of Akt/NF-κB signaling. *Life Sci.* **2018**, *208*, 208–220. [CrossRef]
90. Wang, S.; Chen, K.; Yu, J.; Wang, X.; Li, Q.; Lv, F.; Shen, H.; Pei, L. Presynaptic Caytaxin prevents apoptosis via deactivating DAPK1 in the acute phase of cerebral ischemic stroke. *Exp. Neurol.* **2020**, *329*, 113303. [CrossRef]
91. Chuang, Y.T.; Fang, L.W.; Lin-Feng, M.H.; Chen, R.H.; Lai, M.Z. The tumor suppressor death-associated protein kinase targets to TCR-stimulated NF-kappa B activation. *J. Immunol.* **2008**, *180*, 3238–3249. [CrossRef]
92. Li, T.; Wu, Y.N.; Wang, H.; Ma, J.Y.; Zhai, S.S.; Duan, J. Dapk1 improves inflammation, oxidative stress and autophagy in LPS-induced acute lung injury via p38MAPK/NF-kappaB signaling pathway. *Mol. Immunol.* **2020**, *120*, 13–22. [CrossRef] [PubMed]
93. Lai, M.Z.; Chen, R.H. Regulation of inflammation by DAPK. *Apoptosis* **2014**, *19*, 357–363. [CrossRef] [PubMed]
94. Choi, M.S.; Kim, Y.; Jung, J.Y.; Yang, S.H.; Lee, T.R.; Shin, D.W. Resveratrol induces autophagy through death-associated protein kinase 1 (DAPK1) in human dermal fibroblasts under normal culture conditions. *Exp. Dermatol.* **2013**, *22*, 491–494. [CrossRef] [PubMed]
95. Saiko, P.; Szakmary, A.; Jaeger, W.; Szekeres, T. Resveratrol and its analogs: Defense against cancer, coronary disease and neurodegenerative maladies or just a fad? *Mutat. Res.* **2008**, *658*, 68–94. [CrossRef]
96. Gao, B.; Kong, Q.; Kemp, K.; Zhao, Y.S.; Fang, D. Analysis of sirtuin 1 expression reveals a molecular explanation of IL-2-mediated reversal of T-cell tolerance. *Proc. Natl. Acad. Sci. USA* **2012**, *109*, 899–904. [CrossRef]
97. Zhang, J.; Lee, S.M.; Shannon, S.; Gao, B.; Chen, W.; Chen, A.; Divekar, R.; McBurney, M.W.; Braley-Mullen, H.; Zaghouani, H.; et al. The type III histone deacetylase Sirt1 is essential for maintenance of T cell tolerance in mice. *J. Clin. Invest.* **2009**, *119*, 3048–3058. [CrossRef]
98. Wicinski, M.; Socha, M.; Walczak, M.; Wodkiewicz, E.; Malinowski, B.; Rewerski, S.; Gorski, K.; Pawlak-Osinska, K. Beneficial Effects of Resveratrol Administration-Focus on Potential Biochemical Mechanisms in Cardiovascular Conditions. *Nutrients* **2018**, *10*, 1813. [CrossRef]
99. Fu, Y.; Wang, Y.; Du, L.; Xu, C.; Cao, J.; Fan, T.; Liu, J.; Su, X.; Fan, S.; Liu, Q.; et al. Resveratrol inhibits ionising irradiation-induced inflammation in MSCs by activating SIRT1 and limiting NLRP-3 inflammasome activation. *Int. J. Mol. Sci.* **2013**, *14*, 14105–14118. [CrossRef]
100. Qu, L.; Yu, Y.; Qiu, L.; Yang, D.; Yan, L.; Guo, J.; Jahan, R. Sirtuin 1 regulates matrix metalloproteinase-13 expression induced by Porphyromonas endodontalis lipopolysaccharide via targeting nuclear factor-κB in osteoblasts. *J. Oral Microbiol.* **2017**, *9*, 1317578. [CrossRef]
101. Yeung, F.; Hoberg, J.E.; Ramsey, C.S.; Keller, M.D.; Jones, D.R.; Frye, R.A.; Mayo, M.W. Modulation of NF-κB-dependent transcription and cell survival by the SIRT1 deacetylase. *EMBO J.* **2004**, *23*, 2369–2380. [CrossRef]
102. Bonizzi, G.; Karin, M. The two NF-kappaB activation pathways and their role in innate and adaptive immunity. *Trends Immunol.* **2004**, *25*, 280–288. [CrossRef]
103. Yamamoto, Y.; Gaynor, R.B. Therapeutic potential of inhibition of the NF-kappaB pathway in the treatment of inflammation and cancer. *J. Clin. Investig.* **2001**, *107*, 135–142. [CrossRef]
104. Shakibaei, M.; Buhrmann, C.; Mobasheri, A. Resveratrol-mediated SIRT-1 interactions with p300 modulate receptor activator of NF-kappaB ligand (RANKL) activation of NF-kappaB signaling and inhibit osteoclastogenesis in bone-derived cells. *J. Biol. Chem.* **2011**, *286*, 11492–11505. [CrossRef]
105. Pan, W.; Yu, H.; Huang, S.; Zhu, P. Resveratrol Protects against TNF-alpha-Induced Injury in Human Umbilical Endothelial Cells through Promoting Sirtuin-1-Induced Repression of NF-KB and p38 MAPK. *PLoS ONE* **2016**, *11*, e0147034.
106. Bode, A.M.; Dong, Z. Mitogen-activated protein kinase activation in UV-induced signal transduction. *Sci. STKE* **2003**, *2003*, RE2. [CrossRef]

107. Bode, A.M.; Dong, Z. Targeting signal transduction pathways by chemopreventive agents. *Mutat. Res.* **2004**, *555*, 33–51. [CrossRef] [PubMed]
108. Kim, T.W.; Michniewicz, M.; Bergmann, D.C.; Wang, Z.Y. Brassinosteroid regulates stomatal development by GSK3-mediated inhibition of a MAPK pathway. *Nature* **2012**, *482*, 419–422. [CrossRef] [PubMed]
109. Johnson, G.L.; Lapadat, R. Mitogen-activated protein kinase pathways mediated by ERK, JNK, and p38 protein kinases. *Science* **2002**, *298*, 1911–1912. [CrossRef]
110. Chun, K.S.; Surh, Y.J. Signal transduction pathways regulating cyclooxygenase-2 expression: Potential molecular targets for chemoprevention. *Biochem. Pharmacol.* **2004**, *68*, 1089–1100. [CrossRef]
111. Raingeaud, J.; Gupta, S.; Rogers, J.S.; Dickens, M.; Han, J.; Ulevitch, R.J.; Davis, R.J. Pro-inflammatory cytokines and environmental stress cause p38 mitogen-activated protein kinase activation by dual phosphorylation on tyrosine and threonine. *J. Biol. Chem.* **1995**, *270*, 7420–7426. [CrossRef]
112. Koul, H.K.; Pal, M.; Koul, S. Role of p38 MAP Kinase Signal Transduction in Solid Tumors. *Genes Cancer* **2013**, *4*, 342–359. [CrossRef] [PubMed]
113. Shen, M.Y.; Hsiao, G.; Liu, C.L.; Fong, T.H.; Lin, K.H.; Chou, D.S.; Sheu, J.R. Inhibitory mechanisms of resveratrol in platelet activation: Pivotal roles of p38 MAPK and NO/cyclic GMP. *Br. J. Haematol.* **2007**, *139*, 475–485. [CrossRef]
114. Chen, R.-S.; Ko, J.-C.; Chiu, H.-C.; Wo, T.-Y.; Huang, Y.-J.; Tseng, S.-C.; Chen, H.-J.; Huang, Y.-C.; Jian, Y.-J.; Lee, W.-T.; et al. Pemetrexed downregulates ERCC1 expression and enhances cytotoxicity effected by resveratrol in human nonsmall cell lung cancer cells. *Naunyn Schmiedebergs Arch. Pharmacol.* **2013**, *386*, 1047–1059. [CrossRef] [PubMed]
115. Cao, L.; Chen, X.; Xiao, X.; Ma, Q.; Li, W. Resveratrol inhibits hyperglycemia-driven ROS-induced invasion and migration of pancreatic cancer cells via suppression of the ERK and p38 MAPK signaling pathways. *Int. J. Oncol.* **2016**, *49*, 735–743. [CrossRef]
116. Meng, Q.; Sun, S.; Luo, Z.; Shi, B.; Shan, A.; Cheng, B. Maternal dietary resveratrol alleviates weaning-associated diarrhea and intestinal inflammation in pig offspring by changing intestinal gene expression and microbiota. *Food Funct.* **2019**, *10*, 5626–5643. [CrossRef] [PubMed]
117. Lv, X.C.; Zhou, H.Y. Resveratrol protects H9c2 embryonic rat heart derived cells from oxidative stress by inducing autophagy: Role of p38 mitogen-activated protein kinase. *Can. J. Physiol. Pharmacol.* **2012**, *90*, 655–662. [CrossRef] [PubMed]
118. Li, C.; Hu, W.L.; Lu, M.X.; Xiao, G.F. Resveratrol induces apoptosis of benign prostatic hyperplasia epithelial cell line (BPH-1) through p38 MAPK-FOXO3a pathway. *BMC Complement Altern. Med.* **2019**, *19*, 233. [CrossRef]
119. Lou, Z.; Li, X.; Zhao, X.; Du, K.; Li, X.; Wang, B. Resveratrol attenuates hydrogen peroxide-induced apoptosis, reactive oxygen species generation, and PSGL-1 and VWF activation in human umbilical vein endothelial cells, potentially via MAPK signalling pathways. *Mol. Med. Rep.* **2018**, *17*, 2479–2487. [CrossRef]
120. Yang, G.; Chang, C.C.; Yang, Y.; Yuan, L.; Xu, L.; Ho, C.T.; Li, S. Resveratrol Alleviates Rheumatoid Arthritis via Reducing ROS and Inflammation, Inhibiting MAPK Signaling Pathways, and Suppressing Angiogenesis. *J. Agric. Food Chem.* **2018**, *66*, 12953–12960. [CrossRef]
121. Zhou, H.; Chen, Q.; Kong, D.L.; Guo, J.; Wang, Q.; Yu, S.Y. Effect of Resveratrol on Gliotransmitter Levels and p38 Activities in Cultured Astrocytes. *Neurochem. Res.* **2011**, *36*, 17–26. [CrossRef] [PubMed]
122. Hu, W.; Yang, E.; Ye, J.; Han, W.; Du, Z.-L. Resveratrol protects neuronal cells from isoflurane-induced inflammation and oxidative stress-associated death by attenuating apoptosis via Akt/p38 MAPK signaling. *Exp. Ther. Med.* **2018**, *15*, 1568–1573. [CrossRef]
123. Zhang, X.; Wang, Y.; Xiao, C.; Wei, Z.; Wang, J.; Yang, Z.; Fu, Y. Resveratrol inhibits LPS-induced mice mastitis through attenuating the MAPK and NF-kappa B signaling pathway. *Microb. Pathog.* **2017**, *107*, 462–467. [CrossRef] [PubMed]
124. Wang, G.; Hu, Z.; Fu, Q.; Song, X.; Cui, Q.; Jia, R.; Zou, Y.; He, C.; Li, L.; Yin, Z. Resveratrol mitigates lipopolysaccharide-mediated acute inflammation in rats by inhibiting the TLR4/NF-kappaBp65/MAPKs signaling cascade. *Sci. Rep.* **2017**, *7*, 45006. [CrossRef]
125. Karin, M. The regulation of AP-1 activity by mitogen-activated protein kinases. *Philos Trans. R. Soc. Lond. B Biol. Sci.* **1996**, *351*, 127–134. [CrossRef]
126. Eferl, R.; Wagner, E.F. AP-1: A double-edged sword in tumorigenesis. *Nat. Rev. Cancer* **2003**, *3*, 859–868. [CrossRef]
127. Shen, F.; Chen, S.J.; Dong, X.J.; Zhong, H.; Li, Y.T.; Cheng, G.F. Suppression of IL-8 gene transcription by resveratrol in phorbol ester treated human monocytic cells. *J. Asian Nat. Prod. Res.* **2003**, *5*, 151–157. [CrossRef] [PubMed]
128. Kim, A.L.; Zhu, Y.; Zhu, H.; Han, L.; Kopelovich, L.; Bickers, D.R.; Athar, M. Resveratrol inhibits proliferation of human epidermoid carcinoma A431 cells by modulating MEK1 and AP-1 signalling pathways. *Exp. Dermatol.* **2006**, *15*, 538–546. [CrossRef] [PubMed]
129. Kundu, J.K.; Surh, Y.J. Molecular basis of chemoprevention by resveratrol: NF-kappaB and AP-1 as potential targets. *Mutat. Res.* **2004**, *555*, 65–80. [CrossRef] [PubMed]
130. Surh, Y.-J.; Ferguson, L.R. Dietary and medicinal antimutagens and anticarcinogens: Molecular mechanisms and chemopreventive potential—highlights of a symposium. *Mutat. Res-Fund. Mol. M.* **2003**, *523–524*, 1–8. [CrossRef]
131. Donnelly, L.E.; Newton, R.; Kennedy, G.E.; Fenwick, P.S.; Leung, R.H.; Ito, K.; Russell, R.E.; Barnes, P.J. Anti-inflammatory effects of resveratrol in lung epithelial cells: Molecular mechanisms. *Am. J. Physiol. Lung Cell Mol. Physiol.* **2004**, *287*, L774–L783. [CrossRef] [PubMed]
132. Burkhardt, S.; Reiter, R.J.; Tand, D.X.; Hardeland, R. DNA oxidatively damaged by chromium(III) and H2O2 is protected by the antioxidants melatonin, N1-acetyl-N2-formyl-5-methoxykynuramine, resveratrol and uric acid. *Int. J. Biochem. Cell Biol.* **2001**, *33*, 775–783. [CrossRef]

133. Damianaki, A.; Bakogeorgou, E.; Kampa, M.; Notas, G.; Hatzoglou, A.; Panagiotou, S.; Gemetzi, C.; Kouroumalis, E.; Martin, P.M.; Castanas, E. Potent inhibitory action of red wine polyphenols on human breast cancer cells. *J. Cell Biochem.* **2000**, *78*, 429–441. [CrossRef]
134. Sgambato, A.; Ardito, R.; Faraglia, B.; Boninsegna, A.; Wolf, F.I.; Cittadini, A. Resveratrol, a natural phenolic compound, inhibits cell proliferation and prevents oxidative DNA damage. *Mutat. Res.* **2001**, *496*, 171–180. [CrossRef]
135. Cadenas, S.; Barja, G. Resveratrol, melatonin, vitamin E, and PBN protect against renal oxidative DNA damage induced by the kidney carcinogen KBrO3. *Free Radic. Biol. Med.* **1999**, *26*, 1531–1537. [CrossRef]
136. Cheng, K.; Song, Z.; Li, S.; Yan, E.; Zhang, H.; Zhang, L.; Wang, C.; Wang, T. Effects of resveratrol on intestinal oxidative status and inflammation in heat-stressed rats. *J. Therm. Boil.* **2019**, *85*, 102415. [CrossRef]
137. Ohshima, H.; Bartsch, B. Chronic infections and inflammatory processes as cancer risk factors: Possible role of nitric oxide in carcinogenesis. *Mutat. Res.* **1994**, *305*, 253–264. [CrossRef]
138. Yang, J.; Zhu, C.; Ye, J.; Lv, Y.; Wang, L.; Chen, Z.; Jiang, Z. Protection of Porcine Intestinal-Epithelial Cells from Deoxynivalenol-Induced Damage by Resveratrol via the Nrf2 Signaling Pathway. *J. Agric. Food Chem.* **2018**, *67*, 1726–1735. [CrossRef]
139. Gao, Y.; Fu, R.; Wang, J.; Yang, X.; Wen, L.; Feng, J. Resveratrol mitigates the oxidative stress mediated by hypoxic-ischemic brain injury in neonatal rats via Nrf2/HO-1 pathway. *Pharm. Biol.* **2018**, *56*, 440–449. [CrossRef] [PubMed]
140. Meng, Z.; Jing, H.; Gan, L.; Li, H.; Luo, B. Resveratrol attenuated estrogen-deficient-induced cardiac dysfunction: Role of AMPK, SIRT1, and mitochondrial function. *Am. J. Trans. Res.* **2016**, *8*, 2641–2649.

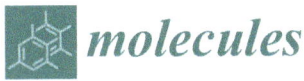

Review

Microbiota-Mediated Immune Regulation in Atherosclerosis

Sahar Eshghjoo [1], Arul Jayaraman [2], Yuxiang Sun [3,*] and Robert C. Alaniz [1,*]

1. Department of Microbial Pathogenesis and Immunology, College of Medicine, Texas A&M University Health Science Center, Bryan, TX 77807, USA; eshghjoo@tamu.edu
2. Artie McFerrin Department of Chemical Engineering, Texas A&M University, College Station, TX 77840, USA; arulj@mail.che.tamu.edu
3. Department of Nutrition, Texas A&M University, College Station, TX 77843, USA
* Correspondence: yuxiangs@tamu.edu (Y.S.); robert_alaniz@tamu.edu (R.C.A.); Tel.: +1-(979)-862-9143 (Y.S.); +1-(206)-818-9450 (R.C.A.)

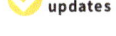

Citation: Eshghjoo, S.; Jayaraman, A.; Sun, Y.; Alaniz, R.C. Microbiota-Mediated Immune Regulation in Atherosclerosis. *Molecules* 2021, 26, 179. https://doi.org/10.3390/molecules26010179

Academic Editors: Sokcheon Pak and Soo Liang Ooi
Received: 1 December 2020
Accepted: 29 December 2020
Published: 1 January 2021

Publisher's Note: MDPI stays neutral with regard to jurisdictional claims in published maps and institutional affiliations.

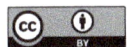

Copyright: © 2021 by the authors. Licensee MDPI, Basel, Switzerland. This article is an open access article distributed under the terms and conditions of the Creative Commons Attribution (CC BY) license (https://creativecommons.org/licenses/by/4.0/).

Abstract: There is a high level of interest in identifying metabolites of endogenously produced or dietary compounds generated by the gastrointestinal (GI) tract microbiota, and determining the functions of these metabolites in health and disease. There is a wealth of compelling evidence that the microbiota is linked with many complex chronic inflammatory diseases, including atherosclerosis. Macrophages are key target immune cells in atherosclerosis. A hallmark of atherosclerosis is the accumulation of pro-inflammatory macrophages in coronary arteries that respond to pro-atherogenic stimuli and failure of digesting lipids that contribute to foam cell formation in atherosclerotic plaques. This review illustrates the role of tryptophan-derived microbiota metabolites as an aryl hydrocarbon receptor (AhR) ligand that has immunomodulatory properties. Also, microbiota-dependent trimethylamine-N-oxide (TMAO) metabolite production is associated with a deleterious effect that promotes atherosclerosis, and metabolite indoxyl sulfate has been shown to exacerbate atherosclerosis. Our objective in this review is to discuss the role of microbiota-derived metabolites in atherosclerosis, specifically the consequences of microbiota-induced effects of innate immunity in response to atherogenic stimuli, and how specific beneficial/detrimental metabolites impact the development of atherosclerosis by regulating chronic endotoxemic and lipotoxic inflammation.

Keywords: microbiota; atherosclerosis; innate immunity; microbiome metabolites; macrophage

1. Introduction

Cardiovascular disease (CVD) is a complex human disease that restricts blood flow in the heart and blood vessels [1]. Atherosclerosis is a major form of CVD, symbolized by excess buildup of arterial plaque (atheroma) along the arterial wall [2]. The arterial plaque in atherosclerosis is composed of lipids (cholesterol and fatty acids), debris, fibrotic material, macrophages (Macs), dendritic cells (DCs), and some other host immune cells [3]. Within the atherosclerotic plaques, Macs polarize to a pro-inflammatory state which ingests and degrade debris and lipids, promoting the formation of foam cells in the plaques, leading to the adverse effects of restricted blood flow [4].

Gut microbiota refers to microorganisms (with gene makeup distinctive from the host) living in the GI tract, which produce various unique metabolites. Metabolites refer to small molecules that result from metabolic processes, produced endogenously by the host and by microorganisms' processing of dietary compounds. Identification of a microbiome profile in the GI tract and the functional determination of microbiome-derived metabolites are very important for health and disease [5–7]. A study demonstrated that tryptophan-derived compounds are depleted in the GI tract and the circulation of germ-free mice, indicating these tryptophan metabolites are dependent on the microbiota [6]. Indole is an important beneficial metabolite produced from tryptophan; it has been shown that indole is not detected in the cecal tissue of germ-free mice [6].

There is now an increasing appreciation that the microbiota is an essential partner in overall gut homeostasis and host health. Furthermore, when the microbiota is perturbed by environmental or dietary stresses (referred to as dysbiosis), it can lead to increased inflammation and altered metabolism in the host [7] (Figure 1). There is a wealth of compelling evidence that the microbiota is linked with multiple complex diseases, including CVD [8]; however, our understanding of the mechanisms of how the microbiota affect CVD is limited. Perhaps the most specific example of the link between the microbiota and CVD is the production of trimethylamine-*N*-oxide (TMAO), the oxidized form of trimethylamine (TMA), a microbiota-dependent detrimental metabolite derived from diets rich in phosphatidylcholine, choline, and L-carnitine, associated with a significantly increased risk of atherosclerosis [9]. Although a number of microbiota-derived metabolites have been identified and studied, the full array of activities for most individual metabolites has not been completely established, further research is needed to better understand the properties and functions of the metabolites, the microbe(s) that produce them, the cellular and molecular targets, and their roles in health and disease. Thus, in this review, we discuss that the microbiota promotes atherosclerosis by the production of specific beneficial (e.g., Indole) and detrimental (e.g., Indoxyl Sulfate, TMA/TMAO) metabolites [10], and their impacts on the development of atherosclerosis in obese patients by regulating chronic endotoxemic/lipotoxic inflammation and metabolic functions.

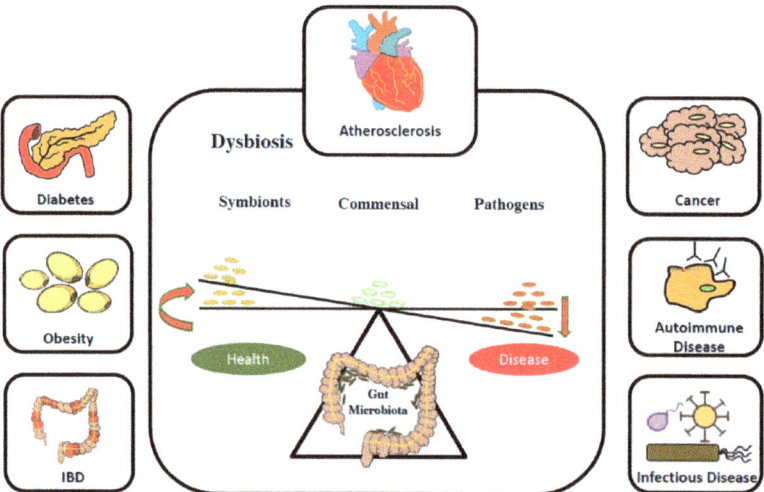

Figure 1. The microbiota is important for overall health. The balance between health and disease is regulated by microbiota in many ways. Microbiota in equilibrium is linked with homeostasis; when it is perturbed, it leads to dysbiosis and diseases.

The published data has investigated the impact of the microbiota as a rich source of potent immunomodulatory metabolites derived from tryptophan (Trp) [11]. In particular, the primary microbiota-derived Trp-metabolite indole (C8H7N), a potent endogenous ligand for the aryl hydrocarbon receptor (AhR), regulates gut inflammation, and microbiota dysbiosis [12]. We specifically discussed the inflammatory and metabolic responses of pro-atherogenic phagocytes, especially macrophages and their polarization, exposed to lipotoxic compounds and their regulation by the microbiota-derived metabolites.

2. Microbiota-Derived Metabolites Associated with Atherosclerosis

The microbiota is recognized for its role in the production of beneficial SCFAs and their functions in the regulation of complex chronic inflammatory diseases such as atherosclerosis. A link between the microbiota and atherosclerosis emerged from studies of TMAO [13–15].

A significant hallmark of atherosclerosis is the accumulation of pro-inflammatory Macs and dendritic cells (DCs) in coronary arteries that respond to pro-atherogenic stimuli, such as free fatty acids (FFAs) and oxidized LDLs (oxLDLs), and the failure to digest lipids that contribute to the formation of foam cells in atherosclerotic plaques [16,17]. Mechanisms that reduce Mac/DC inflammation, increase lipid degradation, and prevent foam cell formation would all decrease atherosclerosis progression.

There is overwhelming evidence that microbiome, microbial metabolism, and microbiota-derived/dependent nutritional metabolites contribute to the pathogenesis of atherosclerosis [18]. The mechanistic links between gut microbiota and health/disease outcome are largely undefined. Indole, TMAO, and Indoxyl sulfate are among the few best-studied microbiome-derived/dependent metabolites that have been reported to have roles in the regulation of atherosclerosis [19].

2.1. TMAO (Trimethylamine-N-Oxide)

TMAO is a microbial dependent metabolite. It is a byproduct of microbial metabolism of L-carnitine and choline in the gut after ingestion of eggs, meat, or fish, and TMAO is directly correlated with atherosclerosis [20]. After metabolizing carnitine and choline to TMA, through the bacteria, TMA is absorbed from the gut and transferred into the circulation [21]. Then, via an enzyme named Flavin monooxygenase, TMA is oxidized into TMAO in the liver. Other than atherosclerosis, plasma levels of TMAO are increased in patients with chronic kidney diseases (CKD) and diabetes as well [22]. The reason for the TMAO increase in these diseases is still unknown. Some studies suggest that reduced clearance of TMAO by kidneys in CKD or increased TMAO metabolism levels by bacteria in the gut are among the possible reasons [23]. Other data suggest that dysbiosis is directly linked to increased serum levels of TMAO. In the CKD patients, the relative abundance of dominant bacteria changes, and the expression of the enzyme that leads to TMAO production increases [24].

Rodent studies also show that TMAO, as a risk factor, enhances atherosclerosis prevalence through increasing the expression of scavenger receptors and reducing cholesterol efflux in Macs, and consequently increases levels of foam cell formation of the aforementioned Macs [25]. This proatherogenic metabolite has a positive correlation with lesion formation and development, as well as the size of the atherosclerotic plaque in arteries [26]. Atherosclerosis starts with the accumulation of foam cells in the arteries. Monocytes in the circulation penetrate the arteries where there are lesions and transform into Macs; by phagocyting modified cholesterol and lipoproteins, these Macs transform into foam cells (Figure 2). Accumulation of foam cells under the artery endothelial cells then form plaques, and the rupture of the plaque can block arteries and cause a stroke [27].

Macs regulate lipoprotein metabolism and are the key cells involved in atherosclerosis because they are the origin of the foam cells. The migration of Macs to the plaque areas and the mechanisms of foam cell transformation have very important implications. There is some evidence suggesting that TMAO is involved [28]. When the LDLs or low-density lipoproteins are oxidized by the free radicals in the arterial walls, the Macs are triggered to phagocytose these modified lipoproteins by increasing the expression of scavenger receptors such as CD36 and SRA-1 that have high sensitivity to modified lipoproteins [29]. TMAO upregulates these scavenger receptors' expression and induces the uptake of these modified LDLs by Macs [30]. TMAO increases Macs' migration and promotes the expression of inflammatory cytokines such as IL-6 and TNF [31].

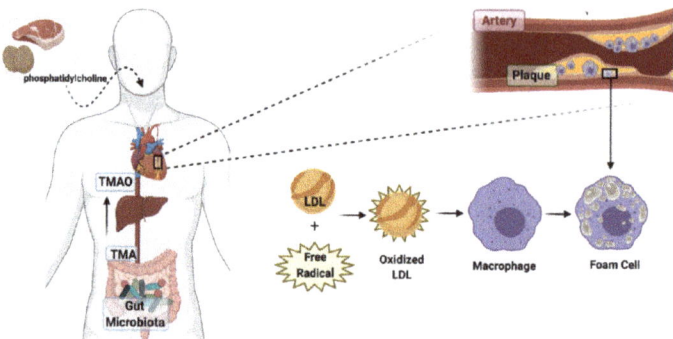

Figure 2. Role of trimethylamine N-oxide in atherosclerosis. Schematic pathway of phosphatidylcholine transformation to TMA and TMAO (trimethylamine N-oxide) via the gut microbiota. Dietary intake of foods like red meat and egg can alter the composition of gut microbiota. It can result in increased TMA production levels, subsequently leading to increased TMAO synthesis in the liver, eventually leading to elevated levels of oxidized LDLs and increased plaque formation. Accumulated foam cells in the plaques are lipid-laden Macs that have ingested modified lipoproteins, having a foamy appearance. In atherosclerosis, inflammatory Macs are converted into foam cells.

2.2. Indoxyl Sulfate (I3S)

Indoxyl sulfate, aka, 3-indoxyl sulfate or 3-indoxylsulfuric acid (I3S), is a bacterial metabolic byproduct of dietary nutrients. I3S plays a role as a uremic toxin and a cardiotoxin [32]. A microbial enzyme, named tryptophanase, catabolizes the tryptophan to indole. Then the indole gets absorbed and converted into indoxyl sulfate in the liver. Dysbiosis and epigenetic alterations of the gut microbiota alter the amino acid metabolism and increase the levels of I3S in the serum (Figure 3) [33]. Also, the amount of tryptophanase expression in the microbiota increases to facilitate Indoxyl sulfate production in CKD and CVD patients [34], and the prevalence of atherosclerosis is higher in CKD patients [35]. Based on the epidemiology studies, CKD patients have a high risk for atherosclerosis beyond traditional risk factors, indicating the possible role of microbiota in the pathogenesis of the diseases, such as CKD and CVD.

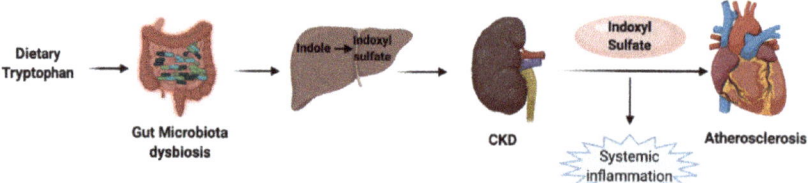

Figure 3. Effect of Indoxyl sulfate in atherosclerosis. Schematic presentation of the Indoxyl sulfate pathway is linked to atherosclerosis. Tryptophan is metabolized by the gut microbiota into indole, and indole is absorbed into the circulation. In the liver, indole is metabolized to indoxyl sulfate. In chronic kidney disease and dysbiosis conditions, kidneys are incapable of clearing indoxyl sulfate. This results in the accumulation of indoxyl sulfate. Systemic inflammation caused by indoxyl sulfate can cause coronary calcification and chronic cardiovascular abnormalities, eventually leading to atherosclerosis.

Plasma concentration of I3S increases in atherosclerosis and CKD patients [36]. I3S has a high affinity to proteins, and therefore it cannot be removed by kidneys easily [37]. In vitro studies show that indoxyl sulfate can enhance leukocyte activation and increase their adhesion to endothelial cells and eventually cause elevated levels of oxidative stress and inflammation [38]. Furthermore, it is hypothesized that indoxyl sulfate reduces Macs' cholesterol efflux and induces foam cell formation [39]. I3S is also related to glucose intolerance by reducing GLUT-1 expression and the hepatic LXR signaling pathway [40]. Thus, increased levels of inflammatory Macs may reflect the severity of atherosclerosis.

Proteomics studies indicate activation of some pathways via I3S in Macs, such as the ubiquitin-proteasome pathway and Notch signaling [41]. Some studies show that membrane transport proteins such as OATP2B1 regulates the uptake of I3S in Macs [42]. I3S is an agonist for AhR, and it can increase cell proliferation of vascular smooth muscle through AhR and activation of NF-κB signaling [43]. Furthermore, I3S is known to increase ROS production [44].

2.3. Indole

Indole is a gut microbiota-derived tryptophan catabolite. It is produced during the tryptophan metabolic process by the tryptophan lyase (tnaA) enzyme (Figure 4) [45]. Indole is an agonist for the aryl hydrocarbon receptor (AhR). There is a high concentration of indole in the GI tract, and it can enter the blood circulation [46]. Indole is detectable in human and mouse luminal contents at 0.1 to 4 mM concentrations and around 0.1 to 10 μM in the circulation [47]. Indole is a very small molecule, and it is easily diffusible and can directly interact with immune cells [48].

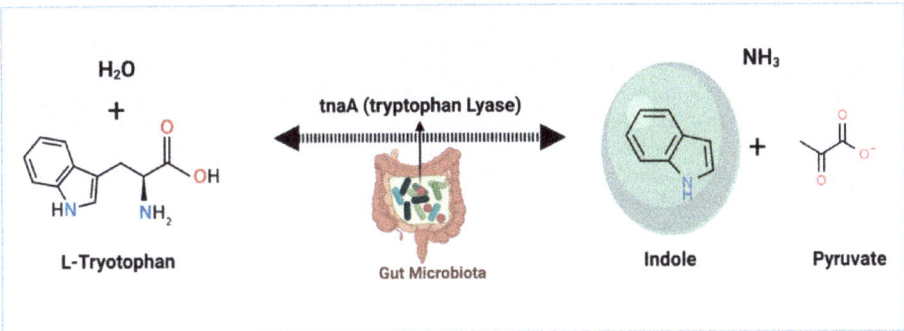

Figure 4. Indole is a gut microbiota-derived metabolite. Indole is produced from tryptophan amino acid through the action of the tryptophan lyase enzyme. Indole is an aromatic heterocyclic organic molecule and has a bicyclic structure. Indole has anti-inflammatory regulatory effects on intestinal epithelial cells and immune cells in the gut and distal organs (through circulation) in the body.

It has been reported that indole has anti-inflammatory effects [49]. Studies show that plasma levels of indole and indole derivatives are negatively correlated to advanced atherosclerosis [50]. Indole is produced by various gram-negative and gram-positive bacteria species, such as *E. coli*, *Bacteroides*, and *Clostridium* [51]. In in vitro studies have indicated that other than immunomodulatory effects, indole promotes health outcomes in intestinal epithelial cells in humans and rodents by preventing colitis induced by dextran sulfate sodium (DSS) and strengthening the epithelial barrier [52]. A study suggested the important positive role of indole supplementation to facilitate anti-inflammatory drugs [53].

Gut bacteria genomic information of the human microbiome suggests that tryptophan metabolites are the most important bioactive microbiota metabolites [54]. Studies demonstrate that in atherosclerotic patients, microbiome tryptophan synthesis takes place; consequently, plasma levels of tryptophan metabolites are reduced [55]. There are some tryptophan derivatives, such as indoxyl sulfate or indole acetate, where increased levels of these metabolites have been reported to have a direct correlation with CVD and other diseases [56]. This suggests the importance and sensitivity of the equilibrium of microbial tryptophan metabolites in the host's gut and overall health. Molecular targets of tryptophan derivatives are still unknown, but some indoles have been reported to have modulatory effects through the AhR [57]. A study proposes the development of antibiotics to control the metabolic changes in atherosclerosis. Data indicated that diminished microbiota metabolism by antibiotics reduced tryptophan metabolism and exacerbated atherosclerosis [55]. Studying the crosstalk between metabolic changes, immune cells, and molecular targets is currently a very important topic in atherosclerosis research.

3. Aryl Hydrocarbon Receptor (AhR)

AhR is a ligand-activated transcription factor. AhR is activated by various endogenous and exogenous polycyclic aromatic hydrocarbon ligands [58]. AhR was first identified as a receptor for industrial toxin, n-dioxin [59]. Now, AhR is recognized as a significant mediator of immune cell activity, particularly in the GI tract [60].

AhR is involved in different cellular activities such as cell differentiation/proliferation, cytokine production, and responses to environmental toxins [61]. AhR has been suggested to have roles in the gut and immune system, such as the regulation of the intraepithelial lymphocytes (IELs) and innate lymphoid cells (ILC) in the gut [62].

AhR has been reported to regulate the induction of T-reg and Th17 [63]. The crosstalk between intestinal microbiota and immunity, and the role of AhR in antigen-presenting cells (APCs) have not been well-characterized. AhR can detect environmental signals such as dietary ligands [64]; it is also present in immune cells [64,65]. AhR is considered a candidate pattern recognition receptor sensor for immune responses driven by nutritional and microbial gut metabolites [65].

AhR exists in the cytosol, binds to the ligand, and then translocates to the nucleus via a nuclear translocator to act as a transcription factor [58,66]. In a study detecting a panel for AhR ligands in BMDCs, some ligands like I3C (indole 3-carbinol) and FICZ (6 formyl indolo carbazole) have been among ligands that induce pro-inflammatory effects in lipopolysaccharides (LPS) induced APCs, which is in contrast with the studies that suggest AhR activation has anti-inflammatory immunomodulatory effects [67]. For example, 4-n-nonylphenol, an agonist for AhR, can induce T-regs [68]. The published data suggest that AhR signaling in monocyte-derived-Macs has an important impact on the function of Macs [69]. A detailed investigation of ligands and their functional dependency on AhR is necessary to unravel the role of AhR in regulating Macs, and how it interacts with endogenous intestinal ligands.

Studies highlight that the expression of AhR is related to atherosclerosis [70], but the effects of AhR activation is dependent on the agonists, species, and cell type. For example, in ApoE-KO mice, increased AhR is linked to increased symptoms of atherosclerosis, but on the other hand, activation of AhR through indoles has modulatory effects on the reduction of CVD [70,71]. Some studies highlight the beneficial role of specific indoles in the prevention of atherosclerosis [72]. Collectively, data regarding AhR in atherosclerosis show that AhR activation has both beneficial and adverse effects depending on the different circumstances. Since the role of AhR is different in species, data from rodent studies may not be an accurate indication of its function in humans.

4. Metabolic Impairment, Inflammation, and Endotoxemia in CVD

Bacterial endotoxins LPS, aka lipoglycans, are macromolecules composed of an O-antigen containing polysaccharide and a lipid, joined by a covalent bond. The outer cell membrane of the gram-negative bacteria has conserved components of LPS [73]. LPS can lead to innate immunity activation and the onset of inflammatory reactions [74]. Usually, plasma endotoxin levels in patients with sepsis are at ~300 pg/mL; high levels of LPS can cause sepsis both in humans and rodents [74–76]. "Metabolic endotoxemia" happens when there is a low but constant level of LPS in blood circulation which can cause innate immune responses and consistent inflammation in the circulation without signs of significant infection [76].

Other than sepsis, there are other diseases that are caused by metabolic and inflammatory dysregulations, e.g., insulin resistance (IR), type 2 diabetes, and atherosclerosis [77]. Many factors in obesity (such as high levels of cholesterol, saturated fatty acids, endotoxins, etc.) can raise the levels of inflammation, reverse cholesterol transport (RCT), and reduce insulin signaling [78]. Macs are the most important cells involved in the process of upregulation and downregulation of metabolic-inflammatory responses. Macs use the induction of metabolic pathways in response to an overabundance of lipids from adipocytes, e.g., saturated fatty acids (particularly palmitate) and circulating modified lipids [79]. AMPK (AMP-activated protein kinase) and PPARs (peroxisome proliferator-activated receptors) are important regulators of metabolic and inflammatory mechanisms through modulating cellular homeostasis (80). Palmitate, a known saturated fatty acid, causes metabolic inflammation through NLRP3 or (NOD)-like receptor protein 3 inflammasome and inhibits AMPK activation [79,80]. In contrast, unsaturated fatty acids normally do not cause metabolic inflammation [81].

Studies show that high levels of LPS in the serum directly affect the onset or exacerbation of CVD, especially atherosclerosis [82]. Experiments in rodents have indicated that endotoxins accelerate the incidence and progression of atherosclerosis [83]. The LPS receptor is toll-like receptor-4 (TLR-4). Mice that are deficient for TLR-4 are more resistant to atherosclerosis development or progression [84]. It is hypothesized that when there is endotoxin alone without infection, LPS from intestinal gram-negative bacteria or nutrients can translocate from the intestinal lumen to the circulation [85]. Furthermore, increased endotoxemia levels have shown a direct correlation with increased levels of dietary fat uptake in rodents and humans [77].

Permeability of the intestinal lumen plays an important role in the severity of endotoxemia because of the high density of endotoxins in the intestine compared to the plasma [86]. Patients with CVD have increased plasma endotoxins, indicating pathological signs of luminal permeability [82]. Microbiota and the metabolites produced by the gut microbiome play an important role in the permeability of the intestinal lumen [87].

5. Conclusions

Since microbiota-derived or dependent metabolites have substantial beneficial or detrimental effects in gut and distal organs, cell-specific investigations are highly valuable. In terms of atherosclerosis, metabolites in macrophages have an important role in preventing foam cell formation. Other than tryptophan metabolites, different microbiota-dependent metabolites such as TMAO metabolism have been reported to have a role in atherosclerosis progression. Overall, this review underscores the importance of microbiota, their dependent metabolites, the effect of metabolites on innate immunity, and the development of atherosclerosis.

Multi-dimensional investigations, both targeted and unbiased approaches, are warranted to further elucidate the mechanistic pathways mediating the effects of microbiome-derived metabolites and to fully unravel the impact of microbiota on pathogenesis and prognosis of atherosclerosis. Both the direct effects of metabolites in the heart as well as the indirect effects via the gut-brain axis and endocrine system should be considered. Modern nanomedical techniques may be proven to be helpful in advancing the microbiome as a feasible therapeutic strategy. In addition, since age, gender, and ethnic background are known to affect disease development, future research investigations and clinical trials of metabolites should be designed to assess the influences of these factors as well.

Although studies have shown that tryptophan metabolism has an essential role in regulating atherosclerosis, the mechanistic role of the indoles through gut microbiota has not been fully unraveled. Future works need to elucidate the mechanisms of actions by which microbiota metabolites induce inflammatory or anti-inflammatory, pro-foam cell or anti-foam cell formation, and pro-autophagic or anti-autophagic functions. Additional perspectives regarding novel endogenous therapeutics that regulate Mac's metabolism will be extremely helpful in atherosclerosis prevention and treatment.

Author Contributions: All authors wrote and revised the manuscript. All authors have read and agreed to the published version of the manuscript.

Funding: The work was supported by the National Institutes of Health (NIH) R01DK118334 (to Sun and Alaniz) and (NIH) R01AI110642 (to Jayaraman and Alaniz).

Conflicts of Interest: The authors declare no conflict of interest.

References

1. Flora, G.D.; Nayak, M.K. A brief review of cardiovascular diseases, associated risk factors and current treatment regimes. *Curr. Pharm. Des.* **2019**, *25*, 4063–4084. [CrossRef]
2. Kocyigit, D.; Gurses, K.M.; Tokgozoglu, L. Anti-inflammatory therapy in atherosclerosis. *Front. Biosci.* **2020**, *25*, 242–269. [CrossRef]
3. Chistiakov, D.A.; Kashirskikh, D.A.; Khotina, V.A.; Grechko, A.V.; Orekhov, A.N. Immune-inflammatory responses in atherosclerosis: The role of myeloid cells. *J. Clin. Med.* **2019**, *8*, 1798. [CrossRef] [PubMed]
4. Shah, P.K. Inflammation, infection and atherosclerosis. *Trends Cardiovasc. Med.* **2019**, *29*, 468–472. [CrossRef] [PubMed]
5. Zangara, M.T.; McDonald, C. How diet and the microbiome shape health or contribute to disease: A mini-review of current models and clinical studies. *Exp. Biol. Med.* **2019**, *244*, 484–493. [CrossRef]
6. Wikoff, W.R.; Anfora, A.T.; Liu, J.; Schultz, P.G.; Lesley, S.A.; Peters, E.C.; Siuzdak, G. Metabolomics analysis reveals large effects of gut microflora on mammalian blood metabolites. *Proc. Natl. Acad. Sci. USA* **2009**, *106*, 3698–3703. [CrossRef] [PubMed]
7. Wilson, A.S.; Koller, K.R.; Ramaboli, M.C.; Nesengani, L.T.; Ocvirk, S.; Chen, C.; Flanagan, C.A.; Sapp, F.R.; Merritt, Z.T.; Bhatti, F. Diet and the human gut microbiome: An international review. *Dig. Dis. Sci.* **2020**, *65*, 723–740. [CrossRef]
8. Anselmi, G.; Gagliardi, L.; Egidi, G.; Leone, S.; Gasbarrini, A.; Miggiano, G.A.D.; Galiuto, L. Gut microbiota and cardiovascular diseases: A critical review. *Cardiol. Rev.* **2020**, in press. [CrossRef]
9. Dehghan, P.; Farhangi, M.A.; Nikniaz, L.; Nikniaz, Z.; Asghari-Jafarabadi, M. Gut microbiota-derived metabolite trimethylamine N-oxide (TMAO) potentially increases the risk of obesity in adults: An exploratory systematic review and dose-response meta-analysis. *Obes. Rev.* **2020**, *21*, e12993. [CrossRef]
10. Zeng, C.; Tan, H. Gut Microbiota and Heart, Vascular Injury. In *Gut Microbiota and Pathogenesis of Organ Injury*; Springer: Berlin/Heidelberg, Germany, 2020.
11. Brown, J.; Robusto, B.; Morel, L. Intestinal Dysbiosis and Tryptophan Metabolism in Autoimmunity. *Front. Immunol.* **2020**, *11*, 1741. [CrossRef]
12. Li, X.; Lu, C.; Fan, D.; Lu, X.; Xia, Y.; Zhao, H.; Xu, H.; Zhu, Y.; Li, J.; Liu, H. Human Umbilical Mesenchymal Stem Cells Display Therapeutic Potential in Rheumatoid Arthritis by Regulating Interactions Between Immunity and Gut Microbiota via the Aryl Hydrocarbon Receptor. *Front. Cell Dev. Biol.* **2020**, *8*, 131. [CrossRef] [PubMed]
13. Collins, S.L.; Patterson, A.D. The gut microbiome: An orchestrator of xenobiotic metabolism. *Acta Pharm. Sin. B* **2020**, *10*, 19–32. [CrossRef] [PubMed]
14. De Angelis, M.; Ferrocino, I.; Calabrese, F.M.; De Filippis, F.; Cavallo, N.; Siragusa, S.; Rampelli, S.; Di Cagno, R.; Rantsiou, K.; Vannini, L. Diet influences the functions of the human intestinal microbiome. *Sci. Rep.* **2020**, *10*, 1–15. [CrossRef] [PubMed]
15. Pieczynska, M.D.; Yang, Y.; Petrykowski, S.; Horbanczuk, O.K.; Atanasov, A.G.; Horbanczuk, J.O. Gut Microbiota and Its Metabolites in Atherosclerosis Development. *Molecules* **2020**, *25*, 594. [CrossRef]
16. Zhu, Y.; Li, Q.; Jiang, H. Gut microbiota in atherosclerosis: Focus on trimethylamine N-oxide. *Apmis* **2020**, *128*, 353–366. [CrossRef]
17. Bisgaard, L.S.; Mogensen, C.K.; Rosendahl, A.; Cucak, H.; Nielsen, L.B.; Rasmussen, S.E.; Pedersen, T.X. Bone marrow-derived and peritoneal macrophages have different inflammatory response to oxLDL and M1/M2 marker expression-implications for atherosclerosis research. *Sci. Rep.* **2016**, *6*, 35234. [CrossRef]
18. Jonsson, A.L.; Bäckhed, F. Role of gut microbiota in atherosclerosis. *Nat. Rev. Cardiol.* **2017**, *14*, 79–87. [CrossRef]
19. Bogiatzi, C.; Gloor, G.; Allen-Vercoe, E.; Reid, G.; Wong, R.G.; Urquhart, B.L.; Dinculescu, V.; Ruetz, K.N.; Velenosi, T.J.; Pignanelli, M. Metabolic products of the intestinal microbiome and extremes of atherosclerosis. *Atherosclerosis* **2018**, *273*, 91–97. [CrossRef]
20. Spence, J.D. Intestinal microbiome and atherosclerosis. *EBioMedicine* **2016**, *13*, 17. [CrossRef]
21. He, Z.; Chen, Z.-Y. What Are Missing Parts in the Research Story of Trimethylamine-N-Oxide (TMAO)? *J. Agric. Food Chem.* **2017**, *65*, 5227–5228. [CrossRef]
22. Roncal, C.; Martínez-Aguilar, E.; Orbe, J.; Ravassa, S.; Fernandez-Montero, A.; Saenz-Pipaon, G.; Ugarte, A.; de Mendoza, A.E.-H.; Rodriguez, J.A.; Fernández-Alonso, S. Trimethylamine-N-Oxide (TMAO) predicts cardiovascular mortality in peripheral artery disease. *Sci. Rep.* **2019**, *9*, 1–8. [CrossRef] [PubMed]
23. Zeisel, S.H.; Warrier, M. Trimethylamine N-oxide, the microbiome, and heart and kidney disease. *Annu. Rev. Nutr.* **2017**, *37*, 157–181. [CrossRef] [PubMed]
24. Lau, K.; Srivatsav, V.; Rizwan, A.; Nashed, A.; Liu, R.; Shen, R.; Akhtar, M. Bridging the gap between gut microbial dysbiosis and cardiovascular diseases. *Nutrients* **2017**, *9*, 859. [CrossRef] [PubMed]
25. Collins, H.L.; Drazul-Schrader, D.; Sulpizio, A.C.; Koster, P.D.; Williamson, Y.; Adelman, S.J.; Owen, K.; Sanli, T.; Bellamine, A. L-Carnitine intake and high trimethylamine N-oxide plasma levels correlate with low aortic lesions in ApoE−/− transgenic mice expressing CETP. *Atherosclerosis* **2016**, *244*, 29–37. [CrossRef] [PubMed]
26. Ding, L.; Chang, M.; Guo, Y.; Zhang, L.; Xue, C.; Yanagita, T.; Zhang, T.; Wang, Y. Trimethylamine-N-oxide (TMAO)-induced atherosclerosis is associated with bile acid metabolism. *Lipids Health Dis.* **2018**, *17*, 286. [CrossRef] [PubMed]

27. Poston, R.N. Atherosclerosis: Integration of its pathogenesis as a self-perpetuating propagating inflammation: A review. *Cardiovasc. Endocrinol. Metab.* **2019**, *8*, 51. [CrossRef] [PubMed]
28. Chistiakov, D.A.; Melnichenko, A.A.; Myasoedova, V.A.; Grechko, A.V.; Orekhov, A.N. Mechanisms of foam cell formation in atherosclerosis. *J. Mol. Med.* **2017**, *95*, 1153–1165. [CrossRef]
29. Chistiakov, D.A.; Melnichenko, A.A.; Orekhov, A.N.; Bobryshev, Y.V. How do macrophages sense modified low-density lipoproteins? *Int. J. Cardiol.* **2017**, *230*, 232–240. [CrossRef]
30. Chen, P.-Y.F.; Ho, C.-T.; Shahidi, F.; Pan, M.-H. Potential effects of natural dietary compounds on trimethylamine Noxide (TMAO) formation and TMAO-induced atherosclerosis. *J. Food Bioact.* **2018**, *3*, 87–94. [CrossRef]
31. Geng, J.; Yang, C.; Wang, B.; Zhang, X.; Hu, T.; Gu, Y.; Li, J. Trimethylamine N-oxide promotes atherosclerosis via CD36-dependent MAPK/JNK pathway. *Biomed. Pharmacother.* **2018**, *97*, 941–947. [CrossRef]
32. Kamiński, T.W.; Pawlak, K.; Karbowska, M.; Myśliwiec, M.; Pawlak, D. Indoxyl sulfate–the uremic toxin linking hemostatic system disturbances with the prevalence of cardiovascular disease in patients with chronic kidney disease. *BMC Nephrol.* **2017**, *18*, 35. [CrossRef] [PubMed]
33. Gao, H.; Liu, S. Role of uremic toxin indoxyl sulfate in the progression of cardiovascular disease. *Life Sci.* **2017**, *185*, 23–29. [CrossRef] [PubMed]
34. Skye, S.M.; Hazen, S.L. Microbial Modulation of a Uremic Toxin. *Cell Host Microbe* **2016**, *20*, 691–692. [CrossRef] [PubMed]
35. Hung, S.C.; Kuo, K.L.; Wu, C.C.; Tarng, D.C. Indoxyl sulfate: A novel cardiovascular risk factor in chronic kidney disease. *J. Am. Heart Assoc.* **2017**, *6*, e005022. [CrossRef] [PubMed]
36. De Brito, J.S.; Borges, N.A.; Dolenga, C.J.R.; Carraro-Eduardo, J.C.; Nakao, L.S.; Mafra, D. Is there a relationship between tryptophan dietary intake and plasma levels of indoxyl sulfate in chronic kidney disease patients on hemodialysis? *Braz. J. Nephrol.* **2016**, *38*, 396–402. [CrossRef] [PubMed]
37. Tan, X.; Cao, X.; Zou, J.; Shen, B.; Zhang, X.; Liu, Z.; Lv, W.; Teng, J.; Ding, X. Indoxyl sulfate, a valuable biomarker in chronic kidney disease and dialysis. *Hemodial. Int.* **2017**, *21*, 161–167. [CrossRef] [PubMed]
38. Ito, S.; Osaka, M.; Edamatsu, T.; Itoh, Y.; Yoshida, M. Crucial role of the aryl hydrocarbon receptor (AhR) in indoxyl sulfate-induced vascular inflammation. *J. Atheroscler. Thromb.* **2016**, *23*, 960–975. [CrossRef]
39. Yamamoto, S. Molecular mechanisms underlying uremic toxin-related systemic disorders in chronic kidney disease: Focused on β 2-microglobulin-related amyloidosis and indoxyl sulfate-induced atherosclerosis—Oshima Award Address 2016. *Clin. Exp. Nephrol.* **2019**, *23*, 151–157. [CrossRef]
40. Opdebeeck, B.; Maudsley, S.; Azmi, A.; De Maré, A.; De Leger, W.; Meijers, B.; Verhulst, A.; Evenepoel, P.; D'Haese, P.C.; Neven, E. Indoxyl sulfate and p-cresyl sulfate promote vascular calcification and associate with glucose intolerance. *J. Am. Soc. Nephrol.* **2019**, *30*, 751–766. [CrossRef]
41. Nakano, T.; Katsuki, S.; Chen, M.; Decano, J.L.; Halu, A.; Lee, L.H.; Pestana, D.V.; Kum, A.S.; Kuromoto, R.K.; Golden, W.S. Uremic toxin indoxyl sulfate promotes proinflammatory macrophage activation via the interplay of OATP2B1 and Dll4-Notch signaling: Potential mechanism for accelerated atherogenesis in chronic kidney disease. *Circulation* **2019**, *139*, 78–96. [CrossRef]
42. Nakano, T. Indoxyl Sulfate and Arteriosclerosis. In *Uremic Toxins and Organ Failure*; Saito, H., Abe, T., Eds.; Springer: Singapore, 2020; pp. 83–93.
43. Ng, H.-Y.; Bolati, W.; Lee, C.-T.; Chien, Y.-S.; Yisireyili, M.; Saito, S.; Pei, S.-N.; Nishijima, F.; Niwa, T. Indoxyl sulfate downregulates Mas receptor via aryl hydrocarbon receptor/nuclear factor-kappa B, and induces cell proliferation and tissue factor expression in vascular smooth muscle cells. *Nephron* **2016**, *133*, 205–212. [CrossRef] [PubMed]
44. Tsutsumi, S.; Tokunaga, Y.; Shimizu, S.; Kinoshita, H.; Ono, M.; Kurogi, K.; Sakakibara, Y.; Suiko, M.; Liu, M.-C.; Yasuda, S. Investigation of the effects of indoxyl sulfate, a uremic toxin, on the intracellular oxidation level and phagocytic activity using an HL-60-differentiated human macrophage cell model. *Biosci. Biotechnol. Biochem.* **2020**, *84*, 1023–1029. [CrossRef] [PubMed]
45. Wang, T.; Zheng, X.; Ji, H.; Wang, T.-L.; Xing, X.-H.; Zhang, C. Dynamics of transcription–translation coordination tune bacterial indole signaling. *Nat. Chem. Biol.* **2020**, *16*, 440–449. [CrossRef] [PubMed]
46. Konopelski, P.; Ufnal, M. Indoles-gut bacteria metabolites of tryptophan with pharmacotherapeutic potential. *Curr. Drug Metab.* **2018**, *19*, 883–890. [CrossRef]
47. Kumar, A.; Sperandio, V. Indole signaling at the host-microbiota-pathogen interface. *mBio* **2019**, *10*, e01031-19. [CrossRef]
48. Chadha, N.; Silakari, O. Indoles as therapeutics of interest in medicinal chemistry: Bird's eye view. *Eur. J. Med. Chem.* **2017**, *134*, 159–184. [CrossRef]
49. Song, Z.; Zhou, Y.; Zhang, W.; Zhan, L.; Yu, Y.; Chen, Y.; Jia, W.; Liu, Z.; Qian, J.; Zhang, Y. Base promoted synthesis of novel indole-dithiocarbamate compounds as potential anti-inflammatory therapeutic agents for treatment of acute lung injury. *Eur. J. Med. Chem.* **2019**, *171*, 54–65. [CrossRef]
50. Cason, C.A.; Dolan, K.T.; Sharma, G.; Tao, M.; Kulkarni, R.; Helenowski, I.B.; Doane, B.M.; Avram, M.J.; McDermott, M.M.; Chang, E.B. Plasma microbiome-modulated indole- and phenyl-derived metabolites associate with advanced atherosclerosis and postoperative outcomes. *J. Vasc. Surg.* **2018**, *68*, 1552–1562.e7. [CrossRef]
51. Lee, J.-H.; Lee, J. Indole as an intercellular signal in microbial communities. *FEMS Microbiol. Rev.* **2010**, *34*, 426–444. [CrossRef]
52. Alexeev, E.E.; Lanis, J.M.; Kao, D.J.; Campbell, E.L.; Kelly, C.J.; Battista, K.D.; Gerich, M.E.; Jenkins, B.R.; Walk, S.T.; Kominsky, D.J. Microbiota-derived indole metabolites promote human and murine intestinal homeostasis through regulation of interleukin-10 receptor. *Am. J. Pathol.* **2018**, *188*, 1183–1194. [CrossRef]

53. Barden, T.C. Indoles: Industrial, agricultural and over-the-counter uses. In *Heterocyclic Scaffolds II*; Springer: Berlin/Heidelberg, Germany, 2010; pp. 31–46.
54. Koh, A.; Bäckhed, F. From Association to Causality: The Role of the Gut Microbiota and Its Functional Products on Host Metabolism. *Mol. Cell* **2020**, *78*, 584–596. [CrossRef] [PubMed]
55. Kappel, B.A.; De Angelis, L.; Heiser, M.; Ballanti, M.; Stoehr, R.; Goettsch, C.; Mavilio, M.; Artati, A.; Paoluzi, O.A.; Adamski, J. Cross-omics analysis revealed gut microbiome-related metabolic pathways underlying atherosclerosis development after antibiotics treatment. *Mol. Metab.* **2020**, 100976. [CrossRef] [PubMed]
56. Addi, T.; Poitevin, S.; McKay, N.; El Mecherfi, K.E.; Kheroua, O.; Jourde-Chiche, N.; de Macedo, A.; Gondouin, B.; Cerini, C.; Brunet, P. Mechanisms of tissue factor induction by the uremic toxin indole-3 acetic acid through aryl hydrocarbon receptor/nuclear factor-kappa B signaling pathway in human endothelial cells. *Arch. Toxicol.* **2019**, *93*, 121–136. [CrossRef] [PubMed]
57. Rannug, A. How the AHR Became Important in Intestinal Homeostasis—A Diurnal FICZ/AHR/CYP1A1 Feedback Controls Both Immunity and Immunopathology. *Int. J. Mol. Sci.* **2020**, *21*, 5681. [CrossRef] [PubMed]
58. Hubbard, T.D.; Murray, I.A.; Perdew, G.H. Indole and tryptophan metabolism: Endogenous and dietary routes to Ah receptor activation. *Drug Metab. Dispos.* **2015**, *43*, 1522–1535. [CrossRef] [PubMed]
59. Denison, M.S.; Deal, R.M. The binding of transformed aromatic hydrocarbon (Ah) receptor to its DNA recognition site is not affected by metal depletion. *Mol. Cell. Endocrinol.* **1990**, *69*, 51–57. [CrossRef]
60. Sun, M.; Ma, N.; He, T.; Johnston, L.J.; Ma, X. Tryptophan (Trp) modulates gut homeostasis via aryl hydrocarbon receptor (AhR). *Crit. Rev. Food Sci. Nutr.* **2020**, *60*, 1760–1768. [CrossRef]
61. Haarmann-Stemmann, T.; Bothe, H.; Abel, J. Growth factors, cytokines and their receptors as downstream targets of arylhydrocarbon receptor (AhR) signaling pathways. *Biochem. Pharmacol.* **2009**, *77*, 508–520. [CrossRef]
62. Kiss, E.A.; Diefenbach, A. Role of the aryl hydrocarbon receptor in controlling maintenance and functional programs of RORγt+ innate lymphoid cells and intraepithelial lymphocytes. *Front. Immunol.* **2012**, *3*, 124. [CrossRef]
63. Ho, P.P.; Steinman, L. The aryl hydrocarbon receptor: A regulator of Th17 and Treg cell development in disease. *Cell Res.* **2008**, *18*, 605–608. [CrossRef]
64. Metidji, A.; Omenetti, S.; Crotta, S.; Li, Y.; Nye, E.; Ross, E.; Li, V.; Maradana, M.R.; Schiering, C.; Stockinger, B. The environmental sensor AHR protects from inflammatory damage by maintaining intestinal stem cell homeostasis and barrier integrity. *Immunity* **2018**, *49*, 353–362.e5. [CrossRef] [PubMed]
65. Rothhammer, V.; Quintana, F.J. The aryl hydrocarbon receptor: An environmental sensor integrating immune responses in health and disease. *Nat. Rev. Immunol.* **2019**, *19*, 184–197. [CrossRef] [PubMed]
66. Gabriely, G.; Quintana, F.J. Role of AHR in the control of GBM-associated myeloid cells. *Semin. Cancer Biol.* **2020**, *64*, 13–18. [CrossRef]
67. Hana'a, A.; Millar, D.G. Effects of aryl-hydrocarbon ligands on dendritic cell maturation. *Int. J. Immunol.* **2013**, *1*, 24–34.
68. Bruhs, A.; Haarmann-Stemmann, T.; Frauenstein, K.; Krutmann, J.; Schwarz, T.; Schwarz, A. Activation of the arylhydrocarbon receptor causes immunosuppression primarily by modulating dendritic cells. *J. Investig. Dermatol.* **2015**, *135*, 435–444. [CrossRef] [PubMed]
69. Goudot, C.; Coillard, A.; Villani, A.-C.; Gueguen, P.; Cros, A.; Sarkizova, S.; Tang-Huau, T.-L.; Bohec, M.; Baulande, S.; Hacohen, N. Aryl hydrocarbon receptor controls monocyte differentiation into dendritic cells versus macrophages. *Immunity* **2017**, *47*, 582–596.e6. [CrossRef]
70. Wu, D.; Nishimura, N.; Kuo, V.; Fiehn, O.; Shahbaz, S.; Van Winkle, L.; Matsumura, F.; Vogel, C.F.A. Activation of aryl hydrocarbon receptor induces vascular inflammation and promotes atherosclerosis in apolipoprotein E−/− mice. *Arterioscler. Thromb. Vasc. Biol.* **2011**, *31*, 1260–1267. [CrossRef] [PubMed]
71. Neavin, D.R.; Liu, D.; Ray, B.; Weinshilboum, R.M. The role of the aryl hydrocarbon receptor (AHR) in immune and inflammatory diseases. *Int. J. Mol. Sci.* **2018**, *19*, 3851. [CrossRef]
72. Zhang, Y.; Li, M.; Li, X.; Zhang, T.; Qin, M.; Ren, L. Isoquinoline alkaloids and indole alkaloids attenuate aortic atherosclerosis in apolipoprotein E deficient mice: A systematic review and meta-analysis. *Front. Pharmacol.* **2018**, *9*, 602. [CrossRef]
73. Domínguez-Medina, C.C.; Pérez-Toledo, M.; Schager, A.E.; Marshall, J.L.; Cook, C.N.; Bobat, S.; Hwang, H.; Chun, B.J.; Logan, E.; Bryant, J.A. Outer membrane protein size and LPS O-antigen define protective antibody targeting to the Salmonella surface. *Nat. Commun.* **2020**, *11*, 851. [CrossRef]
74. Ostareck, D.H.; Ostareck-Lederer, A. RNA-binding proteins in the control of LPS-induced macrophage response. *Front. Genet.* **2019**, *10*, 31. [CrossRef] [PubMed]
75. Napier, B.A.; Andres-Terre, M.; Massis, L.M.; Hryckowian, A.J.; Higginbottom, S.K.; Cumnock, K.; Casey, K.M.; Haileselassie, B.; Lugo, K.A.; Schneider, D.S. Western diet regulates immune status and the response to LPS-driven sepsis independent of diet-associated microbiome. *Proc. Natl. Acad. Sci. USA* **2019**, *116*, 3688–3694. [CrossRef] [PubMed]
76. Fuke, N.; Nagata, N.; Suganuma, H.; Ota, T. Regulation of gut microbiota and metabolic endotoxemia with dietary factors. *Nutrients* **2019**, *11*, 2277. [CrossRef] [PubMed]
77. Li, J.; Lin, S.; Vanhoutte, P.M.; Woo, C.W.; Xu, A. Akkermansia muciniphila protects against atherosclerosis by preventing metabolic endotoxemia-induced inflammation in Apoe−/− mice. *Circulation* **2016**, *133*, 2434–2446. [CrossRef]

78. Wang, H.; Peng, D.-Q. New insights into the mechanism of low high-density lipoprotein cholesterol in obesity. *Lipids Health Dis.* **2011**, *10*, 1–10. [CrossRef]
79. Batista-Gonzalez, A.; Vidal, R.; Criollo, A.; Carreño, L.J. New insights on the role of lipid metabolism in the metabolic reprogramming of macrophages. *Front. Immunol.* **2020**, *10*, 2993. [CrossRef]
80. Claycombe-Larson, K.J.; Alvine, T.; Wu, D.; Kalupahana, N.S.; Moustaid-Moussa, N.; Roemmich, J.N. Nutrients and Immunometabolism: Role of Macrophage NLRP3. *J. Nutr.* **2020**, *150*, 1693–1704. [CrossRef]
81. Pérez-Martínez, P.I.; Rojas-Espinosa, O.; Hernández-Chávez, V.G.; Arce-Paredes, P.; Estrada-Parra, S. Anti-inflammatory effect of omega unsaturated fatty acids and dialysable leucocyte extracts on collagen-induced arthritis in DBA/1 mice. *Int. J. Exp. Pathol.* **2020**, *101*, 55–64. [CrossRef]
82. Moludi, J.; Maleki, V.; Jafari-Vayghyan, H.; Vaghef-Mehrabany, E.; Alizadeh, M. Metabolic endotoxemia and cardiovascular disease: A systematic review about potential roles of prebiotics and probiotics. *Clin. Exp. Pharmacol. Physiol.* **2020**, *47*, 927–939. [CrossRef]
83. Ghosh, S.S.; Wang, J.; Yannie, P.J.; Sandhu, Y.K.; Korzun, W.J.; Ghosh, S. Dietary supplementation with galactooligosaccharides attenuates high-fat, high-cholesterol diet–induced glucose intolerance and disruption of colonic mucin layer in C57BL/6 mice and reduces atherosclerosis in Ldlr−/− mice. *J. Nutr.* **2020**, *150*, 285–293. [CrossRef]
84. Ding, Y.; Subramanian, S.; Montes, V.N.; Goodspeed, L.; Wang, S.; Han, C.; Teresa III, A.S.; Kim, J.; O'Brien, K.D.; Chait, A. Toll-like receptor 4 deficiency decreases atherosclerosis but does not protect against inflammation in obese low-density lipoprotein receptor-deficient mice. *Arterioscler. Thromb. Vasc. Biol.* **2012**, *32*, 1596–1604. [CrossRef] [PubMed]
85. André, P.; Laugerette, F.; Féart, C. Metabolic endocytemia: A potential underlying mechanism of the relationship between dietary fat intake and risk for cognitive impairments in humans? *Nutrients* **2019**, *11*, 1887. [CrossRef] [PubMed]
86. Rohr, M.W.; Narasimhulu, C.A.; Rudeski-Rohr, T.A.; Parthasarathy, S. Negative effects of a high-fat diet on intestinal permeability: A review. *Adv. Nutr.* **2020**, *11*, 77–91. [CrossRef] [PubMed]
87. Allam-Ndoul, B.; Castonguay-Paradis, S.; Veilleux, A. Gut Microbiota and Intestinal Trans-Epithelial Permeability. *Int. J. Mol. Sci.* **2020**, *21*, 6402. [CrossRef] [PubMed]

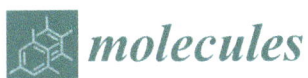

Review

Mini-Review on the Roles of Vitamin C, Vitamin D, and Selenium in the Immune System against COVID-19

Minkyung Bae [1] and Hyeyoung Kim [2,*]

[1] Department of Food and Nutrition, Interdisciplinary Program in Senior Human Ecology, BK21 FOUR, College of Natural Sciences, Changwon National University, Changwon 51140, Korea; mkbae@changwon.ac.kr

[2] Department of Food and Nutrition, BK21 FOUR, College of Human Ecology, Yonsei University, Seoul 03722, Korea

* Correspondence: kim626@yonsei.ac.kr; Tel.: +82-2-2123-3125; Fax: +82-2-364-5781

Received: 29 October 2020; Accepted: 12 November 2020; Published: 16 November 2020

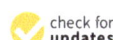

Abstract: Low levels of micronutrients have been associated with adverse clinical outcomes during viral infections. Therefore, to maximize the nutritional defense against infections, a daily allowance of vitamins and trace elements for malnourished patients at risk of or diagnosed with coronavirus disease 2019 (COVID-19) may be beneficial. Recent studies on COVID-19 patients have shown that vitamin D and selenium deficiencies are evident in patients with acute respiratory tract infections. Vitamin D improves the physical barrier against viruses and stimulates the production of antimicrobial peptides. It may prevent cytokine storms by decreasing the production of inflammatory cytokines. Selenium enhances the function of cytotoxic effector cells. Furthermore, selenium is important for maintaining T cell maturation and functions, as well as for T cell-dependent antibody production. Vitamin C is considered an antiviral agent as it increases immunity. Administration of vitamin C increased the survival rate of COVID-19 patients by attenuating excessive activation of the immune response. Vitamin C increases antiviral cytokines and free radical formation, decreasing viral yield. It also attenuates excessive inflammatory responses and hyperactivation of immune cells. In this mini-review, the roles of vitamin C, vitamin D, and selenium in the immune system are discussed in relation to COVID-19.

Keywords: COVID-19; infectious disease; selenium; virus; vitamin C; vitamin D

1. Introduction

Coronavirus disease 2019 (COVID-19) is caused by the severe acute respiratory syndrome coronavirus 2 (SARS-CoV-2). COVID-19 has spread rapidly across the world, with 39,944,882 confirmed cases and 1,111,998 deaths reported to the World Health Organization (WHO), as of 19 October 2020 [1]. It has been reported that the severity of COVID-19 can be influenced by various factors such as age, sex, ethnicity, and underlying comorbidities [2–5]. Although many therapeutic treatments have been suggested, there is no approved antiviral treatment specific for COVID-19.

Recently, the European Society for Clinical Nutrition and Metabolism (ESPEN) proposed 10 practical recommendations for the management of COVID-19 patients [6]. The recommendations include the prevention of malnutrition by providing adequate amounts of macronutrients to maintain energy, protein, fat, and carbohydrate requirements. Moreover, sufficient supplementation with vitamins and minerals is important for the prevention of viral infection.

Low levels of micronutrients such as vitamins A, E, B$_6$, B$_{12}$, zinc, and selenium have been associated with adverse clinical outcomes during viral infections [7]. A recent review by Zhang and

Liu [8] demonstrated that besides vitamins A and D, vitamin B, vitamin C, omega-3 polyunsaturated fatty acids, and trace elements (selenium, zinc, and iron) should be considered in the assessment of micronutrients in COVID-19 patients. A recent small-scale nutritional status study on COVID-19 patients in Korea showed significant deficiency of vitamin D and selenium in patients with and without pneumonia [9]. Serum levels of vitamins B_1, B_6, B_{12}, D, folate, selenium, and zinc were determined in 50 patients with COVID-19. Seventy-six percent of the patients had vitamin D deficiency, and 42% had selenium deficiency [9]. Vitamin D deficiency has been associated with a number of different viral diseases, including influenza [10–12] and hepatitis C [13]. However, other studies have questioned this relationship for influenza [14,15]. Selenium deficiency is associated with mortality in COVID-19 [16], and a sufficient selenium level is important for recovery from the disease [17]. Vitamin C is known to have antiviral effects, and a high-dose treatment shows beneficial effects in COVID-19 patients [18,19].

This mini-review discusses the role of vitamin C, vitamin D, and selenium in immunity, and the beneficial effects of these micronutrients in reducing the risk of infectious diseases, particularly COVID-19.

2. Micronutrients and the Immune System

2.1. The Role of Vitamin C in the Immune System

COVID-19 can develop into acute respiratory distress syndrome, secondary infection, and sepsis [20]. An intravenous treatment with high-dose vitamin C has shown beneficial effects on sepsis and septic shock [18,21]. An intravenous infusion of vitamin C (50 mg/kg body weight) every 6 h for 96 h significantly decreased mortality and increased the number of intensive care unit (ICU)-free days in patients with sepsis and acute respiratory distress syndrome, compared to the control group [19]. In another study, seven months of treatment with intravenous vitamin C, hydrocortisone, and thiamine significantly decreased hospital mortality in septic patients, compared to the control group. In addition, the treatment group had no sepsis-related progressive organ failure, including acute kidney injury [21]. In another case, a 74-year-old woman with COVID-19 developed acute respiratory distress syndrome and septic shock. The patient was treated with high-dose intravenous vitamin C (11 g/d for 10 d) and showed rapid recovery [19].

Vitamin C treatment has antiviral effects. Clinical trials have shown that administration of high doses of vitamin C has beneficial effects against the common cold [22,23]. A high-dose vitamin C (hourly doses of 1000 mg of vitamin C for the first 6 h and then 3 times daily for 3 d) treatment decreased flu and cold symptoms in patients when compared to the control group [22]. A meta-analysis has shown that administration of high doses of vitamin C at the onset of the common cold decreased the duration of the cold and relieved the symptoms, such as chest pain, fever, and chills [23]. An animal study has demonstrated that vitamin C treatment enhances resistance to viral infection. In this study, vitamin C supplementation in drinking water, as 3.3 g/L of sodium L-ascorbate, improved antiviral immune response at the early stage of viral infection, in the lungs of vitamin C-insufficient Gulo (−/−) mice infected with influenza A virus (H3N2/Hong Kong). The administration of vitamin C markedly improved the survival rate, with no death for 7 d, while all vitamin C-insufficient Gulo (−/−) mice infected with influenza A virus died within a week. Moreover, vitamin C supplementation increased interferon-α/β (IFN-α/β) in the lungs of Gulo (−/−) mice infected with influenza A virus, but did not change the levels of inflammatory cytokines, including interleukin $1\alpha/\beta$ (IL-$1\alpha/\beta$) and tumor necrosis factor-α (TNF-α), in the lungs of the mice [24]. Vitamin C and dehydroascorbic acid decreased the yield of influenza virus type A in Madin–Darby canine kidney (MDCK) cells derived from canine kidney cells in vitro [25]. The study suggests that the antiviral effect of vitamin C might be mediated by free radical formation or its binding to the virus or molecules involved in viral replication. Therefore, the antiviral effect of vitamin C may be attributed to the production of antiviral cytokines (IFN-α/β), free radical formation, or direct binding to the virus.

Vitamin C potentially attenuates excessive immune response in patients with COVID-19. Severe COVID-19 infection induces pulmonary and systemic inflammatory responses [26]. The microbial infection causes excessive activation of macrophages for production of inflammatory mediators and nitric oxide (NO) [27], which can be reinforced by oxidative stress and NO itself [28]. COVID-19 patients had significantly higher levels of molecules related to inflammation, such as NO_2^-, NO_3^-, C-reactive protein, and lactate dehydrogenase in blood, compared to healthy individuals. After oral or intravenous administration of vitamin C with methylene blue and a known antioxidant N-acetyl cysteine, the blood levels of NO_3^-, methemoglobin, C-reactive protein, and lactate dehydrogenase were markedly decreased in four out of five patients [28]. This study also demonstrated that pro-oxidant/antioxidant imbalance is present in patients with COVID-19 [28]. In another study, intravenous vitamin C was administered at a dose of 1 g every 8 h for 3 d, to 17 patients infected with COVID-19. After vitamin C treatment, the patients had decreased inflammatory markers, such as ferritin and D-dimer, and a fraction of the earlier inspired oxygen requirements [29]. These studies suggest that the administration of vitamin C may increase the survival rate in COVID-19 patients, by attenuating excessive activation of immune responses.

Vitamin C may prevent the hyperactivation of immune cells by inhibiting glyceraldehyde 3-phosphate dehydrogenase (GAPDH). The glycolytic enzyme GAPDH can regulate the rate of glycolysis in activated myeloid and lymphoid cells [30]. Vitamin C can be oxidized intracellularly and extracellularly into its inactive form dehydroascorbate [31]. Inside cells, dehydroascorbate is reduced to ascorbate, while reduced glutathione (GSH) is oxidized [32]. Oxidized glutathione (glutathione disulfide) can be reduced to GSH by nicotinamide adenine dinucleotide phosphate (NADPH) [32]. Vitamin C has antioxidant capacity; however, high-dose vitamin C can display pro-oxidant activity by decreasing reactive oxygen species (ROS) scavenging systems, including GSH and NADPH [33]. Increased ROS can induce DNA damage, followed by the activation of poly(ADP-ribose) polymerase (PARP) [34]. PARP consumes NAD^+ to synthesize poly(ADP-ribose) for DNA repair [35]. As NAD^+ is needed for GAPDH activity, depletion of NAD^+ decreases the enzymatic activity of GAPDH. Thus, the inhibition of GAPDH by a high dose of vitamin C may reduce the activation of immune cells by decreasing adenosine triphosphate (ATP) production in the cells [30].

Clinical trials are needed to investigate the effect of vitamin C on COVID-19 infection. A clinical trial was conducted from 14 February, 2020 to 30 September, 2020 in Zhongnan Hospital of Wuhan University, China [36]. In the trial, 12 g of vitamin C in 50 mL of sterile water was administered to patients for 4 h, and this was repeated every 12 h; therefore, the total amount of vitamin C administered to each patient was 24 g/d. This study is one of the first clinical trials to administer intravenous vitamin C to treat COVID-19. The study will investigate whether intravenous vitamin C could suppress cytokine storms caused by COVID-19, improve pulmonary function, and reduce the risk of acute respiratory distress syndrome in COVID-19.

2.2. The Role of Vitamin D in the Immune System

Adequate vitamin D levels in the body can be achieved by sufficient vitamin D consumption and sun exposure. The risk factors for vitamin D deficiency are age, smoking, obesity, and chronic diseases such as diabetes and hypertension [37]. 25-hydroxyvitamin D levels were inversely correlated with acute respiratory infection, as reported in the National Health and Nutrition Survey (NHANES) 2001–2006 [38]. Sufficient concentration of 25-hydroxyvitamin D was associated with a reduction in the risk of acute respiratory tract infections in adults [39]. In addition, sufficient levels of 25-hydroxyvitamin D in the serum were inversely correlated with the risk of viral respiratory tract infection in children [40]. Moreover, there was a small case study conducted with 10 COVID-19 patients in Indonesia [41]. On blood analysis, nine patients had vitamin D deficiency, and one patient had insufficient levels of vitamin D. Therefore, there was no patient with adequate vitamin D levels in the study. This indicates that vitamin D deficiency might be a risk factor for viral infection.

Studies have investigated the relationship between vitamin D deficiency and COVID-19 [42,43]. As vitamin D can be synthesized by sunlight exposure on the skin, living at a higher latitude is a risk factor for vitamin D deficiency [44]. The prevalence rate of COVID-19 and the rate of related deaths were significantly higher in high-latitude states (latitude ≥ 37°) than in low-latitude states (latitude < 37°) in the United States [42]. The average annual hours of sunlight exposure was negatively correlated with COVID-19 mortality [45]. It has also been suggested that vitamin D deficiency (serum 25-hydroxy vitamin D level of 20 ng/mL or lower) and insufficiency (serum 25-hydroxy vitamin D level of 21 to 29 ng/mL) are associated with increased mortality in COVID-19 in Indonesia [43]. A meta-analysis of 11 studies covering 360,972 COVID-19 patients was conducted. Among the patients, 37.7% had vitamin D deficiency, and 32.2% had vitamin D insufficiency. Furthermore, the risk of COVID-19 was significantly increased in patients with low levels of vitamin D [46]. Another meta-analysis that covered 1368 COVID-19 patients showed that a low level of vitamin D was significantly associated with worse prognoses in the patients [47]. The mortality rate of hospitalized COVID-19 patients who were vitamin D sufficient (serum 25-hydroxy vitamin D ≥ 30 ng/mL) was 5%; however, patients with severe vitamin D deficiency (serum 25-hydroxy vitamin D < 10 ng/mL) had a 50% mortality rate after 10 d of hospitalization [48]. Vitamin D deficiency was positively correlated with hospitalization within 24 h and ICU admission during hospitalization in COVID-19 patients [49]. The aforementioned studies suggest that vitamin D deficiency can result in poor prognoses in patients with COVID-19. Therefore, vitamin D may be used as an adjunctive therapy for COVID-19 patients.

Vitamin D reduces the risk of viral infections. It improves the body's physical barrier by regulating the production of proteins for tight junctions [50], adherens junctions [51], and gap junctions [52], which can be disturbed by infection by microorganisms, including viruses [53]. In addition, lung epithelial cells express 1α-hydroxylase that converts 25-hydroxyvitamin D3 to 1,25-dihydroxyvitamin D3, the active form of vitamin D [54]. Active vitamin D increases the expression of vitamin D-regulated genes, such as cathelicidin and toll-like receptor co-receptor CD14 in human tracheobronchial epithelial cells [54]. Double-stranded RNA produced by most viruses can increase the expression of 1α-hydroxylase, leading to increased production of active vitamin D and the expression of cathelicidin in human tracheobronchial epithelial cells [54]. Therefore, adequate vitamin D might prevent the invasion of coronaviruses by enhancing physical barriers and increasing the production of antimicrobial peptides in the lung epithelium.

Vitamin D stimulates the production of antimicrobial peptides, such as cathelicidin and defensins [55] that have antimicrobial activities against various microorganisms, including bacteria, viruses, and fungi [56,57]. In a study in mice, cathelicidin LL-37 decreased influenza A virus replication [58]. Human cathelicidin displays antiviral effects by reducing viral particles produced by respiratory syncytial virus in epithelial cells, thus decreasing cell death in HEp-2 human epithelial cells [59]. Human β-defensin 2 displays antiviral activity by destabilizing the viral envelope in respiratory syncytial virus, which inhibits its infection in human lung epithelial cells [60]. Thus, it is important to maintain sufficient vitamin D levels to produce antimicrobial peptides.

Vitamin D modulates helper T cell responses. It reduces T helper type 1 (Th1) immune responses [61] and induces Th2 responses [62]. Th1 cells produce pro-inflammatory cytokines, such as IFN-γ and TNF-β, while Th2 cells produce IL-4, IL-5, IL-10, and IL-13 [63]. As vitamin D induces a shift from Th1 to Th2 phenotype, it decreases Th1 cytokines but increases Th2 cytokines [64].

Vitamin D may prevent cytokine storms in patients with COVID-19. COVID-19 can lead to cytokine storms and immunogenic damage to the endothelium and alveolar membrane [36], which may contribute to mortality in COVID-19 [65]. Severely ill patients with COVID-19 have a high level of pro-inflammatory cytokines, such as IL-6, compared to patients with moderate symptoms [65]. The increased level of IL-6 in critically ill COVID-19 patients was related to the detection of SARS-CoV-2 nucleic acid in serum [66]. Vitamin D can decrease the production of pro-inflammatory cytokines, such as TNF-α, IL-6, IL-1β [67], IL-12, and IFN-γ [68]. The anti-inflammatory effect of vitamin D might be due to the inhibition of nuclear factor κB (NF-κB) activation [69]. The vitamin D receptor interacts with inhibitor of κB (IκB) kinase β to inhibit NF-κB activation, and the interaction is enhanced by vitamin D [69].

Recent studies have shown that vitamin D deficiency is correlated with poor prognosis in COVID-19 patients. However, there was no association between blood concentration of vitamin D and the risk of COVID-19 in the UK biobank [70]. Therefore, large-scale controlled studies are necessary to determine the effect of vitamin D on COVID-19.

2.3. The Role of Selenium in the Immune System

Selenium deficiency may be a risk factor for COVID-19 mortality. A cross-sectional study conducted in Germany showed that the serum level of selenium was significantly higher in the surviving patients with COVID-19 compared to the deceased patients with COVID-19 [16]. Another study also determined that the recovery rate from COVID-19 was significantly associated with selenium levels in patients in China [17].

Selenium deficiency exacerbates virulence and progression of viral infections, such as influenza A [71,72] and Coxsackievirus B3 [73]. Selenium-deficient mice developed more severe lung pathology due to influenza virus infection than selenium-adequate mice [72]. The virus isolated from the lungs of selenium-deficient mice at 5 d after infection had mutations in its genome that made it more virulent [72]. In another study, Coxsackievirus B3, a normally avirulent phenotype, resulted in heart damage in selenium-deficient mice. Coxsackievirus B3 underwent a genetic mutation to a virulent phenotype in the selenium-deficient mice [73]. Selenium deficiency in the host affects the viral genome, leading to the virus becoming more virulent.

Selenium demonstrates antiviral effect by regulating $CD4^+$ T cell response. It increased $CD4^+$ T cell activation, proliferation, and differentiation by maintaining the intracellular level of free thiol in mice fed with a high-selenium diet (1.0 mg/kg body weight) compared to a low-selenium diet (0.08 mg/kg body weight) or medium-selenium diet (0.25 mg/kg body weight) for 8 w [74]. $CD4^+$ T cells isolated from mice fed with a high-selenium diet demonstrated increased T cell receptor (TCR) signaling and TCR-stimulated IL-2 expression. In addition, high consumption of selenium induced the Th1 phenotype with increased IFN-γ in $CD4^+$ T cells [74]. Selenium deficiency induced severe interstitial pneumonitis in mice infected with influenza virus, when compared to selenium-adequate mice [71]. Selenium deficiency decreased the mRNA expression of IFN-γ and IL-2, but increased the mRNA expression of IL-10, IL-13, IL-4, and IL-5 in the mediastinal lymph nodes [71]. As IL-10, IL-13, IL-4, and IL-5 are part of Th2 responses, selenium deficiency may have induced more Th2 responses than Th1 responses in the lungs of mice infected with influenza virus.

Selenium is important for the function of cytotoxic effector cells, such as $CD8^+$ T cells and natural killer (NK) cells. TNF-α and IFN-γ have antiviral effects against influenza virus in $CD8^+$ T cells [75]. Selenium supplementation increased the plasma levels of TNF-α and IFN-γ in mice infected with the influenza virus [76]. The number of $CD8^+$ T cells was lower in the lungs of selenium-deficient mice than in selenium-sufficient mice [71]. Dietary supplementation with selenium (200 μg/d for 8 w) increased the cytotoxicity of $CD8^+$ T cells by increasing the number of cells in the human peripheral blood lymphocyte population [77]. Furthermore, selenium supplementation increased the lytic activity of NK cells from human peripheral blood lymphocytes [77] and mouse spleen [78]. Therefore, selenium supplementation may enhance the function of cytotoxic effector cells in COVID-19.

Selenium plays an important role in the production of antibodies. Selenoprotein deficiency induced impaired T cell maturation, functions, and T cell-dependent antibody response in mice [79]. Selenoprotein synthesis requires selenocysteine tRNA, for inserting the selenocysteine into the protein [80]. T cells deficient in selenocysteine tRNA displayed selenoprotein deficiency, and the selenoprotein-deficient T cells showed markedly reduced proliferation in response to T cell receptor stimulation [80]. Moreover, the serum levels of antibodies, such as immunoglobulin M (IgM), IgG1, IgG2a, IgG2b, and IgG3, were lower in selenoprotein-deficient mice than in control mice [80].

Blood coagulation may increase mortality in patients with COVID-19 [81]. A low plasma selenium concentration was correlated with increased tissue damage, presence of infection, and organ failure, as well as increased mortality in ICU patients. In addition, the plasma selenium level was positively correlated with minimum platelet count, minimum plasma antithrombin activity, and protein C activity in the patients [82]. Venous thromboembolism includes deep vein thrombosis and pulmonary embolism, which are commonly developed in critically ill patients with infection [83]. It has been reported that venous thromboembolism occurred in 27% of COVID-19 patients in the ICU [84]. In another report, the cumulative incidence of venous thromboembolisms in COVID-19 patients at 7, 14, and 21 d after ICU admission was 26%, 47%, and 59%, respectively. The incidences were significantly higher in ICU patients than in patients in the general wards [85]. Selenium deficiency increased the ratio of thromboxane A_2 to prostacyclin I_2 in rats [86], inducing vasoconstriction and blood coagulation [87]. This might explain the mechanism for venous thromboembolism in selenium-deficient COVID-19 patients. Further clinical trials are required to evaluate the beneficial effects of selenium against COVID-19

3. Conclusions

Nutritional therapy should be a part of patient care for survival of this life-threatening disease (COVID-19), as well as for better and shorter recovery. Most importantly, checking malnutrition and providing optimal nutritional supplementation are critical steps for optimal functioning of the immune system in the human body. Patients with malnutrition are more likely to be from lower socioeconomic groups; thus, nutrition supplementation is important for the risk group as well as older adults who have a relatively weak immune system. In this review, we focused on the importance of vitamin C, vitamin D, and selenium for immunity enhancement. The immunomodulatory properties and the consequences of deficiencies or supplementation of these micronutrients against viral infectious diseases, including COVID-19, are summarized in Table 1. Since severely ill COVID-19 patients were reported to be deficient in more than one nutrient, we suggest that nutritional deficiencies may favor the onset of COVID-19 and increase the severity of the disease. Combination of some of these micronutrients (vitamin C, vitamin D, and selenium) may help to boost the immune system, prevent virus spread, and reduce the disease progressing to severe stages.

Table 1. The effect of micronutrients on the immune system against viral infectious diseases.

Micronutrient	Immunomodulatory Properties	Consequences of Deficiency/Effects of Supplementation in Infectious Diseases, including Coronavirus Disease 2019 (COVID-19)
Vitamin C	Increasing antiviral cytokines, such as interferon (IFN)-α/β [24] Increasing free radical formation to decrease viral yield [25] Attenuating excessive inflammatory response [27] Ameliorating hyperactivation of immune cells by altering energy metabolism [30]	Decreased flu or cold symptoms due to treatment with high dose of vitamin C [22,23] Decreased inflammatory mediators/markers due to the administration of vitamin C in COVID-19 patients [28,29]

Table 1. *Cont.*

Micronutrient	Immunomodulatory Properties	Consequences of Deficiency/Effects of Supplementation in Infectious Diseases, including Coronavirus Disease 2019 (COVID-19)
Vitamin D	Improving the physical barriers of the body by regulating the production of proteins for tight junctions [50], adherens junctions [51], and gap junctions [52] Stimulating the production of antimicrobial peptides, such as cathelicidin and defensins [55] Modulating T helper (Th) cell responses to induce a shift from Th1 to Th2 responses [61,62,64] Preventing cytokine storms by decreasing inflammatory cytokines [67,68] and nuclear factor κB (NF-κB) activation [69]	Inverse correlation between vitamin D level and viral respiratory tract infection [38–40] Vitamin D deficiency/insufficiency observed in patients with COVID-19 [41] Inverse correlation between COVID-19 mortality and sunlight exposure [45] or vitamin D level [43,48] Worse prognosis in COVID-19 patients with a low level of vitamin D [47,49]
Selenium	Preventing mutations in viral genome [71–73] Increasing $CD4^+$ T cell activation, proliferation, and differentiation; inducing Th1 phenotype [74] Enhancing the function of cytotoxic effector cells by increasing the cytotoxicity of $CD8^+$ T cells and lytic activity of natural killer (NK) cells [77] Maintaining T cell maturation and functions, including T cell-dependent antibody production [79,80] Preventing vasoconstriction and blood coagulation [87], which may increase COVID-19 mortality [81]	Higher selenium level in surviving COVID-19 patients compared to deceased patients [16] Higher recovery rate from COVID-19 in patients with higher selenium levels [17]

Author Contributions: Conceptualization: H.K.; investigation, writing, and original draft preparation: M.B.; writing, review, and editing: H.K. All authors have read and agreed to the published version of the manuscript.

Funding: This research received no external funding.

Conflicts of Interest: The authors declare no conflict of interest.

Abbreviations

COVID-19	Coronavirus disease 2019
ESPEN	European Society for Clinical Nutrition and Metabolism
GAPDH	Glyceraldehyde 3-phosphate dehydrogenase
GSH	Reduced glutathione
ICU	Intensive care unit
IFN	Interferon
Ig	Immunoglobulin
IL	Interleukin
IκB	Inhibitor of κB
MDCK	Madin–Darby canine kidney cells
NADPH	Nicotinamide adenine dinucleotide phosphate
NF-κB	Nuclear factor κB
NHANES	National Health and Nutrition Survey

NK	Natural killer cells
NO	Nitric oxide
PARP	Poly(ADP-ribose) polymerase
ROS	Reactive oxygen species
TCR	T cell receptor
Th	T helper type
TNF	Tumor necrosis factor

References

1. WHO Coronavirus Disease (COVID-19) Dashboard. Available online: https://covid19.who.int/ (accessed on 19 October 2020).
2. Perez-Saez, J.; Lauer, S.A.; Kaiser, L.; Regard, S.; Delaporte, E.; Guessous, I.; Stringhini, S.; Azman, A.S.; Group, S.-P.S. Serology-informed estimates of SARS-COV-2 infection fatality risk in Geneva, Switzerland. *Lancer Infect Dis.* **2020**. (published online July 14 2020). [CrossRef]
3. Gold, M.S.; Sehayek, D.; Gabrielli, S.; Zhang, X.; McCusker, C.; Ben-Shoshan, M. COVID-19 and comorbidities: A systematic review and meta-analysis. *Postgrad. Med.* **2020**, 1786964. [CrossRef] [PubMed]
4. Jain, V.; Yuan, J.-M. Predictive symptoms and comorbidities for severe COVID-19 and intensive care unit admission: A systematic review and meta-analysis. *Int. J. Public Health* **2020**, *65*, 533–546. [CrossRef] [PubMed]
5. Pan, D.; Sze, S.; Minhas, J.S.; Bangash, M.N.; Pareek, N.; Divall, P.; Williams, C.M.; Oggioni, M.R.; Squire, I.B.; Nellums, L.B. The impact of ethnicity on clinical outcomes in COVID-19: A systematic review. *EClinicalMedicine* **2020**, *23*, 100404. [CrossRef] [PubMed]
6. Barazzoni, R.; Bischoff, S.C.; Breda, J.; Wickramasinghe, K.; Krznaric, Z.; Nitzan, D.; Pirlich, M.; Singer, P. ESPEN expert statements and practical guidance for nutritional management of individuals with SARS-CoV-2 infection. *Clin. Nutr.* **2020**, *39*, 1631–1638. [CrossRef] [PubMed]
7. Semba, R.D.; Tang, A.M. Micronutrients and the pathogenesis of human immunodeficiency virus infection. *Br. J. Nutr.* **1999**, *81*, 181–189. [CrossRef] [PubMed]
8. Zhang, L.; Liu, Y. Potential interventions for novel coronavirus in China: A systematic review. *J. Med. Virol.* **2020**, *92*, 479–490. [CrossRef]
9. Im, J.H.; Je, Y.S.; Baek, J.; Chung, M.-H.; Kwon, H.Y.; Lee, J.-S. Nutritional status of patients with coronavirus disease 2019 (COVID-19). *Int. J. Infect. Dis.* **2020**, *21*, 743.
10. Cannell, J.; Vieth, R.; Umhau, J.; Holick, M.; Grant, W.; Madronich, S.; Garland, C.F.; Giovannucci, E. Epidemic influenza and vitamin D. *Epidemiol. Infect.* **2006**, *134*, 1129–1140. [CrossRef]
11. Mascitelli, L.; Grant, W.B.; Goldstein, M.R. Obesity, influenza virus infection, and hypovitaminosis D. *J. Infect. Dis.* **2012**, *206*, 1481–1482. [CrossRef]
12. Goncalves-Mendes, N.; Talvas, J.; Dualé, C.; Guttmann, A.; Corbin, V.; Marceau, G.; Sapin, V.; Brachet, P.; Evrard, B.; Laurichesse, H.; et al. Impact of vitamin D supplementation on influenza vaccine response and immune functions in deficient elderly persons: A randomized placebo-controlled trial. *Front. Immunol.* **2019**, *10*, 65. [CrossRef] [PubMed]
13. Villar, L.M.; Del Campo, J.A.; Ranchal, I.; Lampe, E.; Romero-Gomez, M. Association between vitamin D and hepatitis C virus infection: A meta-analysis. *World J. Gastroenterol. WJG* **2013**, *19*, 5917–5924. [CrossRef] [PubMed]
14. Nanri, A.; Nakamoto, K.; Sakamoto, N.; Imai, T.; Akter, S.; Nonaka, D.; Mizoue, T. Association of serum 25-hydroxyvitamin D with influenza in case-control study nested in a cohort of Japanese employees. *Clin. Nutr.* **2017**, *36*, 1288–1293. [CrossRef] [PubMed]
15. Lee, M.-D.; Lin, C.-H.; Lei, W.-T.; Chang, H.-Y.; Lee, H.-C.; Yeung, C.-Y.; Chiu, N.-C.; Chi, H.; Liu, J.-M.; Hsu, R.-J.; et al. Does vitamin D deficiency affect the immunogenic responses to influenza vaccination? A systematic review and meta-analysis. *Nutrients* **2018**, *10*, 409. [CrossRef] [PubMed]
16. Moghaddam, A.; Heller, R.A.; Sun, Q.; Seelig, J.; Cherkezov, A.; Seibert, L.; Hackler, J.; Seemann, P.; Diegmann, J.; Pilz, M.; et al. Selenium deficiency is associated with mortality risk from COVID-19. *Nutrients* **2020**, *12*, 2098. [CrossRef]

17. Zhang, J.; Taylor, E.W.; Bennett, K.; Saad, R.; Rayman, M.P. Association between regional selenium status and reported outcome of COVID-19 cases in China. *Am. J. Clin. Nutr.* **2020**, *111*, 1297–1299. [CrossRef]
18. Truwit, J.D.; Hite, R.D.; Morris, P.E.; DeWilde, C.; Priday, A.; Fisher, B.; Thacker, L.R.; Natarajan, R.; Brophy, D.F.; Sculthorpe, R. Effect of vitamin C infusion on organ failure and biomarkers of inflammation and vascular injury in patients with sepsis and severe acute respiratory failure: The CITRIS-ALI randomized clinical trial. *JAMA* **2019**, *322*, 1261–1270.
19. Khan, H.M.W.; Parikh, N.; Megala, S.M.; Predeteanu, G.S. Unusual early recovery of a critical COVID-19 patient after administration of intravenous vitamin C. *Am. J. Case Rep.* **2020**, *21*, e925521-1.
20. Adams, K.K.; Baker, W.L.; Sobieraj, D.M. Myth Busters: Dietary Supplements and COVID-19. *Ann. Pharmacother.* **2020**, *54*, 820–826. [CrossRef]
21. Marik, P.E.; Khangoora, V.; Rivera, R.; Hooper, M.H.; Catravas, J. Hydrocortisone, vitamin C, and thiamine for the treatment of severe sepsis and septic shock: A retrospective before-after study. *Chest* **2017**, *151*, 1229–1238. [CrossRef]
22. Gorton, H.C.; Jarvis, K. The effectiveness of vitamin C in preventing and relieving the symptoms of virus-induced respiratory infections. *J. Manip. Physiol. Ther.* **1999**, *22*, 530–533. [CrossRef]
23. Ran, L.; Zhao, W.; Wang, J.; Wang, H.; Zhao, Y.; Tseng, Y.; Bu, H. Extra dose of vitamin C based on a daily supplementation shortens the common cold: A meta-analysis of 9 randomized controlled trials. *BioMed Res. Int.* **2018**, *2018*, 1837634. [CrossRef] [PubMed]
24. Kim, Y.; Kim, H.; Bae, S.; Choi, J.; Lim, S.Y.; Lee, N.; Kong, J.M.; Hwang, Y.-i.; Kang, J.S.; Lee, W.J. Vitamin C is an essential factor on the anti-viral immune responses through the production of interferon-α/β at the initial stage of influenza A virus (H3N2) infection. *Immune Netw.* **2013**, *13*, 70–74. [CrossRef] [PubMed]
25. Furuya, A.; Uozaki, M.; Yamasaki, H.; Arakawa, T.; Arita, M.; Koyama, A.H. Antiviral effects of ascorbic and dehydroascorbic acids in vitro. *Int. J. Mol. Med.* **2008**, *22*, 541–545.
26. García, L.F. Immune response, inflammation, and the clinical spectrum of COVID-19. *Front. Immunol.* **2020**, *11*, 1441. [CrossRef]
27. Tripathi, P.; Tripathi, P.; Kashyap, L.; Singh, V. The role of nitric oxide in inflammatory reactions. *FEMS Immunol. Med. Microbiol.* **2007**, *51*, 443–452. [CrossRef]
28. Alamdari, D.H.; Moghaddam, A.B.; Amini, S.; Keramati, M.R.; Zarmehri, A.M.; Alamdari, A.H.; Damsaz, M.; Banpour, H.; Yarahmadi, A.; Koliakos, G. Application of methylene blue-vitamin C–N-acetyl cysteine for treatment of critically ill COVID-19 patients, report of a phase-I clinical trial. *Eur. J. Pharmacol.* **2020**, *885*, 173494. [CrossRef]
29. Hiedra, R.; Lo, K.B.; Elbashabsheh, M.; Gul, F.; Wright, R.M.; Albano, J.; Azmaiparashvili, Z.; Patarroyo Aponte, G. The use of IV vitamin C for patients with COVID-19: A case series. *Expert Rev. Anti-Infect. Ther.* **2020**, *1*, 1–3. [CrossRef]
30. Kornberg, M.D.; Bhargava, P.; Kim, P.M.; Putluri, V.; Snowman, A.M.; Putluri, N.; Calabresi, P.A.; Snyder, S.H. Dimethyl fumarate targets GAPDH and aerobic glycolysis to modulate immunity. *Science* **2018**, *360*, 449–453. [CrossRef]
31. Ngo, B.; Van Riper, J.M.; Cantley, L.C.; Yun, J. Targeting cancer vulnerabilities with high-dose vitamin C. *Nat. Rev. Cancer* **2019**, *19*, 271–282. [CrossRef]
32. Wilson, J.X. The physiological role of dehydroascorbic acid. *FEBS Lett.* **2002**, *527*, 5–9. [CrossRef]
33. Yun, J.; Mullarky, E.; Lu, C.; Bosch, K.N.; Kavalier, A.; Rivera, K.; Roper, J.; Chio, I.I.C.; Giannopoulou, E.G.; Rago, C.; et al. Vitamin C selectively kills KRAS and BRAF mutant colorectal cancer cells by targeting GAPDH. *Science* **2015**, *350*, 1391–1396. [CrossRef] [PubMed]
34. Hocsak, E.; Szabo, V.; Kalman, N.; Antus, C.; Cseh, A.; Sumegi, K.; Eros, K.; Hegedus, Z.; Gallyas, F., Jr.; Sumegi, B.; et al. PARP inhibition protects mitochondria and reduces ROS production via PARP-1-ATF4-MKP-1-MAPK retrograde pathway. *Free Radic. Biol. Med.* **2017**, *108*, 770–784. [CrossRef]
35. Fang, E.F.; Bohr, V.A. NAD+: The convergence of DNA repair and mitophagy. *Autophagy* **2017**, *13*, 442–443. [CrossRef]
36. Liu, F.; Zhu, Y.; Zhang, J.; Li, Y.; Peng, Z. Intravenous high-dose vitamin C for the treatment of severe COVID-19: Study protocol for a multicentre randomised controlled trial. *BMJ Open* **2020**, *10*, e039519. [CrossRef] [PubMed]
37. Siuka, D.; Pfeifer, M.; Pinter, B. Vitamin D Supplementation During the COVID-19 Pandemic. *Mayo Clin. Proc.* **2020**, *95*, 1804–1805. [CrossRef] [PubMed]

38. Monlezun, D.J.; Bittner, E.A.; Christopher, K.B.; Camargo, C.A.; Quraishi, S.A. Vitamin D status and acute respiratory infection: Cross sectional results from the United States National Health and Nutrition Examination Survey, 2001–2006. *Nutrients* **2015**, *7*, 1933–1944. [CrossRef] [PubMed]
39. Sabetta, J.R.; DePetrillo, P.; Cipriani, R.J.; Smardin, J.; Burns, L.A.; Landry, M.L. Serum 25-hydroxyvitamin d and the incidence of acute viral respiratory tract infections in healthy adults. *PLoS ONE* **2010**, *5*, e11088. [CrossRef]
40. Science, M.; Maguire, J.L.; Russell, M.L.; Smieja, M.; Walter, S.D.; Loeb, M. Low serum 25-hydroxyvitamin D level and risk of upper respiratory tract infection in children and adolescents. *Clin. Infect. Dis.* **2013**, *57*, 392–397. [CrossRef]
41. Pinzon, R.T.; Angela, A.; Pradana, A.W. Vitamin D Deficiency Among Patients with COVID-19: Case Series and Recent Literature Review. *Res. Sq.* **2020**. [CrossRef]
42. Li, Y.; Li, Q.; Zhang, N.; Liu, Z. Sunlight and vitamin D in the prevention of coronavirus disease (COVID-19) infection and mortality in the United States. *Res. Sq.* **2020**. [CrossRef]
43. Raharusun, P.; Priambada, S.; Budiarti, C.; Agung, E.; Budi, C. Patterns of COVID-19 Mortality and Vitamin D: An Indonesian Study. Available at SSRN 3585561. 2020. Available online: https://ultrasuninternational.com/ (accessed on 26 April 2020).
44. Leary, P.F.; Zamfirova, I.; Au, J.; McCracken, W.H. Effect of latitude on vitamin D levels. *J. Am. Osteopath. Assoc.* **2017**, *117*, 433–439. [CrossRef] [PubMed]
45. Lansiaux, É.; Pébaÿ, P.P.; Picard, J.-L.; Forget, J. Covid-19 and vit-d: Disease mortality negatively correlates with sunlight exposure. *Spat. Spatio-Temporal Epidemiol.* **2020**, *35*, 100362. [CrossRef] [PubMed]
46. Ghasemian, R.; Shamshirian, A.; Heydari, K.; Malekan, M.; Alizadeh-Navaei, R.; Ebrahimzadeh, M.A.; Jafarpour, H.; Shahmirzadi, A.R.; Khodabandeh, M.; Seyfari, B.; et al. The Role of Vitamin D in The Age of COVID-19: A Systematic Review and Meta-Analysis Along with an Ecological Approach. *medRxiv* **2020**. [CrossRef]
47. Munshi, R.; Hussein, M.H.; Toraih, E.A.; Elshazli, R.M.; Jardak, C.; Sultana, N.; Youssef, M.R.; Omar, M.; Attia, A.S.; Fawzy, M.S.; et al. Vitamin D insufficiency as a potential culprit in critical COVID-19 patients. *J. Med. Virol.* **2020**. [CrossRef]
48. Carpagnano, G.E.; Di Lecce, V.; Quaranta, V.N.; Zito, A.; Buonamico, E.; Capozza, E.; Palumbo, A.; Di Gioia, G.; Valerio, V.N.; Resta, O. Vitamin D deficiency as a predictor of poor prognosis in patients with acute respiratory failure due to COVID-19. *J. Endocrinol. Investig.* **2020**, 1–7. [CrossRef]
49. Mendy, A.; Apewokin, S.; Wells, A.A.; Morrow, A.L. Factors associated with hospitalization and disease severity in a racially and ethnically diverse population of COVID-19 patients. *medRxiv* **2020**. [CrossRef]
50. Chen, H.; Lu, R.; Zhang, Y.-g.; Sun, J. Vitamin D receptor deletion leads to the destruction of tight and adherens junctions in lungs. *Tissue Barriers* **2018**, *6*, 1–13. [CrossRef]
51. Gniadecki, R.; Gajkowska, B.; Hansen, M. 1, 25-dihydroxyvitamin D3 stimulates the assembly of adherens junctions in keratinocytes: Involvement of protein kinase C. *Endocrinology* **1997**, *138*, 2241–2248. [CrossRef]
52. Clairmont, A.; Tessmann, D.; Stock, A.; Nicolai, S.; Stahl, W.; Sies, H. Induction of gap junctional intercellular communication by vitamin D in human skin fibroblasts is dependent on the nuclear vitamin D receptor. *Carcinogenesis* **1996**, *17*, 1389–1391. [CrossRef]
53. Kast, J.; McFarlane, A.; Głobińska, A.; Sokolowska, M.; Wawrzyniak, P.; Sanak, M.; Schwarze, J.; Akdis, C.; Wanke, K. Respiratory syncytial virus infection influences tight junction integrity. *Clin. Exp. Immunol.* **2017**, *190*, 351–359. [CrossRef] [PubMed]
54. Hansdottir, S.; Monick, M.M.; Hinde, S.L.; Lovan, N.; Look, D.C.; Hunninghake, G.W. Respiratory epithelial cells convert inactive vitamin D to its active form: Potential effects on host defense. *J. Immunol.* **2008**, *181*, 7090–7099. [CrossRef] [PubMed]
55. Wang, T.-T.; Nestel, F.P.; Bourdeau, V.; Nagai, Y.; Wang, Q.; Liao, J.; Tavera-Mendoza, L.; Lin, R.; Hanrahan, J.W.; Mader, S.; et al. Cutting edge: 1,25-dihydroxyvitamin D3 is a direct inducer of antimicrobial peptide gene expression. *J. Immunol.* **2004**, *173*, 2909–2912. [CrossRef] [PubMed]
56. Kościuczuk, E.M.; Lisowski, P.; Jarczak, J.; Strzałkowska, N.; Jóźwik, A.; Horbańczuk, J.; Krzyżewski, J.; Zwierzchowski, L.; Bagnicka, E. Cathelicidins: Family of antimicrobial peptides. A review. *Mol. Biol. Rep.* **2012**, *39*, 10957–10970. [CrossRef] [PubMed]
57. Raj, P.A.; Dentino, A.R. Current status of defensins and their role in innate and adaptive immunity. *FEMS Microbiol. Lett.* **2002**, *206*, 9–18. [CrossRef]

58. Barlow, P.G.; Svoboda, P.; Mackellar, A.; Nash, A.A.; York, I.A.; Pohl, J.; Davidson, D.J.; Donis, R.O. Antiviral activity and increased host defense against influenza infection elicited by the human cathelicidin LL-37. *PLoS ONE* **2011**, *6*, e25333. [CrossRef]
59. Currie, S.M.; Findlay, E.G.; McHugh, B.J.; Mackellar, A.; Man, T.; Macmillan, D.; Wang, H.; Fitch, P.M.; Schwarze, J.; Davidson, D.J. The human cathelicidin LL-37 has antiviral activity against respiratory syncytial virus. *PLoS ONE* **2013**, *8*, e73659. [CrossRef]
60. Kota, S.; Sabbah, A.; Harnack, R.; Xiang, Y.; Meng, X.; Bose, S. Role of human β-defensin-2 during tumor necrosis factor-α/NF-κB-mediated innate antiviral response against human respiratory syncytial virus. *J. Biol. Chem.* **2008**, *283*, 22417–22429. [CrossRef]
61. Lemire, J.M.; Archer, D.C.; Beck, L.; Spiegelberg, H.L. Immunosuppressive actions of 1,25-dihydroxyvitamin D3: Preferential inhibition of Th1 functions. *J. Nutr.* **1995**, *125* (Suppl. 6), 1704S–1708S.
62. Boonstra, A.; Barrat, F.J.; Crain, C.; Heath, V.L.; Savelkoul, H.F.; O'Garra, A. 1α, 25-Dihydroxyvitamin D3 has a direct effect on naive CD4+ T cells to enhance the development of Th2 cells. *J. Immunol.* **2001**, *167*, 4974–4980. [CrossRef]
63. Kaiko, G.E.; Horvat, J.C.; Beagley, K.W.; Hansbro, P.M. Immunological decision-making: How does the immune system decide to mount a helper T-cell response? *Immunology* **2008**, *123*, 326–338. [CrossRef] [PubMed]
64. Sloka, S.; Silva, C.; Wang, J.; Yong, V.W. Predominance of Th2 polarization by vitamin D through a STAT6-dependent mechanism. *J. Neuroinflamm.* **2011**, *8*, 56. [CrossRef] [PubMed]
65. Tang, Y.; Liu, J.; Zhang, D.; Xu, Z.; Ji, J.; Wen, C. Cytokine storm in COVID-19: The current evidence and treatment strategies. *Front. Immunol.* **2020**, *11*, 1708. [CrossRef] [PubMed]
66. Chen, X.; Zhao, B.; Qu, Y.; Chen, Y.; Xiong, J.; Feng, Y.; Men, D.; Huang, Q.; Liu, Y.; Yang, B. Detectable serum SARS-CoV-2 viral load (RNAaemia) is closely correlated with drastically elevated interleukin 6 (IL-6) level in critically ill COVID-19 patients. *Clin. Infect. Dis.* **2020**, *71*, 1937–1942. [CrossRef]
67. Khare, D.; Godbole, N.M.; Pawar, S.D.; Mohan, V.; Pandey, G.; Gupta, S.; Kumar, D.; Dhole, T.N.; Godbole, M.M. Calcitriol [1,25[OH]$_2$D$_3$] pre- and post-treatment suppresses inflammatory response to influenza A (H1N1) infection in human lung A549 epithelial cells. *Eur. J. Nutr.* **2013**, *52*, 1405–1415. [CrossRef]
68. Sharifi, A.; Vahedi, H.; Nedjat, S.; Rafiei, H.; Hosseinzadeh-Attar, M.J. Effect of single-dose injection of vitamin D on immune cytokines in ulcerative colitis patients: A randomized placebo-controlled trial. *APMIS Acta Pathol. Microbiol. Immunol. Scand.* **2019**, *127*, 681–687. [CrossRef]
69. Chen, Y.; Zhang, J.; Ge, X.; Du, J.; Deb, D.K.; Li, Y.C. Vitamin D receptor inhibits nuclear factor κB activation by interacting with IκB kinase β protein. *J. Biol. Chem.* **2013**, *288*, 19450–19458. [CrossRef]
70. Hastie, C.E.; Mackay, D.F.; Ho, F.; Celis-Morales, C.A.; Katikireddi, S.V.; Niedzwiedz, C.L.; Jani, B.D.; Welsh, P.; Mair, F.S.; Gray, S.R.; et al. Vitamin D concentrations and COVID-19 infection in UK Biobank. *Diabetes Metab. Syndr. Clin. Res. Rev.* **2020**, *14*, 561–565. [CrossRef]
71. Beck, M.A.; Nelson, H.K.; Shi, Q.; Van Dael, P.; Schiffrin, E.J.; Blum, S.; Barclay, D.; Levander, O.A. Selenium deficiency increases the pathology of an influenza virus infection. *FASEB J.* **2001**, *15*, 1481–1483. [CrossRef]
72. Nelson, H.K.; Shi, Q.; Van Dael, P.; Schiffrin, E.J.; Blum, S.; Barclay, D.; Levander, O.A.; Beck, M.A. Host nutritional selenium status as a driving force for influenza virus mutations. *FASEB J.* **2001**, *15*, 1727–1738. [CrossRef]
73. Beck, M.A.; Shi, Q.; Morris, V.C.; Levander, O.A. Rapid genomic evolution of a non-virulent coxsackievirus B3 in selenium-deficient mice results in selection of identical virulent isolates. *Nat. Med.* **1995**, *1*, 433–436. [CrossRef] [PubMed]
74. Hoffmann, F.W.; Hashimoto, A.C.; Shafer, L.A.; Dow, S.; Berry, M.J.; Hoffmann, P.R. Dietary selenium modulates activation and differentiation of CD4+ T cells in mice through a mechanism involving cellular free thiols. *J. Nutr.* **2010**, *140*, 1155–1161. [CrossRef] [PubMed]
75. KUWANO, K.; KAWASHIMA, T.; ARAI, S. Antiviral effect of TNF-α and IFN-γ secreted from a CD8+ influenza virus-specific CTL clone. *Viral Immunol.* **1993**, *6*, 1–11. [CrossRef] [PubMed]
76. Yu, L.; Sun, L.; Nan, Y.; Zhu, L.-Y. Protection from H1N1 influenza virus infections in mice by supplementation with selenium: A comparison with selenium-deficient mice. *Biol. Trace Elem. Res.* **2011**, *141*, 254–261. [CrossRef] [PubMed]
77. Kiremidjian-Schumacher, L.; Roy, M.; Wishe, H.I.; Cohen, M.W.; Stotzky, G. Supplementation with selenium and human immune cell functions. *Biol. Trace Elem. Res.* **1994**, *41*, 115. [CrossRef]

78. Kiremidjian-Schumacher, L.; Roy, M.; Wishe, H.I.; Cohen, M.W.; Stotzky, G. Supplementation with selenium augments the functions of natural killer and lymphokine-activated killer cells. *Biol. Trace Elem. Res.* **1996**, *52*, 227–239. [CrossRef]
79. Carlson, B.A.; Yoo, M.-H.; Shrimali, R.K.; Irons, R.; Gladyshev, V.N.; Hatfield, D.L.; Park, J.M. Role of selenium-containing proteins in T-cell and macrophage function. *Proc. Nutr. Soc.* **2010**, *69*, 300–310. [CrossRef]
80. Commans, S.; Böck, A. Selenocysteine inserting tRNAs: An overview. *FEMS Microbiol. Rev.* **1999**, *23*, 335–351. [CrossRef]
81. Zhou, F.; Yu, T.; Du, R.; Fan, G.; Liu, Y.; Liu, Z.; Xiang, J.; Wang, Y.; Song, B.; Gu, X.; et al. Clinical course and risk factors for mortality of adult inpatients with COVID-19 in Wuhan, China: A retrospective cohort study. *Lancet* **2020**, *395*, 1054–1062. [CrossRef]
82. Sakr, Y.; Reinhart, K.; Bloos, F.; Marx, G.; Russwurm, S.; Bauer, M.; Brunkhorst, F. Time course and relationship between plasma selenium concentrations, systemic inflammatory response, sepsis, and multiorgan failure. *Br. J. Anaesth.* **2007**, *98*, 775–784. [CrossRef]
83. Spyropoulos, A.C.; Weitz, J.I. Hospitalized COVID-19 patients and venous thromboembolism: A perfect storm. *Am. Heart Assoc.* **2020**, *142*, 129–132. [CrossRef] [PubMed]
84. Klok, F.; Kruip, M.; Van der Meer, N.; Arbous, M.; Gommers, D.; Kant, K.; Kaptein, F.; van Paassen, J.; Stals, M.; Huisman, M.; et al. Incidence of thrombotic complications in critically ill ICU patients with COVID-19. *Thromb. Res.* **2020**, *191*, 145–147. [CrossRef] [PubMed]
85. Middeldorp, S.; Coppens, M.; van Haaps, T.F.; Foppen, M.; Vlaar, A.P.; Müller, M.C.; Bouman, C.C.; Beenen, L.F.; Kootte, R.S.; Heijmans, J.; et al. Incidence of venous thromboembolism in hospitalized patients with COVID-19. *J. Thromb. Haemost.* **2020**, *18*, 1995–2002. [CrossRef] [PubMed]
86. Haberland, A.; Neubert, K.; Kruse, I.; Behne, D.; Schimke, I. Consequences of long-term selenium-deficient diet on the prostacyclin and thromboxane release from rat aorta. *Biol. Trace Elem. Res.* **2001**, *81*, 71–78. [CrossRef]
87. Miller, S.B. Prostaglandins in health and disease: An overview. *Semin. Arthritis Rheum.* **2006**, *36*, 37–49. [CrossRef] [PubMed]

Publisher's Note: MDPI stays neutral with regard to jurisdictional claims in published maps and institutional affiliations.

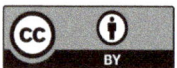

© 2020 by the authors. Licensee MDPI, Basel, Switzerland. This article is an open access article distributed under the terms and conditions of the Creative Commons Attribution (CC BY) license (http://creativecommons.org/licenses/by/4.0/).

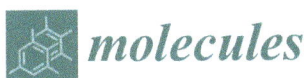

Review

Astaxanthin and its Effects in Inflammatory Responses and Inflammation-Associated Diseases: Recent Advances and Future Directions

Ming Xian Chang [1,2,3,*] **and Fan Xiong** [1]

1. State Key Laboratory of Freshwater Ecology and Biotechnology, Key Laboratory of Aquaculture Disease Control, Institute of Hydrobiology, Chinese Academy of Sciences, Wuhan 430072, China; xiongfan@ihb.ac.cn
2. Innovation Academy for Seed Design, Chinese Academy of Sciences, Wuhan 430072, China
3. University of Chinese Academy of Sciences, Beijing 100049, China
* Correspondence: mingxianchang@ihb.ac.cn; Tel.: +86-1862-797-0488

Academic Editors: Sokcheon Pak and Soo Liang Ooi
Received: 24 October 2020; Accepted: 9 November 2020; Published: 16 November 2020

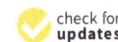

Abstract: Astaxanthin is a natural lipid-soluble and red-orange carotenoid. Due to its strong antioxidant property, anti-inflammatory, anti-apoptotic, and immune modulation, astaxanthin has gained growing interest as a multi-target pharmacological agent against various diseases. In the current review, the anti-inflammation mechanisms of astaxanthin involved in targeting for inflammatory biomarkers and multiple signaling pathways, including PI3K/AKT, Nrf2, NF-κB, ERK1/2, JNK, p38 MAPK, and JAK-2/STAT-3, have been described. Furthermore, the applications of anti-inflammatory effects of astaxanthin in neurological diseases, diabetes, gastrointestinal diseases, hepatic and renal diseases, eye and skin disorders, are highlighted. In addition to the protective effects of astaxanthin in various chronic and acute diseases, we also summarize recent advances for the inconsistent roles of astaxanthin in infectious diseases, and give our view that the exact function of astaxanthin in response to different pathogen infection and the potential protective effects of astaxanthin in viral infectious diseases should be important research directions in the future.

Keywords: astaxanthin; oxidative stress; anti-inflammatory; inflammation-associated diseases

1. Introduction

Astaxanthin is a natural lipid-soluble and red-orange oxycarotenoid pigment, and belongs to a group of carotenoids called xanthophylls, which include β-cryptoxanthin, β-carotene, lycopene, and zeaxanthin (Figure 1) [1,2]. Astaxanthin was firstly discovered in lobsters and employed in aquaculture [3]. Owing to its anti-oxidative features, astaxanthin has gained the approval as a supplement for food in 1991 [4,5]. Astaxanthin is primarily biosynthesized by microalgae, phytoplankton, yeast and bacteria [6,7], and then accumulated in zooplankton, crustaceans and subsequently fish [8,9]. Astaxanthin can be extracted in sundry seafood including algae, shrimp, krill, lobster, asteroidean, crustacean, trout, red sea bream, and salmon [10].

Astaxanthin is derived from β-carotene by 3-hydroxylation and 4-ketolation, and catalyzed by β-carotene hydroxylase and β-carotene ketolase respectively [11]. It has a molecular structure similar to that of β-carotene, with the polar ionone rings at either end of the molecule and a nonpolar zone in the middle [12]. However, in contrast to 11 in β-carotene, the possession of 13 conjugated double polyunsaturated bonds gives astaxanthin unique chemical properties, molecular structure and light absorption characteristics [10], which makes astaxanthin more polar and greatly enhances its antioxidant property [13,14]. Astaxanthin exists in three different stereoisomers, namely (3S, 3'S), (3R, 3'R) and (3R, 3'S), that differ in the configuration of two hydroxyl groups on the molecule.

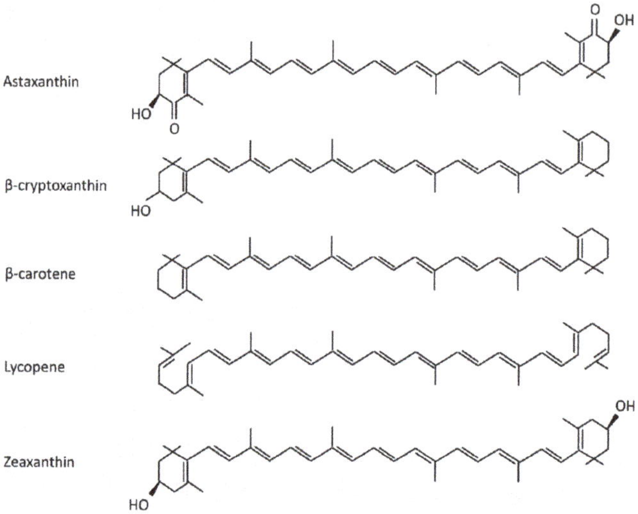

Figure 1. Chemical structures of selected carotenoids.

Nowadays, most of available astaxanthin on the market is synthetically produced for the usages in the feeds. Synthetic astaxanthin starts from the ketoisophorone obtained from petroleum, which yields more different stereoisomers than that is naturally found [15]. Only a small part of commercial astaxanthin is extracted from *Haematococcus pluvialis* (algal production), *Xanthophyllomyces dendrorhous* (yeast production) or other astaxanthin-producing biological organisms [16]. In those organisms, the free form of astaxanthin is relatively uncommon, and most of astaxanthin is either conjugated with proteins or esterified with one or two fatty acids. In *H. pluvialis*, 99% of astaxanthin exist in the way of acyl esters, which make up nearly all the astaxanthin currently available in commercial dietary supplements [12]. However due to the early scare report, which showed that petrochemicals for astaxanthin synthesis could cause cancer, only the astaxanthin made from algal and yeast is approved for human consumption [17,18]. Synthetic forms of astaxanthin are predominantly used for animal feed.

Similar to other carotenoids, astaxanthin has numerous metabolic and physiological functions. However, astaxanthin is more bioactive than other carotenoids such as zeaxanthin, lutein, and carotene. Astaxanthin has attracted considerable interest due to its potential pharmacological effects, including a strong antioxidant property, DNA repair, stress forbearance, cell regeneration, neuroprotective, antiproliferative, anti-inflammatory, anti-apoptotic, antidiabetic, anticancer, and skin-protective effects [6,19,20]. The aim of this review is to highlight and summarize the advances toward understanding the effects of astaxanthin on inflammatory responses and inflammation-associated diseases.

2. The Anti-Inflammation Mechanisms of Astaxanthin

Inflammation is a biological response to harmful stimuli, such as pathogens, damaged cells, toxic compounds or irradiation, and acts by removing injurious stimuli and initiating the healing process [21]. Usually, inflammation is a defense mechanism that is vital to host health, when cellular and molecular events efficiently minimize impending injury or infection and contribute to restoration of tissue homeostasis [22]. However, nonresolving inflammation is not a primary cause but contributes to their pathogenesis for a variety of chronic diseases including chronic obstructive pulmonary disease, inflammatory bowel disease, neurodegenerative disease, atherosclerosis, or rheumatoid arthritis and so on [22]. In recent decades, a great number of inflammatory biomarkers including kinins, acute phase proteins (APPs), platelet-activating factor (PAF), prostaglandins, leukotrienes, amines, purines, cytokines, chemokines, adhesion molecules, and inflammatory signaling pathways including NF-κB, MAPK, and JAK-STAT pathways have been found [23,24].

The various mechanisms of astaxanthin in the anti-inflammatory response have been demonstrated (Figure 2). Many APPs in mammals, such as C-reactive protein (CRP), lipopolysaccharide-binding protein (LBP), caeruloplasmin, haptoglobin, serum amyloid A, transferrin, collectin, fibrinogen and alpha 1-acid glycoprotein, have been used as biomarkers of inflammation and disease, which contribute to repair of tissue damage, kill infectious microbes and restore homeostasis [25,26]. Furthermore, chronic and abnormal activation of some inducible enzymes, including NADPH oxidase (NOX), inducible nitric oxide synthase (iNOS), cyclooxygenase (COX)-2, high-mobility group box 1 (HMGB1), superoxide dismutase (SOD), and glutathione peroxidase (GPx), have been shown to play vital roles in the development of some inflammatory diseases such as oncogenesis and cardiovascular disease [24,27]. In LPS-stimulated BV-2 microglial cells, astaxanthin inhibited the production of inflammatory mediators via suppressing the activation and protein degradation of iNOS and COX-2 [28]. In the streptozotocin (STZ)-induced diabetic rats, the administration of astaxanthin significantly decreased the protein expressions of COX-2, iNOS and ICAM-1, which suggested that the inhibitory effect of astaxanthin on diabetes-induced hepatic dysfunction could be derived from the inhibition of the inflammatory responses [29]. In young soccer players, astaxanthin supplementation prevented inflammation induced by rigorous physical training [30]. In human keratinocytes, astaxanthin effectively protected against UV-induced inflammation by decreasing the mRNA and protein expressions of iNOS and COX-2 [31]. All these data suggest that astaxanthin can exhibit its anti-inflammatory action by targeting for APPs and certain inducible enzymes.

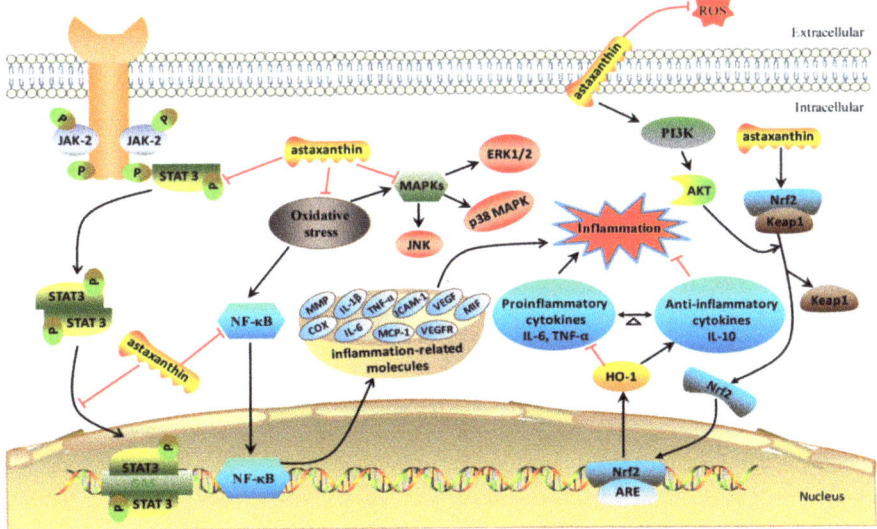

Figure 2. The anti-inflammation mechanisms of astaxanthin. Inflammatory biomarkers, such as many acute phase proteins (APPs), inducible enzymes, chemokines and cytokines, are target genes regulated by astaxanthin. In addition to inflammatory molecules, astaxanthin can promote PI3K/AkT and nuclear factor erythroid 2-like 2 (Nrf2) signaling pathways, but block NF-κB, extracellular-signal-regulated kinase (ERK1/2), c-Jun N-terminal kinases (JNK), p38 MAPK, and JAK-2/STAT-3 signaling pathways to attenuate inflammation. Red arrows indicate inhibitory action, and black arrows show enhancement action.

Chemokines and cytokines are also target genes regulated by astaxanthin (Figure 2). The monocyte chemotactic protein 1 (MCP-1) is known to be an important chemokine for macrophage recruitment.

In mouse adipose tissue, targeting for MCP-1 may prevent the perturbations associated with macrophage-induced inflammation [32]. Astaxanthin was found to suppress IκB-α degradation and NF-κB nuclear translocation, which led to significant inhibition of expression of MCP-1 and other inflammation-related molecules, including IL-6, vascular endothelial growth factors (VEGFs), intercellular adhesion molecule-1 (ICAM-1), VEGF receptor (VEGFR)-1 and VEGFR-2 [33]. Interferon-gamma (IFN-γ) is a pleiotropic cytokine involved in antiproliferative, pro-apoptotic, antitumor, autoinflammatory, and autoimmune diseases [34,35]. In ovalbumin-induced allergic asthma mice, astaxanthin treatment attenuated their airway inflammation, reduced the levels of total IgE and IgG1, and regulate the Th1/Th2 imbalance via inhibiting the release of IL-4 and IL-5 Th2 cytokines and increasing the release of IFN-γ Th1 cytokine [36]. The mRNA expression levels of IL-1β, IL-6, CCL2, and CXCL2 were significantly decreased by astaxanthin in the colonic mucosa of azoxymethane-treated mice [37]. Astaxanthin administration was found to improve the dermatitis and pruritus via the suppression of mRNA and protein expressions of eotaxin, macrophage migration inhibitory factor (MIF), IL-4, and IL-5 [38].

In addition to inflammatory biomarkers, it is most widely reported that astaxanthin can block the NF-κB-dependent signaling pathway and forestall gene expression of downstream inflammatory mediators such as IL-1β, IL-6, and tumor necrosis factor-α (TNF-α) [39,40]. Furthermore, in vivo and in vitro studies revealed that astaxanthin could influence the MAPK signaling pathway via modulating the expression and activity of extracellular-signal-regulated kinase (ERK1/2), c-Jun N-terminal kinases (JNK) and p38 MAP Kinase [41,42]. Several studies also demonstrated that the nuclear factor erythroid 2-like 2 (Nrf2) signaling plays an important role in inflammatory diseases [43,44]. In Adriamycin-induced focal segmental glomerulosclerosis (FSGS) mice, astaxanthin treatment could exert anti-inflammatory and antioxidant effects by promoting Nrf2 expression [45]. As regards in the diabetes rat model, dietary supplementation of astaxanthin improved cognitive deficits from oxidative stress, nitric oxide synthase and inflammation via promoting the expression of PI3K/AkT in the brain [46]. Astaxanthin also prevented the development and progression of hamster buccal pouch (HBP) carcinomas through the inhibition of JAK-2/STAT-3 signaling and its downstream targets cyclin D1, MMP-2, -9 and VEGF [47].

3. The Anti-Inflammatory Effects of Astaxanthin in Chronic and Acute Diseases

3.1. The Anti-Inflammatory Effects of Astaxanthin in Neurological Diseases

Alzheimer's disease is one of the most severe chronic neurodegenerative disorders. Astaxanthin is able to act against Alzheimer's disease. In Wistar rats with Alzheimer's disease, astaxanthin powder from shrimp (*Litopenaeus vannamei*) shells showed a significant alleviation of cognitive functions (Table 1) [48]. In APP/PSEN1 (APP/PS1) double-transgenic mice, the administration of synthesized docosahexaenoic-acid-acylated astaxanthin diesters (AST-DHA) attenuated cognitive disorders by regulating the parameters of oxidative stress and suppressing neuroinflammation (Table 1) [49].

Parkinson's disease (PD), which is an age-related disorder mainly caused by neuroinflammation and oxidative stress, is the second most common cause of neurodegenerative disorders. Astaxanthin was found to multi-target drug in preventing PD disease progression. In a mouse PD model from both young and aged mice, a natural compound astaxanthin was less efficacious in the aged animals, since astaxanthin failed in protecting against 1-methyl-4-phenyl-1,2,3,6-tetrahydropyridine (MPTP) neurotoxicity in aged animals (Table 1) [50]. Alpha synuclein (SNCA) is a major causative gene that responsible for the onset of PD. Astaxanthin could protect against PD-caused neuron damage by targeting miR-7/SNCA axis to suppress endoplasmic reticulum (ER) stress (Table 1) [51]. The effects of DHA-astaxanthin (DHA-acylated astaxanthin ester), non-esterified astaxanthin and DHA + astaxanthin (combination of non-esterified astaxanthin with DHA) on PD were investigated in mice with PD. The results revealed that DHA-astaxanthin significantly suppressed the PD development in MPTP-induced mice, which was better than the effects of astaxanthin and DHA + astaxanthin.

Although all three astaxanthin supplements could inhibit oxidative stress, DHA-astaxanthin group had the highest inhibiting effect for the apoptosis of dopaminergic neurons through JNK and P38 MAPK pathway, which suggested that DHA-astaxanthin was superior to astaxanthin in preventing behavioral deficits via apoptosis rather than oxidative stress (Table 1) [52].

Cerebral ischemia/reperfusion (IR) can cause irreversible neuronal injuries. Several studies have investigated the effect of astaxanthin treatment in preventing the risk of ischemia on brain recovery. In a mouse model of vascular cognitive impairment (VCI), astaxanthin treatment improved learning and memory deficits after repeated cerebral IR injury, with the reduced damage of hippocampal neurons and the inhibition of neuronal apoptosis (Table 1) [53]. Preventive treatment of astaxanthin also prevented neurological deficits and reduced cerebral infarction volume through multiple mechanisms, which included the suppression of ROS (reactive oxygen species), prevention of apoptosis, activation of Nrf2–ARE defense pathway, and promotion of neural regeneration (Table 1) [54]. Compared with those in the cerebral ischemia model group (MCAO group), astaxanthin treatment can promote the axonal regeneration and improve the motor function via activating the cAMP/PKA/CREB signaling pathway (Table 1) [55]. For acute cerebral infarction (ACI) rat, the treatment with astaxanthin notably inhibited oxidative stress and increased the mRNA expression of brain-derived neurotrophic factor (BDNF) and nerve growth factor (NGF), which led to ameliorate ACI (Table 1) [56]. Astaxanthin also protected the brain from oxidative damage and reduced neuronal deficits due to cerebral ischemia reperfusion injury (IRI) (Table 1) [57]. The mechanisms of astaxanthin in neuroprotective properties against cerebral ischemia-induced apoptosis were investigated, and the in vitro data revealed that astaxanthin could confer neuroprotection against the oxygen and glucose deprivation (OGD)-induced apoptosis via the PI3K/Akt/GSK3β/Nrf2 signaling pathway (Table 1) [58].

Neuropathic pain (NP) is caused by a disease or a lesion in the somatosensory nervous system [59]. In the carrageenan-induced mice paw edema and pain, the treatment with astaxanthin from *Litopenaeus vannamei* exhibited the anti-inflammatory activities and the decreased pain (Table 1) [60]. In the in vitro and/or in vivo model of NP, astaxanthin could significantly attenuate behavioral and biochemical alterations with the decreased oxidative stress (Table 1) [61], and chronic trans-astaxanthin treatment could exert therapeutic effects on thermal hyperalgesia and co-morbid depressive-like behaviors in mice with chronic pain via its potent anti-inflammatory property (Table 1) [62]. It was also found that astaxanthin attenuated neuroinflammation and mechanical allodynia via decreasing the expression of inflammatory signaling mediators (NR2B and p-p38MAPK) and inflammatory cytokine TNF-α (Table 1) [63]. Astaxanthin was also found to decrease mechanical and thermal pain through the inhibition of ERK1/2 and the activation of AKT (Table 1) [64].

Table 1. The anti-inflammatory effects of astaxanthin in neurological diseases.

Model	Dosage	Biomarkers	Disease	Ref
Wistar rats	10 mg/kg body weight	Oxidative markers	Alzheimer's Disease	[48]
APP/PS1 mice	/	Oxidative markers; inflammasome expression	Alzheimer's Disease	[49]
Mice	Bioastin® at a dose of 30 mg/kg bodyweight	MPTP neurotoxin	Parkinson's disease	[50]
Human neuroblastoma SH-SY5Y cell line and C57BL/6 mice	5, 10, 25, and 50 μM in cell line	miR-7/SNCA axis	Parkinson's disease	[51]
Mice with Parkinson's disease (PD),	/	The mitochondria-mediated pathway; JNK and P38 MAPK pathway	Parkinson's disease	[52]
Male ICR mice	10 mg/kg/day	Oxidative stress parameters; Cytochrome C, cleaved Caspase-3 and Bax	Cerebral ischemia/ reperfusion (IR)	[53]
Male SD (Sprague-Dawley) rats	10 mg/kg or 5 mg/kg	Oxidative stress; antioxidant genes; assessment of cell death; cell regeneration genes	Cerebral ischemia	[54]
MCAO mice	30 mg/kg	cAMP concentration	Cerebral ischemia	[55]

Table 1. Cont.

Model	Dosage	Biomarkers	Disease	Ref
Male Sprague Dawley rats	20, 40, and 80 mg/kg	Oxidative stress	Acute cerebral infarction	[56]
Adult male Sprague-Dawley rats	/	Oxidant parameter	Cerebral ischemia reperfusion injury	[57]
Human SH-SY5Y cells	5, 10, 20 and 40 μmol/L	PI3K/Akt/GSK3β/ Nrf2 signaling	Cerebral ischemia	[58]
Male ICR mice	50, 100, 150 mg/kg	ROS	Edema and pain	[60]
Rat C6 glial cells; Adult male Sprague Dawley rats	5 and 10 mg/kg	ROS	Neuropathic pain	[61]
Chronic constriction injury (CCI) mice	80 mg/kg	IL-1β, IL-6 and TNF-α	Neuropathic pain	[62]
Adult male Wistar rats	10 μL of 0.2 mM	NR2B, p-p38MAPK and TNF-α	Neuropathic pain	[63]
Spinal cord injury (SCI) rats	/	ERK1/2, AKT	Neuropathic pain	[64]

3.2. The Anti-Inflammatory Effects of Astaxanthin in Diabetes

Diabetes mellitus (DM) is the most common metabolic disease, and the underlying factors that lead to the development of pathologies in diabetes are involved in oxidative stress and chronic inflammation [65]. Landon et al. have reviewed the biological effects and the underlying mechanisms of astaxanthin on the prevention and the treatment of DM-associated pathologies [66]. Although the exact mechanism remains elusive, astaxanthin has been found to reduce inflammation, oxidative stress and apoptosis through the regulation of different pathways. The protective effects of astaxanthin on diabetic retinopathy (DR) and diabetic neuropathy were suggested for the inhibitory effect of astaxanthin on the inflammation through the NF-κB pathway, microvascular damages through VEGF production and apoptosis through the regulation of MAPK and PI3K/Akt pathways. The protective effects of astaxanthin on diabetic nephropathy (DN) were suggested for the inhibitory effect of astaxanthin on NF-κB translocation, transforming growth factor beta (TGF-β) production, inflammation and fibrosis. The protective effects of astaxanthin on diabetic cardiovascular complications were suggested for the inhibitory effect of astaxanthin on the inflammation through the NF-κB pathway, oxidative stress regulation through thrombosis and vasoconstriction, the levels of the oxidized low-density lipoprotein (oxLDL) and vasoconstriction [66].

3.3. The Anti-Inflammatory Effects of Astaxanthin in Gastrointestinal Diseases

Inflammatory bowel disease is a chronic inflammatory disease with increased risk for colorectal cancer. In the dextran sulfate sodium (DSS)-induced colitis, dietary astaxanthin significantly inhibited the occurrence of colonic mucosal ulcers and adenocarcinoma partly through inhibition of the expression of inflammatory cytokines, which included IL-1β, IL-6, COX-2 (Table 2) [67]. In C57BL/6J mice, the mRNA expression of IL-1β, IL-6, TNF-α, IL-36α, and IL-36γ, and the activation of NF-κB, AP-1, and MAPK were suppressed by dietary astaxanthin (Table 2) [68]. In C57BL/KsJ-db/db (db/db) obese mice, astaxanthin inhibited the development of colonic premalignant lesions by reducing oxidative stress, attenuating chronic inflammation, and inhibiting NF-κB activation and cell proliferation in the colonic mucosa (Table 2) [37].

Table 2. The anti-inflammatory effects of astaxanthin in gastrointestinal diseases.

Model	Dosage	Biomarkers	Disease	Ref
Male ICR mice	50, 100, 200 ppm in diet	NF-κB, IL-1β, IL-6, COX-2	dextran sulfate sodium (DSS)-induced colitis	[67]
C57BL/6J mice	0.02 or 0.04% in diet	IL-1β, IL-6, TNF-α, IL-36α, IL-36γ, NF-κB, AP-1, ERK1/2, p38 MAPK, JNK	dextran sulfate sodium (DSS)-induced colitis	[68]
C57BL/KsJ-db/db obese mice	200 ppm in diet	IL-1β, IL-6, CCL2, CXCL2, NF-κB	azoxymethane-induced colonic premalignant lesions	[37]

3.4. The Anti-Inflammatory Effects of Astaxanthin in Hepatic and Renal Diseases

Several studies have reported the roles of astaxanthin in hepatic and renal diseases (Table 3). Focal segmental glomerulosclerosis (FSGS) is a specific pattern of chronic renal injury. Astaxanthin treatment exhibited significant improvements in renal functional parameters and exerted anti-inflammatory and antioxidant effects by increasing the expression of Nrf2 and inhibiting the activation of nucleotide-binding oligomerization domain-like receptor protein 3 (NLRP3) inflammasome in FSGS mouse models [45]. Astaxanthin has effects in protecting cells and/or organs from ischemia/reperfusion (IR) induced injury by the reduced oxidative stress and inflammation in kidney [69], and contrast-induced acute kidney injury (CI-AKI) by SIRT1-p53 and SIRT1/FOXO3a pathways [70,71]. In the hepatic IR injury model, astaxanthin pretreatment attenuates apoptosis and autophagy via the ROS/MAPK pathway [41], or may be involved in the inhibitory mechanism through the decrease of ROS production and inflammatory cytokine expression, and inactivation of MAPK [72]. Astaxanthin also has a protective effect in ConA-induced autoimmune hepatitis through the down-regulation of JNK/p-JNK-mediated apoptosis and autophagy [73].

Table 3. The anti-inflammatory effects of astaxanthin in hepatic and renal diseases.

Model	Dosage	Biomarkers	Disease	Ref
Male Balb/c mice	50 mg/kg	Nrf2, NLRP3, IL-1β, IL-18	Adriamycin-induced FSGS	[45]
Male ICR mice	5 mg/kg/day	TNF-α, IL-1β, IL-6	Ischemia/reperfusion (IR) induced injury	[69]
Male Sprague Dawley (SD) rats	/	Oxidative stress indicators, antioxidant stress indicators	Contrast-induced acute kidney injury (CI-AKI)	[70]
Male Sprague Dawley rats	50 and 100 mg/kg	Oxidative stress markers and apoptosis-related proteins	Contrast-induced acute kidney injury (CI-AKI)	[71]
Male Balb/C mice	30 mg/kg or 60 mg/kg	ROS, inflammatory cytokines and MAPK proteins	Hepatic ischemia reperfusion (IR)	[41]
Male C57BL/6 mice	25 mg/kg	ROS, inflammatory cytokines, MAPK and apoptosis-related proteins	Hepatic ischemia reperfusion (IR)	[72]
Male Balb/c mice	20 mg/kg and 40 mg/kg	NF-κB p65, TNF-α, IL-6, IL-1β, IFN-γ, autophagy and apoptotic proteins	ConA-induced autoimmune hepatitis	[73]

3.5. The Anti-Inflammatory Effects of Astaxanthin in Eye and Skin Disorders

Dry eye disease (DED) has become a chronic ocular surface disease. The protective effect and potential mechanism of astaxanthin on DED were characterized, and suggested that PI3K/Akt signaling pathway may be involved in the protection of astaxanthin in dry eye via regulating the expression of HMGB1 (Table 4) [74]. Furthermore, a study showed that astaxanthin encapsulated in liposomes was effective in preventing DED through promoting antioxidative effects (Table 4) [75].

Table 4. The anti-inflammatory effects of astaxanthin in skin and eye disorders.

Model	Dosage	Biomarkers	Disease	Ref
BALB/c mice	1-μL drop of 5 μM	HMGB1, TNF-α, IL-1β, PI3K/Akt	Dry eye disease	[74]
Male Sprague-Dawley rats	200 μM	DED-related factors	Dry eye disease	[75]
Male NC/Nga mice	100 mg/kg	Eotaxin, MIF, IL-4, IL-5 and L-histidine decarboxylase	Atopic dermatitis	[38]
HR-1 mice	10 μg or 20 μg/cm^2	IL-1β, IL-6, TNF-α, IgE, COX-2, NF-κB, iNOS	Atopic dermatitis	[76]

Atopic dermatitis (AD) is a common chronic inflammatory skin disease. The administration of astaxanthin can reduce the clinical skin severity score and the spontaneous scratching in AD mice via the regulation of the inflammatory effects (Table 4) [38], reduce the skin inflammation and allergic responses induced by PA treatment via inhibition of NF-κB signaling (Table 4) [76].

4. The Anti-Inflammatory Effects of Astaxanthin in Bacterial Infectious Diseases

Infection with *Helicobacter pylori* is a critical cause of gastrointestinal diseases, which stimulates the production of ROS and leads to the expression of inflammatory mediators in tissues [77]. The treatment of astaxanthin from shrimp cephalothorax influences cytokine release of splenocytes in *H. pylori*-infected mice with the increasing expression of IFN-γ, IL-10, and IL-2 (Table 5) [78]. Astaxanthin-rich algal meal showed an inhibitory effect on *H. pylori* growth and lower inflammation scores in a BALB/cA mouse model (Table 5) [79–81]. In human gastric epithelial cells, astaxanthin inhibited *H. pylori*-induced mitochondrial dysfunction and ROS-mediated IL-8 expression via activating peroxisome proliferator-activated receptors-γ (PPAR-γ) (Table 5) [82]. However, in patients with *H. pylori*, the treatment of astaxanthin had no significant effect on *H. pylori* growth or the expression of any of the interleukins, but with a significant up-regulation of CD4 and down-regulation of CD8 (Table 5) [83]. Although the inflammatory biomarkers regulated by astaxanthin are different between human and mice infected with *H. pylori*, all these data suggest the protective effects of astaxanthin against *H. pylori* infection.

Table 5. The anti-inflammatory effects of astaxanthin in infectious diseases.

Model	Dosage	Biomarkers	Disease	Ref
BALB/c female mice	10 or 40 mg/d	IFN-γ, IL-2 and IL-10	*Helicobacter pylori* infection	[78]
BALB/cA mice	10, 50, and 100 mg/kg	Bacterial load, the numbers of inflammatory cells	*Helicobacter pylori* infection	[79]
Balb/cA mice	200 mg per kg body weight per day	IFN-γ, IL-4, IL-2, bacterial load	*Helicobacter pylori* infection	[80]
Female BALB/c mice	100 mg/kg	IFN-γ, IL-4, bacterial load	*Helicobacter pylori* infection	[81]
Human gastric epithelial cell line AGS	5 μM	ROS, NF-κB, IL-8, PPAR-γ	*Helicobacter pylori* infection	[82]
Patients	40 mg daily	CD4, CD8	*Helicobacter pylori* infected	[83]

5. Conclusions and Future Directions

Massive evidences in vivo and in vitro have showed the anti-inflammatory effects and mechanisms of astaxanthin in mammals. Astaxanthin has been confirmed to alleviate chronic and acute inflammation invarious diseases, including neurodegenerative disorders, diabetes, gastrointestinal disease, renal inflammation, as well as skin and eye diseases in different experimental models, which demonstrate that astaxanthin can be an excellent candidate for treating inflammation-related diseases. Significantly, many clinical studies and reports also prove the effects of astaxanthin in cardioprotection, immune modulation, skin and cosmetic benefits, sport performance, ophthalmology and safety [84]. All these data suggest that astaxanthin will be a suitable multi-target pharmacological agent.

In addition to in mammals, astaxanthin is reported to play an important role in non-mammalian models. A dietary supplementation with astaxanthin was found to lessen immunopathology of mealworm beetle (*Tenebrio molitor*) through an immune depressive effect. The larvae fed with astaxanthin were more sensitive to the infection with *Bacillus cereus* and *B. thuringiensis* infection [85]. In common carp (*Cyprinus carpio*), dietary astaxanthin significantly increased the growth rate, respiratory burst activity, lysozyme activity and bactericidal activity. *C. carpio* fed with all astaxanthin enriched diets were more resistant for *Aeromonas hydrophila* infection [86]. The inconsistent roles of astaxanthin in infectious diseases suggest that more studies are needed to investigate the exact function of astaxanthin in response to different pathogen infection, especially in aquaculture animals.

Compared with the researches of astaxanthin in various chronic and acute diseases, only a few attempts have been made to elucidate the anti-inflammatory effects of astaxanthin in bacterial infectious diseases. There are few reports about the effect of astaxanthin in viral infection. A research showed that astaxanthin did not affect antiviral effects of IFN or ribavirin (RBV) against hepatitis C virus [87]. However, another research showed that astaxanthin has the potential antiviral effect via protecting cells from HPV L1 binding [88]. In Pacific white shrimp, astaxanthin could promote the mRNA expression of antioxidant enzyme gene and increase the resistance to white spot syndrome virus (WSSV) [89]. Significantly, since the pathogenesis and complications of many viral infectious diseases such as coronavirus disease 2019 (COVID-19) are also involved in the role of oxidative stress, inflammation, apoptosis, and autophagy [90–92], astaxanthin may be a promising candidate in combating viral infectious diseases. However, it's not clear at present whether the anti-inflammatory effects of astaxanthin or other functions of astaxanthin, such as antioxidative, anti-apoptosis, and autophagy-modulatory activities, have a protective effect for viral infectious diseases, especially for COVID-19 infection. More studies are needed to investigate the potential protective effects of astaxanthin in viral infectious diseases.

Author Contributions: Conceptualization, F.X. and M.X.C.; designing the structure of the paper, M.X.C. and F.X.; drafting the manuscript, M.X.C. and F.X.; review and editing the paper: M.X.C.; revising the manuscript, M.X.C. All authors have read and agreed to the published version of the manuscript.

Funding: This research did not receive any specific grant from funding agencies in the public, commercial, or not-for-profit sectors.

Conflicts of Interest: The authors declare no conflict of interest.

References

1. Zarneshan, S.N.; Fakhri, S.; Farzaei, M.H.; Khan, H.; Saso, L. Astaxanthin targets PI3K/Akt signaling pathway toward potential therapeutic applications. *Food Chem. Toxicol.* **2020**, *145*, 111714. [CrossRef] [PubMed]
2. Zheng, Y.F.; Bae, S.H.; Kwon, M.J.; Park, J.B.; Choi, H.D.; Shin, W.G.; Bae, S.K. Inhibitory effects of astaxanthin, β-cryptoxanthin, canthaxanthin, lutein, and zeaxanthin on cytochrome P450 enzyme activities. *Food Chem. Toxicol.* **2013**, *59*, 78–85. [CrossRef] [PubMed]
3. Bjerkeng, B.; Peisker, M.; Schwartzenberg, K.V.; Ytrestøyl, T.; Åsgård, T. Digestibility and muscle retention of astaxanthin in Atlantic salmon, Salmo salar, fed diets with the red yeast Phaffia rhodozyma in comparison with synthetic formulated astaxanthin. *Aquaculture* **2007**, *269*, 476–489. [CrossRef]
4. Wang, C.; Armstrong, D.W.; Chang, C.D. Rapid baseline separation of enantiomers and a mesoform of all-trans-astaxanthin, 13-cis-astaxanthin, adonirubin, and adonixanthin in standards and commercial supplements. *J. Chromatogr. A* **2008**, *1194*, 172–177. [CrossRef] [PubMed]
5. Stewart, J.S.; Lignell, A.; Pettersson, A.; Elfving, E.; Soni, M.G. Safety assessment of astaxanthin-rich microalgae biomass: Acute and subchronic toxicity studies in rats. *Food Chem. Toxicol.* **2008**, *46*, 3030–3036. [CrossRef]
6. Yuan, J.P.; Peng, J.; Yin, K.; Wang, J.H. Potential health-promoting effects of astaxanthin: A high-value carotenoid mostly from microalgae. *Mol. Nutr. Food Res.* **2011**, *55*, 150–165. [CrossRef]
7. Yuan, J.P.; Chen, F.; Liu, X.; Li, X.Z. Carotenoid composition in the green microalga Chlorococcum. *Food Chem.* **2002**, *76*, 319–325. [CrossRef]
8. Ambati, R.R.; Phang, S.M.; Ravi, S.; Aswathanarayana, R.G. Astaxanthin: Sources, extraction, stability, biological activities and its commercial applications—A review. *Mar. Drugs* **2014**, *12*, 128–152. [CrossRef]
9. Balietti, M.; Giannubilo, S.R.; Giorgetti, B.; Solazzi, M.; Turi, A.; Casoli, T.; Ciavattini, A.; Fattorettia, P. The effect of astaxanthin on the aging rat brain: Gender-related differences in modulating inflammation. *J. Sci. Food Agric.* **2016**, *96*, 615–618. [CrossRef]
10. Kurashige, M.; Okimasu, E.; Inoue, M.; Utsumi, K. Inhibition of oxidative injury of biological membranes by astaxanthin. *Physiol. Chem. Phys. Med. NMR* **1990**, *22*, 27–38.

11. Cai, X.; Chen, Y.; Xie, X.; Yao, D.; Ding, C.; Chen, M. Astaxanthin prevents against lipopolysaccharide-induced acute lung injury and sepsis via inhibiting activation of MAPK/NF-κB. *Am. J. Transl. Res.* **2019**, *11*, 1884–1894. [PubMed]
12. Kidd, P. Astaxanthin, cell membrane nutrient with diverse clinical benefits and anti-aging potential. *Altern. Med. Rev.* **2011**, *16*, 355–364. [PubMed]
13. Curek, G.D.; Cort, A.; Yucel, G.; Demir, N.; Ozturk, S.; Elpek, G.O.; Savas, B.; Aslan, M. Effect of astaxanthin on hepatocellular injury following ischemia/reperfusion. *Toxicology* **2010**, *267*, 147–153. [CrossRef] [PubMed]
14. Martin, H.D.; Jäger, C.; Ruck, C.; Schmidt, M. Anti- and prooxidant properties of carotenoids. *J. Fur Prakt. Chem.-Chem.-Ztg.* **1999**, *341*, 302–308. [CrossRef]
15. Seabra, L.M.J.; Pedrosa, L.F.C. Astaxanthin: Structural and functional aspects. *Rev. De Nutr.-Braz. J. Nutr.* **2010**, *23*, 1041–1050. [CrossRef]
16. Zhou, P.; Li, M.; Shen, B.; Yao, Z.; Bian, Q.; Ye, L.; Yu, H. Directed Coevolution of β-Carotene Ketolase and Hydroxylase and Its Application in Temperature-Regulated Biosynthesis of Astaxanthin. *J. Agric. Food Chem.* **2019**, *67*, 1072–1080. [CrossRef]
17. Newsome, R. Food colors. *Food Technol.* **1986**, *40*, 49–56.
18. Nguyen, K.D. Astaxanthin: A Comparative Case of Synthetic VS. Natural Production. Chemical and Biomolecular Engineering Publications and Other Works. 2013. Available online: http://trace.tennessee.edu/utk_chembiopubs/94.2013 (accessed on 6 May 2013).
19. Galasso, C.; Orefice, I.; Pellone, P.; Cirino, P.; Miele, R.; Ianora, A.; Brunet, C.; Sansone, C. On the Neuroprotective Role of Astaxanthin: New Perspectives? *Mar. Drugs* **2018**, *16*, 247. [CrossRef]
20. Davinelli, S.; Nielsen, M.E.; Scapagnini, G. Astaxanthin in Skin Health, Repair, and Disease: A Comprehensive Review. *Nutrients* **2018**, *10*, 522. [CrossRef]
21. Medzhitov, R. Inflammation 2010: New adventures of an old flame. *Cell* **2010**, *140*, 771–776. [CrossRef]
22. Nathan, C.; Ding, A. Nonresolving inflammation. *Cell* **2010**, *140*, 871–882. [CrossRef] [PubMed]
23. Kim, Y.S.; Young, M.R.; Bobe, G.; Colburn, N.H.; Milner, J.A. Bioactive food components, inflammatory targets, and cancer prevention. *Cancer Prev. Res.* **2009**, *2*, 200–208. [CrossRef] [PubMed]
24. Chen, L.; Deng, H.; Cui, H.; Fang, J.; Zuo, Z.; Deng, J.; Li, Y.; Wang, X.; Zhao, L. Inflammatory responses and inflammation-associated diseases in organs. *Oncotarget* **2017**, *9*, 7204–7218. [CrossRef] [PubMed]
25. Eckersall, P.D.; Bell, R. Acute phase proteins: Biomarkers of infection and inflammation in veterinary medicine. *Vet. J.* **2010**, *185*, 23–27. [CrossRef]
26. Murata, H.; Shimada, N.; Yoshioka, M. Current research on acute phase proteins in veterinary diagnosis: An overview. *Vet. J.* **2004**, *168*, 28–40. [CrossRef]
27. Murakami, A.; Ohigashi, H. Targeting NOX, INOS and COX-2 in inflammatory cells: Chemoprevention using food phytochemicals. *Int. J. Cancer* **2007**, *121*, 2357–2363. [CrossRef]
28. Choi, S.K.; Park, Y.S.; Choi, D.K.; Chang, H.I. Effects of astaxanthin on the production of NO and the expression of COX-2 and iNOS in LPS-stimulated BV2 microglial cells. *J. Microbiol. Biotechnol.* **2008**, *18*, 1990–1996.
29. Park, C.H.; Xu, F.H.; Roh, S.S.; Song, Y.O.; Uebaba, K.; Noh, J.S.; Yokozawa, T. Astaxanthin and Corni Fructus protect against diabetes-induced oxidative stress, inflammation, and advanced glycation end product in livers of streptozotocin-induced diabetic rats. *J. Med. Food* **2015**, *18*, 337–344. [CrossRef]
30. Baralic, I.; Andjelkovic, M.; Djordjevic, B.; Dikic, N.; Radivojevic, N.; Suzin-Zivkovic, V.; Radojevic-Skodric, S.; Pejic, S. Effect of Astaxanthin Supplementation on Salivary IgA, Oxidative Stress, and Inflammation in Young Soccer Players. *Evid. Based Complement. Alternat. Med.* **2015**, *2015*, 783761. [CrossRef]
31. Yoshihisa, Y.; Rehman, M.U.; Shimizu, T. Astaxanthin, a xanthophyll carotenoid, inhibits ultraviolet-induced apoptosis in keratinocytes. *Exp. Dermatol.* **2014**, *23*, 178–183. [CrossRef]
32. Cranford, T.L.; Enos, R.T.; Velázquez, K.T.; McClellan, J.L.; Davis, J.M.; Singh, U.P.; Nagarkatti, M.; Nagarkatti, P.S.; Robinson, C.M.; Murphy, E.A. Role of MCP-1 on inflammatory processes and metabolic dysfunction following high-fat feedings in the FVB/N strain. *Int. J. Obes.* **2016**, *40*, 844–851. [CrossRef] [PubMed]
33. Izumi-Nagai, K.; Nagai, N.; Ohgami, K.; Satofuka, S.; Ozawa, Y.; Tsubota, K.; Ohno, S.; Oike, Y.; Ishida, S. Inhibition of choroidal neovascularization with an anti-inflammatory carotenoid astaxanthin. *Invest. Ophthalmol. Vis. Sci.* **2008**, *49*, 1679–1685. [CrossRef] [PubMed]

34. Schoenborn, J.R.; Wilson, C.B. Regulation of interferon-gamma during innate and adaptive immune responses. *Adv. Immunol.* **2007**, *96*, 41–101. [PubMed]
35. Castro, F.; Cardoso, A.P.; Gonçalves, R.M.; Serre, K.; Oliveira, M.J. Interferon-Gamma at the Crossroads of Tumor Immune Surveillance or Evasion. *Front. Immunol.* **2018**, *9*, 847. [CrossRef]
36. Hwang, Y.H.; Hong, S.G.; Mun, S.K.; Kim, S.J.; Lee, S.J.; Kim, J.J.; Kang, K.Y.; Yee, S.T. The Protective Effects of Astaxanthin on the OVA-Induced Asthma Mice Model. *Molecules* **2017**, *22*, 2019. [CrossRef]
37. Kochi, T.; Shimizu, M.; Sumi, T.; Kubota, M.; Shirakami, Y.; Tanaka, T.; Moriwaki, H. Inhibitory effects of astaxanthin on azoxymethane-induced colonic preneoplastic lesions in C57/BL/KsJ-db/db mice. *BMC Gastroenterol.* **2014**, *14*, 212. [CrossRef]
38. Yoshihisa, Y.; Andoh, T.; Matsunaga, K.; Rehman, M.U.; Maoka, T.; Shimizu, T. Efficacy of Astaxanthin for the Treatment of Atopic Dermatitis in a Murine Model. *PLoS ONE* **2016**, *11*, e0152288. [CrossRef]
39. Speranza, L.; Pesce, M.; Patruno, A.; Franceschelli, S.; De Lutiis, M.A.; Grilli, A.; Felaco, M. Astaxanthin treatment reduced oxidative induced pro-inflammatory cytokines secretion in U937: SHP-1 as a novel biological target. *Mar. Drugs* **2012**, *10*, 890–899. [CrossRef]
40. Suzuki, Y.; Ohgami, K.; Shiratori, K.; Jin, X.H.; Ilieva, I.; Koyama, Y.; Yazawa, K.; Yoshida, K.; Kase, S.; Ohno, S. Suppressive effects of astaxanthin against rat endotoxin-induced uveitis by inhibiting the NF-kappaB signaling pathway. *Exp. Eye Res.* **2006**, *82*, 275–281. [CrossRef]
41. Li, J.; Wang, F.; Xia, Y.; Dai, W.; Chen, K.; Li, S.; Liu, T.; Zheng, Y.; Wang, J.; Lu, W.; et al. Astaxanthin Pretreatment Attenuates Hepatic Ischemia Reperfusion-Induced Apoptosis and Autophagy via the ROS/MAPK Pathway in Mice. *Mar. Drugs* **2015**, *13*, 3368–3387. [CrossRef]
42. Yang, X.; Guo, A.L.; Pang, Y.P.; Cheng, X.J.; Xu, T.; Li, X.R.; Liu, J.; Zhang, Y.Y.; Liu, Y. Astaxanthin Attenuates Environmental Tobacco Smoke-Induced Cognitive Deficits: A Critical Role of p38 MAPK. *Mar. Drugs* **2019**, *17*, 24. [CrossRef]
43. Vomund, S.; Schäfer, A.; Parnham, M.J.; Brüne, B.; Von Knethen, A. Nrf2, the Master Regulator of Anti-Oxidative Responses. *Int. J. Mol. Sci.* **2017**, *18*, 2772. [CrossRef] [PubMed]
44. Ahmed, S.M.; Luo, L.; Namani, A.; Wang, X.J.; Tang, X. Nrf2 signaling pathway: Pivotal roles in inflammation. *Biochim. Biophys. Acta Mol. Basis Dis.* **2017**, *1863*, 585–597. [CrossRef] [PubMed]
45. Liu, G.; Shi, Y.; Peng, X.; Liu, H.; Peng, Y.; He, L. Astaxanthin attenuates adriamycin-induced focal segmental glomerulosclerosis. *Pharmacology* **2015**, *95*, 193–200. [CrossRef] [PubMed]
46. Xu, L.; Zhu, J.; Yin, W.; Ding, X. Astaxanthin improves cognitive deficits from oxidative stress, nitric oxide synthase and inflammation through upregulation of PI3K/Akt in diabetes rat. *Int. J. Clin. Exp. Pathol.* **2015**, *8*, 6083–6094.
47. Kowshik, J.; Baba, A.B.; Giri, H.; Deepak Reddy, G.; Dixit, M.; Nagini, S. Astaxanthin inhibits JAK/STAT-3 signaling to abrogate cell proliferation, invasion and angiogenesis in a hamster model of oral cancer. *PLoS ONE* **2014**, *9*, e109114. [CrossRef]
48. Taksima, T.; Chonpathompikunlert, P.; Sroyraya, M.; Hutamekalin, P.; Limpawattana, M.; Klaypradit, W. Effects of Astaxanthin from Shrimp Shell on Oxidative Stress and Behavior in Animal Model of Alzheimer's Disease. *Mar. Drugs* **2019**, *17*, 628. [CrossRef]
49. Che, H.; Li, Q.; Zhang, T.; Wang, D.; Yang, L.; Xu, J.; Yanagita, T.; Xue, C.; Chang, Y.; Wang, Y. Effects of Astaxanthin and Docosahexaenoic-Acid-Acylated Astaxanthin on Alzheimer's Disease in APP/PS1 Double-Transgenic Mice. *J. Agric. Food Chem.* **2018**, *66*, 4948–4957. [CrossRef]
50. Grimmig, B.; Daly, L.; Subbarayan, M.; Hudson, C.; Williamson, R.; Nash, K.; Bickford, P.C. Astaxanthin is neuroprotective in an aged mouse model of Parkinson's disease. *Oncotarget* **2017**, *9*, 10388–10401. [CrossRef]
51. Shen, D.F.; Qi, H.P.; Ma, C.; Chang, M.X.; Zhang, W.N.; Song, R.R. Astaxanthin suppresses endoplasmic reticulum stress and protects against neuron damage in Parkinson's disease by regulating miR-7/SNCA axis. *Neurosci. Res.* **2020**, in press. [CrossRef]
52. Wang, C.C.; Shi, H.H.; Xu, J.; Yanagita, T.; Xue, C.H.; Zhang, T.T.; Wang, Y.M. Docosahexaenoic acid-acylated astaxanthin ester exhibits superior performance over non-esterified astaxanthin in preventing behavioral deficits coupled with apoptosis in MPTP-induced mice with Parkinson's disease. *Food Funct.* **2020**, *11*, 8038–8050. [CrossRef] [PubMed]

53. Xue, Y.; Qu, Z.; Fu, J.; Zhen, J.; Wang, W.; Cai, Y.; Wang, W. The protective effect of astaxanthin on learning and memory deficits and oxidative stress in a mouse model of repeated cerebral ischemia/reperfusion. *Brain Res. Bull.* **2017**, *131*, 221–228. [CrossRef] [PubMed]
54. Pan, L.; Zhou, Y.; Li, X.F.; Wan, Q.J.; Yu, L.H. Preventive treatment of astaxanthin provides neuroprotection through suppression of reactive oxygen species and activation of antioxidant defense pathway after stroke in rats. *Brain Res. Bull.* **2017**, *130*, 211–220. [CrossRef] [PubMed]
55. Wang, Y.L.; Zhu, X.L.; Sun, M.H.; Dang, Y.K. Effects of astaxanthin on axonal regeneration via cAMP/PKA signaling pathway in mice with focal cerebral infarction. *Eur. Rev. Med. Pharmacol. Sci.* **2019**, *23*, 135–143.
56. Nai, Y.; Liu, H.; Bi, X.; Gao, H.; Ren, C. Protective effect of astaxanthin on acute cerebral infarction in rats. *Hum. Exp. Toxicol.* **2018**, *37*, 929–936. [CrossRef]
57. Cakir, E.; Cakir, U.; Tayman, C.; Turkmenoglu, T.T.; Gonel, A.; Turan, I.O. Favorable Effects of Astaxanthin on Brain Damage due to Ischemia- Reperfusion Injury. *Comb. Chem. High Throughput Screen.* **2020**, *23*, 214–224. [CrossRef]
58. Zhang, J.; Ding, C.; Zhang, S.; Xu, Y. Neuroprotective effects of astaxanthin against oxygen and glucose deprivation damage via the PI3K/Akt/GSK3β/Nrf2 signaling pathway in vitro. *J. Cell Mol. Med.* **2020**, *24*, 8977–8985. [CrossRef]
59. Finnerup, N.B.; Haroutounian, S.; Kamerman, P.; Baron, R.; Bennett, D.L.; Bouhassira, D.; Cruccu, G.; Freeman, R.; Hansson, P.; Nurmikko, T.; et al. Neuropathic pain: An updated grading system for research and clinical practice. *Pain* **2016**, *157*, 1599–1606. [CrossRef]
60. Kuedo, Z.; Sangsuriyawong, A.; Klaypradit, W.; Tipmanee, V.; Chonpathompikunlert, P. Effects of Astaxanthin from *Litopenaeus Vannamei* on Carrageenan-Induced Edema and Pain Behavior in Mice. *Molecules* **2016**, *21*, 382. [CrossRef]
61. Sharma, K.; Sharma, D.; Sharma, M.; Sharma, N.; Bidve, P.; Prajapati, N.; Kalia, K.; Tiwari, V. Astaxanthin ameliorates behavioral and biochemical alterations in in-vitro and in-vivo model of neuropathic pain. *Neurosci. Lett.* **2018**, *674*, 162–170. [CrossRef]
62. Jiang, X.; Yan, Q.; Liu, F.; Jing, C.; Ding, L.; Zhang, L.; Pang, C. Chronic trans-astaxanthin treatment exerts antihyperalgesic effect and corrects co-morbid depressive like behaviors in mice with chronic pain. *Neurosci. Lett.* **2018**, *662*, 36–43. [CrossRef]
63. Fakhri, S.; Dargahi, L.; Abbaszadeh, F.; Jorjani, M. Astaxanthin attenuates neuroinflammation contributed to the neuropathic pain and motor dysfunction following compression spinal cord injury. *Brain Res. Bull.* **2018**, *143*, 217–224. [CrossRef]
64. Fakhri, S.; Dargahi, L.; Abbaszadeh, F.; Jorjani, M. Effects of astaxanthin on sensory-motor function in a compression model of spinal cord injury: Involvement of ERK and AKT signaling pathway. *Eur. J. Pain.* **2019**, *23*, 750–764. [CrossRef] [PubMed]
65. Newsholme, P.; Cruzat, V.F.; Keane, K.N.; Carlessi, R.; De Bittencourt, P.I., Jr. Molecular mechanisms of ROS production and oxidative stress in diabetes. *Biochem. J.* **2016**, *473*, 4527–4550. [CrossRef] [PubMed]
66. Landon, R.; Gueguen, V.; Petite, H.; Letourneur, D.; Pavon-Djavid, G.; Anagnostou, F. Impact of Astaxanthin on Diabetes Pathogenesis and Chronic Complications. *Mar. Drugs* **2020**, *18*, 357. [CrossRef] [PubMed]
67. Yasui, Y.; Hosokawa, M.; Mikami, N.; Miyashita, K.; Tanaka, T. Dietary astaxanthin inhibits colitis and colitis-associated colon carcinogenesis in mice via modulation of the inflammatory cytokines. *Chem. Biol. Interact.* **2011**, *193*, 79–87. [CrossRef]
68. Sakai, S.; Nishida, A.; Ohno, M.; Inatomi, O.; Bamba, S.; Sugimoto, M.; Kawahara, M.; Andoh, A. Astaxanthin, a xanthophyll carotenoid, prevents development of dextran sulphate sodium-induced murine colitis. *J. Clin. Biochem. Nutr.* **2019**, *64*, 66–72. [CrossRef]
69. Qiu, X.; Fu, K.; Zhao, X.; Zhang, Y.; Yuan, Y.; Zhang, S.; Gu, X.; Guo, H. Protective effects of astaxanthin against ischemia/reperfusion induced renal injury in mice. *J. Transl. Med.* **2015**, *13*, 28. [CrossRef]
70. Gao, D.; Wang, H.; Xu, Y.; Zheng, D.; Zhang, Q.; Li, W. Protective effect of astaxanthin against contrast-induced acute kidney injury via SIRT1-p53 pathway in rats. *Int. Urol. Nephrol.* **2019**, *51*, 351–358. [CrossRef]
71. Liu, N.; Chen, J.; Gao, D.; Li, W.; Zheng, D. Astaxanthin attenuates contrast agent-induced acute kidney injury in vitro and in vivo via the regulation of SIRT1/FOXO3a expression. *Int. Urol. Nephrol.* **2018**, *50*, 1171–1180. [CrossRef]

72. Li, S.; Takahara, T.; Fujino, M.; Fukuhara, Y.; Sugiyama, T.; Li, X.K.; Takahara, S. Astaxanthin prevents ischemia-reperfusion injury of the steatotic liver in mice. *PLoS ONE* **2017**, *12*, e0187810. [CrossRef] [PubMed]
73. Li, J.; Xia, Y.; Liu, T.; Wang, J.; Dai, W.; Wang, F.; Zheng, Y.; Chen, K.; Li, S.; Abudumijiti, H.; et al. Protective effects of astaxanthin on ConA-induced autoimmune hepatitis by the JNK/p-JNK pathway-mediated inhibition of autophagy and apoptosis. *PLoS ONE* **2015**, *10*, e0120440. [CrossRef] [PubMed]
74. Li, H.; Li, J.; Hou, C.; Li, J.; Peng, H.; Wang, Q. The effect of astaxanthin on inflammation in hyperosmolarity of experimental dry eye model in vitro and in vivo. *Exp. Eye Res.* **2020**, *197*, 108113. [CrossRef] [PubMed]
75. Shimokawa, T.; Fukuta, T.; Inagi, T.; Kogure, K. Protective effect of high-affinity liposomes encapsulating astaxanthin against corneal disorder in the in vivo rat dry eye disease model. *J. Clin. Biochem. Nutr.* **2020**, *66*, 224–232. [CrossRef]
76. Park, J.H.; Yeo, I.J.; Han, J.H.; Suh, J.W.; Lee, H.P.; Hong, J.T. Anti-inflammatory effect of astaxanthin in phthalic anhydride-induced atopic dermatitis animal model. *Exp. Dermatol.* **2018**, *27*, 378–385. [CrossRef]
77. Polk, D.B.; Peek, R.M., Jr. *Helicobacter pylori*: Gastric cancer and beyond. *Nat. Rev. Cancer* **2010**, *10*, 403–414. [CrossRef]
78. Davinelli, S.; Melvang, H.M.; Andersen, L.P.; Scapagnini, G.; Nielsen, M.E. Astaxanthin from Shrimp Cephalothorax Stimulates the Immune Response by Enhancing IFN-γ, IL-10, and IL-2 Secretion in Splenocytes of Helicobacter Pylori-Infected Mice. *Mar. Drugs* **2019**, *17*, 382. [CrossRef]
79. Wang, X.; Willén, R.; Wadström, T. Astaxanthin-rich algal meal and vitamin C inhibit *Helicobacter pylori* infection in BALB/cA mice. *Antimicrob. Agents Chemother.* **2000**, *44*, 2452–2457. [CrossRef]
80. Bennedsen, M.; Wang, X.; Willén, R.; Wadström, T.; Andersen, L.P. Treatment of H. pylori infected mice with antioxidant astaxanthin reduces gastric inflammation, bacterial load and modulates cytokine release by splenocytes. *Immunol. Lett.* **1999**, *70*, 185–189. [CrossRef]
81. Liu, B.H.; Lee, Y.K. Effect of total secondary carotenoids extracts from Chlorococcum sp on Helicobacter pylori-infected BALB/c mice. *Int. Immunopharmacol.* **2003**, *3*, 979–986. [CrossRef]
82. Kim, S.H.; Lim, J.W.; Kim, H. Astaxanthin Inhibits Mitochondrial Dysfunction and Interleukin-8 Expression in *Helicobacter pylori*-Infected Gastric Epithelial Cells. *Nutrients* **2018**, *10*, 1320. [CrossRef] [PubMed]
83. Andersen, L.P.; Holck, S.; Kupcinskas, L.; Kiudelis, G.; Jonaitis, L.; Janciauskas, D.; Permin, H.; Wadström, T. Gastric inflammatory markers and interleukins in patients with functional dyspepsia treated with astaxanthin. *FEMS Immunol. Med. Microbiol.* **2007**, *50*, 244–248. [CrossRef] [PubMed]
84. Fakhri, S.; Abbaszadeh, F.; Dargahi, L.; Jorjani, M. Astaxanthin: A mechanistic review on its biological activities and health benefits. *Pharmacol. Res.* **2018**, *136*, 1–20. [CrossRef] [PubMed]
85. Dhinaut, J.; Balourdet, A.; Teixeira, M.; Chogne, M.; Moret, Y. A dietary carotenoid reduces immunopathology and enhances longevity through an immune depressive effect in an insect model. *Sci. Rep.* **2017**, *7*, 12429. [CrossRef] [PubMed]
86. Jagruthi, C.; Yogeshwari, G.; Anbazahan, S.M.; Mari, L.S.; Arockiaraj, J.; Mariappan, P.; Sudhakar, G.R.; Balasundaram, C.; Harikrishnan, R. Effect of dietary astaxanthin against Aeromonas hydrophila infection in common carp, *Cyprinus carpio*. *Fish Shellfish Immunol.* **2014**, *41*, 674–680. [CrossRef]
87. Nakamura, M.; Saito, H.; Ikeda, M.; Hokari, R.; Kato, N.; Hibi, T.; Miura, S. An antioxidant resveratrol significantly enhanced replication of hepatitis C virus. *World J. Gastroenterol.* **2010**, *16*, 184–192. [CrossRef]
88. Donà, G.; Andrisani, A.; Tibaldi, E.; Brunati, A.M.; Sabbadin, C.; Armanini, D.; Ambrosini, G.; Ragazzi, E.; Bordin, L. Astaxanthin Prevents Human Papillomavirus L1 Protein Binding in Human Sperm Membranes. *Mar. Drugs* **2018**, *16*, 427. [CrossRef]
89. Wang, H.; Dai, A.; Liu, F.; Guan, Y. Effects of dietary astaxanthin on the immune response, resistance to white spot syndrome virus and transcription of antioxidant enzyme genes in Pacific white shrimp *Litopenaeus vannamei*. *Iran. J. Fish. Sci.* **2015**, *14*, 699–718.
90. Nasi, A.; McArdle, S.; Gaudernack, G.; Westman, G.; Melief, C.; Rockberg, J.; Arens, R.; Kouretas, D.; Sjölin, J.; Mangsbo, S. Reactive oxygen species as an initiator of toxic innate immune responses in retort to SARS-CoV-2 in an ageing population, consider N-acetylcysteine as early therapeutic intervention. *Toxicol. Rep.* **2020**, *7*, 768–771. [CrossRef]

91. Blanco-Melo, D.; Nilsson-Payant, B.E.; Liu, W.C.; Uhl, S.; Hoagland, D.; Møller, R.; Jordan, T.X.; Oishi, K.; Panis, M.; Sachs, D.; et al. Imbalanced Host Response to SARS-CoV-2 Drives Development of COVID-19. *Cell* **2020**, *181*, 1036–1045. [CrossRef]
92. Pehote, G.; Vij, N. Autophagy Augmentation to Alleviate Immune Response Dysfunction, and Resolve Respiratory and COVID-19 Exacerbations. *Cells* **2020**, *9*, 1952. [CrossRef] [PubMed]

Sample Availability: Samples of the compounds are not available from the authors.

Publisher's Note: MDPI stays neutral with regard to jurisdictional claims in published maps and institutional affiliations.

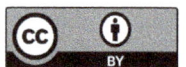

© 2020 by the authors. Licensee MDPI, Basel, Switzerland. This article is an open access article distributed under the terms and conditions of the Creative Commons Attribution (CC BY) license (http://creativecommons.org/licenses/by/4.0/).

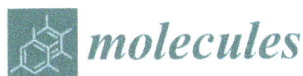

Review

Mast Cell Regulation and Irritable Bowel Syndrome: Effects of Food Components with Potential Nutraceutical Use

José Antonio Uranga [1], Vicente Martínez [2,3] and Raquel Abalo [1,4,*]

[1] High Performance Research Group in Physiopathology and Pharmacology of the Digestive System NeuGut-URJC, Department of Basic Health Sciences, Faculty of Health Sciences, Universidad Rey Juan Carlos (URJC), Campus de Alcorcón, Avda. de Atenas s/n, 28022 Madrid, Spain; jose.uranga@urjc.es

[2] Department of Cell Biology, Physiology and Immunology, Neurosciences Institute, Universitat Autònoma de Barcelona, 08193 Barcelona, Spain; vicente.martinez@uab.es

[3] Center for Networked Biomedical Research on Liver and Digestive Diseases (Centro de Investigación Biomédica en Red de Enfermedades Hepáticas y Digestivas, CIBERehd), Instituto de Salud Carlos III, 28029 Madrid, Spain

[4] Associated Unit to Institute of Medicinal Chemistry (Unidad Asociada I+D+i del Instituto de Química Médica, IQM), Spanish National Research Council (Consejo Superior de Investigaciones Científicas, CSIC), 28006 Madrid, Spain

* Correspondence: raquel.abalo@urjc.es; Tel.: +34-914-888854

Academic Editors: Sokcheon Pak and Soo Liang Ooi
Received: 30 July 2020; Accepted: 17 September 2020; Published: 20 September 2020

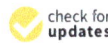

Abstract: Mast cells are key actors in inflammatory reactions. Upon activation, they release histamine, heparin and nerve growth factor, among many other mediators that modulate immune response and neuron sensitization. One important feature of mast cells is that their population is usually increased in animal models and biopsies from patients with irritable bowel syndrome (IBS). Therefore, mast cells and mast cell mediators are regarded as key components in IBS pathophysiology. IBS is a common functional gastrointestinal disorder affecting the quality of life of up to 20% of the population worldwide. It is characterized by abdominal pain and altered bowel habits, with heterogeneous phenotypes ranging from constipation to diarrhea, with a mixed subtype and even an unclassified form. Nutrient intake is one of the triggering factors of IBS. In this respect, certain components of the daily food, such as fatty acids, amino acids or plant-derived substances like flavonoids, have been described to modulate mast cells' activity. In this review, we will focus on the effect of these molecules, either stimulatory or inhibitory, on mast cell degranulation, looking for a nutraceutical capable of decreasing IBS symptoms.

Keywords: cannabidiol; fatty acids; heparin; histamine; irritable bowel syndrome; mast cells; nerve growth factor; nutraceuticals; polyphenols; visceral pain

1. Introduction

Amongst the many non-communicable chronic diseases, irritable bowel syndrome (IBS) is remarkable for its worldwide prevalence, variety of symptoms, diversity of etiologies, complicated diagnosis and high economic burden [1–4]. IBS has been classically described as a functional disorder of the gastrointestinal (GI) tract, in contrast with organic GI diseases (like inflammatory bowel disease, IBD), in which symptoms are explained by clear underlying pathogenic findings (namely, overt inflammation), although some overlapping has also been suggested [5]. Whereas the contribution of oxidative imbalances has been proposed more recently [6], low-grade/subtle inflammation is currently widely recognized to occur in IBS [7], leading to sensitization of local nerve fibers and, more importantly, to central sensitization [8]. Thus, IBS (like other functional GI disorders) is considered as a brain–gut axis disorder [9,10].

Although other immune cells may be involved in the pathophysiology of IBS, mast cells have been highlighted as important cell mediators of local nerve fiber sensitization [9]. Interestingly, these cells are well known for their role in the development of type 1 hypersensitization reactions, i.e., allergies, including those to different foods in particular patients [11]. However, it has been shown that specific components of food, i.e. some nutraceuticals, exert modulatory effects on these cells that may influence (increase or reduce) IBS symptoms. These nutraceuticals have been tested mostly in vitro, although some evidences have also been accumulated recently in preclinical in vivo models.

In this review, we will first describe the general features of mast cells, with particular focus on their pathophysiologic involvement in IBS. Thereafter, we will describe different nutraceuticals that have been studied for their possible modulatory effects on mast cell activity and, therefore, their potential role in triggering or inhibiting IBS symptoms. Importantly, their most likely molecular mechanisms of action will be discussed.

2. Mast Cells

Mast cells are immune cells with a widespread distribution. They are found in most vascularized tissues, although they are more abundant in the connective tissue of skin and mucosae, like those from respiratory, digestive and genitourinary tracts, where pathogens, allergens and other environmental agents may be encountered. In these locations, mast cells are mainly seen surrounding blood vessels, neurons or nerve fibers, muscle cells, glands and hair follicles [12,13].

Unlike other cells of hematopoietic origin derived from multipotent progenitors, mast cells do not differentiate in the bone marrow. Instead, they recapitulate the dual origin of macrophages and differentiate from yolk sac and bone marrow precursors, completing their maturation in a tissue-specific manner. This implies that there are several mast cells subtypes, depending not only on their origin but also on their final destination and expression profile [14–17]. Migration to tissues involves the expression of surface receptors and adhesion molecules, in coordination with cytoskeletal changes, to promote cell attachment to specialized regions of vascular endothelium and extravasation to particular areas of tissues. These changes vary in a tissue-specific manner according to the microenvironment of their final destination [16–18]. Regarding this, the gut and the respiratory tract have been the best-studied systems, with clear homing differences between them. Mast cells are abundant in the intestine, thanks to their constitutive expression of $\alpha 4\beta 7$ integrin that bind to the endothelial adhesion molecule VCAM-1 (vascular cell adhesion molecule 1). On the contrary, under physiological conditions, the lung does not have a significant number of mast cell progenitors, but their numbers greatly increase during allergen-induced pulmonary inflammation, when they are actively recruited [12]. In fact, the number of mast cells in the tissues does not only depend on recruitment from blood vessels, since they can enter mitosis and proliferate in their final destinations following appropriate stimulation [19].

Although no mast cell-specific chemokine has been described so far, mast cells express several chemokine receptors which could direct their migration. Similarly, the expression of receptors like CXCR2 (chemokine (C-X-C motif) ligand 2 (Interleukin 8 receptor beta)) by endothelial cells leads to an increase of VCAM-1, which facilitates the recruitment of mast cell progenitors [18]. Another crucial factor in mast cell function is the stem cell factor (SCF) or c-kit ligand (CD117). C-kit is expressed throughout all mast cell developmental stages, from progenitors to mature cells. However, it does not seem to be involved in cell recruitment to tissues but in survival [20] and maturation of mast cells following chemotactic gradients once they reach their target organ [18]. Likewise, fibroblast membrane-bound SCF induces mast cell maturation [21]. Apart from that, other growth factors and cytokines can regulate mast cell migration and proliferation. Thus, the Th1-specific transcription factor T-bet is necessary for mast cell homing to the lung and gut. Other factors, like the Th-2-associated cytokine interleukin (IL) 4 (IL-4) and the regulatory T cells (Treg) transforming growth factor (TGF) β1 (TGF-β1) are mutually antagonistic on mast cell survival and migration; whereas IL-4 promotes survival and proliferation, TGF-β1 suppresses these processes and induces apoptosis. Other factors like IL-10, tumor necrosis factor α (TNF-α) and nerve growth factor (NGF) are also involved in mast cell physiology in an ambivalent way, since the former limits the cell migration led by TNF-α and NGF [13,18,22]. Finally, lipid mediators have also been described to play a role in mast cell maturation and homing. Bone marrow-derived mast cell (BMMC) progenitors respond chemotactically to leukotriene (LT) B4 (LTB4) but become unresponsive to LTB4 after maturation. On the contrary, prostaglandin (PG) E2 (PGE2) is an active chemotactic agent for more mature mast cells and may be involved in localization within tissues, rather than in the recruitment of progenitors from the circulation [18,23].

Once mast cells become mature, they show a distinctive feature: their large electron-dense cytoplasmic granules. The content of such granules was firstly identified as heparin and histamine [12], although mature mast cells can store and secrete a much wider variety of active products, from cytokines to proteases (Table 1). Interestingly, mast cells have been classified in humans according to their protease content: those containing predominantly tryptase (T type), which are mainly located in mucosae (i.e., colon), also known as mucosal mast cells, and connective tissue mast cells, with both tryptase and chymase as major proteases (TC type) [16,24]. It is important to note that these subtypes, and their specific proteases, may differ substantially between species, and especially between humans and rodents. This is something to consider when working with animal models [16,25]. Similarly, some plasticity can be seen between both types. In vitro studies have shown that T mast cells can alter their cytokine and protease profile after incubation with IL-4, IL-6, lipopolysaccharide (LPS) or TGF-β1 in the presence of SCF [24,26]. Also, production of heparin can be modified according to cell microenvironment in a reversible way [27,28]. Thus, the composition of granules is not homogenous, but influenced by genetic or environmental factors that modify the functional properties of mast cells [13].

Table 1. Molecules that may be secreted by mast cells [a].

Category	Specific Molecules
Biogenic amines	Histamine, 5-HT, Dopamine, Polyamines
Lysosomal Enzymes	β-hexosaminidase, β-glucuronidase, β-D-galactosidase, Arylsulphatase A, Cathepsins
Proteases	Chymase, Tryptase, Carboxypeptidase A, Granzyme B, MMPs, Renin
Other Enzymes	Kinogenases, Heparanase, Angiogenin, Caspase-3, COX 1 and 2
Proteoglycans/Glycosaminoglycans	Serglycin, Heparin
Cytokines	TNF, IL-1, IL-2, IL-3, IL-4, IL-5, IL-6, IL-8, IL-9, IL-10, IL-11, IL-12, IL-13IL-15, IL-16 IL-17, IL-18, IL-25, IL-33, IFN, MIP-1α and 2β
Chemokines	RANTES (CCL5), eotaxin (CCL11), MCP-1 (CCL2), MCP-3 (CCL7), MCP-4
Growth Factors	TGF-β, VEGF, NGF, SCF, GM-CSF, FGF, NGF, PDGF, LIF
Peptides	CRF, Endorphin, ET-1, Cathelicidin (LL37), Defensins, SP, VIP
Phospholipid Metabolites	PGD2, PGE2, LTB4, LTC4, PAF
Reactive Oxygen Species	NO
Others	MBP, Complement Factors C3 and C5

[a] Adapted from References [12,29]. See abbreviations at the end of the article.

In order to carry out their functions, mast cells can recognize antigens thanks to a wide range of receptors, including toll-like receptors (TLRs, indirect receptors that recognize pathogen-associated molecular patterns, PAMPs), immunoglobulin (Ig) receptors and complement, but also specific G-coupled receptors (MRGPRX2, MAS-related G protein coupled receptor-X2) for a wide range of neuropeptides and basic molecules [30–32]. The expression of these receptors depends on the subtype of mast cell. For example, MRGPRX2 is barely expressed in mucosal mast cells [30]. Expression of some receptors might even be inducible, as seems to be the case for TLRs (although reports on this are somehow conflicting [32,33]). After antigen binding, the response of mast cells will be also specific according to the specific receptor activated and the subtype of mast cell affected [30]. Regarding TLRs, their activation induces the nuclear translocation of nuclear factor κβ (NFκβ) in the nucleus to induce the transcription of cytokines. Particularly, TLR2 recognizes mainly PAMPs from Gram-positive bacteria, which causes the release of cytokines, such as IL-4, and histamine. LPS from Gram-negative bacteria binds to TLR4, which induces the release of pro-inflammatory cytokines (TNF-α, IL-1, IL-6) [32,34,35].

Similarly, MRGPRX2 are receptors for sensing molecules from Gram-positive bacteria triggering mast cell degranulation [35].

However, the best-studied mechanism of mast cell activation is that mediated by the IgE receptor (FcεRI, high-affinity IgE receptor) pathway. IgE antibodies are produced by mature B cells in response to CD4+ Th2 cells. They are mostly found bound to FcεRI receptors on the mast cell surface. These receptors are constitutively expressed as tetrameric receptors composed of an IgE-binding α chain, a membrane β chain and two γ chains, found as a disulfide-linked homodimer. IgE binding to FcεRI initiates phosphorylation cascades that cause degranulation, activation of transcription factors and synthesis of cytokines. Similarly, intracellular calcium concentration is increased by inositol-1,4,5-triphosphate (IP3) production, which releases calcium from the endoplasmic reticulum. Calcium activates and causes NFκB to translocate to the cell nucleus, which results again in transcription of cytokines. In addition, mast cells also express Fc receptors for IgA and IgG, although with less sensitivity [29,36,37].

The variety and specificity of the secreted products after the stimulation of mast cell receptors make these cells a main actor of the immune response. In fact, it is considered that enhancing host resistance to toxins and acute inflammation in response to pathogens might be the original function of these cells [13]. This goes beyond mast cells just being effectors of hypersensitivity reactions classically associated with allergy. They release mediators that increase vascular permeability, fluid accumulation and recruitment of immune cells, such as eosinophils, natural killer (NK) cells, neutrophils and additional mast cells [30,38], but also stimulate, through their ILs, the antigen presentation activity of dendritic cells to cytotoxic T cells. Additionally, they may also activate cytotoxic T cells directly [39]. Moreover, mast cells produce antibacterial products, such as cathelicidins and defensins, and also contribute to antiviral responses by recruiting CD8+ T cells, which produce interferon α (IFN-α) and β (IFN-β) [38]. Thus, mast cells may be considered multifunctional immune cells that, after the appropriate stimuli, mediate pro- or anti-inflammatory and/or immunosuppressive activities, both innate and adaptive, against viral, microbial and parasitic pathogens, autoimmunity and response to graft rejection, among others.

Apart from this, the variety of products that mast cells may release makes them important effectors of other non-immune functions. For instance, they stimulate keratinocytes and fibroblast during scar remodeling and reepithelization in wound healing [40]. Also, mast cells are implicated in the pathogenesis of inflammatory disorders, like atherosclerosis and aortic aneurysms, by releasing IL-6 and IFN-γ that increase the expression of matrix proteases and elastase, leading to muscle apoptosis and vascular wall remodeling [41]. During systemic hypoxia, mast cells degranulate and mediate vascular inflammatory response after reactive oxygen species (ROS) generation [38]. This mechanism of activation is also responsible for mast cell activation during the reperfusion phase after ischemia. During this process, mast cells release mediators like histamine, tryptase and chymase that increase leukocyte adhesion to endothelium and vascular permeability [42]. Their effect on endothelial cells has also been shown in certain cancers, like skin or pancreatic tumors, where they induce angiogenesis [43]. In these regards, Gounaris and collaborators have studied the effect of mast cells in colorectal cancer using an animal model defective for the adenomatous polyposis coli (APC) gene [44], a commonly mutated gene in this kind of tumors [45]. They found an increased number of mast cells at the place of polyp formation and an important remission of the lesions after mast cell depletion. However, conflicting results were obtained when APC-deficient mice were crossed with Sash mice, a mouse strain deficient for mast cells. In this case, the lack of mast cells was associated to an increase in the number and size of polyps [46]. The exact role of mast cell secretome in cancer is yet to be elucidated. However, these authors speculate that the stage of tumors could explain this result since a protective effect of the inflammatory system, by means of promoting apoptosis, is observed in early stages of tumorigenesis, while the opposite is observed at later stages, when inflammatory mediators would promote tumor progression stimulating angiogenesis [46].

Overall, mast cells display important roles in immune and non-immune functions throughout the body. Their involvement in IBS will be succinctly described next.

3. Mast Cells and Irritable Bowel Syndrome

Irritable bowel syndrome (IBS) is a common digestive functional disorder that seriously affects the quality of life of up to 20% of the population worldwide [1,3,47]. It is characterized by abdominal pain and altered bowel habits with heterogeneous phenotypes that range from IBS with predominant constipation (IBS-C) to IBS with predominant diarrhea (IBS-D), with a mixed subtype (IBS-M) and even an unclassified form (IBS-U) in patients who do not meet the previous criteria [2,48]. The pathogenesis of IBS is hardly understood, and the lack of tissue or molecular markers, on the one side, and that of animal models expressing all the symptoms, on the other, constitute main challenges that hamper the development of effective therapeutic approaches. However, experimental and clinical work during the last two decades has shown that altered mucosal and immune functions, enteric microbiota and nervous communication between gut and brain, play a central role in the perceptions described by patients [49].

The enteric immune system comprises a large diversity of immune cells, like mast cells, that may be sensitized and activate the inflammatory cascade in response to both extrinsic (parasites, viruses, bacteria and food) and intrinsic factors (hormones and neurotransmitters from the central nervous system, CNS). Exposure of the GI tract to an antigen also may increase fluid secretion, smooth muscle contraction and peristalsis. This highlights the intimate relationship between immune cells and enteric neurons [38].

The enteric nervous system (ENS) comprises two ganglionic plexuses. The myenteric plexus is located between the longitudinal and the circular muscle layers and is the main responsible agent controlling gut motility. The submucous plexus is located between the inner muscle layer and the mucosa and is mainly involved in interganglion communication and secretory functions. The ENS is in contact with the CNS through afferent sensory neurons and sympathetic and parasympathetic efferent neurons. Both efferent and afferent nerve fibers ramify substantially and make contact not only with enteric neurons but also with immune cells [50,51].

When an antigen permeates through the mucosa, a direct or indirect activation of mast cells' receptors may happen, leading to degranulation and release of their mediators, as described above. The importance of mast cells in the regulation and recruitment of immune cells to the gut became highlighted when using mast cell-deficient animal models. In these animals, oral antigen sensitization did not cause immune cell infiltration in the digestive tract, unlike that observed in wild-type animals [52]. Moreover, histamine, one of the more important products secreted by mast cells, is increased in GI diseases like IBD and modulates functions of the submucous plexus, such as ion transport and neuron excitation [53,54]. Cytokines released from mast cells have pro-secretory effects in the colon [55], and the serine protease tryptase, one of the more abundant elements of mast cells secretome [56], induces the production of inflammatory mediators in IBD patients [50]. These mediators increase the excitability of enteric sensory nerves [57], which is facilitated by the close proximity between nerve endings and mast cells [58]. Indeed, it has been estimated that 90% of intestinal mucosal mast cells are in direct contact with or very close to nerves [50,58]. Similarly, mast cells can be activated by neuropeptides such as substance P (SP), resulting in the release of proteases, i.e., as a conditioned response to cold pain stress [57]. In fact, a CNS interaction with mast cells may be considered the link between stress and GI symptoms. Interestingly, in vitro observations suggest that acetylcholine promotes histamine release from mast cells, whereas degranulation and mast cell proliferation is suppressed by sympathetic activation and β2 adrenoreceptor activation [59]. Indeed, mast cells are relevant for maintaining gut homeostasis and a correct response to injury, environmental pathogens and stress [50,60]. Regarding this, stress and early adverse life events are tightly associated with IBS and even animal models of IBS have been developed under these bases [61]. In particular, rats subjected to wrap restraint stress (WRS), and pups separated from their mother, known as the maternal separation (MS) model, develop some of the typical findings of IBS, including mast cell hyperplasia close to mucosal nerve endings [62]. These effects are related to the stress-mediated release of corticotropin-releasing factor (CRF) and the subsequent activation of CRF-mediated responses. In fact, in humans, CRF acting on mast cells induces degranulation and the release of tryptase, TNF-α and histamine, resulting in visceral hypersensitivity and increased intestinal permeability, distinctive components of IBS pathophysiology. On the contrary, GI effects of stress are reduced by administration of selective CRF receptor antagonists, mast cell stabilizers and protease inhibitors [60,63,64].

Two main in vitro approaches have been assayed to study IBS: biopsies from IBS patients or cultured cells or organoids treated with extracts from human biopsies or fecal supernatants from IBS patients [61]. IBS biopsies show an increased occurrence of mast cells in the *lamina propria* compared with healthy controls [65]. Accordingly, the concentration of products from mast cells, like histamine, proteases, cytokines and PGs, is increased in mucosal biopsies and stool of IBS patients [66–69]. Interestingly, this correlates with IBS symptoms and may be the cause of the sensitization of enteric neurons and visceral afferents [66–74]. Similarly, mast cell mediators have also been observed to correlate with signal intensity in mesenteric afferent nerve recordings of isolated rat jejunum previously perfused with human IBS supernatants [75,76]. Sensitization has also been shown in dorsal root ganglia (DRG) neurons cultured with serine proteases or mast cell mediators released from human colonic IBS-D biopsies [76–78].

The importance of mast cells in intestinal nerve sensitization can be appreciated using mast cell stabilizers, like ketotifen or disodium cromoglycate (DSCG). Indeed, treatment with ketotifen significantly decreased abdominal pain, bloating, flatulence and diarrhea in IBS patients [79]. Similarly, DSCG administration resulted in a clinical improvement of symptoms in IBS-D patients after decreasing the expression of TLRs and the release of tryptase [80,81]. However, no clinical trials using these drugs are found in the ClinicalTrial.gov registry. Anti-inflammatory drugs like 5-aminosalicylic acid (5-ASA, also known as mesalamine or mesalazine) decreased the number of mast cells and their associated products of secretion, although some reports also indicate a lack of effects modulating mast cell density [82]. Despite that mesalazine has been tested in several formally registered clinical trials, its effects on colonic symptoms are not consistent [83,84]. However, the topic still raises interest and a new meta-analysis has been recently prospectively registered in PROSPERO (CRD42019147860) with the intention to provide high-quality synthesis on existing evidence for the usefulness of mesalazine on IBS [85]. Interestingly, other alternatives are being explored, like AST-10 (a carbon adsorbent capable of adsorbing low molecular substances like histamine and serotonin; ClinicalTrial.gov identifier: NCT00583128), with relatively modest results [86], or, more recently, zeolite (a volcanic mineral with absorptive properties; amongst others, the researchers will study histamine-associated readouts; ClinicalTrial.gov identifier: NCT03817645), with no results yet (currently in recruitment phase). The interference with mast cell mediators may also be an alternative for IBS patients. In this sense, the most convincing (and specific) results are those obtained with the H_1 histamine-receptor antagonist ebastine, which decreased abdominal pain and visceral hypersensitivity in a clinical trial with 50 patients (ClinicalTrials.gov identifier: NCT01144832), whose results were published in 2016 [87]. More recently, an additional multi-center clinical trial with 200 patients was registered (ClinicalTrials.gov identifier: NCT01908465), although no further information is yet available. Although promising, the scarce number of patients in these trials preclude definitive answers and makes further replication necessary [60,88]. The message is, though, that some beneficial effects might be offered by other substances with similar mechanisms of action, including food components.

Apart from their effect on enteric nerve endings, proteases released by mast cells may also affect the integrity of the colonic mucosa. The mucosal barrier acts as a semipermeable barrier allowing the absorption of nutrients but limiting the transport of potentially harmful antigens and microorganisms. A number of studies have suggested that an increase in intestinal permeability could be a key factor of IBS progression. Indeed, the permeability of biopsies from IBS patients is increased compared to normal individuals [89,90], as also occurs with the permeability of animal mucosa samples treated with fecal supernatants from IBS patients [91]. Likewise, permeability of human cultured colonic cells was increased after incubation with supernatants of human IBS biopsies [89–93] or fecal supernatants from IBS patients [94].

Interestingly, the effects of proteases may be different depending on the type of IBS considered. Specifically, serine proteases levels are elevated in IBS-D patients [91]. On the contrary, cysteine proteases are predominant in the feces of the constipation variant [94]. Both degrade different adhesive proteins. Likewise, release of tryptase from mast cells increases permeability in vivo and in vitro, opening tight junctions after degrading junctional adhesion molecule (JAM), a key adhesive molecule [89,95,96]. The effect of mucosal damage may also be seen in patients suffering from post-infectious IBS (PI-IBS), a form of IBS that may occur after acute infectious gastroenteritis [97]. In this case, patients exhibit greater expression of proinflammatory products from mast cells, like IL-1β [98].

Overall, these studies clearly suggest that barrier function breakdown, with the possibility of bacterial invasion and low-grade immune system activation, plays an important role in the development of IBS symptoms, including pain hypersensitivity. This effect can be reinforced by the direct activation of mast cells in stress situations [99]. This highlights the consideration of IBS as a brain–gut axis disorder [10].

Besides the factors mentioned above, and strengthening a pivotal role of diet in IBS, compelling evidences show a link between food components, mast cells and IBS-related pathophysiology. In particular, gluten and diets rich in fermentable oligosaccharides, disaccharides, monosaccharides and polyols (FODMAPs) have received significant attention. FODMAPs are associated with the development of IBS or, at least, IBS-related symptoms, since short-chain carbohydrates pass unaltered into the colon, where they are fermented, generating gas and distention [99–101] and, subsequently, low FODMAPs diets have been successfully used to reduce IBS symptoms [101–105]. FODMAPs-induced IBS symptomatology might involve the recruitment and activation of mast cells [99]. Indeed, recent pre-clinical data show that the effects of FODMAPs diets in different animal models of IBS might be related to an increase in colonic mast cells [106,107]. Moreover, changes in histamine levels, one of the key mediators released during mast cell activation, are reduced in IBS patients under a low FODMAPs diet, thus indicating a potential modulation of mast cell activity [104].

A role for gluten in IBS pathophysiology is supported by the fact that a gluten-free diet ameliorates IBS symptomatology, while IBS symptoms are induced following the ingestion of gluten in patients with IBS [100,108]. However, there are questions regarding which components of wheat are implicated in these responses and the underlying mechanisms. In any case, mast cells have a relevant role in the pathophysiology of celiac disease [109], thus indicating that they might also be involved in the generation of IBS symptomatology.

Other dietary interventions have focused on different carbohydrates or fiber composition (like the paleo diet, the specific carbohydrate diet and the diet for sucrose-isomaltase deficiency), on proteins (such as the reduced resistant protein diet), or on bioactive molecules (such as the low amine/histamine diet, the low capsaicin diet and the low food chemical diet). Although further investigation is needed for the use of these diets in the clinical practice, it seems clear that there is a large array of potential harmful molecules for patients with IBS [110].

Altogether, these observations further support the view that mast cells should be regarded as a target in the treatment of IBS, subjected to potential diet/nutraceutical interventions.

4. Nutraceuticals Affecting Mast Cell Activity

Mast cells' activity can be modulated by different stimuli, with stimulation via the FcεRI being the best-established activation signal. Since aggregation of IgE and subsequent FcεRI activation on mast cells initiates type I allergic reactions, nutrient-associated modulation of mast cells has been directed mainly towards allergic reactions [111,112]. However, mast cell activation and degranulation, as well as synthesis of mediators, can also be modulated by several IgE-FcεRI-independent mechanisms [113]. In any case, although functional and inflammatory GI disorders are not allergic processes, immune-related mechanisms linked to dietary antigens might have relevance in their pathophysiology [114–118]. Moreover, connection between IgE-mediated responses and IBS may be not only local, but also systemic. Indeed, IBS prevalence is higher in patients suffering from atopic IgE-dependent diseases than in healthy populations, and atopic diseases could predispose to developing IBS [118].

Numerous food components have been shown to manifest immunomodulatory capacities as it relates to mast cell functioning, acting as modulators of mast cell activation/degranulation or/and modulating the synthesis of mediators (see Tables 2–8). The bioactivity of these nutrients could be used by applying them as nutraceuticals in the context of diverse mast cell-associated diseases through the downregulation of mast cell activation. Given the key role played by mast cells in GI functional, particularly IBS [119,120], and inflammatory disorders [121,122], a potential application of these nutraceuticals is envisaged in the management of these conditions. It is important to note that most of the data available so far derives from in vitro observations in relevant systems (different human- and rodent-derived mast cell lines and isolated mast cells), with only a few in vivo studies in relevant animal models or clinical trials. Indeed, the clinical trials performed so far are very limited and a direct relationship between mast cells and the possible positive effects observed at a clinical level cannot be established. Thus, such a link can only be hypothesized, so far, taking into account preclinical, in vitro and in vivo, observations.

4.1. Lipids

Lipid-rich enteral feeding significantly decreased circulatory levels of mouse mast cell protease, compared with isocaloric low-lipid nutrition or fasting, thus indicating a potential role for diet-derived lipids as immunomodulatory agents with effects on intestinal mast cells' activity [123]. Although the mechanisms of action are not fully elucidated, direct effects of immunomodulatory lipids on mast cells' degranulation, changes in local lipid composition and changes in lipid transport affecting mast cells' reactivity are possible mechanisms by which the function of mast cells might be modulated by diet-derived lipidic compounds [124]. These actions open the use of specific lipids as nutraceuticals with the aim of reducing mast cell activity and therefore the undesired neuro-immune-endocrine responses associated.

4.1.1. Fatty Acids

Evidences indicate that different fatty acids are able to modulate the synthesis and release of mast cell mediators [125]. Effects observed were fatty-acid-specific and included both facilitation and inhibition of release, depending upon the mediators considered (Table 2). Main evidences derive from in vitro studies based on the incubation of human mast cell lines (mainly LAD-2 and HMC-1) or BMMCs with different fatty acids, assessing the release of different mediators. In this respect, the n-6 long-chain polyunsaturated fatty acid (PUFA) arachidonic acid (AA) or the n-3 long-chain PUFAs eicosapentaenoic acid (EPA) or docosahexaenoic acid (DHA) affected mast cell activation, although they did not affect IgE-mediated mast cell degranulation [126]. Similarly, α-linolenic acid (ALA) and its metabolites, including EPA and DHA, decreased the in vitro production of ILs [127] and PGD2 [128]. In a different study, EPA and DHA reduced TNF-α release from HMC-1 cells but did not affect degranulation [129]. Overall, n-3 long-chain PUFAs were associated with anti-inflammatory/antiallergic effects, while n-6 long-chain PUFAs seem to be related with proinflammatory/proallergic responses.

Similar modulatory activity was observed in a canine mastocytoma cell line (C2). Specifically, γ-linolenic acid (GLA) (n-6) increased tryptase activity and decreased histamine release in stimulated C2 cells and DHA (n-3) reduced PGE2 production. On the other hand, ALA (n-3) caused a reduction of tryptase activity, PGE2 production as well as histamine release, while linoleic acid or AA (n-6) increased them [130–132]. No effects were observed on chymase activity. Thus, ALA (n-3) exhibited specific anti-inflammatory effects, at least as it relates to cultured canine mastocytoma cells.

In an in vivo approach, a diet rich in n-6 linoleic acid, saturated fatty acids (safflower oil), but not monounsaturated fatty acids (coconut oil) or n-3 PUFAs (fish oil), reduced circulatory release of chymase II, as a marker for degranulation of mucosal mast cells, in an intestinal mast cell-IgE-mediated inflammatory reaction model in rats [133]. These effects were associated with an enrichment of linoleic acid in the mast cell membrane, which altered the membrane structure and resulted in a reduced number and/or affinity of IgE receptors. However, a direct inhibitory effect of linoleic acid or its metabolites on IgE-mediated degranulation might also be possible [133]. These observations were further confirmed in a murine atopic model in which oral administration of fish oil, containing high levels of omega-3 fatty acids, significantly reduced the severity of dermatitis and the thickening of epidermis/dermis [127]. However, in a model of stress-induced visceral hypersensitivity in maternally-separated rats, a model associated with mast cell hyperactivity and, as previously mentioned, regarded as relevant for the study of IBS pathophysiology, a diet enriched in n-3 PUFAs (tuna oil) did not affect hypersensitivity nor mast cell degranulation [129].

Short-chain fatty acids (namely acetate, propionate and butyrate) have been suggested to modulate inflammatory responses within the gut, including the inhibition of the release of mast cell-derived proinflammatory mediators [134,135]. Following these observations, in an in vivo study, sodium butyrate supplementation improved intestinal health in pigs, an effect associated with a reduction in the percentage of degranulated mast cells and the content of its inflammatory mediators (histamine, tryptase, TNF-α and IL-6) in the mucosa of the jejunum. Moreover, a reduction in mast cell expression of tryptase, TNF-α and IL-6 was also observed [136].

Table 2. Immunomodulatory effects of fatty acids on mast cell activity.

Compound	System	Effect [a]	Mechanism of Action	Reference
\multicolumn{5}{c}{In Vitro Studies}				
AA (20:4n-6)	LAD2 HMC-1	↑ PGD2 ↑ TNF-α	ROS generation and MAPK signaling	[126]
AA (20:4n-6)	C2	↑ Tryptase activity ↑ PGE2 production ↑ Histamine release	Changes in cellular redox state and lipid peroxidation (suggested)	[132]
ALA (18:3n-3)	MC/9, BMMCs	↓ IL-4, IL-5 and IL-13 production	Modulation of nuclear expression of GATA-1 and GATA-2	[127]
ALA (18:3n-3)	C2	↓ Tryptase activity ↓ PGE2 production ↓ Histamine release		[130,131]
DHA (226n-3)	LAD2 HMC-1	↓ Il-4 ↓ IL-13 ↓ ROS generation	MAPK signaling	[126]
DHA (22:6n-3)	HMC-1	↓ TNF-α release	PPARγ-dependent activation	[129]
EPA (20:5n-3)	LAD2 HMC-1	↓ Il-4 ↓ IL-13 ↓ ROS generation	MAPK signaling	[126]
EPA (20:5n-3)	Mast cells cultured from human umbilical cord mononuclear cells	↓ PGD2 generation	Inhibition of COX-1 and COX-2 activities	[128]
EPA (20:5n-3)	MC/9, BMMCs	↓ IL-4, Il-5 and IL-13 production	Modulation of nuclear expression of GATA-1 and GATA-2	[127]
EPA (20:5n-3)	HMC-1	↓ TNF-α release	PPARγ-dependent activation	[129]
EPA (20:5n-3)	MC/9, BMMCs	↓ IL-4, Il-5 and IL-13 production	Modulation of nuclear expression of GATA-1 and GATA-2	[127]
EPA (20:5n-3)	C2	↑ PGE2 production ↑ Histamine release	Changes in cellular redox state and lipid peroxidation (suggested)	[132]
GLA (18:3n-6)	C2	↑ Tryptase activity ↑ Histamine release		[130,131]

Table 2. Cont.

Compound	System	Effect ᵃ	Mechanism of Action	Reference
In Vivo Studies				
Diet rich in n-6 linoleic acid, saturated fatty acids (safflower oil)	Intestinal mast cell-IgE-mediated inflammatory reaction model in rats	↓ Rat chymase II		[133]
Fish oil containing high level of omega-3 fatty acids	NC/Nga murine atopic model.	↓ Severity of dermatitis ↓ Thickening of epidermis/dermis ↓ Histamine content		[127]
Sodium butyrate (SCFA)	Pig	↓ Tryptase content/expression ↓ TNF-α content/expression ↓ IL-6 content/expression	JNK signaling pathways	[136]

ᵃ: ↑: Facilitation; ↓: Inhibition. See abbreviations at the end of the article.

4.1.2. Cannabinoids, Cannabinoid-Related Compounds and Other Lipidic Molecules

Cannabidiol is a non-psychoactive cannabinoid with positive effects on intestinal health that has been suggested as a potential nutraceutical because of its effects on the endocannabinoid system (see Reference [137] for a recent review on the topic). In a murine model of LPS-induced intestinal inflammation, cannabidiol prevented the associated upregulation of mast cell chymase and matrix metalloproteinase (MMP) 9 (MMP9), thus suggesting a potential anti-inflammatory effect mediated, at least partially, through the modulation of mast cell activity [138].

Palmithoylethanolamide, the saturated fatty acid amide of palmitic acid, is a dietary component commonly found in egg yolk and peanuts, structurally related to the endocannabinoid anandamide. Palmithoylethanolamide has been considered as an endogenous modulator of mast cell activation (see Reference [139] for review). Palmithoylethanolamide modulated the activity of the endocannabinoid system in mast cells, thus potentiating its beneficial effects on inflammation. Moreover, palmithoylethanolamide has been shown to prevent IgE-induced degranulation in isolated canine skin mast cells (histamine, PGD2 and TNF-α release) [140]. Similar results were also observed in human mast cells (HMC-1), where palmithoylethanolamide prevented NGF release [141]. These in vitro evidences agree with in vivo observations showing that palmithoylethanolamide was able to control mast cell-derived inflammation in immunogenic and non-immunogenic animal models of disease [142–145]. Overall, positive effects of palmithoylethanolamide were associated with a reduction of the production and release (degranulation) of several mediators, such as TNF-α and neurotrophic factors, like NGF, and proteases (tryptase and chymase) [146,147]. From these evidences, several studies have assessed the utility of palmithoylethanolamide in inflammatory and pain syndromes in both animals and humans (see Reference [139] for review). In some cases, the clinical improvement of symptoms was clearly correlated with the control of mast cell activation [148]. A recent clinical trial assessed the analgesic properties of dietary supplementation with palmitoylethanolamide and polydatin in IBS, reporting an improvement of abdominal pain severity (ClinicalTrials.gov number, NCT01370720) [149]. However, no changes in mast cells numbers or in the mast cell activation profile were observed [149]. Therefore, the link between the positive clinical effects and the potential modulation of mast cells is still a question and further studies are required to elucidate the mechanism of action of palmitoylethanolamide/polydatin in IBS.

Sphingolipids, and particularly ceramide and sphingosine, have been shown to negatively regulate mast cell signals and function [150]. In particular, they inhibited cytokine production from mast cells in culture [151] and induced apoptotic cell death in mouse BMMCs [150]. On the other hand, sphingosine-1-phosphate exhibits positive regulatory actions, enhancing mast cell function, including LT synthesis, TNF-α production, chemokine production and β-hexosaminidase release [150,152].

Table 3 offers a summary of the compounds mentioned in this section and their effects on mast cells' activity.

Table 3. Immunomodulatory effects of cannabinoids, cannabinoid-related compounds and other lipidic molecules on mast cell activity.

Compound	System	Effect [a]	Mechanism of Action	Reference
Cannabinoids and Cannabinoid-Related Compounds				
Cannabidiol	LPS-induced intestinal inflammation in mice	↓ Chymase up-regulation ↓ MMP9 up-regulation	Involvement of astroglial signaling neurotrophin S100B and PPARγ-dependent mechanisms	[138]
Palmithoylethanolamide	Canine skin mast cells	↓ Histamine release ↓ PGD2 release ↓ TNF-α release		[140]
Palmithoylethanolamide	HMC-1	↓ NGF release	GPR55-mediated	[141]
Palmithoylethanolamide	Neuropathic pain (chronic constriction injury of sciatic nerve in mice)	↓ TNF-α release ↓ NGF release		[146]
Palmithoylethanolamide	Spinal cord injury (mice)	↓ Proteases (tryptase and chymase) release		[147]
Palmithoylethanolamide/Polydatin	Clinical trial in IBS patients (NCT01370720)	Without changes in mast cell counts		[149]
Other Lipidic Molecules				
Ceramide/sphingosine	Mouse BMMCs	↓ IL-5, IL-10 and IL-13 production ↑ LT synthesis	Inhibition of PI3K-Akt pathway	[151]
Sphingosine-1-phosphate	Mouse BMMCs RBL-2H3 cells (rat)	↑ TNF-production ↑ Chemokines production ↑ β-hexosaminidase release	FcεRI-mediated activation of SphK-S1P1/S1P2 pathway	[150,152]

[a]: ↑: Facilitation; ↓: Inhibition. See abbreviations at the end of the article.

4.1.3. Fat-Soluble Vitamins

Table 4 summarizes the immunomodulatory effects exerted by vitamins D and E on mast cell activity.

Vitamin D is necessary to maintain the stability of mast cells, which activate automatically in a vitamin D-deficient environment, in the absence of specific activators. Exposure to vitamin D3 (calcitriol) resulted in an increased expression of vitamin D receptors and repressed the expression of TNF-α in different mast cell lines [153]. In accordance with these observations, sensitized mice receiving a vitamin D-supplemented diet showed reduced levels of serum histamine and TNF-α when challenged with the sensitizing antigen, thus indicating a hampered mast cell activation and a protective role for vitamin D [153].

Inefficiently absorbed vitamin E analogues could be considered as preventive nutraceuticals against intestinal inflammatory and allergic events and colon cancer. Vitamin E, and in general tocopherol analogues, have been shown to inhibit proliferation and survival of mast cells, likely affecting components of the c-kit/PI3K/PKB signaling cascade [154]. Several in vitro studies using different mast cell lines have also demonstrated that vitamin E modulates degranulation of mast cells, leading to a reduction in proinflammatory mediators, including histamine and PGD2 release, and a decrease in chymase activity, whereas tryptase activity was not affected [155,156]. Overall, these effects might be associated with the anti-free-radical and antioxidative stress actions of tocopherols [154].

Table 4. Immunomodulatory effects of fat-soluble vitamins on mast cell activity.

Compound	System	Effect [a]	Mechanism of Action	Reference
Vitamin D3 (calcitriol)	HMC-1 cells (human) RBL-2H3 cells (rat) p815 cells (mouse) Mouse BMMCs	↓ TNF-α expression ↓ TNF-α production ↓ Histamine release	Inhibition of FcεRI and MyD88, associated to decreased Syk phosphorylation and MAPK and NFκB levels. VDR binding to the TNF-α promoter leading to decreased acetylation of histone H3/H4, RNA polymerase II and OCT1 (a transcription factor of TNF-α) at the promoter locus, repressing TNF-α expression	[153]
Vitamin D3 (calcitriol)	Ovalbumin –sensitized mice with vitamin D-supplemented diet	↓ Serum TNF-α ↓ Serum histamine		[153]
Vitamin E (tocopherols)	C2 (canine)	↓ Histamine release ↓ PGD2 release ↓ Chymase activity		[155]
Vitamin E (tocopherols)	Rat peritoneal mast cells	↓ Histamine release	Changes in lipid peroxidation through the lipoxygenase pathway	[156]

[a]: ↑: Facilitation; ↓: Inhibition. See abbreviations at the end of the article.

4.2. Amino Acids

Experimental data have shown that human intestinal mast cells respond to the stimulation with specific amino acids, namely arginine and glutamine (Table 5). Arginine and glutamine are considered conditionally essential amino acids, mainly in stages of metabolic stress in the gut. In particular, it has been shown that pharmacological doses of arginine in combination with glutamine exert protective effects, for example, in Crohn's disease (CD), by reducing the production of proinflammatory cytokines such as TNF-α, IL-6 and IL-8 [157]. Studies in mature human mast cells isolated from normal surgery tissue specimens showed that a combination of both amino acids at pharmacological doses reduced LTC4 secretion and the expression of the chemokines CCL2, CCL4, IL-8 and TNF-α [158]. These observations suggest that the beneficial effects previously observed might be associated, at least partially, to a direct effect modulating intestinal mast cells' activity.

Recent data showed that dietary asparagine supplementation ameliorated LPS-induced intestinal dysfunction in pigs in in vivo conditions [159]. Although a direct effect on mast cells was not assessed, a reversion in the increase in intestinal mast cells triggered by LPS was observed, thus indicating a potential effect preventing mast cell-mediated actions within the gut. Further studies are needed to determine if asparagine, in addition to mast cell density, is able to also modulate mast cell activity/degranulation.

Table 5. Immunomodulatory effects of amino acids on mast cell activity.

Compound	System	Effect [a]	Mechanism of Action	Reference
Arginine + Glutamine	Human intestinal mast cells	↓ LT C4 secretion ↓ CCL2 expression ↓ CCL4 expression ↓ IL-8 expression	Decreased activation levels of signaling molecules of the MAPK family (extracellular signal-regulated kinase, JNK and p38) and the Akt	[158]
Glycine	Murine model of allergy to cow's milk	↓ Plasma levels of mouse mast cell protease-1		[160]

[a]: ↑: Facilitation; ↓: Inhibition. See abbreviations at the end of the article.

Table 6. Immunomodulatory effects of carotenoids on mast cell activity.

Compound	System	Effect [a]	Mechanism of Action	Reference
Carotenoids (fucoxanthin, astaxanthin, zeaxanthin and β-carotene)	Rat RBL-2H3 cells Mouse BMMCs	↓ β-hexosaminidase release	Inhibition of FcεRI-mediated intracellular signaling: phosphorylation of Lyn kinase and Fyn kinase	[161]
α- and β-carotene	Ovalbumin–sensitized mice	↓ Histamine release		[163]
Astaxanthin	DNFB-induced contact dermatitis in mice	↓ TNF-α levels ↓ IFN-γ levels		[162]
Astaxanthin	Rat RBL-2H3 cells	↓ Histamine release ↓ β-hexosaminidase		[162]

[a]: ↑: Facilitation; ↓: Inhibition. See abbreviations at the end of the article.

In a murine model of allergy to cow's milk, oral administration of glycine modulated mast cell-dependent allergic responses (as denoted by a reduction in plasma levels of mouse mast cell protease-1) and normalized the intestinal density of mast cells [160]. These effects on allergic mechanisms suggest that glycine might have a potential nutraceutical application modulating mast cell activity within the gut.

4.3. Carotenoids

Carotenoids are a heterogeneous group of natural pigments with diverse biological functions, including anti-oxidative and anti-inflammatory activities, which might affect mast cell function and, therefore, have an impact on GI physiology and pathophysiology. Numerous carotenoid compounds have been shown to modulate the activity of mast cell-related cell lines in in vitro conditions (Table 6). These include compounds such as fucoxanthin, astaxanthin, zeaxanthin or α- and β-carotene. Overall, these compounds inhibited antigen-induced degranulation [161] and histamine release [162]. These in vitro findings correlate with in vivo observations showing negative modulatory effects on mast cell function. For instance, α- and β-carotene treatment inhibited allergic responses, including the rise in serum histamine associated with mast cell activation [163]. Similarly, astaxanthin reduced signs of inflammation and the levels of TNF-α and IFN-γ in a dinitrofluorobenzene (DNFB)-induced contact dermatitis mouse model [162].

Retinol has been suggested as a negative regulator for the differentiation of human mast cells [164–166]. However, no effect [165] or enhanced degranulation has been observed upon incubation of mature mast cells with vitamin A [167]. Therefore, additional studies are necessary to determine the potential nutraceutical effects of retinol modulating the activity of intestinal mast cells and/or the maturation/differentiation process of mast cells arriving to the gut.

4.4. Polyphenolic Compounds

4.4.1. Flavonoids

Flavonoids (or bioflavonoids) are a family of naturally occurring polyphenolic plant and fungus substances with antioxidative, anti-cancer and anti-inflammatory properties. They are naturally found in fruits, vegetables, herbs, nuts, spices and red wine, with low toxicity compared to other active plant compounds. One group of flavonoids, the flavonols (3-hydroxyflavone), has been shown to have beneficial effects on mast cells (Table 7).

Several flavonoids (such as flavone, luteolin, fisetin, quercetin, rutin, kaempferol, myricetin, caffeic acid, nobiletin or morin) decreased the expression and/or inhibited the release of pro-inflammatory cytokines (TNF-α, IL-1, IL-6, and CXCL8, CCL2, CCL3 and CCL4), cysteinyl LTs and PGD2, as well as of tryptase, β-hexosaminidase and histamine in human and rodent mast cells in in vitro conditions [168–178]. These modulatory effects were both IgE-dependent and independent and exhibited compound-dependent selectivity and potency; for instance, morin was significantly less potent than other flavonoids modulating the activity of rat basophilic leukemia (RBL) cells [170].

In the murine IL-10 knockout model of colitis, treatment with the citrus flavonoid nobiletin resulted in a reduction of clinical colitis and a reduction of mast cell number and degranulation, which correlated positively with disease activity indexes [179].

Fermented soy germ-derived phytoestrogens, containing daidzein, glycitein and genistein present in aglycone forms, represent gut absorbable isoflavone forms structurally related to 17β-estradiol, but with higher affinity for estrogen receptors [180]. In a model of stress-induced IBS-like symptoms in female rats, supplementation with these soy germ fermented ingredients prevented the development of visceral hypersensitivity and intestinal barrier alterations characteristic of IBS. A reduction in colonic mast cell density and fecal proteolytic activity was also observed, thus suggesting that the functional changes observed might be associated with a modulation of mast cell activity [181].

Catechins (a family of flavonols) also play a critical role influencing mast cell activation, especially their derivative epigallocatechin-3-gallate (EGCG), a major green tea polyphenol [182–184]. Both, IgE-dependent and independent effects have been implicated in catechins effects, with some contradictory observations. EGCG inhibited histamine release from RBL-2H3 cells [185,186] and reduced degranulation (β-hexosaminidase release) and LTC4 secretion from RBL-2H3 cells as well as BMMCs upon IgE-dependent stimulation [182]. However, EGCG induced cytokine production (IL-13 and TNF-α) in mast cells (RBL-2H3 cells and BMMCs) via Ca^{2+} influx and ROS generation [183].

Flavanones, particularly hesperetin and naringenin, are also important bioactive components of citric fruits. Hesperetin and naringenin suppressed degranulation in RBL-2H3 cells, leading to the suppression of cytokines [187].

Table 7. Immunomodulatory effects of polyphenolic compounds on mast cell activity.

Compound	System	Effect [a]	Mechanism of Action	Reference
Quercitin	RBL-2H3 cells	↑ Rat mast cell protease II synthesis ↑ Accumulation of secretory granules ↓ Histamine release ↓ β-hexosaminidase release		[168, 171]
Flavone	RBL-2H3 cells	↑ Accumulation of secretory granules ↓ β-hexosaminidase release		[68]
Kaempferol	RBL-2H3 cells	↓ β-hexosaminidase release		[68]
Myricetin	RBL-2H3 cells	↓ β-hexosaminidase release		[68]
Luteolin, baicalein, quercetin	BMMCs Rat peritoneal mast cells	↓ Histamine release ↓ IL-6 production ↓ TNF-α production		[171]
Luteolin, baicalein, quercetin	Human cultured mast cells	↓ Histamine release ↓ LTs release ↓ PGD2 release	Inhibition of Ca^{2+} influx and PKC, ERKs and JNK signaling pathways	[172]
Kaempferol, myrecitin, quercetin, rutin, fisetin	RBL-2H3 cells HMC-1 cells	↓ Histamine release ↓ TNF-α expression and release ↓ IL-1β expression and release ↓ IL-6 expression and release ↓ IL-8 expression and release	Suppression of NFκB activation (fisetin, myricetin and rutin)	[174]
Quercetin, kaempferol, 14yricetin, morin	Human umbilical cord BMMCs	↓ TNF-α release ↓ IL-6 release ↓ IL-8 release ↓ CXCL8 expression ↓ CCL3 expression ↓ CCL4 expression	Suppression of intracellular Ca^{2+}, inhibition of PKC θ phosphorylation	[175]
Nobiletin, tangeretin	Human intestinal mast cells	↓ IL-1β expression (tangeretin) ↓ TNF-α expression ↓ β-hexosaminidase release (nobiletin) ↓ cysteinyl LTC4 (nobiletin) ↓ Mast cell density (colon)	Reduced phosphorylation of ERK1/2	[177]
Nobiletin	Murine IL-10 knockout model of colitis	↓ Mast cell degranulation (colon) ↓ Colonic mast cell density		[177]
Daidzein, glycitein and genistein	Restraint stress-induced IBS-like alterations in rats		Estrogen receptor-mediated	[181]
Green tea polyphenols	RBL-2H3 cells	↓ Histamine release	Metabolic events associated to the elevation of intracellular Ca^{2+}, inhibition of tyrosine phosphorylation of cellular proteins including pp125(FAK)	[185, 186]
Green tea polyphenols	RBL-2H3 cells BMMCs	↓ β-hexosaminidase release ↓ LTC4 secretion	Changes in ROS production and mitochondrial membrane potential	[182]
Green tea polyphenols (EGCG)	RBL-2H3 cells BMMCs	↓ IL-13 production ↑ TNF-α production	SOC-dependent Ca^{2+} influx and ROS generation	[183]

[a]: ↑: Facilitation; ↓: Inhibition. See abbreviations at the end of the article.

4.4.2. Other Polyphenolic Compounds

Not yet characterized polyphenolic compounds [188] are likely to mediate the beneficial effects observed in vivo for royal jelly in a murine model of cow milk allergy [189]. In this model, oral administration of royal jelly reduced histamine levels and prevented the associated intestinal damage, at least partially due to the activation of mast cells [189].

4.5. Spices

Two spices or their derived compounds have shown interesting roles related with immunomodulation of mast cell activity (Table 8): curcumin and cinnamon.

4.5.1. Curcumin

Curcumin is a diarylheptanoid phytochemical, belonging to the group of curcuminoids, which are natural bioactive phenols derived from the rhizome (turmeric) of *Curcuma longa* plants [190]. In vitro (BMMCs and RBL-2H3 cells) and in vivo studies (passive cutaneous anaphylaxis in mice) have shown that curcumin inhibited antigen-mediated activation of mast cells by suppressing degranulation and secretion of TNF-α and IL-4 [191]. Similar positive effects were also observed in a model of food-induced, IgE-mediated intestinal inflammatory reaction in rats, in which curcumin supplementation reduced mast cell activity [133]. Several clinical studies support a role for curcumin in inflammatory and functional GI diseases. In a randomized, double-blind placebo-controlled study in patients with ulcerative colitis, curcumin (plus sulfasalazine or mesalamine) improved the clinical activity index and the endoscopic score and prevented acute ulcerative colitis flares [192]. Similarly, in a randomized controlled clinical trial, curcumin (plus mesalazine) induced remission in patients with mild-to-moderate ulcerative colitis (ClinicalTrials.gov identifier: NCT01320436) [193]. As it relates to IBS, in a small group of patients [194], curcumin decreased abdominal pain intensity and improved quality of life. A combination of curcumin with fennel essential oil (with anethole as the active component) has also shown an improvement of symptoms and quality of life in IBS patients [195]. However, there is no evidence linking these positive clinical effects with the modulation of mast cell activity. The interest in curcumin is also highlighted by the fact that, according to the ClinicalTrial.gov registry, two additional clinical trials on IBS have been completed (ClinicalTrials.gov identifiers: NCT00779493 and NCT01418066), although no data have been released.

4.5.2. Cinnamon Extract—Cinnamaldehyde

Cinnamon extract treatment on IgE-stimulated RBL-2H3 cells as well as on human intestinal mast cells caused a downregulation of degranulation and *de novo* synthesis of proinflammatory mediators (CXCL8, CCL2, CCL3, CCL4 and TNF), β-hexosaminidase and cysteinyl LTs, as well as tryptase expression [196]. For RBL-2H3 cells, the IgE-independent activation was also detected, although to a lower extent [196]. Moreover, oral cinnamon extract treatment caused a downregulation of tryptase and carboxypeptidase A3 (MC-CPA) expression [196] and reduced expression of mast cell proteases (MC-CPA, MCP-1 and MCP-4) and pro-inflammatory mediators (CXCL8, CCL2, CCL3 and CCL4) during colitis in IL-10 knockout mice [197]. A subsequent study identified cinnamaldehyde as the main mediator of cinnamon extract in mast cell inhibition [198].

Table 8. Immunomodulatory effects of spices on mast cell activity.

Compound	System	Effect [a]	Mechanism of Action	Reference
Curcumin	Intestinal mast cell-IgE-mediated inflammatory reaction model in rats	↓ Rat chymase II	Inhibition of Syk activity, inhibition of phosphorylation of Akt and MAPKs p38, p44/42 and JNK	[133]
Curcumin	RBL-2H3 cells BMMCs	↓ TNF-α expression and release ↓ IL-4 expression and release ↓ β-hexosaminidase release		[191]
Curcumin	Passive cutaneous anaphylaxis model in mice	↓ Mast cell-dependent passive cutaneous anaphylaxis responses (Evans blue extravasation) ↓ Tryptase expression ↓ β-hexosaminidase release ↓ cysLt release ↓ CXCL8 release		[191]
Cinnamon extract/Cinnamaldehyde	Human intestinal mast cells RBL-2H3 cells	↓ CXCL8 expression ↓ CCL2 expression ↓ CCL3 expression ↓ CCL4 expression ↓ TNF-α expression	Inhibition of Akt and the MAPKs ERK, JNK, and p38; inhibition of PLCγ1 phosphorilation	[196,198]
Cinnamon extract/Cinnamaldehyde	Mouse duodenal tissue	↓ MCP6 and MC-CPA expression ↓ Proteases expression (MC-CPA, MCP-1 and MCP-4)		[196]
Cinnamon extract/Cinnamaldehyde	Murine IL-10 knockout model of colitis	↓ Expression of pro-inflammatory mediators (CXCL8, CCL2, CCL3 and CCL4, IL-1β, TNF, INFγ)	Inhibition of NFκB signaling	[197]

[a]: ↑: Facilitation; ↓: Inhibition. See abbreviations at the end of the article.

5. Conclusions

Mast cells play a prominent role in the pathophysiology of functional GI disorders, particularly IBS. Therefore, they have been regarded for a long time as a pharmacological target for the control of IBS. However, the paucity in the development of specific drugs targeting mast cells, or affecting IBS pathophysiology in general, has increased the interest in the search of alternative treatments. In this context, nutrient-derived bioactive compounds, administered as nutraceuticals, might represent a feasible alternative to the traditional pharmacological approach. Consistent in vivo and in vitro evidences indicate that numerous nutrient-derived bioactive compounds (including a variety of lipidic compounds, amino acids or numerous polyphenolic compounds) have the ability to modulate mast cell activity in a specific manner, reducing the release (mast cell degranulation) and the *de novo* synthesis of mast cells' mediators considered to mediate, at least in part, the neuro-immune-endocrine alterations present in IBS (Figure 1). Nevertheless, the clinical evidences are still scarce and additional studies are necessary to clearly show validity of this approach and the efficacy of nutraceuticals for the treatment of IBS, and, in particular, modulating mast cell activity. Moreover, it is expected that during the coming years, additional studies, both in vitro, in cellular systems and organoid human cell cultures, and in vivo, in disease-relevant animal models, will contribute to the identification of new food-derived bioactive compounds with potential nutraceutical applications, including the negative modulation of mast cells.

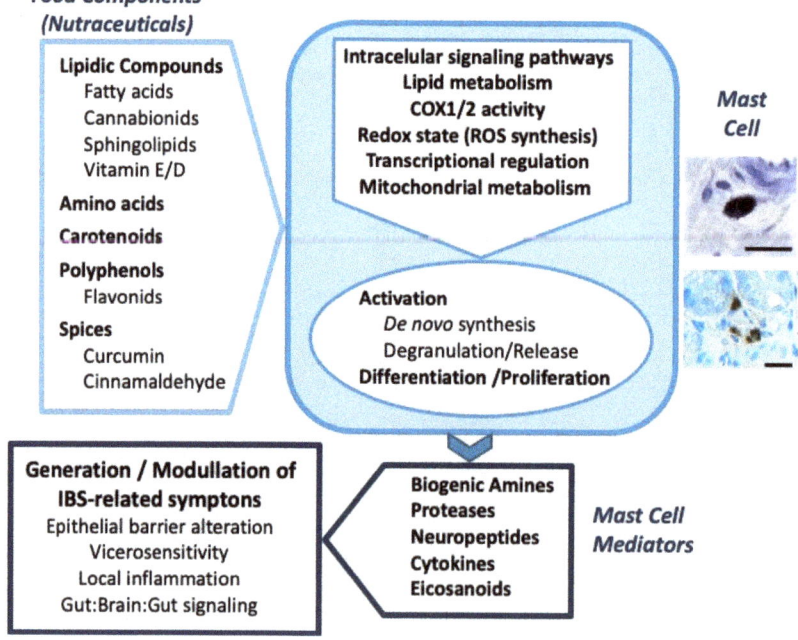

Figure 1. Schematic representation of the modulatory activity of food components on mast cells and their relationship with the generation and modulation of irritable bowel syndrome (IBS)-related symptoms. The figure integrates the main bioactive food components with potential nutraceutical use (as discussed in the text), the main mechanisms of action proposed on mast cells and some of the key symptoms related to IBS that can be modulated through the action of mast cell-derived mediators. See text for details. The photomicrographs (right) show mast cells in the rat intestine, identified with toluidine blue staining (upper photomicrograph) and rat mast cell protease 2 immunohistochemistry (lower photomicrograph). Scale bar: 20 μm.

Author Contributions: Conceptualization, R.A.; writing—original draft preparation, J.A.U. and V.M.; writing—review and editing, R.A.; funding acquisition, R.A. All authors have read and agreed to the published version of the manuscript.

Funding: This research was funded by Ministerio de Ciencia, Innovación y Universidades, grant number PID2019-111510RB-I00.

Conflicts of Interest: The authors declare no conflict of interest. The funders had no role in the design of the study; in the collection, analyses, or interpretation of data; in the writing of the manuscript, or in the decision to publish the results.

Abbreviations

5-ASA	5-aminosalicylic acid
5-HT	serotonin
AA	arachidonic acid
ALA	α-linolenic acid
Akt	protein kinase B
APC	adenomatous polyposis coli
BMMCs	bone marrow-derived mast cells
C2	canine mastocytoma cell line
CCL	C-C motif chemokine ligand
CD	Crohn's disease
CNS	central nervous system
COX	cyclooxygenase
CRF	corticotropin releasing factor
CXCL	Chemokine (C-X-C motif) ligand
CXCR2	chemokine (C-X-C motif) ligand 2 (Interleukin 8 receptor beta)
DHA	docosahexaenoic acid
DNFB	dinitrofluorobenzene
DRG	dorsal root ganglia
DSCG	disodium cromoglicate
EGCG	epigallocatechin-3-gallate
ENS	enteric nervous system
EPA	eicosapentaenoic acid
ERK	extracellular signal-regulated kinase
ET-1	endothelin 1
FcεRI	high-affinity IgE receptor
FGF	fibroblast growth factor
FODMAPs	fermentable oligosaccharides, disaccharides, monosaccharides and polyols
GATA-1	GATA binding protein-1
GATA-2	GATA binding protein-2
GI	gastrointestinal
GLA	γ-linolenic acid
GM-CSF	granulocyte macrophage colony-stimulating factor
IBD	inflammatory bowel disease
IBS	irritable bowel syndrome
IBS-C	IBS with predominant constipation
IBS-D	IBS with predominant diarrhea
IBS-M	mixed IBS
IBS-U	unclassified IBS
IFN	interferon
Ig	immunoglobulin
IL	interleukin
IP3	inositol-1,4,5-triphosphate
JAM	junctional adhesion molecule
JNK	c-Jun NH2–terminal kinase
LIF	leukemia inhibitory factor
LPS	lipopolysaccharide
LT	leukotriene
MAPK	mitogen-activated protein kinase
MBP	eosinophil major basic protein
MC-CPA	carboxypeptidase A3
MCP	monocyte chemotactic protein
MIP	macrophage inflammatory protein
MMP	matrix metalloproteinase
MMP9	matrix metallopeptidase 9
MRGPRX2	MAS-related G-protein-coupled receptor X2
MS	maternal separation test
MyD88	myeloid differentiation primary response 88

NFκβ	nuclear factor κβ
NGF	nerve growth factor
NK	natural killer
NO	nitric oxide
PAF	platelet activating factor
PAMP	pathogen-associated molecular pattern
PDGF	platelet-derived growth factor
PG	prostaglandin
PI-IBS	post-infectious IBS
PI3K-Akt	phosphoinositide 3-OH kinase-protein kinase B
PKC	protein kinase C
PKC θ	calcium-insensitive protein kinase C theta
PLCγ1	phosphoinositide-specific phospholipase C
pp125 (FAK)	focal adhesion kinase
PPARγ	peroxisome proliferator-activated receptor γ
PUFA	polyunsaturated fatty acid
RANTES	regulated upon activation, normal T cell expressed and secreted
RBL	Rat basophilic leukemia
RBL-2H3	rat basophilic leukemia mast cell line
ROS	reactive oxygen species
S1P1	sphingosine-1-phosphate (S1P) receptor 1
S1P2	sphingosine-1-phosphate (S1P) receptor 2
SCF	stem cell factor
SCFA	short chain fatty acid
SOC	store-operated Ca^{2+} channels
SP	substance P
SphK	sphingosine kinase
SyK	tyrosine-protein kinase SYK or spleen tyrosine kinase
TGF	transforming growth factor
TLR	toll-like receptors
TNF	tumor necrosis factor
Treg	regulatory T cells
VCAM-1	vascular cell adhesion molecule 1
VEGF	vascular endothelial growth factor
VIP	vasoactive intestinal peptide
VDR	vitamin D receptor
WRS	wrap restraint stress

References

1. Black, C.J.; Ford, A.C. Global burden of irritable bowel syndrome: Trends, predictions and risk factors. *Nat. Rev. Gastro. Hepat.* **2020**, *17*, 473–486. [CrossRef] [PubMed]
2. Grad, S.; Dumitrascu, D.L. Irritable Bowel Syndrome Subtypes: New Names for Old Medical Conditions. *Dig. Dis.* **2020**, *38*, 122–127. [CrossRef] [PubMed]
3. Creed, F. Review article: The incidence and risk factors for irritable bowel syndrome in population-based studies. *Aliment Pharm. Therap.* **2019**, *50*, 507–516. [CrossRef] [PubMed]
4. Canavan, C.; West, J.; Card, T. Review article: The economic impact of the irritable bowel syndrome. *Aliment Pharm. Therap.* **2014**, *40*, 1023–1034. [CrossRef] [PubMed]
5. Spiller, R.; Major, G. IBS and IBD-separate entities or on a spectrum? *Nat. Rev. Gastro. Hepat.* **2016**, *13*, 613–621. [CrossRef] [PubMed]
6. Balmus, I.M.; Ciobica, A.; Cojocariu, R.; Luca, A.C.; Gorgan, L. Irritable Bowel Syndrome and Neurological Deficiencies: Is There A Relationship? The Possible Relevance of the Oxidative Stress Status. *Medicina* **2020**, *56*, 175. [CrossRef]
7. Ng, Q.X.; Soh, A.Y.S.; Loke, W.; Lim, D.Y.; Yeo, W.S. The role of inflammation in irritable bowel syndrome (IBS). *J. Inflamm. Res.* **2018**, *11*, 345–349. [CrossRef]
8. Verne, G.N.; Price, D.D. Irritable bowel syndrome as a common precipitant of central sensitization. *Curr. Rheumatol. Rep.* **2002**, *4*, 322–328. [CrossRef]
9. Casado-Bedmar, M.; Keita, Å.V. Potential neuro-immune therapeutic targets in irritable bowel syndrome. *Therap. Adv. Gastroenter.* **2020**, *13*, 1756284820910630. [CrossRef]
10. Labanski, A.; Langhorst, J.; Engler, H.; Elsenbruch, S. Stress and the brain-gut axis in functional and chronic-inflammatory gastrointestinal diseases: A transdisciplinary challenge. *Psychoneuroendocrinology* **2020**, *111*, 104501. [CrossRef]

11. Thangam, E.B.; Jemima, E.A.; Singh, H.; Baig, M.S.; Khan, M.; Mathias, C.B.; Church, M.K.; Saluja, R. The Role of Histamine and Histamine Receptors in Mast Cell-Mediated Allergy and Inflammation: The Hunt for New Therapeutic Targets. *Front Immunol.* **2018**, *9*, 1873. [CrossRef] [PubMed]
12. da Silva, E.Z.; Jamur, M.C.; Oliver, C. Mast Cell Function: A New Vision of an Old Cell. Journal of Histochem. *Cytochem* **2014**, *62*, 698–738. [CrossRef] [PubMed]
13. Galli, S.J.; Borregaard, N.; Wynn, T.A. Phenotypic and functional plasticity of cells of innate immunity: Macrophages, mast cells and neutrophils. *Nat. Immunol.* **2011**, *12*, 1035–1044. [CrossRef] [PubMed]
14. Gentek, R.; Ghigo, C.; Hoeffel, G.; Bulle, M.J.; Msallam, R.; Gautier, G.; Launay, P.; Chen, J.; Ginhoux, F.; Bajénoff, M. Hemogenic Endothelial Fate Mapping Reveals Dual Developmental Origin of Mast Cells. *Immunity* **2018**, *48*, 1160–1171. [CrossRef] [PubMed]
15. Li, Z.; Liu, S.; Xu, J.; Zhang, X.; Han, D.; Liu, J.; Xia, M.; Yi, L.; Shen, Q.; Xu, S.; et al. Adult Connective Tissue-Resident Mast Cells Originate from Late Erythro-Myeloid Progenitors. *Immunity* **2018**, *49*, 640–653. [CrossRef]
16. Dwyer, D.F.; Barrett, N.A.; Austen, K.F. Expression profiling of constitutive mast cells reveals a unique identity within the immune system. *Nat. Immunol.* **2016**, *17*, 878–887. [CrossRef]
17. Gurish, M.F.; Austen, K.F. Developmental Origin and Functional Specialization of Mast Cell Subsets. *Immunity* **2012**, *37*, 25–33. [CrossRef]
18. Collington, S.J.; Timothy, J.; Williams, T.J.; Weller, C.L. Mechanisms underlying the localisation of mast cells in tissues. *Trends Immunol.* **2011**, *32*, 478–485. [CrossRef]
19. Galli, S.J.; Grimbaldeston, M.; Tsai, M. Immunomodulatory mast cells: Negative, as well as positive, regulators of innate and acquired immunity. *Nat. Rev. Immunol.* **2008**, *8*, 478–486. [CrossRef]
20. Iemura, A.; Tsai, M.; Ando, A.; Wershi, B.K.; Galli, S.J. The c-kit Ligand, Stem Cell Factor, Promotes Mast Cell Survival by Suppressing Apoptosis. *Am. J. Pathol.* **1994**, *144*, 321–328.
21. Hogaboam, C.; Kunkel, S.L.; Strieter, R.M.; Taub, D.D.; Lincoln, P.; Standiford, T.J.; Lukacs, N.W. Novel Role of Transmembrane SCF for Mast Cell Activation and Eotaxin Production in Mast Cell-Fibroblast Interactions. *J. Immunol.* **1998**, *160*, 6166–6171. [PubMed]
22. Macey, M.R.; Sturgill, J.L.; Johanna, K.; Morales, J.K.; Falanga, Y.T.; Morales, J.; Sarah, K.; Norton, S.K.; Yerram, N.; Shim, H.; et al. IL-4 and TGF-b1 Counterbalance One Another while Regulating Mast Cell Homeostasis. *J. Immunol.* **2010**, *184*, 4688–4695. [CrossRef] [PubMed]
23. Weller, C.L.; Collington, S.J.; Hartnell, A.; Conroy, D.M.; Kaise, T.; Barker, J.E.; Wilson, M.S.; Taylor, G.W.; Jose, P.J.; Williams, T.J. Chemotactic action of prostaglandin E2 on mouse mast cells acting via the PGE2 receptor 3. *Proc. Nat. Acad. Sci. USA* **2007**, *104*, 11712–11717. [CrossRef] [PubMed]
24. Irani, A.A.; Schechter, N.M.; Craig, S.S.; Deblois, G.; Schwartz, L.B. Two types of human mast cells that have distinct neutral protease compositions. *Proc. Nat. Acad. Sci. USA* **1986**, *83*, 4464–4468. [CrossRef]
25. Pejler, G.; Rönnberg, E.; Waern, I.; Wernersson, S. Mast cell proteases: Multifaceted regulators of inflammatory disease. *Blood* **2010**, *115*, 4981–4990. [CrossRef]
26. Kirshenbaum, A.S.; Swindle, E.; Kulka, M.; Wu, Y.; Metcalfe, D.D. Effect of lipopolysaccharide (LPS) and peptidoglycan (PGN) on human mast cell numbers, cytokine production, and protease composition. *BMC Immunol.* **2008**, *9*, 45. [CrossRef]
27. Gebhardt, T.; Lorentz, A.; Detmer, F.; Trautwein, C.; Bektas, H.; Manns, M.P.; Bischoff, S.C. Growth, phenotype, and function of human intestinal mast cells are tightly regulated by transforming growth factor β1. *Gut* **2005**, *54*, 928–934. [CrossRef]
28. Kanakura, Y.; Thompson, H.; Nakano, T.; Yamamura, T.; Asai, H.; Kitamura, Y.; Metcalfe, D.D.; Galli, S.J. Multiple bidirectional alterations of phenotype and changes in proliferative potential during the in vitro and in vivo passage of clonal mast cell populations derived from mouse peritoneal mast cells. *Blood* **1988**, *72*, 877–885. [CrossRef]
29. Galli, S.J.; Kalesnikoff, J.; Grimbaldeston, M.A.; Piliponsky, A.M.; Williams, C.; Tsai, M. Mast cells as "tunable" effector and immunoregulatory cells: Recent Advances. *Annu. Rev. Immunol.* **2005**, *23*, 749–786. [CrossRef]
30. Subramanian, H.; Gupta, K.; Ali, H. Roles of MAS-related G protein coupled receptor-X2 (MRGPRX2) on mast cell-mediated host defense, pseudoallergic drug reactions and chronic inflammatory diseases. *Allergy Clin. Immunol.* **2016**, *138*, 700–710. [CrossRef]
31. McNeil, B.D.; Pundir, P.; Meeker, S.; Han, L.; Undem, B.J.; Kulka, M.; Dong, X. Identification of a mast cell specific receptor crucial for pseudo-allergic drug reactions. *Nature* **2015**, *519*, 237–241. [CrossRef] [PubMed]

32. Marshall, J.S. Mast-cell responses to pathogens. *Nat. Rev. Immunol.* **2004**, *4*, 787–799. [CrossRef] [PubMed]
33. Plum, T.; Xi Wang, W.; Rettel, M.; Krijgsveld, J.; Thorsten, B.; Feyerabend, T.B.; Rodewald, H.R. Human Mast Cell Proteome Reveals Unique Lineage, Putative Functions, and Structural Basis for Cell Ablation. *Immunity* **2020**, *52*, 404–416. [CrossRef] [PubMed]
34. Metz, M.; Siebenhaar, F.; Maurer, M. Mast cell functions in the innate skin immune system. *Immunobiology* **2008**, *213*, 251–260. [CrossRef]
35. Pundir, P.; Liu, R.; Vasavda, C.; Serhan, N.; Limjunyawong, N.; Yee, R.; Zhan, Y.; Dong, X.; Wu, X.; Zhang, Y.; et al. A Connective Tissue Mast Cell-Specific Receptor Detects Bacterial Quorum Sensing Molecules and Mediates Antibacterial Immunity. *Cell Host Microbe* **2019**, *26*, 114–122. [CrossRef]
36. Sibilano, R.; Fross, B.; Pucillo, C.E. Mast cell activation: A complex interplay of positive and negative signaling pathways. *Eur. J. Immunol.* **2014**, *44*, 2558–2566. [CrossRef]
37. MacGlashan, D. IgE receptor and signal transduction in mast cells and basophils. *Cur. Op. Immunol.* **2008**, *20*, 717–723. [CrossRef]
38. Krystel-Whittemore, M.; Dileepan, K.N.; Wood, J.G. Mast Cell: A Multi-Functional Master Cell. *Front Immunol.* **2016**, *6*, 620. [CrossRef]
39. Nakae, S.; Suto, H.; Iikura, M.; Kakurai, M.; Sedgwick, J.D.; Tsai, M.; Galli, S.J. Mast Cells Enhance T Cell Activation: Importance of Mast Cell Costimulatory Molecules and Secreted TNF. *J. Immunol.* **2006**, *176*, 2238–2248. [CrossRef]
40. Wulff, B.C.; Wilgus, T.A. Mast cell activity in the healing wound: More than meets the eye? *Exp. Dermatol.* **2013**, *22*, 507–510. [CrossRef]
41. Sun, J.; Sukhova, G.K.; Yang, M.; Wolters, P.J.; MacFarlane, L.A.; Libby, P.; Sun, C.; Zhang, Y.; Liu, J.; Ennis, T.L.; et al. Mast cells modulate the pathogenesis of elastase-induced abdominal aortic aneurysms in mice. *J. Clin. Investig.* **2007**, *117*, 3359–3368. [CrossRef] [PubMed]
42. Yang, M.Q.; Ma, Y.Y.; Tao, S.F.; Ding, J.; Rao, L.H.; Jiang, H.; Li, J.Y. Mast cell degranulation promotes ischemia reperfusion injury in rat liver. *J. Surg. Res.* **2014**, *186*, 170–178. [CrossRef] [PubMed]
43. Kalesnikoff, J.; Galli, S.J. New developments in mast cell biology. *Nat. Immunol.* **2008**, *9*, 1215–1223. [CrossRef] [PubMed]
44. Gounaris, E.; Erdman, S.E.; Restaino, C.; Gurish, M.F.; Friend, D.S.; Gounari, F.; Lee, D.M.; Zhang, G.; Glickman, J.N.; Shin, K.; et al. Mast cells are an essential hematopoietic component for polyp development. *Proc. Natl. Acad. Sci. USA* **2007**, *104*, 19977–19982. [CrossRef] [PubMed]
45. Uranga, J.A.; Cámara, J.C.; Herradón, E.; Vera, G.; Jagerovic, N.; Quesada, E.; Fernández, J.; Lombó, F.; Abalo, R. New strategies for treatment and prevention of colorectal cancer. In *Gastrointestinal Cancers*; Tyagi, A., Prasad, S., Eds.; Nova publishers: New York, NY, USA, 2017; pp. 103–170. ISBN 978-1-53610-168-3.
46. Sinnamon, M.J.; Carter, K.J.; Sims, L.P.; Lafleur, B.; Fingleton, B.; Matrisian, L.M. A protective role of mast cells in intestinal tumorigenesis. *Carcinogenesis* **2008**, *29*, 880–886. [CrossRef]
47. Lovell, R.M.; Ford, A.C. Global prevalence of and risk factors for irritable bowel syndrome: A meta-analysis. *Clin. Gastroenterol. Hepatol.* **2012**, *10*, 712–721. [CrossRef]
48. Schmulson, M.J.; Drossman, D.A. What Is New in Rome IV. *J. Neurogastroenterol.* **2017**, *23*, 151–163. [CrossRef]
49. Fichna, J. *A Comprehensive Overview of Irritable Bowel Syndrome-Clinical and Basic Science Aspects*; Fichna, J., Ed.; Academic Press-Elsevier: London, UK, 2020; ISBN 978-0-12-821324-7.
50. Buhner, S.; Schemann, M. Mast cell–nerve axis with a focus on the human gut. *BBA-Mol. Basis. Dis.* **2012**, *1822*, 85–92. [CrossRef]
51. Costa, M.; Brookes, S.J.H.; Hennig, G.W. Anatomy and physiology of the enteric nervous System. *Gut* **2000**, *47*, iv15–iv19. [CrossRef]
52. Yu, L.C.; Perdue, M.H. Role of mast cells in intestinal mucosal function: Studies in models of hypersensitivity and stress. *Immunol. Rev.* **2001**, *179*, 61–73. [CrossRef]
53. Breunig, E.; Michel, K.; Florian Zeller, F.; Stefan Seidl, S.; Weyhern, C.W.H.V.; Schemann, M. Histamine excites neurones in the human submucous plexus through activation of H1, H2, H3 and H4 receptors. *J. Physiol.* **2007**, *583*, 731–742. [CrossRef] [PubMed]
54. Keely, S.J.; Stack, W.A.; O'Donoghue, D.P.; Baird, A.W. Regulation of ion transport by histamine in human colon. *Eur. J. Pharmacol.* **1995**, *279*, 203–209. [CrossRef]

55. Bode, H.; Schmitz, H.; Fromm, M.; Scholz, P.; Riecken, E.O.; Schulzke, J.D. IL-1beta and TNF-alpha, but not IFN-alpha, IFN-gamma, IL-6 or IL-8, are secretory mediators in human distal colon. *Cytokine* **1998**, *10*, 457–465. [CrossRef] [PubMed]
56. Schwartz, L.B.; Lewis, R.A.; Austen, K.F. Tryptase from Human Pulmonary Mast Cells. *J. Biol. Chem.* **1981**, *256*, 11939–11943.
57. van der Kleij, H.P.M.; Bienenstock, J. Significance of conversation between mast cells and nerves. *Allergy Asthma Clin. Immunol.* **2005**, *1*, 65–80. [CrossRef]
58. Stead, R.H.; Dixon, M.F.; Bramwell, N.H.; Riddell, R.H.; Biennenstock, J. Mast cells are closely apposed to nerves in the human gastrointestinal mucosa. *Gastroenterology* **1989**, *97*, 575–585. [CrossRef]
59. Gebhardt, T.; Gerhard, R.; Bedoui, S.; Erpenbeck, V.J.; Hoffmann, M.W.; Manns, M.P.; Bischoff, S.C. β2-Adrenoceptor-mediated suppression of human intestinal mast cell functions is caused by disruption of filamentous actin dynamics. *Eur. J. Immunol.* **2005**, *35*, 1124–1132. [CrossRef]
60. Zhang, L.; Song, J.; Hou, X. Mast Cells and Irritable Bowel Syndrome: From the Bench to the Bedside. *J. Neurogastroent. Motil.* **2016**, *22*, 181–192. [CrossRef]
61. López Gómez, L.; Bagués, A.; Uranga, J.A.; Abalo, R. Preclinical models of irritable bowel syndrome. In *A Comprehensive Overview of Irritable Bowel Syndrome-Clinical and Basic Science Aspects*; Fichna, J., Ed.; Academic Press-Elsevier: London, UK, 2020; ISBN 978-0-12-821324-7.
62. Vannucchi, M.G.; Evangelista, S. Experimental Models of Irritable Bowel Syndrome and the Role of the Enteric Neurotransmission. *J. Clin. Med.* **2018**, *7*, 4. [CrossRef]
63. Overman, E.L.; Rivier, J.E.; Moeser, A.J. CRF induces intestinal epithelial barrier injury via the release of mast cell proteases and TNF-α. *PLoS ONE* **2012**, *7*, e39935. [CrossRef]
64. Taché, Y.; Larauche, M.; Yuan, P.Q.; Million, M. Brain and gut CRF signaling: Biological actions and role in the gastrointestinal tract. *Curr. Mol. Pharmacol.* **2018**, *11*, 51–71. [CrossRef] [PubMed]
65. Krammer, L.; Sowa, A.S.; Lorentz, A. Mast cells in irritable bowel syndrome: A systematic review. *J. Gastroint. Liver. Dis.* **2019**, *28*, 463–472. [CrossRef]
66. Buhner, S.; Li, Q.; Vignali, S.; Barbara, G.; De Giorgio, R.; Stanghellini, V.; Cremon, C.; Zeller, F.; Langer, R.; Daniel, H.; et al. Activation of human enteric neurons by supernatants of colonic biopsy specimens from patients with irritable bowel syndrome. *Gastroenterology* **2009**, *137*, 1425–1434. [CrossRef] [PubMed]
67. Guilarte, M.; Santos, J.; de Torres, I.; Alonso, C.; Vicario, M.; Ramos, L.; Martínez, C.; Casellas, F.; Saperas, E.; Malagelada, J.R. Diarrhoea-predominant IBS patients show mast cell activation and hyperplasia in the jejunum. *Gut* **2007**, *56*, 203–209. [CrossRef] [PubMed]
68. Balestra, B.; Vicini, R.; Cremon, C.; Zecchi, L.; Dothel, G.; Vasina, V.; De Giorgio, R.; Paccapelo, A.; Pastoris, O.; Stanghellini, V.; et al. Colonic mucosal mediators from patients with irritable bowel syndrome excite enteric cholinergic motor neurons. *Neurogastroent. Motil.* **2012**, *24*, 1118-e570. [CrossRef]
69. Barbara, G.; Stanghellini, V.; De Giorgio, R.; Cremon, C.; Cottrell, G.S.; Santini, D.; Pasquinelli, G.; Morselli-Labate, A.M.; Grady, E.F.; Bunnett, N.W.; et al. Activated mast cells in proximity to colonic nerves correlate with abdominal pain in irritable bowel syndrome. *Gastroenterology* **2004**, *126*, 693–702. [CrossRef]
70. Liang, W.J.; Zhang, G.; Luo, H.S.; Liang, L.X.; Huang, D.; Zhang, F.C. Tryptase and Protease-Activated Receptor 2 Expression Levels in Irritable Bowel Syndrome. *Gut Liver* **2016**, *10*, 382–390. [CrossRef]
71. Nasser, Y.; Boeckxstaens, G.E.; Wouters, M.M.; Schemann, M.; Vanner, S. Using human intestinal biopsies to study the pathogenesis of irritable bowel syndrome. *Neurogastroent. Motil.* **2014**, *26*, 455–469. [CrossRef]
72. Camilleri, M.; Lasch, K.; Zhou, W. Irritable bowel syndrome: Methods, mechanisms, and pathophysiology. The confluence of increased permeability, inflammation, and pain in irritable bowel syndrome. *Am. J. Physiol. Gastrointest. Liver. Physiol.* **2012**, *303*, G775–G785. [CrossRef]
73. Park, J.H.; Rhee, P.L.; Kim, H.S.; Lee, J.H.; Kim, Y.H.; Kim, J.J.; Rhee, J.C. Mucosal mast cell counts correlate with visceral hypersensitivity in patients with diarrhea predominant irritable bowel syndrome. *J. Gastroen. Hepatol.* **2006**, *21*, 71–78. [CrossRef]
74. O'Sullivan, M.; Clayton, N.; Breslin, N.P.; Harman, I.; Bountra, C.; McLaren, A.; O'Morain, C.A. Increased mast cells in the irritable bowel syndrome. *Neurogastroent. Motil.* **2000**, *12*, 449–457. [CrossRef] [PubMed]
75. Cremon, C.; Carini, G.; Wang, B.; Vasina, V.; Cogliandro, R.F.; De Giorgio, R.; Stanghellini, V.; Grundy, D.; Tonini, M.; De Ponti, F.; et al. Intestinal serotonin release, sensory neuron activation, and abdominal pain in irritable bowel syndrome. *Am. J. Gastroenterol.* **2011**, *106*, 1290–1298. [CrossRef] [PubMed]

76. Barbara, G.; Wang, B.; Stanghellini, V.; de Giorgio, R.; Cremon, C.; Di Nardo, G.; Trevisani, M.; Campi, B.; Geppetti, P.; Tonini, M.; et al. Mast cell-dependent excitation of visceral-nociceptive sensory neurons in irritable bowel syndrome. *Gastroenterology* **2007**, *132*, 26–37. [CrossRef] [PubMed]
77. Valdez-Morales, E.E.; Overington, J.; Guerrero-Alba, R.; Ochoa-Cortes, F.; Ibeakanma, C.O.; Spreadbury, I.; Bunnett, N.W.; Beyak, M.; Vanner, S.J. Sensitization of peripheral sensory nerves by mediators from colonic biopsies of diarrhea-predominant irritable bowel syndrome patients: A role for PAR2. *Am. J. Gastroenterol.* **2013**, *108*, 1634–1643. [CrossRef]
78. Cenac, N.; Andrews, C.N.; Holzhausen, M.; Chapman, K.; Cottrell, G.; Andrade-Gordon, P.; Steinhoff, M.; Barbara, G.; Beck, P.; Bunnett, N.W.; et al. Role for protease activity in visceral pain in irritable bowel syndrome. *J. Clin. Invest.* **2007**, *117*, 636–647. [CrossRef]
79. Klooker, T.K.; Braak, B.; Koopman, K.; Welting, O.; Wouters, M.M.; van der Heide, S.; Schemann, M.; Bischoff, S.C.; van den Wijngaard, R.N.; Boeckxstaens, G.E. The mast cell stabiliser ketotifen decreases visceral hypersensitivity and improves intestinal symptoms in patients with irritable bowel syndrome. *Gut* **2010**, *59*, 1213–1221. [CrossRef]
80. Stefanini, G.F.; Prati, E.; Albini, M.C.; Piccinini, G.; Capelli, S.; Castelli, E.; Mazzetti, M.; Gasbarrini, G. Oral disodium cromoglycate treatment on irritable bowel syndrome: An open study on 101 subjects with diarrheic type. *Am. J. Gastroenterol.* **1992**, *87*, 55–57.
81. Stefanini, G.F.; Saggioro, A.; Alvisi, V.; Angelini, G.; Capurso, L.; di Lorenzo, G.; Dobrilla, G.; Dodero, M.; Galimberti, M.; Gasbarrini, G.; et al. Oral cromolyn sodium in comparison with elimination diet in the irritable bowel syndrome, diarrheic type. Multicenter study of 428 patients. *Scand. J. Gastroenterol.* **1995**, *30*, 535–541. [CrossRef]
82. Ghadir, M.R.; Poradineh, M.; Sotodeh, M.; Ansari, R.; Kolahdoozan, S.; Hormati, A.; Yousefi, M.H.; Mirzaei, S.; Vahedi, H. Mesalazine Has No Effect on Mucosal Immune Biomarkers in Patients with Diarrhea-Dominant Irritable Bowel Syndrome Referred to Shariati Hospital: A Randomized Double-Blind, Placebo-Controlled Trial. *Middle East J. Dig. Dis.* **2017**, *9*, 20–25. [CrossRef]
83. Camilleri, M. Current and future pharmacological treatments for diarrhea-predominant irritable bowel syndrome. *Expert Opin. Pharmaco.* **2013**, *14*, 1151–1160. [CrossRef]
84. Zhang, F.M.; Li, S.; Ding, L.; Xiang, S.H.; Zhu, H.T.; Yu, J.H.; Xu, G.Q. Effectiveness of mesalazine to treat irritable bowel syndrome: A meta-analysis. *Medicine* **2019**, *98*, e16297. [CrossRef] [PubMed]
85. Cheng, W.; Li, J.; Liu, X. 5-Aminosalicylic acid for treatment of irritable bowel syndrome: A protocol for a systematic review and meta-analysis. *Medicine* **2020**, *99*, e19351. [CrossRef] [PubMed]
86. Tack, J.F.; Jr Miner, P.B.; Fischer, L.; Harris, M.S. Randomised clinical trial: The safety and efficacy of AST-120 in non-constipating irritable bowel syndrome—a double-blind, placebo-controlled study. *Aliment Pharmacol. Ther.* **2011**, *34*, 868–877. [CrossRef] [PubMed]
87. Wouters, M.M.; Balemans, D.; Van Wanrooy, S.; Dooley, J.; Cibert-Goton, V.; Alpizar, Y.A.; Valdez-Morales, E.E.; Nasser, Y.; Van Veldhoven, P.P.; Vanbrabant, W.; et al. Histamine receptor H1-mediated sensitization of TRPV1 mediates visceral hypersensitivity and symptoms in patients with irritable bowel syndrome. *Gastroenterology* **2016**, *150*, 875–887. [CrossRef]
88. Fabisiak, A.; Włodarczyk, J.; Fabisiak, N.; Storr, M.; Fichna, J. Targeting Histamine Receptors in Irritable Bowel Syndrome: A Critical Appraisal. *J. Neurogastroent. Motil.* **2017**, *23*, 341–348. [CrossRef]
89. Vivinus-Nébot, M.; Dainese, R.; Anty, R.; Saint-Paul, M.C.; Nano, J.L.; Gonthie, N.R.; Marjoux, S.; Frin-Mathy, G.; Bernard, G.; Hébuterne, X.; et al. Combination of allergic factors can worsen diarrheic irritable bowel syndrome: Role of barrier defects and mast cells. *Am. J. Gastroenterol.* **2012**, *107*, 75–81. [CrossRef]
90. Piche, T.; Barbara, G.; Aubert, P.; des Varannes, S.B.; Dainese, R.; Nano, J.L.; Cremon, C.; Stanghellini, V.; de Giorgio, R.; Galmiche, J.P.; et al. Impaired intestinal barrier integrity in the colon of patients with irritable bowel syndrome: Involvement of soluble mediators. *Gut* **2009**, *58*, 196–201. [CrossRef]
91. Gecse, K.; Roka, R.; Ferrier, L.; Leveque, M.; Eutamene, H.; Cartier, C.; Ait-Belgnaoui, A.; Rosztoczy, A.; Izbeki, F.; Fioramonti, J.; et al. Increased faecal serine protease activity in diarrhoeic IBS patients: A colonic lumenal factor impairing colonic permeability and sensitivity. *Gut* **2008**, *57*, 591–598. [CrossRef]
92. Barbaro, M.R.; Fuschi, D.; Cremon, C.; Carapelle, M.; Dino, P.; Marcellini, M.M.; Dothel, G.; de Ponti, F.; Stanghellini, V.; Barbara, G. Escherichia coli Nissle 1917 restores epithelial permeability alterations induced by irritable bowel syndrome mediators. *Neurogastroent. Motil.* **2018**, e13388. [CrossRef]

93. Nébot-Vivinus, M.; Harkat, C.; Bzioueche, H.; Cartier, C.; Plichon-Dainese, R.; Moussa, L.; Eutamene, H.; Pishvaie, D.; Holowacz, S.; Seyrig, C.; et al. Multispecies probiotic protects gut barrier function in experimental models. *World J. Gastroenterol.* **2014**, *20*, 6832–6843. [CrossRef]
94. Annaházi, A.; Ferrier, L.; Bézirard, V.; Levêque, M.; Eutamène, H.; AitBelgnaoui, A.; Coëffier, M.; Ducrotté, P.; Roka, R.; Inczefi, O.; et al. Luminal cysteine-proteases degrade colonic tight junction structure and are responsible for abdominal pain in constipation-predominant IBS. *Am. J. Gastroenterol.* **2013**, *108*, 1322–1331. [CrossRef] [PubMed]
95. Wilcz-Villega, E.M.; McClean, S.; O'Sullivan, M.A. Mast cell tryptase reduces junctional adhesion molecule-A (JAM-A) expression in intestinal epithelial cells: Implications for the mechanisms of barrier dysfunction in irritable bowel syndrome. *Am. J. Gastroenterol.* **2013**, *108*, 1140–1151. [CrossRef] [PubMed]
96. Jacob, C.; Yang, P.C.; Darmoul, D.; Amadesi, S.; Saito, T.; Cottrell, G.S.; Coelho, A.M.; Singh, P.; Grady, E.F.; Perdue, M.; et al. Mast cell tryptase controls paracellular permeability of the intestine. Role of protease-activated receptor 2 and beta-arrestins. *J. Biol. Chem.* **2005**, *280*, 31936–31948. [CrossRef] [PubMed]
97. Spiller, R.; Campbell, E. Post-infectious irritable bowel syndrome. *Curr. Opin. Gastroenterol.* **2006**, *22*, 13–17. [CrossRef]
98. Gwee, K.A.; Collins, S.M.; Read, N.W.; Rajnakova, A.; Deng, Y.; Graham, J.C.; McKendrick, M.W.; Moochhala, S.M. Increased rectal mucosal expression of interleukin 1β in recently acquired post-infectious irritable bowel syndrome. *Gut* **2003**, *52*, 523–526. [CrossRef]
99. Uno, Y. Hypothesis: Mechanism of irritable bowel syndrome in inflammatory bowel disease. *Med. Hypotheses* **2019**, *132*, 109324. [CrossRef]
100. Rej, A.; Sanders, D.S. Gluten-Free Diet and Its 'Cousins' in Irritable Bowel Syndrome. *Nutrients* **2018**, *10*, 1727. [CrossRef]
101. Halmos, E.P.; Power, V.A.; Shepherd, S.J.; Gibson, P.R.; Muir, J.G. A diet low in FODMAPs reduces symptoms of irritable bowel syndrome. *Gastroenterolog.* **2014**, *146*, 67–75. [CrossRef]
102. Mansueto, P.; Seidita, A.; D'Alcamo, A.; Carroccio, A. Role of FODMAPs in Patients With Irritable Bowel Syndrome. *Nutr. Clin. Pract.* **2015**, *30*, 665–682. [CrossRef]
103. Altobelli, E.; Del Negro, V.; Angeletti, P.M.; Latella, G. Low-FODMAP Diet Improves Irritable Bowel Syndrome Symptoms: A Meta-Analysis. *Nutrient.* **2017**, *9*, 940. [CrossRef]
104. McIntosh, K.; Reed, D.E.; Schneider, T.; Dang, F.; Keshteli, A.H.; De Palma, G.; Madsen, K.; Bercik, P.; Vanner, S. FODMAPs alter symptoms and the metabolome of patients with IBS: A randomised controlled trial. *Gut* **2017**, *66*, 1241–1251. [CrossRef] [PubMed]
105. Whelan, K.; Martin, L.D.; Staudacher, H.M.; Lomer, M.C.E. The low FODMAP diet in the management of irritable bowel syndrome: An evidence-based review of FODMAP restriction, reintroduction and personalisation in clinical practice. *J. Hum. Nutr. Diet.* **2018**, *31*, 239–255. [CrossRef] [PubMed]
106. Kamphuis, J.B.; Guiard, B.; Leveque, M.; Olier, M.; Jouanin, I.; Yvon, S.; Tondereau, V.; Rivière, P.; Guéraud, F.; Chevolleau, S.; et al. Lactose and fructo-oligosaccharides increase visceral sensitivity in mice via glycation processes, increasing mast cell density in colonic mucosa. *Gastroenterology* **2020**, *158*, 652–663. [CrossRef]
107. Chen, B.R.; Du, L.J.; He, H.Q.; Kim, J.J.; Zhao, Y.; Zhang, Y.W.; Luo, L.; Dai, N. Fructo-oligosaccharide intensifies visceral hypersensitivity and intestinal inflammation in a stress-induced irritable bowel syndrome mouse model. *World J. Gastroenterol.* **2017**, *23*, 8321–8333. [CrossRef] [PubMed]
108. Rej, A.; Sanders, D.S. The overlap of irritable bowel syndrome and noncoeliac gluten sensitivity. *Curr. Opin. Gastroenterol.* **2019**, *35*, 199–205. [CrossRef] [PubMed]
109. Frossi, B.; De Carli, M.; Calabrò, A. Coeliac Disease and Mast Cells. *Int. J. Mol. Sci.* **2019**, *20*, 3400. [CrossRef] [PubMed]
110. Tuck, C.J.; Vanner, S.J. Dietary therapies for functional bowel symptoms: Recent advances, challenges, and future directions. *Neurogastroent. Motil.* **2017**, e13238. [CrossRef]
111. Bischoff, S.C. Role of mast cells in allergic and non-allergic immune responses: Comparison of human and murine data. *Nat. Rev. Immunol.* **2007**, *7*, 93–104. [CrossRef]
112. Siebenhaar, F.; Redegeld, F.A.; Bischoff, S.C.; Gibbs, B.F.; Maurer, M. Mast cells as drivers of disease and therapeutic targets. *Trends Immunol.* **2018**, *39*, 151–162. [CrossRef]
113. Yu, Y.; Blokhuis, B.R.; Garssen, J.; Redegeld, F.A. Non-IgE mediated mast cell activation. *Eur. J. Pharmacol.* **2016**, *778*, 33–43. [CrossRef]

114. Simren, M.; Månsson, A.; Langkilde, A.M.; Svedlund, J.; Abrahamsson, H.; Bengtsson, U.; Björnsson, E.S. Food-related gastrointestinal symptoms in the irritable bowel syndrome. *Digestion* **2001**, *63*, 108–115. [CrossRef] [PubMed]
115. Choung, R.S.; Talley, N.J. Food allergy and intolerance in IBS. *Gastroen Hepatol.* **2006**, *2*, 756–760.
116. Virta, L.J.; Ashorn, M.; Kolho, K.L. Cow's milk allergy, asthma, and pediatric IBD. *J. Pediatr. Gastroen. Nutr.* **2013**, *56*, 649–651. [CrossRef] [PubMed]
117. Walker, M.M.; Powell, N.; Talley, N.J. Atopy and the gastrointestinal tract—a review of a common association in unexplained gastrointestinal disease. *Expert Rev. Gastroen. Hepatol.* **2014**, *8*, 289–299. [CrossRef] [PubMed]
118. Mansueto, P.; D'Alcamo, A.; Seidita, A.; Carroccio, A. Food allergy in irritable bowel syndrome: The case of non-celiac wheat sensitivity. *World J. Gastroenterol.* **2015**, *21*, 7089–7109. [CrossRef] [PubMed]
119. Bashashati, M.; Moossavi, S.; Cremon, C.; Barbaro, M.R.; Moraveji, S.; Talmon, G.; Rezaei, N.; Hughes, P.A.; Bian, Z.X.; Choi, C.H.; et al. Colonic immune cells in irritable bowel syndrome: A systematic review and meta-analysis. *Neurogastroent. Motil.* **2018**, *30*, e13192. [CrossRef]
120. Robles, A.; Perez Ingles, D.; Myneedu, K.; Deoker, A.; Sarosiek, I.; Zuckerman, M.J.; Schmulson, M.J.; Bashashati, M. Mast cells are increased in the small intestinal mucosa of patients with irritable bowel syndrome: A systematic review and meta-analysis. *Neurogastroent. Motil.* **2019**, *31*, e13718. [CrossRef]
121. Boeckxstaens, G. Mast cells and inflammatory bowel disease. *Curr. Opin. Pharmacol.* **2015**, *25*, 45–49. [CrossRef]
122. De Zuani, M.; Dal Secco, C.; Frossi, B. Mast cells at the crossroads of microbiota and IBD. *Eur. J. Immunol.* **2018**, *48*, 1929–1937. [CrossRef]
123. de Haan, J.J.; Hadfoune, M.; Lubbers, T.; Hodin, C.; Lenaerts, K.; Ito, A.; Verbaeys, I.; Skynner, M.J.; Cailotto, C.; van der Vliet, J.; et al. Lipid-rich enteral nutrition regulates mucosal mast cell activation via the vagal anti-inflammatory reflex. *Am. J. Physiol. Gastrointest. Liver. Physiol.* **2013**, *305*, G383–G391. [CrossRef]
124. Hagemann, P.M.; Nsiah-Dosu, S.; Hundt, J.E.; Hartmann, K.; Orinska, Z. Modulation of mast cell reactivity by lipids: The neglected side of allergic diseases. *Front Immunol.* **2019**, *10*, 1174. [CrossRef] [PubMed]
125. Schumann, J.; Basiouni, S.; Gück, T.; Fuhrmann, H. Treating canine atopic dermatitis with unsaturated fatty acids: The role of mast cells and potential mechanisms of action. *J. Anim. Physiol. Anim. Nutr.* **2014**, *98*, 1013–1020. [CrossRef] [PubMed]
126. van den Elsen, L.W.; Nusse, Y.; Balvers, M.; Redegeld, F.A.; Knol, E.F.; Garssen, J.; Willemsen, L.E. n-3 Long-chain PUFA reduce allergy-related mediator release by human mast cells in vitro via inhibition of reactive oxygen species. *Br. J. Nutr.* **2013**, *109*, 1821–1831. [CrossRef] [PubMed]
127. Park, B.; Park, S.; Park, J.; Park, M.; Min, T.; Jin, M. Omega-3 fatty acids suppress Th2-associated cytokine gene expressions and GATA transcription factors in mast cells. *J. Nut. Biochem.* **2013**, *24*, 868–876. [CrossRef]
128. Obata, T.; Nagakura, T.; Masaki, T.; Maekawa, K.; Yamashita, K. Eicosapentaenoic acid inhibits prostaglandin D2 generation by inhibiting cyclo-oxygenase-2 in cultured human mast cells. *Clin. Exp. Allergy* **1999**, *29*, 1129–1135. [CrossRef] [PubMed]
129. van Diest, S.A.; van den Elsen, L.W.; Klok, A.J.; Welting, O.; Hilbers, F.W.; van de Heijning, B.J.; Gaemers, I.C.; Boeckxstaens, G.E.; Werner, M.F.; Willemsen, L.E.; et al. Dietary marine n-3 PUFAs do not affect stress-induced visceral hypersensitivity in a rat maternal separation model. *J. Nutr.* **2015**, *145*, 915–922. [CrossRef] [PubMed]
130. Gueck, T.; Seidel, A.; Fuhrmann, H. Effects of essential fatty acids on mediators of mast cells in culture. *Prostag. Leukotr. Ess.* **2003**, *68*, 317–322. [CrossRef]
131. Gueck, T.; Seidel, A.; Baumann, D.; Meister, A.; Fuhrmann, H. Alterations of mast cell mediator production and release by gamma-linolenic and docosahexaenoic acid. *Vet. Dermatol.* **2004**, *15*, 309–314. [CrossRef]
132. Gueck, T.; Seidel, A.; Fuhrmann, H. Consequences of eicosapentaenoic acid (n-3) and arachidonic acid (n-6) supplementation on mast cell mediators. *J. Anim. Physiol. Anim. Nutr.* **2004**, *88*, 259–265. [CrossRef]
133. Ju, H.R.; Wu, H.Y.; Nishizono, S.; Sakono, M.; Ikeda, I.; Sugano, M.; Imaizumi, K. Effects of dietary fats and curcumin on IgE-mediated degranulation of intestinal mast cells in brown Norway rats. *Biosci. Biotechnol. Biochem.* **1996**, *60*, 1856–1860. [CrossRef]
134. Vinolo, M.A.; Rodrigues, H.G.; Nachbar, R.T.; Curi, R. Regulation of inflammation by short chain fatty acids. *Nutrients* **2011**, *3*, 858–876. [CrossRef] [PubMed]
135. Leonel, A.J.; Alvarez-Leite, J.I. Butyrate: Implications for intestinal function. *Curr. Opin. Clin. Nutr. Metab. Care.* **2012**, *15*, 474–479. [CrossRef] [PubMed]

136. Wang, C.C.; Wu, H.; Lin, F.H.; Gong, R.; Xie, F.; Peng, Y.; Feng, J.; Hu, C.H. Sodium butyrate enhances intestinal integrity, inhibits mast cell activation, inflammatory mediator production and JNK signaling pathway in weaned pigs. *Innate. Immun.* **2018**, *24*, 40–46. [CrossRef] [PubMed]
137. Martínez, V.; Iriondo De-Hond, A.; Borrelli, F.; Capasso, R.; Del Castillo, M.D.; Abalo, R. Cannabidiol and Other Non-Psychoactive Cannabinoids for Prevention and Treatment of Gastrointestinal Disorders: Useful Nutraceuticals? *Int. J. Mol. Sci.* **2020**, *21*, 3067. [CrossRef] [PubMed]
138. De Filippis, D.; Esposito, G.; Cirillo, C.; Cipriano, M.; de Winter, B.; Scuderi, C.; Sarnelli, G.; Cuomo, R.; Steardo, L.; de Man, J.; et al. Cannabidiol reduces intestinal inflammation through the control of neuroimmune axis. *PLoS ONE* **2011**, *6*, 1–8. [CrossRef]
139. De Filippis, D.; Negro, L.; Vaia, M.; Cinelli, M.P.; Iuvone, T. New insights in mast cell modulation by palmitoylethanolamide. *CNS Neurol. Disord. Drug Targets* **2013**, *12*, 78–83. [CrossRef]
140. Cerrato, S.; Brazis, P.; della Valle, M.F.; Miolo, A.; Puigdemont, A. Effects of palmitoylethanolamide on immunologically induced histamine, PGD2 and TNFalpha release from canine skin mast cells. *Vet. Immunol. Immunopathol.* **2010**, *133*, 9–15. [CrossRef]
141. Cantarella, G.; Scollo, M.; Lempereur, L.; Saccani-Jotti, G.; Basile, F.; Bernardini, R. Endocannabinoids inhibit release of nerve growth factor by inflammation-activated mast cells. *Biochem. Pharmacol.* **2011**, *82*, 380–388. [CrossRef]
142. Mazzari, S.; Canella, R.; Petrelli, L.; Marcolongo, G.; Leon, A. N-(2-hydroxyethyl) hexadecanamide is orally active in reducing edema formation and inflammatory hyperalgesia by down-modulating mast cell activation. *Eur. J. Pharmacol.* **1996**, *300*, 227–236. [CrossRef]
143. De Filippis, D.; D'Amico, A.; Cinelli, M.P.; Esposito, G.; Di Marzo, V.; Iuvone, T. Adelmidrol, a palmitoylethanolamide analogue, reduces chronic inflammation in carrageenin granuloma model in rat. *J. Cell Mol. Med.* **2009**, *13*, 1086–1095. [CrossRef]
144. De Filippis, D.; D'Amico, A.; Cipriano, M.; Petrosino, S.; Orlando, P.; Di Marzo, V.; Iuvone, T. Levels of endocannabinoids and palmitoylethanolamide and their pharmacological manipulation in chronic granulomatous inflammation in rats. *Pharmacol. Res.* **2010**, *61*, 321–328. [CrossRef] [PubMed]
145. De Filippis, D.; Luongo, L.; Cipriano, M.; Palazzo, E.; Cinelli, M.P.; de Novellis, V.; Maione, S.; Iuvone, T. Palmitoylethanolamide reduces granuloma-induced hyperalgesia by modulation of mast cell activation in rats. *Mol. Pain.* **2011**, *7*, 3. [CrossRef] [PubMed]
146. Costa, B.; Comelli, F.; Bettoni, I.; Colleoni, M.P.; Giagnoni, G. The endogenous fatty acid amide, palmitoylethanolamide, has anti-allodynic and anti-hyperalgesic effects in a murine model of neuropathic pain: Involvement of CB1, TRPV1 and PPARgamma receptors and neurotrophic factors. *Pain* **2008**, *139*, 541–550. [CrossRef] [PubMed]
147. Esposito, E.; Paterniti, I.; Mazzon, E.; Genovese, T.; Di Paola, R.; Galuppo, M.; Cuzzocrea, S. Effects of palmitoylethanolamide on release of mast cell peptidases and neurotrophic factors after spinal cord injury. *Brain. Behav. Immun.* **2011**, *25*, 1099–1112. [CrossRef] [PubMed]
148. Scarampella, F.; Abramo, F.; Noli, C. Clinical and histological evaluation of an analogue of palmitoylethanolamide, PLR 120 (comicronized Palmidrol INN) in cats with eosinophilic granuloma and eosinophilic plaque: A pilot study. *Vet. Dermatol.* **2001**, *12*, 29–39. [CrossRef] [PubMed]
149. Cremon, C.; Stanghellini, V.; Barbaro, M.; Cogliandro, R.; Bellacosa, L.; Santos, J.; Vicario, M.; Pigrau, M.; Alonso Cotoner, C.; Lobo, B.; et al. Randomised clinical trial: The analgesic properties of dietary supplementation with palmitoylethanolamide and polydatin in irritable bowel syndrome. *Alim. Pharmacol. Ther.* **2017**, *45*, 909–922. [CrossRef]
150. Olivera, A.; Rivera, J. Sphingolipids and the balancing of immune cell function: Lessons from the mast cell. *J. Immunol.* **2005**, *174*, 1153–1158. [CrossRef]
151. Chiba, N.; Masuda, A.; Yoshikai, Y.; Matsuguchi, T. Ceramide inhibits LPS-induced production of IL-5, IL-10, and IL-13 from mast cells. *J. Cell. Physiol.* **2007**, *213*, 126–136. [CrossRef]
152. Jolly, P.S.; Bektas, M.; Olivera, A.; Gonzalez-Espinosa, C.; Proia, R.L.; Rivera, J.; Milstien, S.; Spiegel, S. Transactivation of sphingosine-1-phosphate receptors by FcepsilonRI triggering is required for normal mast cell degranulation and chemotaxis. *J. Exp. Med.* **2004**, *199*, 959–970. [CrossRef]
153. Liu, Z.Q.; Li, X.X.; Qiu, S.Q.; Yu, Y.; Li, M.G.; Yang, L.T.; Li, L.J.; Wang, S.; Zheng, P.Y.; Liu, Z.G.; et al. Vitamin D contributes to mast cell stabilization. *Allergy* **2017**, *72*, 1184–1192. [CrossRef]
154. Zingg, J. Vitamin E and mast cells. *Vitam. Horm.* **2007**, *76*, 393–418. [PubMed]

155. Gueck, T.; Aschenbach, J.R.; Fuhrmann, H. Influence of vitamin E on mast cell mediator release. *Vet. Dermatol.* **2002**, *13*, 301–305. [CrossRef] [PubMed]
156. Ranadive, N.S.; Lewis, R. Differential effects of antioxidants and indomethacin on compound 48/80 induced histamine release and Ca2+ uptake in rat mast cells. *Immunol. Lett.* **1982**, *5*, 145–150. [CrossRef]
157. Lecleire, S.; Hassan, A.; Marion-Letellier, R.; Antonietti, M.; Savoye, G.; Bole-Feysot, C.; Lerebours, E.; Ducrotte, P.; Dechelotte, P.; Coeffier, M. Combined glutamine and arginine decrease proinflammatory cytokine production by biopsies from Crohn's patients in association with changes in nuclear factor-kappa B and p38 mito-gen-activated protein kinase pathways. *J. Nutr.* **2008**, *138*, 2481–2486. [CrossRef]
158. Lechowski, S.; Feilhauer, K.; Staib, L.; Coeffier, M.; Bischoff, S.C.; Lorentz, A. Combined arginine and glutamine decrease release of de novo synthesized leukotrienes and expression of proinflammatory cytokines in activated human intestinal mast cells. *Eur. J. Nutr.* **2013**, *52*, 505–512. [CrossRef] [PubMed]
159. Zhu, H.; Pi, D.; Leng, W.; Wang, X.; Hu, C.A.; Hou, Y.; Xiong, J.; Wang, C.; Qin, Q.; Liu, Y. Asparagine preserves intestinal barrier function from LPS-induced injury and regulates CRF/CRFR signaling pathway. *Innate. Immun.* **2017**, *23*, 546–556. [CrossRef]
160. van Bergenhenegouwen, J.; Braber, S.; Loonstra, R.; Buurman, N.; Rutten, L.; Knipping, K.; Savelkoul, P.; Harthoorn, L.; Jahnsen, F.; Garssen, J.; et al. Oral exposure to the free amino acid glycine inhibits the acute allergic response in a model of cow's milk allergy in mice. *Nut. Res.* **2018**, *58*, 95–105. [CrossRef]
161. Sakai, S.; Sugawara, T.; Matsubara, K.; Hirata, T. Inhibitory effect of carotenoids on the degranulation of mast cells via suppression of antigen-induced aggregation of high affinity IgE receptors. *J. Biol. Chem.* **2009**, *284*, 28172–28179. [CrossRef]
162. Kim, H.; Ahn, Y.; Lee, G.; Cho, S.; Kim, J.; Lee, C.; Lim, B.; Ju, S.; An, W. Effects of astaxanthin on dinitrofluorobenzene-induced contact dermatitis in mice. *Mol. Med. Rep.* **2015**, *12*, 3632–3638. [CrossRef]
163. Sato, Y.; Akiyama, H.; Suganuma, H.; Watanabe, T.; Nagaoka, M.H.; Inakuma, T.; Goda, Y.; Maitani, T. The feeding of -carotene down-regulates serum IgE levels and inhibits the type I allergic response in mice. *Biol. Pharm. Bull.* **2004**, *27*, 978–984. [CrossRef]
164. Kinoshita, T.; Koike, K.; Mwamtemi, H.H.; Ito, S.; Ishida, S.; Nakazawa, Y.; Kurokawa, Y.; Sakashita, K.; Higuchi, T.; Takeuchi, K.; et al. Retinoic acid is a negative regulator for the differentiation of cord blood-derived human mast cell progenitors. *Blood* **2000**, *95*, 2821–2828. [CrossRef] [PubMed]
165. Hjertson, M.; Kivinen, P.; Dimberg, L.; Nilsson, K.; Harvima, I.; Nilsson, G. Retinoic acid inhibits in vitro development of mast cells but has no marked effect on mature human skin tryptase- and chymase-positive mast cells. *J. Investig. Dermatol.* **2003**, *120*, 239–245. [CrossRef] [PubMed]
166. Ishida, S.; Kinoshita, T.; Sugawara, N.; Yamashita, T.; Koike, K. Serum inhibitors for human mast cell growth: Possible role of retinol. *Eur. J. Allergy. Clin. Immunol.* **2003**, *58*, 1044–1052. [CrossRef] [PubMed]
167. Astorquiza, M.I.; Helle, B.; Vergara, R.E. Effect of vitamin A onthe in vitro degranulation of mouse mastcells. *Allergol. Immunopathol.* **1980**, *8*, 87–90.
168. Middleton, E., Jr.; Drzewiecki, G. Flavonoid inhibition of human basophil histamine release stimulated by various agents. *Biochem. Pharmacol.* **1984**, *33*, 3333–3338. [CrossRef]
169. Trnovsky, J.; Letourneau, R.; Haggag, E.; Boucher, W.; Theoharides, T.C. Quercetin-induced expression of rat mast cell protease II and accumulation of secretory granules in rat basophilic leukemia cells. *Biochem. Pharmacol.* **1993**, *46*, 2315–2326. [CrossRef]
170. Alexandrakis, M.; Singh, L.; Boucher, W.; Letourneau, R.; Theofilopoulos, P.; Theoharides, T.C. Differential effect of flavonoids on inhibition of secretion and accumulation of secretory granules in rat basophilic leukemia cells. *Int. J. Immunopharmacol.* **1999**, *21*, 379–390. [CrossRef]
171. Kimata, M.; Inagaki, N.; Nagai, H. Effects of luteolin and other flavonoids on IgE-mediated allergic reactions. *Planta. Med.* **2000**, *66*, 25–29. [CrossRef]
172. Kimata, M.; Shichijo, S.; Miura, T.; Serizawa, I.; Inagaki, N.; Nagai, H. Effects of luteolin, quercetin and baicalein on immunoglobulin E-mediated mediator release from human cultured mast cells. *Clin. Exp. Allergy* **2000**, *30*, 501–508. [CrossRef]
173. Seelinger, G.; Merfort, I.; Schempp, C.M. Anti-oxidant, anti-inflammatory and anti-allergic activities of luteolin. *Planta. Med.* **2008**, *74*, 1667–1677. [CrossRef]
174. Park, H.H.; Lee, S.; Son, K.Y.; Park, S.B.; Kim, M.S.; Choi, E.J.; Singh, T.S.; Ha, J.H.; Lee, M.G.; Kim, J.E.; et al. Flavonoids inhibit histamine release and expression of proinflammatory cytokines in mast cells. *Arch. Pharm. Res.* **2008**, *31*, 1303–1311. [CrossRef] [PubMed]

175. Kempuraj, D.; Madhappan, B.; Chrístodoulou, S.; Boucher, W.; Cao, J.; Papadopoulou, N.; Cetrulo, C.L.; Theoharides, T.C. Flavonols inhibit proinflammatory mediator release, intracellular calcium ion levels and protein kinase C phosphorylation in human mast cells. *Br. J. Pharmacol.* **2005**, *145*, 934–944. [CrossRef] [PubMed]
176. Yang, Y.; Oh, J.M.; Heo, P.; Shin, J.Y.; Kong, B.; Shin, J.; Lee, J.C.; Oh, J.S.; Park, K.W.; Lee, C.H.; et al. Polyphenols differentially inhibit degranulation of distinct subsets of vesicles in mast cells by specific interaction with granule-type-dependent SNARE complexes. *Biochem. J.* **2013**, *450*, 537–546. [CrossRef] [PubMed]
177. Hagenlocher, Y.; Feilhauer, K.; Schäffer, M.; Bischoff, S.C.; Lorentz, A. Citrus peel polymethoxyflavones nobiletin and tangeretin suppress LPS- and IgE-mediated activation of human intestinal mast cells. *Eur. J. Nutr.* **2017**, *56*, 1609–1620. [CrossRef]
178. Tanaka, T.; Iuchi, A.; Harada, H.; Hashimoto, S. Potential Beneficial Effects of Wine Flavonoids on Allergic Diseases. *Diseases* **2019**, *7*, 8. [CrossRef]
179. Hagenlocher, Y.; Gommeringer, S.; Held, A.; Feilhauer, K.; Köninger, J.; Bischoff, S.C.; Lorentz, A. Nobiletin acts anti-inflammatory on murine IL-10-/- colitis and human intestinal fibroblasts. *Eur. J. Nutr.* **2019**, *58*, 1391–1401. [CrossRef]
180. Hubert, J.; Berger, M.; Nepveu, F.; Paul, F.; Daydé, J. Effects of fermentation on the phytochemical composition and antioxidant properties of soy germ. *Food Chem.* **2008**, *109*, 709–721. [CrossRef]
181. Moussa, L.; Bézirard, V.; Salvador-Cartier, C.; Bacquié, V.; Houdeau, E.; Théodorou, V. A new soy germ fermented ingredient displays estrogenic and protease inhibitor activities able to prevent irritable bowel syndrome-like symptoms in stressed female rats. *Clin. Nutr.* **2013**, *32*, 51–58. [CrossRef]
182. Inoue, T.; Suzuki, Y.; Ra, C. Epigallocatechin-3-gallate inhibits mast cell degranulation, leukotriene C4 secretion, and calcium influx via mitochondrial calcium dysfunction. *Free Radic. Biol. Med.* **2010**, *49*, 632–640. [CrossRef]
183. Inoue, T.; Suzuki, Y.; Ra, C. Epigallocatechin-3-gallate induces cytokine production in mast cells by stimulating an extracellular superoxide-mediated calcium influx. *Biochem. Pharmacol.* **2011**, *82*, 1930–1939. [CrossRef]
184. Khan, N.; Mukhtar, H. Tea Polyphenols in promotion of human health. *Nutrients* **2018**, *11*, 39. [CrossRef] [PubMed]
185. Matsuo, N.; Yamada, K.; Shoji, K.; Mori, M.; Sugano, M. Effect of tea polyphenols on histamine release from rat basophilic leukemia (RBL-2H3) cells: The structure-inhibitory activity relationship. *Allergy* **1997**, *52*, 58–64. [CrossRef] [PubMed]
186. Yamashita, K.; Suzuki, Y.; Matsui, T.; Yoshimaru, T.; Yamaki, M.; Suzuki-Karasaki, M.; Hayakawa, S.; Shimizu, K. Epigallocatechin gallate inhibits histamine release from rat basophilic leukemia (RBL-2H3) cells: Role of tyrosine phosphorylation. *Biochem. Biophys. Res. Commun.* **2000**, *274*, 603–608. [CrossRef] [PubMed]
187. Murata, K.; Takano, S.; Masuda, M.; Iinuma, M.; Matsuda, H. Anti-degranulating activity in rat basophilic leukemia RBL-2H3 cells of flavanone glycosides and their aglycones in citrus fruits. *J. Nat. Med.* **2013**, *67*, 643–646. [CrossRef]
188. Fiorani, M.; Accorsi, A.; Blasa, M.; Diamantini, G.; Piatti, E. Flavonoids from Italian multi-floral honeys reduce the extracellular ferricyanide in human red blood cells. *J. Agric. Food Chem.* **2006**, *54*, 8328–8334. [CrossRef]
189. Guendouz, M.; Haddi, A.; Grar, H.; Kheroua, O.; Saidi, D.; Kaddouri, H. Preventive effects of royal jelly against anaphylactic response in a murine model of cow's milk allergy. *Pharm. Biol.* **2017**, *55*, 2145–2152. [CrossRef]
190. Gupta, S.C.; Kismali, G.; Aggarwal, B.B. Curcumin, a component of turmeric: From farm to pharmacy. *Biofactors* **2013**, *39*, 2–13. [CrossRef]
191. Lee, J.H.; Kim, J.W.; Ko, N.Y.; Mun, S.H.; Her, E.; Kim, B.K.; Han, J.W.; Lee, H.Y.; Beaven, M.A.; Kim, Y.M.; et al. Curcumin, a constituent of curry, suppresses IgE-mediated allergic response and mast cell activation at the level of Syk. *J. Allergy Clin. Immunol.* **2008**, *121*, 1225–1231. [CrossRef]
192. Hanai, H.; Iida, T.; Takeuchi, K.; Watanabe, F.; Maruyama, Y.; Andoh, A.; Tsujikawa, T.; Fujiyama, Y.; Mitsuyama, K.; Sata, M.; et al. Curcumin maintenance therapy for ulcerative colitis: Randomized, multicenter, double-blind, placebo-controlled trial. *Clin. Gastroen. Hepatol.* **2006**, *4*, 1502–1506. [CrossRef]

193. Lang, A.; Salomon, N.; Wu, J.C.; Kopylov, U.; Lahat, A.; Har-Noy, O.; Ching, J.Y.; Cheong, P.K.; Avidan, B.; Gamus, D.; et al. Curcumin in combination with mesalamine induces remission in patients with mild-to-moderate ulcerative colitis in a randomized controlled trial. *Clin. Gastroen. Hepatol.* **2015**, *13*, 1444–1449. [CrossRef]
194. Bundy, R.; Walker, A.F.; Middleton, R.W.; Booth, J. Turmeric extract may improve irritable bowel syndrome symptomology in otherwise healthy adults: A pilot study. *J. Altern. Complement. Med.* **2004**, *10*, 1015–1018. [CrossRef] [PubMed]
195. Portincasa, P.; Bonfrate, L.; Scribano, M.L.; Kohn, A.; Caporaso, N.; Festi, D.; Campanale, M.C.; Di Rienzo, T.; Guarino, M.; Taddia, M.; et al. Curcumin and Fennel Essential Oil Improve Symptoms and Quality of Life in Patients with Irritable Bowel Syndrome. *J. Gastrointestin. Liver. Dis.* **2016**, *25*, 151–157. [CrossRef] [PubMed]
196. Hagenlocher, Y.; Bergheim, I.; Zacheja, S.; Schäffer, M.; Bischoff, S.C.; Lorentz, A. Cinnamon extract inhibits degranulation and de novo synthesis of inflammatory mediators in mast cells. *Allergy* **2013**, *68*, 490–497. [CrossRef] [PubMed]
197. Hagenlocher, Y.; Hösel, A.; Bischoff, S.; Lorentz, A. Cinnamon extract reduces symptoms, inflammatory mediators and mast cell markers in murine IL-10−/− colitis. *J. Nut. Biochem.* **2016**, *30*, 85–92. [CrossRef]
198. Hagenlocher, Y.; Kiessling, K.; Schäffer, M.; Bischoff, S.C.; Lorentz, A. Cinnamaldehyde is the main mediator of cinnamon extract in mast cell inhibition. *Eur. J. Nutr.* **2015**, *54*, 1297–1309. [CrossRef]

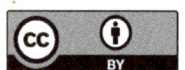

© 2020 by the authors. Licensee MDPI, Basel, Switzerland. This article is an open access article distributed under the terms and conditions of the Creative Commons Attribution (CC BY) license (http://creativecommons.org/licenses/by/4.0/).

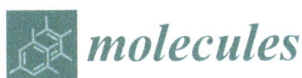

Review

Hormesis and Ginseng: Ginseng Mixtures and Individual Constituents Commonly Display Hormesis Dose Responses, Especially for Neuroprotective Effects

Edward J. Calabrese

Department of Environmental Health Sciences, School of Public Health and Health Sciences, University of Massachusetts, Amherst, MA 01003, USA; edwardc@schoolph.umass.edu; Tel.: +1-413-545-3164

Academic Editors: Sokcheon Pak and Soo Liang Ooi
Received: 14 May 2020; Accepted: 8 June 2020; Published: 11 June 2020

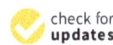

Abstract: This paper demonstrates that ginseng mixtures and individual ginseng chemical constituents commonly induce hormetic dose responses in numerous biological models for endpoints of biomedical and clinical relevance, typically providing a mechanistic framework. The principal focus of ginseng hormesis-related research has been directed toward enhancing neuroprotection against conditions such as Alzheimer's and Parkinson's Diseases, stroke damage, as well as enhancing spinal cord and peripheral neuronal damage repair and reducing pain. Ginseng was also shown to reduce symptoms of diabetes, prevent cardiovascular system damage, protect the kidney from toxicities due to immune suppressant drugs, and prevent corneal damage, amongst other examples. These findings complement similar hormetic-based chemoprotective reports for other widely used dietary-type supplements such as curcumin, ginkgo biloba, and green tea. These findings, which provide further support for the generality of the hormetic dose response in the biomedical literature, have potentially important public health and clinical implications.

Keywords: hormesis; hormetic; ginseng; biphasic; neuroprotection; aging; Alzheimer's Disease; Parkinson's Disease; wound healing; preconditioning

1. Introduction

Ginseng is a widely consumed nutritional supplement with a long history of use in traditional Asian medicine for a range of conditions. Publications in the scientific literature on the pharmacology of ginseng were first listed in the Web of Science in 1905 on the pharmacology of ginseng [1]. While scientific research on ginseng was low through the first 70 years of the 20th century, there was a multidisciplinary resurgent interest in the biological properties of ginseng starting in the 1970s. In 1976, the Journal of *Ginseng Research* was started, reflecting progressive and broadening interest to the present. The range of publications has been highly varied, but with a strong biomedical orientation, with the general goal of assessing whether ginseng might enhance public health and medical prevention/treatment of a wide range of harmful conditions. The present paper provides the first integrative assessment concerning the capacity of ginseng mixtures and some of its specific constituents to induce hormetic dose responses by documenting their occurrence, generality, mechanistic basis, and potential biomedical significance.

Hormesis is a biphasic dose–response relationship that is characterized by low-dose stimulation and high-dose inhibition [2,3]. The magnitude of the low dose stimulation is modest with the maximum stimulation typically being in the 130–160% range (compared to control groups: 100%) [4]. The dose width of the low-dose stimulation is usually less than a 50-fold starting from the estimated toxic/pharmacological threshold (Figure 1). Hormetic responses may occur either by a direct stimulation or an overcompensation to a disruption in homeostasis/slight to modest toxicity.

Preconditioning-mediated biological responses are examples of hormesis, displaying the typical hormetic dose response when sufficient conditioning doses are used in the experiment [5–7]. Hormetic dose responses are general, being independent of biological model, inducing agent, endpoint, level of biological organization, and mechanism [8]. A series of recent publications have documented hormetic dose responses in the biomedical literature for curcumin [9], Ginkgo biloba [10], and green tea [11]. The present findings show that ginseng-induced hormetic effects are also commonly reported that are broadly generalizable, affecting numerous organ systems, cell types, and endpoints, showing capacity to induce acquired resilience for various durations, within multiple and diverse experimental settings, with particular research focus directed toward neuroprotective effects (Tables 1–3). The paper assesses the published literature of individual ginseng constituents as well as various types of ginseng extract mixtures. The paper will also relate the hormetic dose response findings for ginseng to the broader hormetic literature and highlight their potential biomedical and clinical implications.

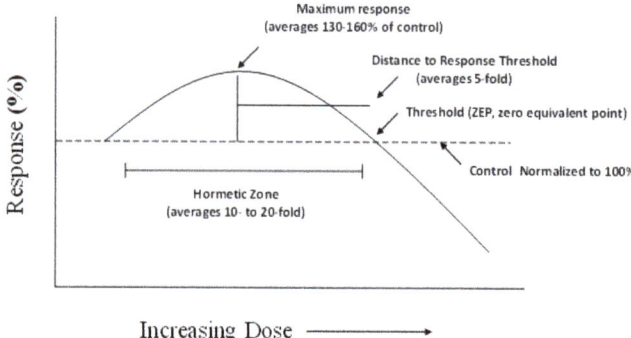

Figure 1. Dose–response curve representing the quantitative features of hormesis (Source: [7]).

Table 1. Hormetic effect with ginseng mixtures/specific constituents and biological models.

Non-Neural Models	
	References
Muscle fiber damage-exercise	Voces et al. [12,13]
HEPG2 cell proliferation	Li et al. [14]
HUVEC	Sung et al. [15]
A549-human pulmonary epithelial cells	Son et al. [16]
Ovary-hormone production	Seghinsara et al. [17]
Diabetes-STZ-model	Lim et al. [18]
Human skin fibroblasts	Kanzaki et al. [19]
PAI-1- PAI-1 (Plasminogen activator inhibitor)	Morisaki et al. [20]
Neural Models	
SH-SY-5Y-Neural	Shi et al. [21]
Brain-TBI studies-Neural	Hu et al. [22]; Xia et al. [23]
Neurite outgrowth-Sprague Dawley- E-16-Neural	Liao et al. [24]
Zebrafish-neuron loss/behavior-Neural	Zhang et al. [25]
Hippocampus, dentate gryus-Neural	Hu et al. [22]; Lim et al. [18]
Astrocytes, preconditioning-Neural	Naval et al. [26]
NSC-Cell proliferation/differentiation-Neural	Gao et al. [27]
IRC mice/female-behavior-Neural-prefrontal cortex	Boonlert et al. [28]
Spinal cord survival	Liao et al. [24]

Table 2. Ginseng-induced hormetic dose responses by constituent/mixtures.

Rg1	Rb1	Rd	Rg3	Polyacetylenes	Gentonin	Ginseng Mixtures
Stem cells	Neuroprotection	Neuroprotection	Neuronal injury	Nerve repair	Wound healing	Neuroprotection
Proliferation/differentiation	AD/PD	PD	Neuronal regeneration	AD	Corneal damage	Learning/memory Behaviors
Neuroprotection	Stroke	Stroke	Atherosclerosis		AD	Hippocampal cell
AD/PD	Neuronal Repair	Neurosphere production			Glycogenolysis	Neurite outgrowth
Stroke	Other: Heart, Diabetes	Glutamate toxicity.				NSC proliferation
Neonatal brain hypoxia		Spinal Cord				
Neuronal wound healing		Other: Heart-cardiomyocytes, Kidney-FK506				Brain Injury
Nerve regeneration						Other: Muscle injury, Osteogenesis, Kidney damage, Hormone production
Other: Heart cardiomyocytes, Immune enhancement, Diabetes						

Table 3. Ginseng-induced hormetic dose response disease and endpoint.

Alzheimer's Disease Prevention: Rg1
Parkinson's Disease Prevention: Rg1
Stroke Damage Prevention: Rg1
Kidney Damage Prevention: Rd
Heart Related Damage Prevention: Rg1
Nerve Cell Damage Prevention/Regeneration: Rg1
Diabetes Prevention: Rg1, Rb1, Rg3
Stem Cell Proliferation/Differential: Rg1 and mixtures.
Brain Traumatic Injury: Mixtures

2. Search Strategy

PubMed, Web of Science, and Google Scholar databases were searched for articles using the terms "hormesis or hormetic and ginseng, and specific ginseng constituents (e.g., Rg1, Rb1, Rc, Rd, Re, ginseng mixtures, ginseng saponins, gintonin, polyacetylenes), dose response and ginseng; U-shaped dose response and ginseng; biphasic dose response and ginseng; preconditioning and ginseng; adaptive response and ginseng; stem cells and ginseng; ginseng and biphasic concentration response; ginseng and conditioning response". All relevant articles were evaluated for the references cited and for all papers citing these papers. All research groups publishing ginseng dose–response relationships were assessed for possible relevant publications in the above databases.

3. Ginseng Constituent RG1

3.1. Rg1-Stem Cell Proliferation and Differentiation

That ginsenoside Rg1 could enhance the proliferation and differentiation of stem cells is a relatively new development. For example, Rg1 treatment enhanced neural progenitor cell (NPC) proliferation in hippocampal tissue [29], endothelial cells [30], and enhanced proliferation and neuro-phenotype differentiation of human adipose-derived stem cells (ASC) [31,32]. These studies, along with an hormetic dose response for NPC by Liu et al. [33] with Rg5 (Figure 2), provide the supportive publications for a framework for subsequent research described below to clarify the nature of the Rg1-mediated hormesis dose response, dose optimization, and underlying mechanisms of stem cell proliferation and differentiation.

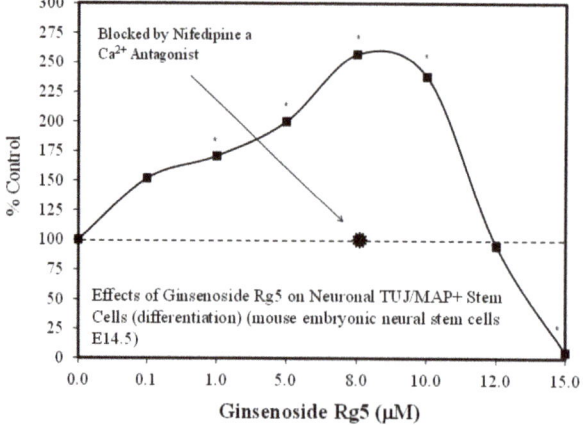

Figure 2. Effects of ginsenoside Rg5 on neuronal TUJ/MAP+ stem cells (differentiation) (mouse embryonic neural stem cells E14.5) (source: [33]). * = statistically significant

Researchers from four stem cell areas have published hormetic dose responses with Rg1. In these studies, the authors assessed both cell proliferation and differentiation. With this dual endpoint consideration, hormetic dose responses were reported for cell proliferation for each of the four papers. Only Liang et al. [34] also showed hormetic dose responses for differentiation endpoints. In the remaining three papers, differentiation endpoints had only one dose, precluding a hormetic dose response evaluation. The four stem cell publications involved the following study subjects: Adipose Stem Cells/ASC: a 23-year-old female [34], neural stem cells: Sprague–Dawley rats—four pregnant females (E-17), with the number of fetuses not reported (Figure 3) [35]; human derived pulp stem cells—50 third impacted molars from subjects 19–28 years of age (gender not mentioned) [36]; human periodontal ligament stem cells, with 10 adults (gender not given) [37]. Each study differed in the number of concentrations tested, ranging from a low of four concentrations with two concentrations below the threshold (ASC) [34] to a high of 10 concentrations with five concentrations below the threshold (NSC) [35].

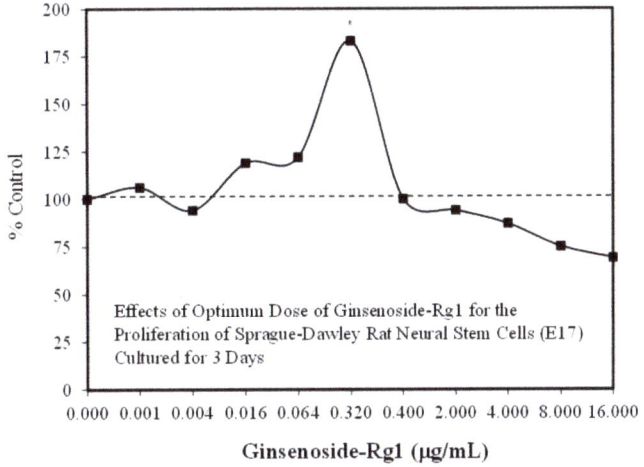

Figure 3. Effects of optimum dose of ginsenoside-Rg1 for the proliferation of Sprague–Dawley rat neural stem cells (E17) cultured for 3 days (source: [35]). * = statistically significant.

Despite these study differences, each displayed consistent evidence of hormetic dose responses (Figures 2–7). The maximum stimulation responses ranged from 130–250% while the stimulation concentration ranged from about 2 [36] to 100-fold [37]. The quantitative features of stem cell proliferation (Figure 4), stem cell paracrine activity (Figure 5a,b), and differentiation responses (e.g., adipocytes/chondrocytres) (Figure 6) reflected the quantitative features of the hormetic dose response [34]. The implications of hormetic–biphasic dose responses of Rg1 for the different stem cells remains to be explored. However, Yin et al. [37] suggests that Rg1 be further assessed as a possible medication for osteogenesis treatment since it enhances the proliferation of human periodontal ligament stem cells in an hormetic-like biphasic dose–response manner (Figure 7). Showing similar biphasic dose–response features, Wang et al. [36] suggested that Rg1 has potential as a pulp-capping agent to enhance pulp healing and preserve pulp vitality. Furthermore, porcine blastocyte hormetic findings were consistent with the above reports as Rg1 mediated protection via decreasing oxidative stress and increasing the cellular uptake of glucose that reduced apoptosis-induced cell death [38]. Finally, additional neural stem cell/hormesis findings are presented on neonatal brain hypoxia within the Rg1 neuroprotection section [39].

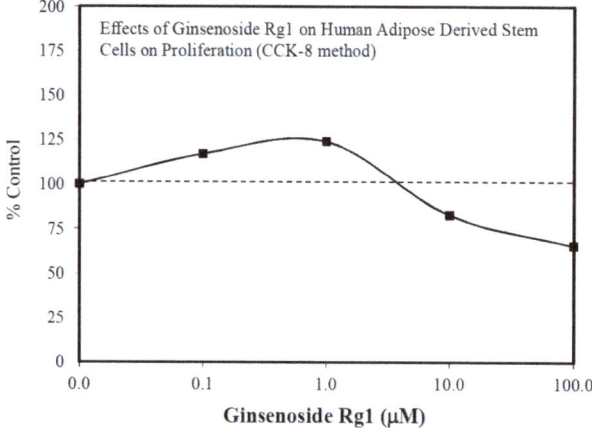

Figure 4. Effects of ginsenoside Rg1 on human adipose-derived stem cells on proliferation (CCK-8 method) (source: [34]).

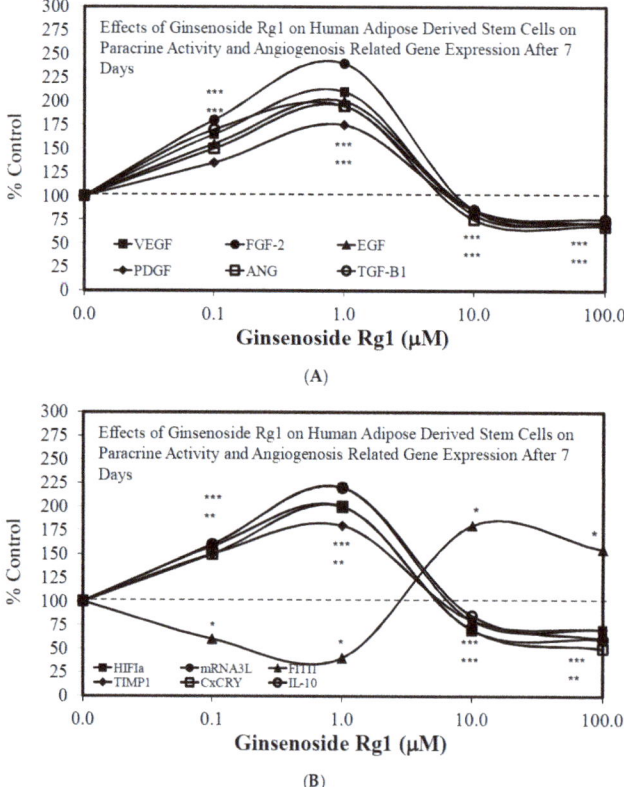

Figure 5. (**A**) Effects of ginsenoside Rg1 on human adipose-derived stem cells on paracrine activity and angiogenosis-related gene expression after 7 days (source: [34]). (**B**) Effects of ginsenoside Rg1 on human adipose-derived stem cells on paracrine activity and angiogenosis-related gene expression after 7 days (source: [34]). Each * represent statistical significance for a data point.

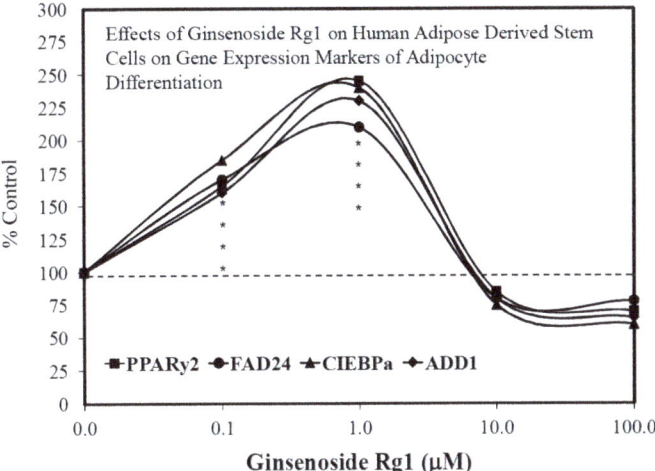

Figure 6. Effects of ginsenoside Rg1 on human adipose-derived stem cells on gene expression markers of adipocyte differentiation (source: [34]). Each * represent statistical significance for a data point.

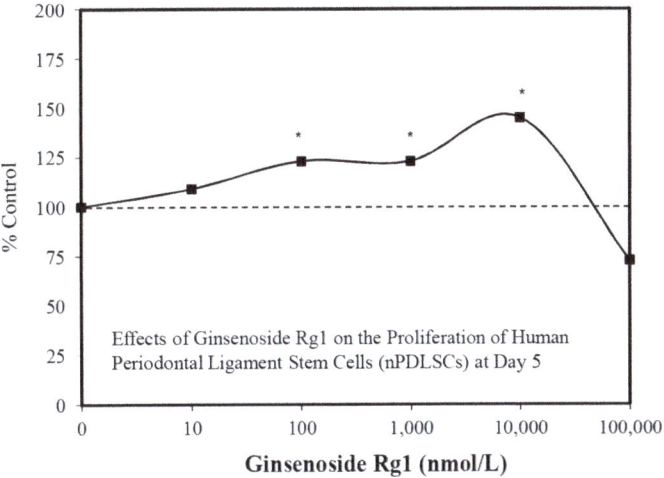

Figure 7. Effects of ginsenoside Rg1 on the proliferation of human periodontal ligament stem cells (nPDLSCs) at Day 5 (Source: [37]). Each * represent statistical significance for a data point.

3.2. Rg1 Neuroprotection

Rg1 affects neuroprotection responses across a spectrum of neurological diseases and injury/damage conditions. These include Parkinson's and Alzheimer's Diseases, stroke, neonatal brain hypoxia-induced injury, and recovery/healing following spinal cord and peripheral nerve injuries and pain. The research approach has emphasized a combination of pre- and post-conditioning experimental protocols, co-administration of the protective/harmful agents, as well as the direct stimulation of neuronal tissue to enhance neuronal survival, neurite outgrowth, and cell migration activities in neuronal wound-healing studies. Furthermore, most of these investigations incorporate mechanistic features that clarified aspects of neuroprotective pathway components and their functions.

3.3. Parkinson's Disease

3.3.1. Introduction

In the case of Parkinson's Disease (PD) and Rg1, three experimental models have been employed, including one in vivo mouse model study [40] and two in vitro models using the SK-N-SH (human neuroblastoma cell line that can express dopamine markers) [41] and the MES23.5 cell line (i.e., a dopaminergic cell line) [42], with each using a preconditioning protocol. Furthermore, the PD symptoms/endpoints were induced by standard/classical chemical agents. In the case of the in vitro experiments, 6-OHDA [41,42] and rotenone [43] were employed, whereas MPTP induced PD symptoms in the in vivo mouse study [40].

3.3.2. In Vitro Studies

In the in vitro studies, the SK-N-SH cell line investigations [41,43] employed a one-hour pretreatment while the MES23.5 cell line study [42] used a 24 h pretreatment. Two in vitro studies [41,42] used the same 6-ODHA concentration of 100 μM with one administering it for 24 h (i.e., SK-N-SH), while the other did so for 48 h (i.e., MES23.5). In the case of the MES23.5 cells, there were 1000 cells/well that were grown for 24 h and then treated. In the SK-N-SH study of Gao et al. [41], cells were grown to 80–90% confluence prior to treatment. Since PD is less common in women than men, the thought that estrogen may protect the brain from developing PD has been widely discussed. Of relevance to the present assessment is that Rg1 was shown to be a phytoestrogen by Chan et al. [44] by enhancing the proliferation of MCF-7 cells in a hormetic manner. These hormetic findings were extended by Gao et al. [41], who reported that pretreatment with Rg1 prevented 6-ODHA induced neurotoxicity in SK-N-SH cells. This protection was blocked by the insulin-like growth factor 1-receptor (IGF-IR) antagonist JB-1 as well as by the estrogen receptor (ER) antagonist ICI 182780. Furthermore, a decrease in BCL-2 induced by 6-OHDA was reversed by the Rg1 pretreatment.

The findings indicated that the protective effects of Rg1 are mediated, at least in part, by its activation of the IGF-IR and ER signaling pathways. The study by Gao et al. [41] also revealed that 6-OHDA affected a downregulation of ER protein expression in SK-N-SH cells and that these effects were prevented by Rg1 preconditioning. Further, experimental evidence suggests that the ER and IGF-IR pathways interact, affecting multiple functions such as neuronal differentiation, plasticity, and neurodegeneration. While these findings support a conclusion that the protective effects of Rg1 on SK-N-SH cells depend on IGF-IR and ER, the research of Ge et al. [42] with MES23.5 cells indicated that Rg1 pretreatment mediated protection via the upregulation of BCL-2 gene expression, the activation of AKT phosphorylation, and the inhibition of ERK1/2 phosphorylation induced by 6-OHDA. However, Ge et al. [42] did not explore the role of IGF-IR and ER in the MES23.5 cell line research. Finally, the Fernandez-Mariano et al. [43] in vitro study, which used the SK-N-SH cell line with retonone as the stressor, also demonstrated a hormetic dose response. The mechanistic focus indicated a key role involving the upregulation of the NrF2 pathway that contributed to the neuroprotective response.

3.3.3. In Vivo Studies

The in vivo (IP) mouse study of Chen et al. [40], which utilized a three-day preconditioning period, limited its hormetic-mediated neuroprotective effects to the enhanced formation of GSH in the substantia nigra and blockage of MPTP upregulation of JNK and cJUN at lower doses. The JNK signaling pathway mediates MPTP-induced neurotoxicity. These protective findings were also linked to increases in the BCL-2/BAX ratio, which estimates cellular ROS levels, providing a redox rheostat function.

3.3.4. Summary

These findings indicate that Rg1 has the capacity to prevent the occurrence of Parkinson's Disease-like processes in a hormetic dose–response manner via multiple complementary means in both in vitro and in vivo experimental protocols that both enhance adaptive capacities as well blunting agent-induced toxicities, with dose and the duration of exposure affecting the outcome.

3.4. Alzheimer's Disease

Since Rg1 was used as a potential neuroprotective agent against PD, it is not surprising that it has also been applied to other neuronal diseases such as AD, since estrogen can reduce the production of beta-amyloid and diminish beta-amyloid-induced toxicity [45–47]. Using primary hippocampal neurons from the embryonic brain of Wistar rats (E-16-18) in a beta-amyloid toxicity study, Rg1 hormetically enhanced cell viability, reduced LDH release, and reduced apoptosis/caspase 3 activity [48]. Rg1 treatment also increased the BCL-2/BAX ratio, suggesting that the neuroprotective effect involves the regulation of caspase 3 levels. The authors raised the question of whether estrogen receptors may affect Rg1-induced neuroprotection. While these findings used an embryonic rat model for a disease of aging in human adults, the mechanistic concept is of potential significance. Subsequent research has supported these estrogen-mediated findings in models of AD using both mouse [49] and rat [50] studies.

3.5. Stroke

Publications linking stroke and Rg1-induced hormetic dose responses were framed differentially than those of PD/AD with no consideration given to its phytoestrogen properties either in hypothesis generation or mechanistic evaluation. In the case of stroke-Rg1 and hormesis, there were three papers, two using PC12 cells with either oxygen glucose deprivation (OGD)/Reperfusion (R) [51] (Figure 8) or CoCl2-inducing stroke-like symptoms/damage [52] and mouse NSC [53] and ODG. In the stroke model studies, the mouse NSC experimentation involved co-treatment with the Rg1 and OGD/R [54], whereas in the two PC12 cell studies, post-conditioning protocols were employed [51,52]. The concentration responses of each experiment were generally similar with optimal hormetic protective responses occurring in the 1–5 µM concentration range. However, the mechanistic experimental strategies involved considerably different approaches. In the case of the mouse NSC study [54], the Rg1 reduced OGD-induced cell damage by the inhibition of p-p38 and p-JNK2 expression, enhancing the BCL-2/BAX ratio and reducing caspase activities. The two PC12 cell studies extended the mechanistic involvement to include SIRT 1 activation and the inhibition of Toll-like receptor 4 (TLR-4)/myeloid differentiation factor 88 (MYD88) [40,51]. These two complementary processes affected the inhibitions of NF-kB transcription activity and the expression of multiple pro-inflammatory cytokines (e.g., IL-1B, TNFa, and IL-6). The anti-inflammatory effects also occurred with other ginsenosides but were more strongly seen with Rb1 and Rb3.

A third stroke approach explored the Rg1 neuroprotective mechanism by the MiR-144/NrF2/ARE pathway (Figure 8) [51]. The Rg1-induced protection was mediated by prolonging the nuclear accumulation of NrF2 and enhancing the expression of ARE target genes. The Rg1 effect was independent of dissociation of Keap-1 but involved post-translational processes. Further, Rg1 suppressed the expression of MiR-144 while increasing Nrf2 production. These findings indicate that Rg1 reduced oxidative stress after ischemic reperfusion (IR) via the inhibition of MiR-144 activity and the subsequent activation of the NRF2/ARE pathway at the post-translational level.

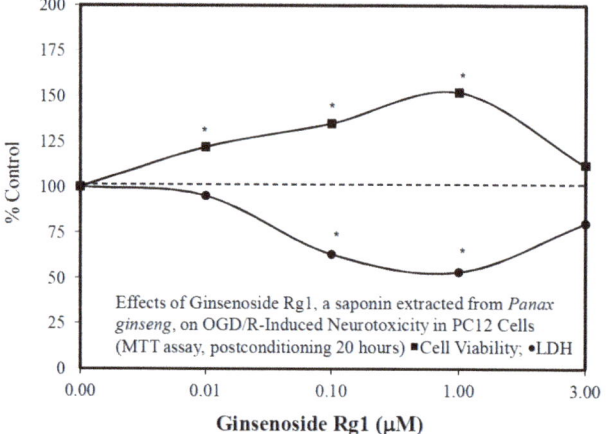

Figure 8. Effects of ginsenoside Rg1, a saponin extracted from *Panax ginseng*, on oxygen glucose deprivation(OGD)/reperfusion (R)-induced neurotoxicity in PC12 cells (MTT assay, postconditioning 20 h) (Source: [51]). Each * represent statistical significance for a data point.

3.6. Neonatal Brain Hypoxia

Another neurological application of Rg1 treatment has involved protection against the hypoxia–ischemia encephalopathy in newborns and other age groups. In their study, Li et al. [39] reported that Rg1 biphasically enhanced the differentiation of NSC into neurons, stromal cells, and oligodendrocytes (Figure 9). In addition to optimizing the hormetic dose, they also placed the dose response within a temporal and developmental context. In these studies, developing neonatal rats receiving transplanted Rg1-induced NSCs at optimized hormetic doses displayed fewer pathological lesions along with significantly improved behavioral performance for multiple parameters (e.g., learning/memory endpoints). These findings are significant, since the Rg1 treatment not only affected the capacity to differentiate stem cells but also displayed enhanced functional intercellular communication capabilities.

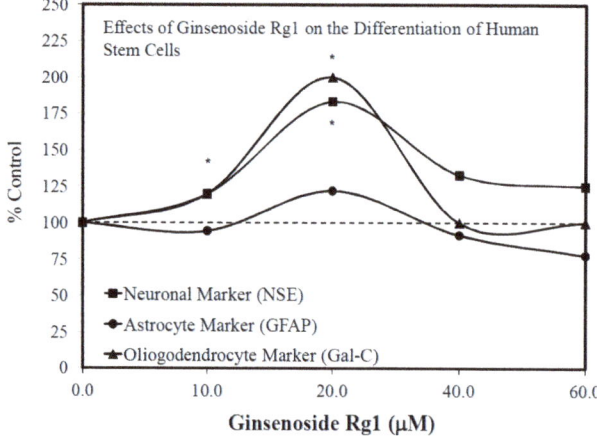

Figure 9. Effects of ginsenoside Rg1 on the differentiation of human stem cells (source: [39]). Each * represent statistical significance for a data point.

4. Neuronal Wound Healing

4.1. Role of Schwann Cells

Several studies assessed the role of Rg1 on spinal cord and peripheral neurons [24,55] within an hormetic dose response context. The Liao et al. [24] experiments showed dose-dependent hormetic dose responses for the Sprague–Dawley rat spinal cord and neurons. Similar findings were reported for Rb1 and ginseng extracts, which are assessed in their respective sections and in the discussion section with a comparison figure. Using a commercial Schwann cell model (RSC96 cells), Lu et al. [55] reported that Rg1 induced hormetic biphasic dose responses for both cell viability and cell migration. Follow-up mechanistic efforts linked the enhanced cell proliferation to the upregulation of the IGF-1 and MAPK pathways and cell cycle proteins. The Rg1-enhanced cell migration activity was mediated by the FGF–2uPA–MMP-9 migration pathway. The respective pathway involvements were elucidated by specific pathway inhibitors. These findings suggest the potential utility of Rg1 to enhance neuron regeneration.

4.2. Role of Angiogenesis

An additional factor that may enhance the capacity for Rg1 to promote recovery from pathological conditions such as hypoxia/ischemia-induced brain damage, nerve injury, and/or myocardial infarction may be via the enhancement of angiogenesis, since it is a common factor of these diverse conditions. Rg1 is an effective inducer of angiogenesis involving cell migration and tubulogenesis via vascular endothelial growth factor receptor-2 (VEGFR-2) in studies with human umbilical vein endothelial cells (HUVEC) (Figure 10) [56]. The VEGFR-2 stimulation was mediated via the RG1 inhibition of MiR-15b expression. These findings suggest that Rg1 affects multiple MiRNAs and mediates different angiogenic mechanisms, including the production of angiogenic factors that enhance cell survival linked to angiogenesis.

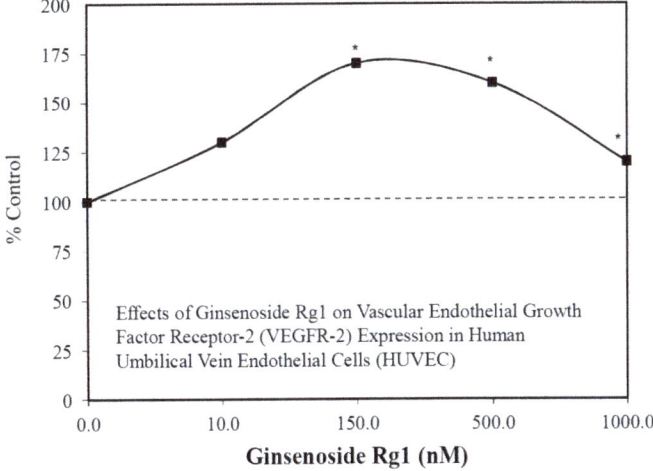

Figure 10. Effects of ginsenoside Rg1 on vascular endothelial growth factor receptor-2 (VEGFR-2) expression in human umbilical vein endothelial cells (HUVEC) (Source: [56]). Each * represent statistical significance for a data point.

4.3. Nerve Regeneration-Role of Schwann Cells

Ginseng has been employed to enhance neuronal protection in a range of experimental research contexts. In such studies, Rg1 displayed neuroprotective properties both reducing the magnitude of damage and facilitating the repair of nerve fiber injuries [57]. Follow-up studies revealed that Rg1 enhanced cultured Schwann cell proliferation and migration in response to peripheral nerve injuries [58,59]. The protective responses were mediated, in part, by the increased expression of glial-derived neurotrophic factor (GDNF) and BCL-2 [60]. Rg1 also enhanced repair and regeneration following sciatic nerve injury, restored the conductivity of regenerative fibers involved in limb motor function, and prevented skeletal muscle atrophy [61]. Follow-up investigations by Huo et al. [62] not only confirmed the findings of Zhou et al. [61] but extended the dose evaluation range, which revealed an hormetic biphasic dose response for nerve conduction velocity, the re-myelination of nerves, and nerve growth factor (NGF) neuronal expression.

4.4. Heart

Rg1 has also displayed hormetic dose responses in protecting embryonic rat heart-derived cells (H9cs) under conditions of nutrition-induced stress [63]. In the case of the cardiac nutritional stress, the experimental approach involved a preconditioning protocol in which the Rg1 was administered 12 h before the nutrition stress-induced injury, which involved incubation in a glucose-free medium. Cell viability was used as an indicator of the chemoprotective response. The Rg1 treatment rescued declining ATP levels and restored mitochondrial membrane potential. These effects were mediated via the activation of PTEN-induced kinase-1 (PINK 1), pAMPK, and aldolase signaling. Such actions of Rg1 are biomedically significant since they are part of an integrated mechanism to prevent mitochondrial damage, enhancing mitochondrial mediated autophagy and the regulation of mitochondrial fusion and fission.

4.5. Immune Responses

There has been surprisingly little hormesis-related research concerning the effects of Rg1 on immune responses. However, two relatively old papers have shown evidence of hormesis in this area. Both papers were unusual in that the 1980 paper of Tong and Chao [64] explored the capacity for Rg1 to induce a low-dose stimulation within the context of a circadian rhythm experimental framework. The hormesis findings were reported throughout the day at 11:00, 12:30, 14:00, and 15:30. In each case, the low-dose stimulation maximized at the same dose for each time period. The capacity of Rg1 to stimulate lymphocyte proliferation required the presence of mitogenic lectins such as phytohemagglutinin (PHA) or Con A. Thus, Rg1 was not able to stimulate proliferation in resting lymphocytes. Similar findings were later reported by Liu et al. [65] with lymphocytes from elderly subjects (65–78 years old) (Figure 11). In both studies, the Rg1 stimulation required the co-presence of PHA with the two agents acting in a synergistic fashion. In contrast to the stimulatory effects in the elderly, the joint exposure to young adults was inhibitory. These findings remain to be further explored.

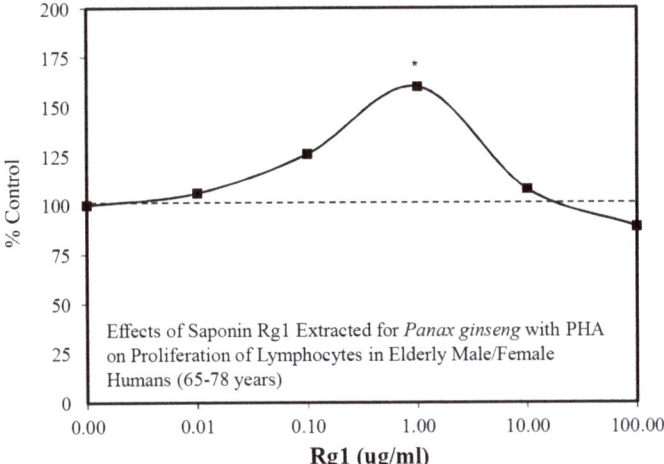

Figure 11. Effects of saponin Rg1 Extracted for *Panax ginseng* with phytohemagglutinin (PHA) on the proliferation of lymphocytes in elderly male/female humans (65–78 years) (source: [65]). Each * represent statistical significance for a data point.

4.6. Diabetes

In the STZ mouse diabetic model, Rg1 oral treatment reduced many diabetes-related conditions. The findings indicated reduced elevated blood glucose, diminished inflammatory factors such as Il-1B and Il-18, and decreased the NLRP3 inflammasome levels in the liver and pancreas [27]. Hormetic-like biphasic dose responses were reported for serum ALT/AST and insulin secretion with the responses being optimized at the intermediate dose.

These manifestations of inflammatory processes were blocked, at least, in part, via the upregulation of the NrF2/ARE pathways, decreasing the STZ induced inflammatory endpoint spectrum. It was also of interest that the Rg1 treatment decreased the capacity of STZ to affect the methylation of hepatic H3K9 in the liver and pancreas.

5. Ginseng Constituent RB1

5.1. Rb1: Neuroprotection

Alzheimer's and Parkinson's Diseases and Stroke Models

The ginsenoside Rb1 has been widely assessed for its neuroprotective features [66]. While most experiments used a limited number of doses, several papers reported hormetic–biphasic dose responses for Rb1. Of the eight in vitro hormetic studies, four utilized pre/post-conditioning and co-treatment experimental protocols. Of these preconditioning studies, two used cell lines (i.e., PC12 and SH-SY5Y), while the remainder employed embryonic Sprague–Dawley rat cortical tissue. The Rb1 preconditioning experiments used different preconditioning periods (1 h, 24 h) with a broad spectrum of stressor agents (i.e., Rotenone-SH-SY5Y cell line) (Figure 12) [43], AB-(25–35)- Sprague–Dawley cortical cells (Figure 13) [67], glutamine-Sprague–Dawley embryonic cortex cells (Figure 14) [68], CoCl2-PC 12 cells (Figure 15) [52] and tert-butylhydroperoxide (tBHT)-Sprague–Dawley embryonic neuroprogenitor cells (Figure 16) [69]. There was also considerable variation of stressor agent toxicity induction rates, ranging from a low of 35–45% (tBHT) [69] to 75–80% (CoCl2) [52]. Despite the range of model conditioning periods, stressor agents, and toxicity induction rates, each experimental setting displayed an hormetic–biphasic dose response with similar quantitative features. Furthermore, the magnitude of protection was also generally similar with optimal protection typically between 0.01 and 10 μM. Three of the preconditioning studies [43,52,69] provided relevant mechanistic findings for the Rb1-induced chemoprotection. In the cases of the rat NPC [69] and SY-SH5Y cell models [43], a neuroprotection role based on the upregulation of Nrf2 was reported. In the PC12 study of Cheng et al. [52], the Rb1 activated SIRT1 and inhibited TLR4/MYD88 protein expression. The activation of SIRT1 affected the deaceylation of NF-kB, which then lead to a reduction of TNFa, IL-2, and IL-6 inflammatory factor production. The parallel inhibition of the expression of TLR4 and MY88 protein expression in the penumbra converged with the effects of the SIRT1 activation to affect a type of molecular pincer action, reducing cellular inflammatory processes. Thus, the integrated activities of Nrf2/ARE and SIRT 1/TLR4 provide a mechanistic foundation by which Rb1 affects chemoprotection.

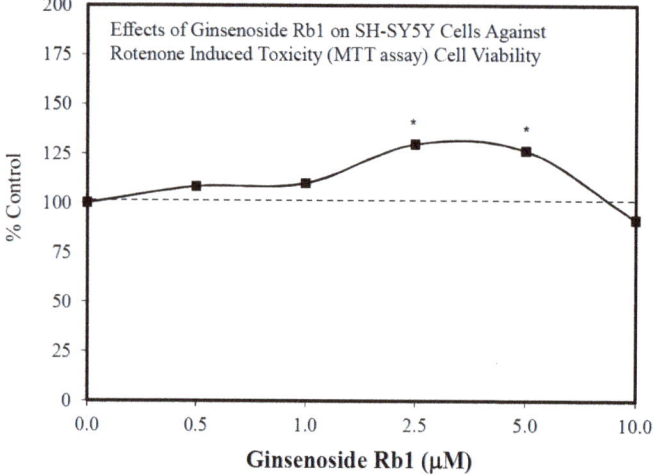

Figure 12. Effects of ginsenoside Rb1 on SH-SY5Y cells against rotenone-induced toxicity (MTT assay) cell viability (source: [43]). Each * represent statistical significance for a data point.

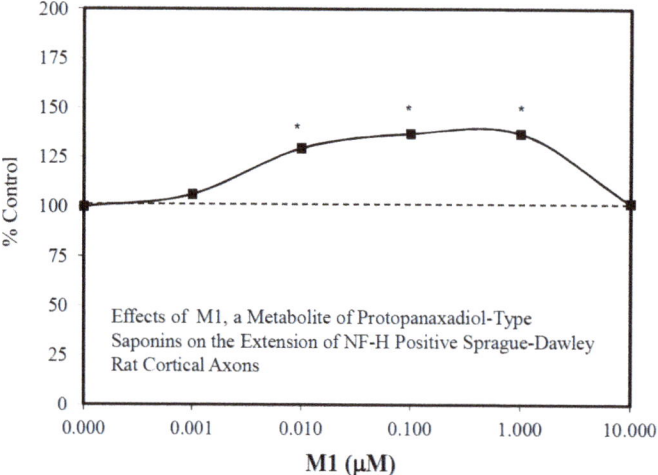

Figure 13. Effects of M1, a metabolite of protopanaxadiol-type saponins on the extension of NF-H positive Sprague–Dawley rat cortical axons (source: [67]). Each * represent statistical significance for a data point.

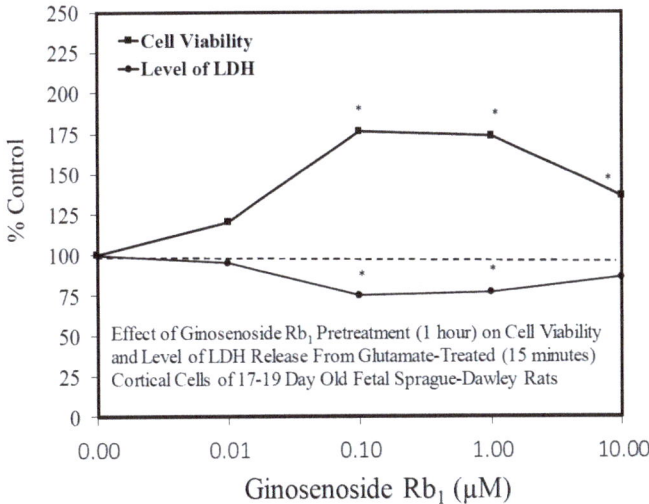

Figure 14. Effect of ginosenoside Rb$_1$ pretreatment (1 h) on cell viability and level of LDH release from glutamate-treated (15 min cortical cells of 17–19-day-old fetal Sprague–Dawley rats (source: [68]). Each * represent statistical significance for a data point.

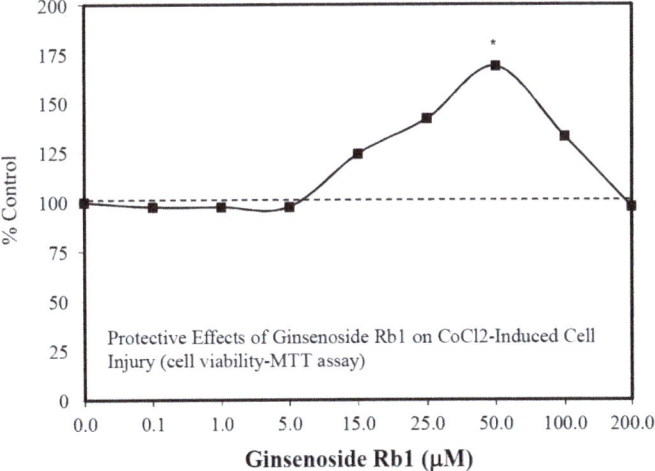

Figure 15. Protective effects of ginsenoside Rb1 on CoCl2-induced cell injury (cell viability: MTT assay) (source: [52]). Each * represent statistical significance for a data point.

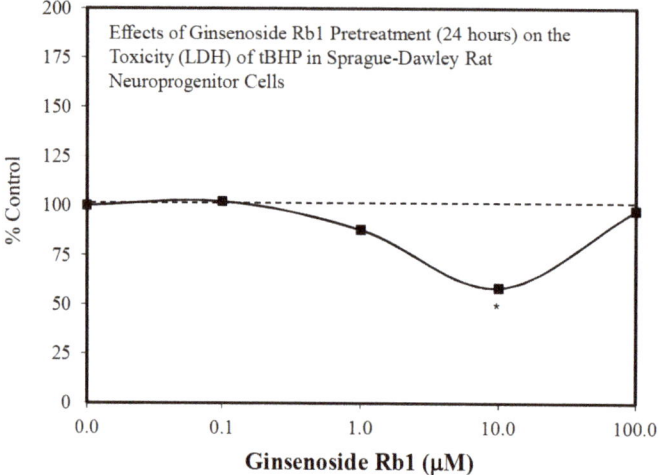

Figure 16. Effects of ginsenoside Rb1 pretreatment (24 h) on the toxicity (LDH) of tBHP in Sprague–Dawley rat neuroprogenitor cells (source: [69]). Each * represent statistical significance for a data point.

5.2. Neuronal Repair/Regeneration Role of Schwann Cells

Schwann cells, glial cells of the peripheral nervous system, have generated considerable interest for their potential application in neural tissue engineering. Schwann cells secrete bio-activation agents that enhance axonal outgrowth and migration. In fact, Schwann cells enhanced nerve cell regeneration in large nerve gap lesions [70,71]. Such observations have resulted in Schwann cells becoming an important addition to tissue engineering nerve grafting activities. However, the biological properties of Schwann cells typically diminish significantly during their preparation time, limiting their practical application in the construction of artificial nerve grafts. As a result of such issues, efforts have been made to upregulate key nerve repair properties of Schwann cells by electrical stimulation [72,73] and via drug treatment [74]. Exploring this issue further, Liang et al. [75] assessed the possible capacity of Rb1 and Rg1 to enhance Schwann cell reparative functions across a 10-fold concentration range. The authors justified their study on the basis that Rb1 and Rg1 promoted neurite outgrowth along with enhancing protection in various preconditioning studies, which are assessed in the present paper. In their study, Liang et al. [75] measured the effects of Rb1/Rg1 on Schwann cell number, intracellular cAMP, PKA activity, and B-NGF and brain-derived neurotrophic factor (BDNF) protein levels. In each case, there was a biphasic dose response for both Rb1 and Rg1. Likewise, the use of a PHA inhibitor (H89) blocked each stimulated endpoint. While these findings demonstrated that Rb1 and Rg1 enhance the proliferation of Schwann cells, there has not been a significant clinical follow up. While the reasons are not clear for this lack of application, it should be pointed out that there is much competition for technology and agents, which may affect subsequent research activities.

5.3. Heart: Cardiomyocytes

Ginsenoside Rb1 was shown to protect heart cells in a series of experimental studies [76–78]. These investigations involved the protection of cardiomyocytes from hydrogen peroxide-induced oxidative stress. The Rb1-induced protective effects were mediated via the suppression of JNK activation [77]. A second report displayed Rb1-induced protection against damage from ischemia-reperfusion (i.e., myocardial infarction/reperfusion) injury in diabetic rats via activation of the P13K/AKT pathway [78]. Rb1 also protected against myocardial ischemia injury via the enhanced expression of eNOS [76]. These initial findings lead to follow-up investigations concerning whether Rb1 could protect neonate rat cardiomyocytes from hypoxia/ischemia (HI) oxygen (10%) induced damage using either a preconditioning or co-exposure protocol [79–81]. The HI experimental study utilized a six-hour preconditioning period followed by a 12 h HI exposure period. Rb1, which was tested over a concentration range of 3–160 µM, demonstrated a biphasic concentration response with protection being optimized at 40 µM, dropping significantly off from 80–160 µM (Figure 17) [80]. An assessment of five MiRNA, at the optimal Rb1 concentration (i.e., 40 µM) revealed that three MiR (Mir-1, Mir 29a, and Mir 208) were markedly increased. However, Mir 21 and Mir 320 were notably decreased. The authors particularly focused on the responses of Mir 21 and Mir 208 based on their specificity for heart tissue. A follow-up investigation extended the initial findings to another stressor, OGD, without a conditioning protocol [81]. The concentration range was reduced to 4–64 µM. As in the previous experiment, the dose response was biphasic, with the optimal response being 32 µM. Of interest was that the OGD-induced damage affected an increase in its target gene, programmed cell death protein 4 (PDCD4), which was the downstream target protein of Mir 21. This increase in PDCD4 was markedly reduced by Rb1. The effect of the Rb1 was blocked by an Mir 21 inhibitor, clarifying a mechanistic foundation for the Rb1-induced protective effects.

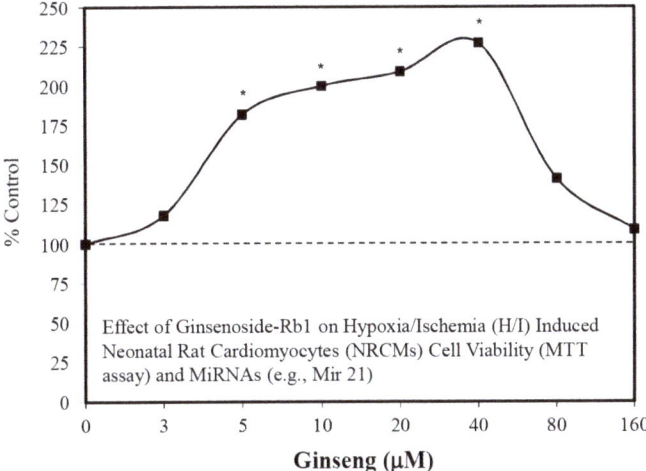

Figure 17. Effect of ginsenoside-Rb1 on hypoxia/ischemia (H/I)-induced neonatal rat cardiomyocytes (NRCMs) cell viability (MTT assay) and MiRNAs (e.g., Mir 21) (Source: [80]). Each * represent statistical significance for a data point.

5.4. Diabetes

Ginseng has long been used in traditional Chinese medicine to treat type 2 diabetes. Various studies confirm that ginseng and some of its principal constituents induce hypoglycemia and insulin sensitizing effects. These findings raised further scientific questions concerning whether ginseng and/or its specific components may affect underlying factors such as adipocyte differentiation, glucose uptake into adipocytes and muscle cells, and insulin sensitivity. Since Rb1 is one of the most common ginseng constituents in multiple plant sources, it was selected for experimental evaluation related to the above question.

5.5. Adipocyte Differentiation

In their research, Shang et al. [82,83] reported that Rb1 enhanced the differentiation of 3T3-L1 pre-adipocytes to adipocytes. During the enhanced differentiation process, the Rb1 also increased the expression of mRNA and proteins of PPARγ2, C/EBPa, and GLUT4. The Rb1 treatment biphasically enhanced basal and insulin mediated glucose uptake by adipocytes (Figure 18) and C2C12 myotubles

(Figure 19). The quantitative features of these two biphasic dose responses were consistent with the hormetic dose response.

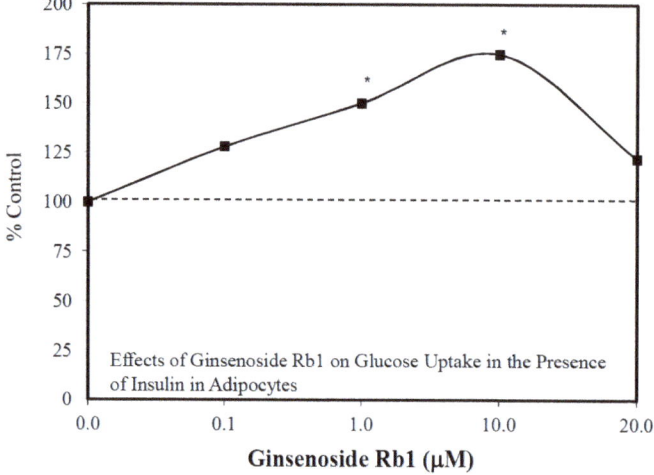

Figure 18. Effects of ginsenoside Rb1 on glucose uptake in the presence of insulin in adipocytes (source: [82]). Each * represent statistical significance for a data point.

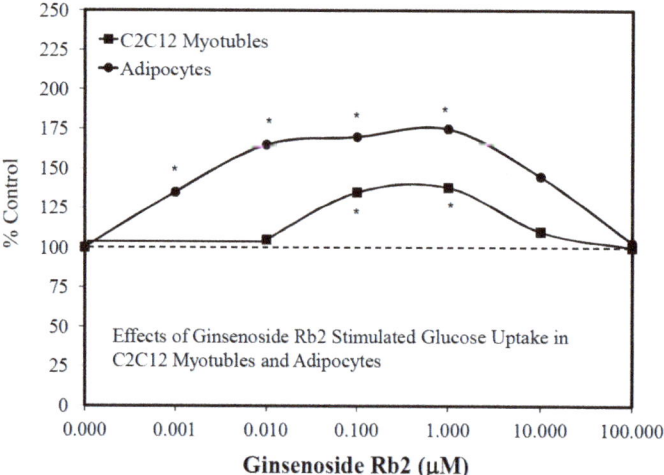

Figure 19. Effects of ginsenoside Rb2 stimulated glucose uptake in C2C12 myotubules and adipocytes (source: [83]). Each * represent statistical significance for a data point.

The mechanisms underlying the adipocyte differentiation and enhanced glucose uptake by the 3T3-1 adipocytes and C2C12 myotubes have been addressed to some extent. Shang et al. [82] proposed that Rb1 may directly bind to PPARγ2, affecting the over expression of PPARγ2 and C/EBPα, enhancing adipocyte differentiation. In fact, PPARγ2 is expressed selectively in adipocytes and is essential for the differentiation process. In addition, Rb1 also enhances glucose transport in mature adipocytes by the insulin signaling pathway. These findings suggest that Rb1 may affect insulin signaling via multiple processes.

5.6. White to Brown Adipocyte Transformation

The above findings have stimulated further research using 3T3-L1 adipocytes, especially in the area of transforming white adipocyte tissue (WAT) into brown [84]. This is of public health interest, since the so-called browning of WAT has been related to reducing obesity and insulin resistance. Using the 3T3-L1 adipocyte cell model, the Rb1 enhanced basal glucose uptake and the browning response based on the induction of multiple biomarkers. This Rb1-induced browning process also displayed the quantitative features of the hormetic dose response. This process was blocked by a PPAPγ antagonist.

Of particular interest was a study by Hosseini et al. [85] concerning an hormetic dose response for Rb1 on GLU4 gene expression in C2C12 cells after 12 h (Figure 20). The C2C12 cells have the capacity to develop into skeletal and cardiac muscle and are widely used as an effective predictive model. The concentration range over which the stimulation occurred was broad, being over five orders of magnitude. However, the maximal increase was distributed over about a 100-fold (0.1–10 µM) concentration range.

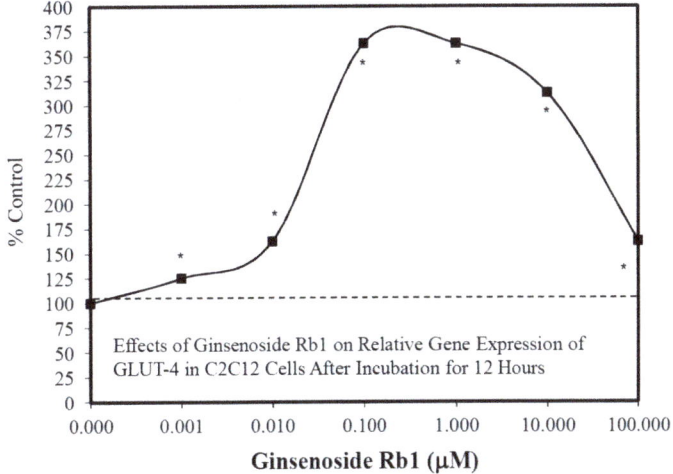

Figure 20. Effects of ginsenoside Rb1 on relative gene expression of GLUT-4 in C2C12 cells after incubation for 12 hours (source: [85]). Each * represent statistical significance for a data point.

5.7. Wound Healing

Another aspect of the diabetes–ginseng interaction is that a local administration of saponin extract significantly enhanced wound healing in diabetic and aging rats [20]. In follow-up clinical trials, oral ginseng enhanced the repair of intractable skin ulcers in patients with diabetes mellitus [19]. Mechanistic follow-up studies have shown that the ginseng treatment enhances would healing via the stimulation of fibronectin synthesis in a hormetic dose response manner through changes in the TGF-β receptor in fibroblasts [19]. More recent experimental studies have shown the Rb1 biphasically enhances human dermal fibroblast proliferation and collagen synthesis (Figure 21) [86]. The authors suggested that their findings may be clinically applicable to wound-dressing strategies, suggesting the possibility impregnating ginseng mixtures into bandages. In fact, ginseng extracts have been reported to protect skin in mouse models from acute UVB irradiation [87] as well as to significantly enhance healing after laser burn injury and excisional wounding [88–90]. Multiple patents are listed in the Web of Science for products containing ginseng for use in wound healing. However, it does not appear that these developments have taken advantage of knowledge of the hormetic dose response.

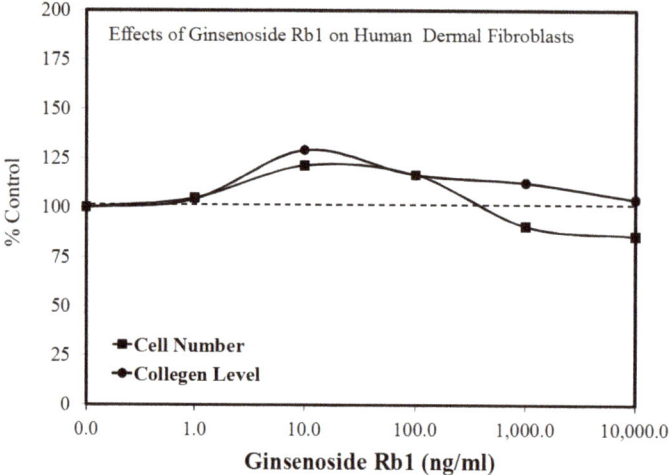

Figure 21. Effects of ginsenoside Rb1 on human dermal fibroblasts (source: [86]).

5.8. Hair Growth

In 2020, Calabrese [91] provided detailed assessment of the occurrence of stimulating hair growth within experimental and clinical frameworks for almost 200 agents, including ginseng. The initial publication showing that ginseng could enhance hair growth was reported by Kubo et al. [92] with the ddy mouse strain, using the findings to obtain a patent in 1986. A spate of hormetic effects of ginseng constituents, including ginsenoside Rb, some its constituents such as Rb1, its metabolite F2, and Rb2 in the growth of hair was reported only within the past few years, following the development of several in vitro models such as human keratinocyte cells, mouse vibrissae hair follicles, and other cellular models (e.g., [93–96]). These hormetic studies with ginseng involved experiments with human hair dermal papilla cells (HHDPs), human keratinocyte cells (HaCaTs) (Figure 22), and other experimental models.

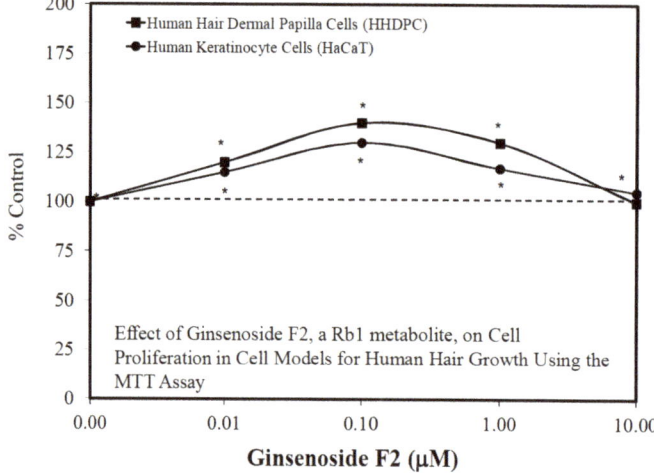

Figure 22. Effect of ginsenoside F2, a Rb1 metabolite, on cell proliferation in cell models for human hair growth using the MTT assay (Source: [93]). Each * represent statistical significance for a data point.

Amongst these findings were observations that hair growth was enhanced in a hormetic fashion; likewise, the Rb treatment prevented the occurrence of hair growth inhibition by dihydrotestosterone (DHT) within a preconditioning experimental framework (Figure 23). Whole animals studies using young adult C57BL/6 male mice extended these hormetic dose responses. These whole animal studies used an oral dosing protocol, making the study of particular relevance to humans, since the doses used are commonly ingested by people. The findings of mouse in vivo studies were consistent with the clinical findings of Kim et al. [97], who reported that orally administered Korean Red Ginseng enhanced hair density and thickness in alopecia patients with a dosage of 3000 mg/day for 24 weeks.

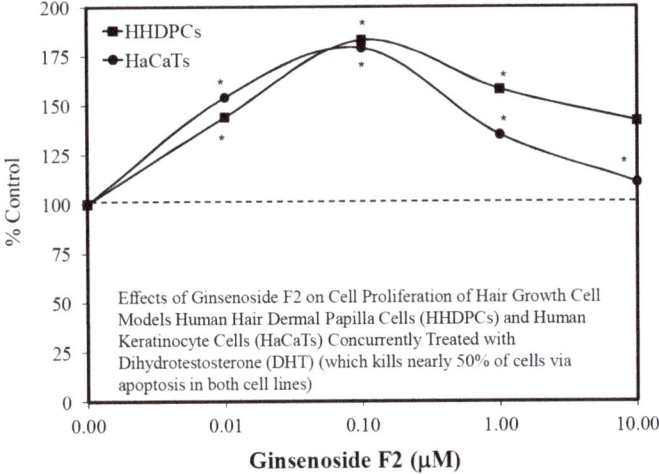

Figure 23. Effects of ginsenoside F2 on cell proliferation of hair growth cell models human hair dermal papilla cells (HHDPCs) and human keratinocyte cells (HaCaTs) concurrently treated with dihydrotestosterone (DHT) (which kills nearly 50% of cells via apoptosis in both cell lines) (Source: [94]). Each * represent statistical significance for a data point.

5.9. Ginseng-Rd

There has been growing interest in the assessment of the principal constituents of ginseng. This section will address the ginseng constituent Rd and how some of its biomedical effects are mediated via hormesis. Interest in Rd originated with the findings of Yokozawa et al. [98–100], showing that Rd displayed antioxidant effects in kidney injury models of senescence-accelerated mice. These initial findings would stimulate research interest in Rd but with a particular focus on neuronal cellular systems starting with the work of Lopez et al. [101], showing that Rd decreased ROS formation in cultured astrocytes.

5.10. Stroke

The first report of a hormetic dose response for Rd was made by Ye et al. [102] using PC 12 cells (Figure 24). In this study, the Rd was administered at the same time as the oxidant stressor, hydrogen peroxide. The Rd treatment displayed hormetic concentration responses for LDH release and cell survival. Low Rd concentrations prevented a complex set of mitochondrial damages by hydrogen peroxide. Linked to the induced protective responses were increases in antioxidant enzymatic activities of SOD and GPx. Several years later, the same researchers extended their hormetic research findings with Rd to in vivo stroke outcomes with an aged male mouse model. Using 16–18-month-old male C57BL/6 mice, the Rd protected against stroke-induced damage within pre- and post-conditioning protocols [103]. The preconditioning protocol utilized five doses (i.e., ranging from 0.1 to 200 mg/kg) (Figure 25), whereas the post-conditioning protocol used only the optimal dose of the preconditioning protocol but applied it at four different times after the induced stroke. In this study, the Rd was highly effective in reducing stroke damage both before (preconditioning) and after induction (post-conditioning). Follow-up mechanistic experiments by Ye et al. [103] confirmed that Rd mediated protection by preventing mitochondrial damage in the cortex and striatum by the upregulation of antioxidant enzyme activities linked to the enhancement of mitochondrial stability.

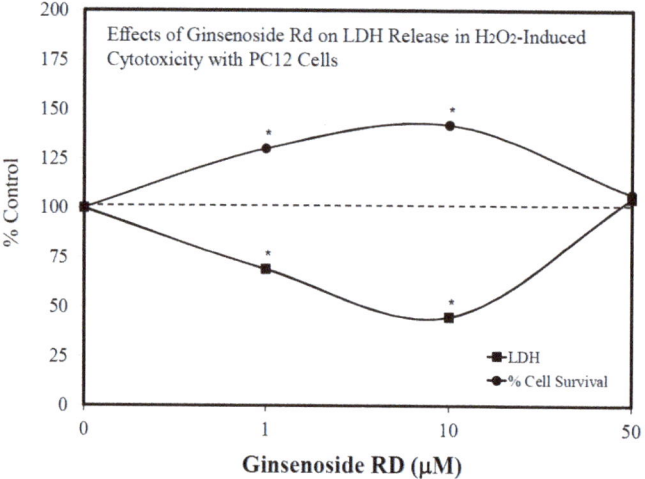

Figure 24. Effects of ginsenoside Rd on LDH release in H2O2-induced cytotoxicity with PC12 cells (source: [102]). Each * represent statistical significance for a data point.

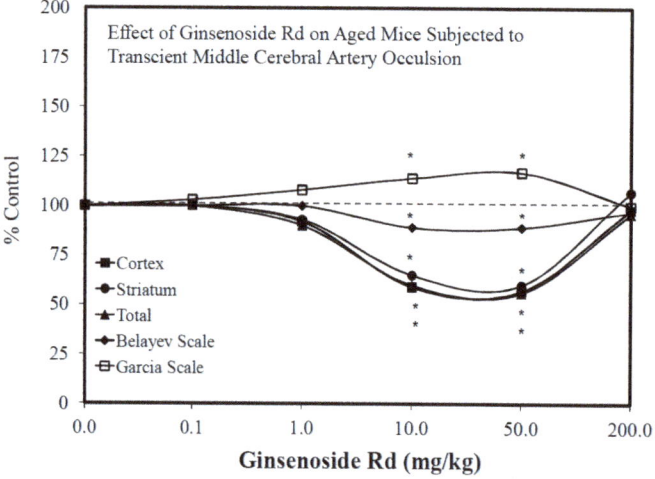

Figure 25. Effect of ginsenoside Rd on aged mice subjected to transcient middle cerebral artery occulsion (source: [103]). Each * represent statistical significance for a data point.

5.11. Other Neuroprotective Studies

Since the initial hormetic studies of Ye and colleagues, there has been a progressive stream of investigations with Rd on a spectrum of neuronal related experimental systems. Follow up studies with Rd revealed hormetic dose responses with (1) the embryonic mouse (Embryonic day—4.5) for neurosphere development [104] (Figure 26), (2) in SH-SY5Y neuronal cells in a preconditioning protocol (2 h) preventing MPP-induced toxicity (Figure 27) [105], (3) in HT22 mouse-derived hippocampal cells that prevented glutamate toxicity in a preconditioning protocol (2 h) (Figure 28) [106] and (4) in an in vivo preconditioning protocol with Sprague–Dawley rat spinal cord tissue preventing ischemia-induced injury (Figure 29) [107]. This complex array of experimental studies demonstrating Rd-induced hormetic dose responses revealed that the protective concentration range was similar, optimizing in the 1–10 µM range. Hormetic pathway analysis revealed that the protection could be blocked by inhibiting the P13K/AKT pathway [105].

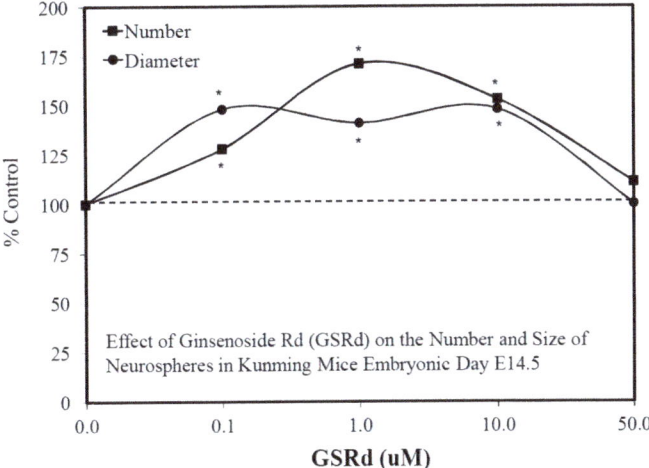

Figure 26. Effect of ginsenoside Rd (GSRd) on the number and size of neurospheres in kunming mice embryonic day E14.5 (Source: [104]). Each * represent statistical significance for a data point.

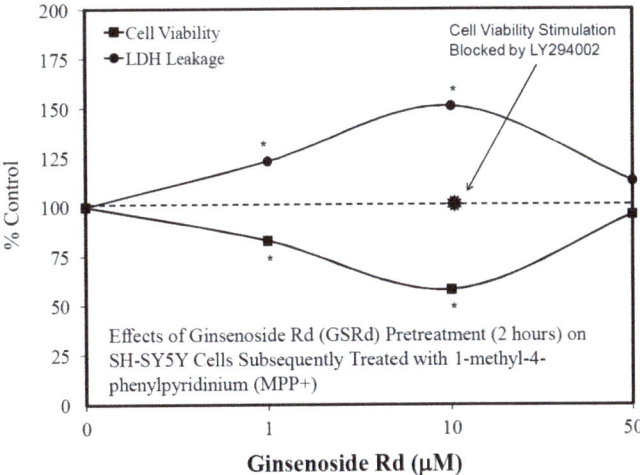

Figure 27. Effects of ginsenoside Rd (GSRd) pretreatment (2 h) on SH-SY5Y cells subsequently treated with 1-methyl-4-phenylpyridinium (MPP+) (source: [105]). Each * represent statistical significance for a data point.

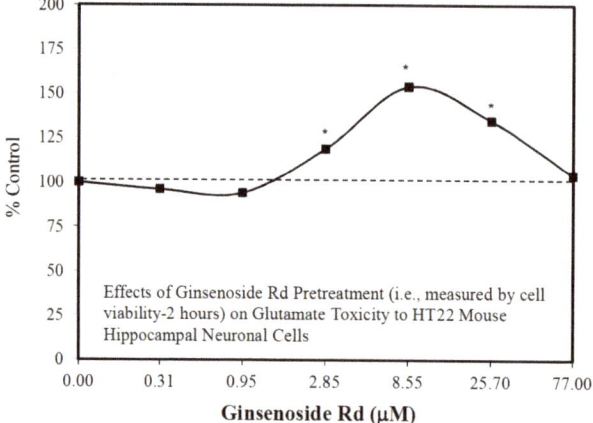

Figure 28. Effects of ginsenoside Rd pretreatment (i.e., measured by cell viability: 2 h) on glutamate toxicity to HT22 mouse hippocampal neuronal cells (source: [106]). Each * represent statistical significance for a data point.

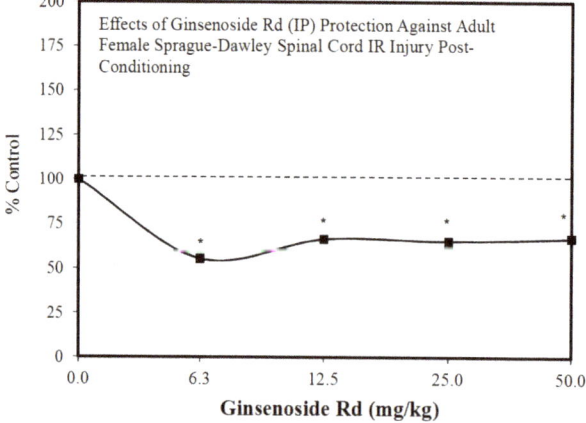

Figure 29. Effects of ginsenoside Rd (IP) protection against adult female sprague-dawley spinal cord IR injury post-conditioning (Source: [107]). Each * represent statistical significance for a data point.

Multiple research teams emphasized that RD is highly lipophilic and readily passes across the blood–brain barrier. It also has a long plasma half-life, being about 50–60 h in humans, and nearly 20 h in rats [108]. These factors are likely to encourage further research and possible clinical application considerations.

5.12. Heart

While the above research focused on the neuroprotective potential of Rd, Wang et al. [109] reported that Rd attenuated myocardial ischemia/reperfusion injury in both in vitro and in vivo studies. In in vitro experimentation, neonatal rat cardiomyocytes from two-day-old Sprague–Dawley rats were assessed in a preconditioning protocol to determine if Rd could protect against ischemia/reperfusion injury. The four concentration-based (0.1–50 µM) study revealed a hormetic concentration response with significant protection reported over the 0.1 to 10.0 µM range based on cell viability and LDH leakage (Figure 30). Extensive follow-up experiments demonstrated that Rd mediated the protection via enhancing mitochondrial membrane potential and preventing mitochondrial-mediated apoptosis. In a complementary in vivo study, the single dose preconditioning protocol reduced the cardiac damage by nearly 50%. The Rd exposure was via an IP administration that would be equivalent to 3500 mg per 70 kg person.

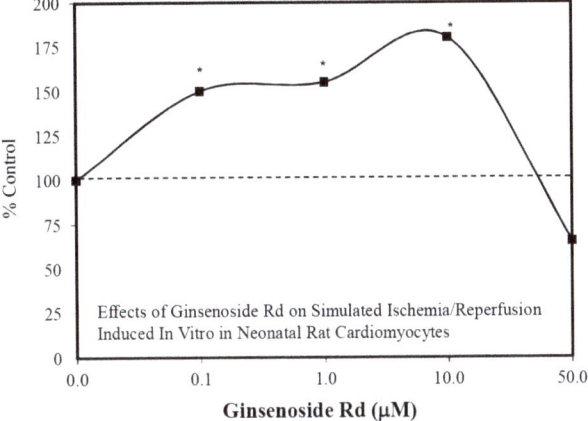

Figure 30. Effects of ginsenoside Rd on simulated ischemia/reperfusion induced in vitro in neonatal rat cardiomyocytes (source: [109]). Each * represent statistical significance for a data point.

5.13. Kidney

In 2018, Lee et al. [110] assessed the capacity of Rb1, Rb2, Rc, Rd, Rg1, and R3 to prevent FK506 toxicity to LLC-PK cells, which is a porcine kidney epithelial cell model. This was undertaken since FK506 is highly nephrotoxic and widely used by humans to prevent organ rejection in transplantation procedures. Of interest to the present section is that Rb2, Rc, and Rd displayed hormetic dose responses in a preconditioning (2 h) protocol (Figure 31) [110]. The ginseng constituents were effective in preventing kidney damage by blocking intoxication pathways such as p38, KIM-1, and caspase 3.

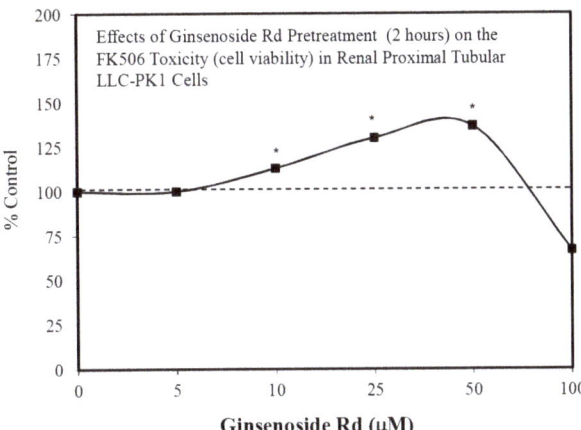

Figure 31. Effects of ginsenoside Rd pretreatment (2 h) on the FK506 toxicity (cell viability) in renal proximal tubular LLC-PK1 cells (Source: [110]). Each * represent statistical significance for a data point.

5.14. Polyacetylenes

Introduction

Aliphatic C17-polyacetylenes of the falcarinol-type are commonly found in carrots and related vegetables such as parsely, celery, parsnip, and fennel. They are also present in the lipophilic fraction of ginseng. Such polyacetylenes may display anti-inflammatory activities [111]. Of particular relevance is that hormetic dose responses have been reported in the areas of neuroprotection [74,112] and tumor cell biology (Figure 32) [112] with several polyacetylenes [e.g., panaxydol (PND) and panaxyol (PNN)].

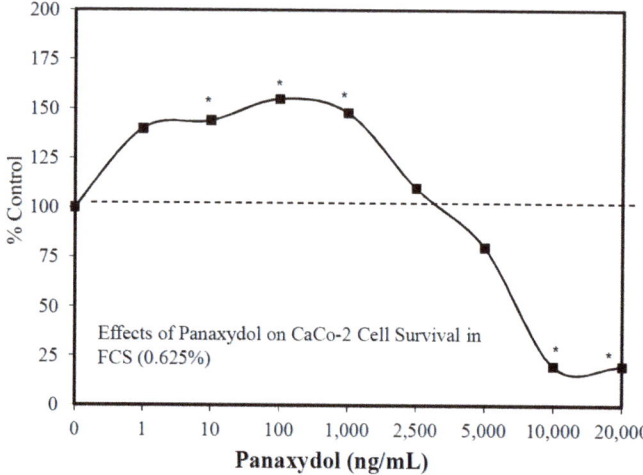

Figure 32. Effects of panaxydol on CaCo-2 cell survival in FCS (0.625%) (Source: [111]). Each * represent statistical significance for a data point.

5.15. Alzheimer's Disease

Nie et al. [112] reported that the pretreatment of primary cultured Sprague–Dawley rat embryonic (E-16) cortical neurons with PND or PNN prior (24 h) to beta-amyloid (25–35) exposure significantly enhanced cell survival as measured by the MTT assay (Figure 33). This protection was dose-related and displayed an hormetic dose response. Similar protection also occurred with PND and PNN when given at the same time as the AB 25–35 treatment. The protective effects were related to a suppression of apoptosis that was mediated by increases in the BCL-2/Bax ratio and enhancement of mitochondrial membrane stability. PND and PNN also reversed AB 25–35 induced calcium influx and intracellular free radical generation. The authors suggested that antioxidants with good blood–brain barrier permeability are needed for use in the prevention of neurodegenerative diseases such as AD. They noted that since PND and PNN are lipophilic and found in many food plants, that ingestion of such plants may offer benefit against such neurodegenerative diseases.

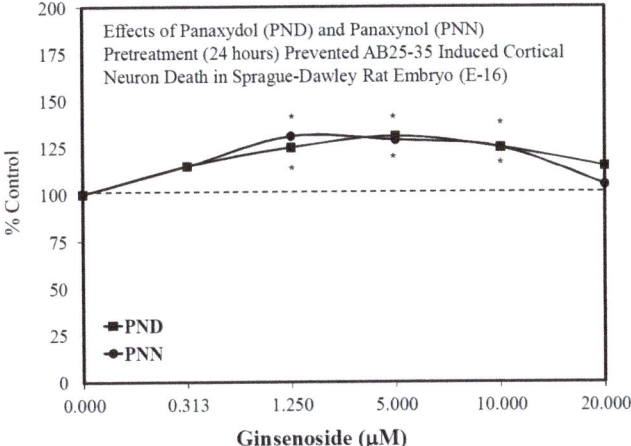

Figure 33. Effects of panaxydol (PND) and panaxynol (PNN) pretreatment (24 h) prevented AB25-35-induced cortical neuron death in Sprague–Dawley rat embryo (E-16) (source: [112]). Each * represent statistical significance for a data point.

5.16. Nerve Regeneration

As a result of the neuroprotective findings of PND/PNN, He et al. [74] assessed whether PND might enhance the capacity of Schwann cells for growth and healing following damage. Using Schwann cells from the sciatic nerve of newborn (1–3-day-old Sprague–Dawley) rats, it was determined that PND enhanced the expression and secretion of nerve growth factor (NGF) and brain-derived neurotrophic factor (BDNF) displaying hormetic dose responses (Figure 34). At the peak level of NGF and BDNF secretion, the Schwann cells also enhanced the synthesis of actin, which is an important component of the cytoskeletin. Similar studies also revealed that the optimal concentration for NGF/BDNF secretion also improved mitochrondrial transmembrane potential. The authors concluded that PND had the potential to enhance repair in neurons by its actions with Schwann cells.

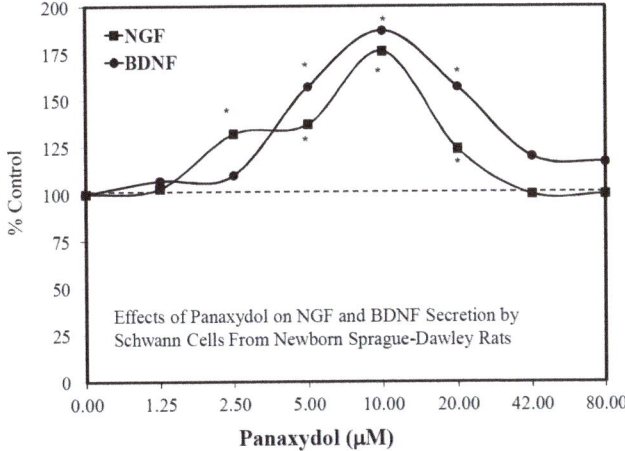

Figure 34. Effects of panaxydol on nerve growth factor (NGF) and brain-derived neurotrophic factor (BDNF) secretion by Schwann cells from newborn Sprague–Dawley rats (Source: [74]). Each * represent statistical significance for a data point.

5.17. Rg3

Pain/Tobacco Toxicity/Diabetes/Vero Cells

A limited number of hormetic dose responses have been reported for Rg3. These include the effects of R3 (20(s)-Rg3 isomer) on plantar incisional pain in an adult Sprague–Dawley rat model. Inflammatory cytokines levels closely correlated with the pain response (Figure 35) [113], protection against cigarette smoke extract-induced cell injury in a preconditioning protocol [114], the biphasic enhancement of glucose-stimulated insulin secretion, and AMPK activities by both the 20R and 20S isomers [115] and protection against glutamate-mediated neuronal cell death to HT22 cells, a mouse hippocampal cell line (Figure 36) [106], and protected against ginsenoside induced cell toxicity in Sprague–Dawley fetal cortical cells. With respect to the biphasic dose response for plantar incision pain, the authors suggested that this could make it more challenging for use in a therapeutic application, noting further the need to document the biphasic dose response in humans. In the present study, the mechanism of pain reduction was not related to opioid, nicotinic, or muscarinic acetylcholine receptors based on experiments with antagonists. However, alpha-2 adrenergic receptors were involved with the pain modulation of Rg3. For example, yohimbine, an alpha 2-adrenergic receptor antagonist, blocked the analgesic effect of Rg3. Finally, 20(S)-Rg3 enhanced the cell proliferation of Vero cells in an hometic dose response manner (Figure 37) [116]. The experiment was designed to assess the capacity of 20(s)-Rg3 to inhibit the growth of herpes simplex viruses (types 1 or 2). In the presence of this evaluation, the hormetic effects on Vero cells were observed. A similar hormetic effect on Vero cells was reported earlier by Song et al. [117] for multiple ginsenosides but only using three concentrations rather than the six concentrations of the Wright and Altman [116] study.

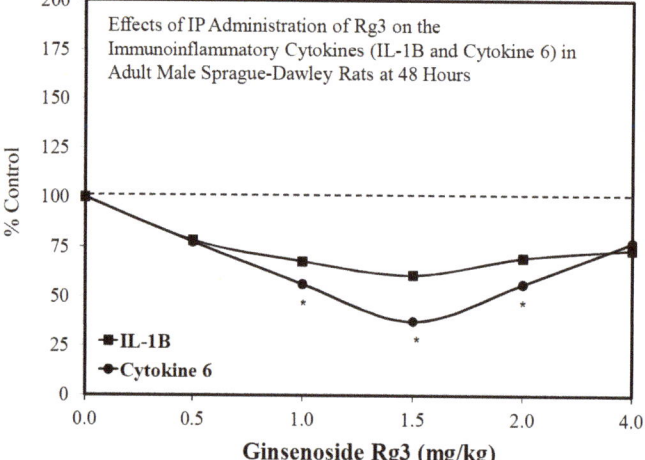

Figure 35. Effects of IP administration of Rg3 on the immunoinflammatory cytokines (IL-1B and cytokine 6) in adult male Sprague–Dawley Rats at 48 hours (source: [113]). Each * represent statistical significance for a data point.

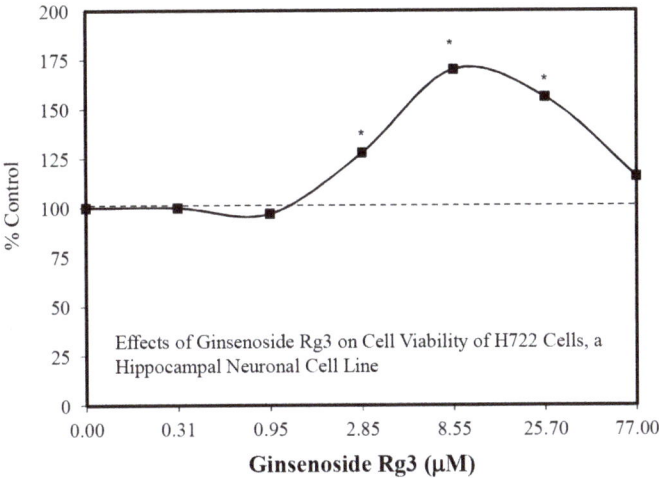

Figure 36. Effects of ginsenoside Rg3 on cell viability of H722 cells, a hippocampal neuronal cell line (source: [106]). Each * represent statistical significance for a data point.

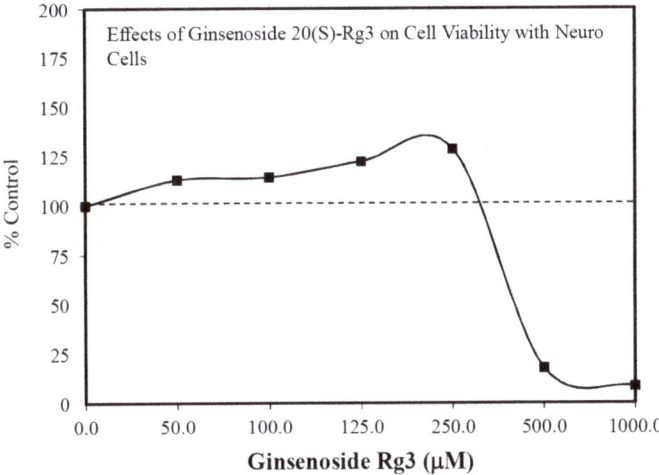

Figure 37. Effects of ginsenoside 20(S)-Rg3 on cell viability with neuro cells (source: [116]).

6. Ginseng Constituent Re

6.1. Introduction

The ginsenoside Re has been reported to display hormetic dose responses, but to a more limited extent than Rg1, Rb1, and Rd. Amongst these hormetic publications were two papers using HUVEC to assess whether Re may reduce oxidative stress and its potential value in diminishing the risk of developing atherosclerosis [118,119]. The remaining three hormetic papers dealt with (1) the capacity of Re to promote nerve cell regeneration by enhancing the proliferation, differentiation, and migration of Schwann cells in the Sprague–Dawley rat model of sciatic nerve crush injury [120], (2) the capacity of Re to prevent toxicity induced by beta amyloid in SH-SY5Y cells [121], and (3) whether Re could block I/R toxicity using PC 12 cells [52].

6.2. Nerve Injury and Regeneration

Using as its rationale the results of a series of a studies with Re on gastric muosal lesions [122], renal ischemia–reperfusion injury [120], and several other only tangentially related protective activities, a sciatic nerve study was undertaken using adult male Sprague–Dawley rats. In this study, six doses served as pretreatment ranging from 0.5 to 3.0 mg/kg [120]. Only the data for the 2.0 mg/kg treatment group were shown, being referred to as the optimal pain-relieving dose. However, the entire dose range response was provided for changes in PCNA expression. For this endpoint, the 1.0–2.0 mg/kg dose range response was significantly increased with the 2.0 mg/kg group showing the largest gain (133% versus 100% control) (Figure 38). This study demonstrated that Re enhanced sciatic nerve repair via multiple hormetic processes.

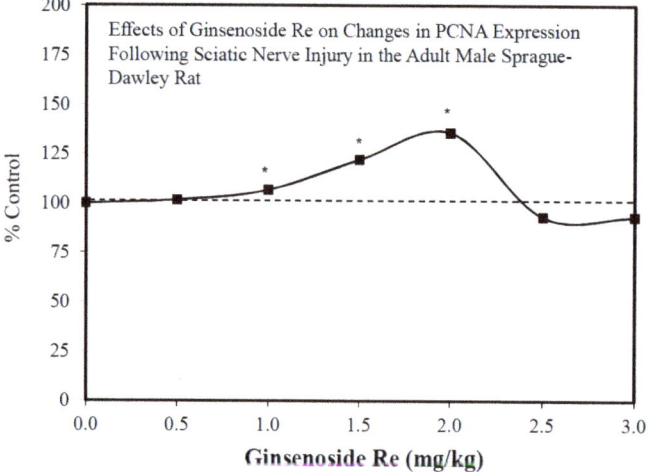

Figure 38. Effects of ginsenoside Re on changes in PCNA expression following sciatic nerve injury in the adult Male Sprague–Dawley rat (source: [120]). Each * represent statistical significance for a data point.

6.3. Alzheimer's Disease

With respect to the beta-amyloid induced toxicity in SH-SY5Y cells, the Re prevented cytotoxicity (Figure 39) and apoptosis by inhibiting the beta-amyloid-activated mitochondrial apoptosis pathway (as inferred by its effects on mitochondrial functions, BCL-2/Bax ratio, cytochrome c release, and caspase 3/9 activities [121]. Re treatment also blocked JNK activation while upregulating NrF2. Furthermore, blocking NrF2 by interfering RNA abolished the protective effects of Re.

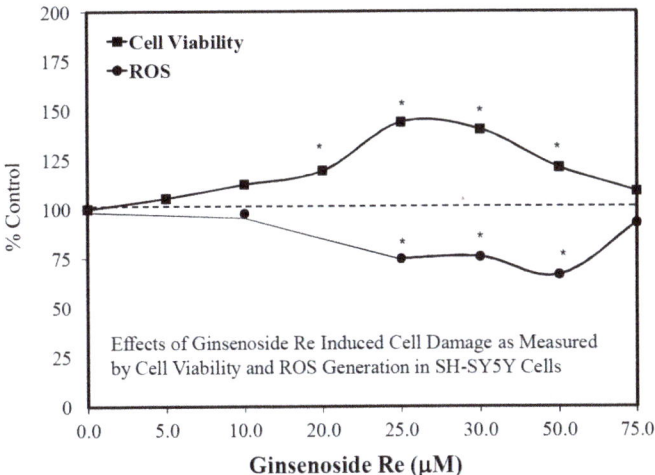

Figure 39. Effects of ginsenoside Re-induced cell damage as measured by cell viability and ROS generation in SH-SY5Y cells (source: [121]). Each * represent statistical significance for a data point.

6.4. Atherosclerosis

Two papers concerning Re and HUVEC displayed hormetic doses responses relating to reducing risks of developing atherosclerosis. However, both studies did so within the context of addressing complementary research questions. The Huang et al. [118] study increased cell proliferation in both direct stimulation and preconditioning experimental protocols. In the case of the preconditioning protocol, the range of conditioning doses displayed the low dose stimulation but was not evaluated at higher doses to sufficiently assess possible inhibitory effects.

The Yang et al. [119] study did not address the issue of a direct low dose stimulation but demonstrated an hormetic dose response in a preconditioning protocol using a broader dose range which had a 3.5-fold higher maximum dose tested than in the Huang et al. [118] study. This study also used Ox-LDL as the stressor rather than hydrogen peroxide. Nonetheless, both studies used the same cell model, offering complementary perspectives. Finally, the study by Cheng et al. [52] was unique as it assessed five ginsenosides using the PC 12 cell model with pre- and post-conditioning protocols with hormetic dose responses being shown for each ginsenoside (Figure 40). This study is discussed in greater detail in the Rg1 and Rb1 sections of this paper.

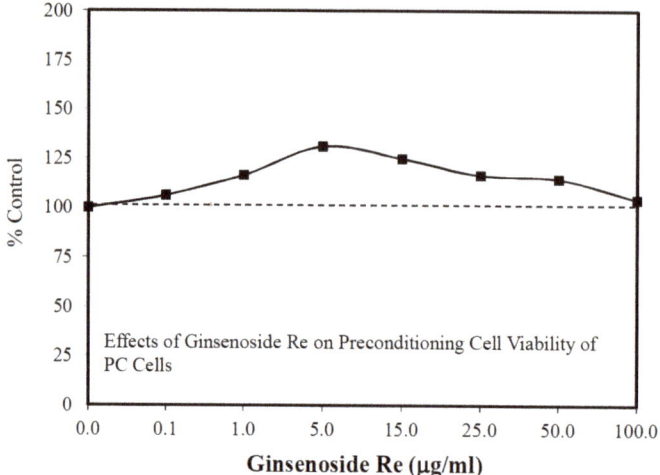

Figure 40. Effects of ginsenoside Re on preconditioning cell viability of PC cells (source: [52]).

6.5. Gintonin

Introduction

Gintonin, a component of ginseng, is an exogenous ligand for G-protein-coupled lysophosphatidic acid (LPA) receptors. Gintonin is a non-saponin and non-acidic carbohydrate polymer. The gintonin-enriched extract (GEF) is comprised of a large proportion of gintonin, linoleic acid, phosphatidic acid (Pa), and other bio-reactive lysophospholipids. The unique feature of gintonin is that it uses G-protein-coupled LPA receptor signaling pathways by which gintonin induces a broad spectrum of hormetic dose responses that affect (1) human dermal fibroblast cell proliferation [123,124], (2) human/rabbit corneal cell repair [125], (3) modulation of the mouse blood brain barrier [126], (4) angiogenesis and wound healing using HUVEC models [127], (5) glycogenolysis and astrocyte preconditioning [128], and (6) beta-amyloid-induced dysfunction in mouse models via cholinergic stimulation of ACH release [129].

6.6. Corneal Injury

Of particular interest was research that employed human corneal epithelium (HCE) cells to evaluate the capacity of gentonin to affect healing-related processes. Kim et al. [125] demonstrated hormetic dose responses for ERK1/2 phosphorylation for epithelial cell proliferation and migration. These effects were blocked by the LPA1/3 receptor antagonist Ki16425, phospholipase C (PLC) inhibitor U73122, inositol 1,4,5-triphosphate receptor antagonist 2 APB and intracellular Ca2+ chelator BAPTA-AM. Of significance was the potential capacity to enhance corneal wound healing when applied to in vivo rabbit models with induced corneal damage. Using an ocular dose of 200 µg gentonin, the healing process was significantly enhanced several fold, depending on the endpoint measured.

6.7. Alzheimer's Disease

In vitro and in vivo studies assessed the area of scopolamine and beta amyloid-protein mouse models of AD [129]. Since the LPA receptor has an important role in learning and memory in aged animals, gintonin was assessed for its capacity to block effects of beta-amyloid on brain functioning. Research with male ICR mice demonstrated that gentonin stimulates the release of ACH from cells expressing an endogenous LPA receptor in a hormetic dose–response manner. These findings complemented studies showing that the oral administration of gintonin reversed scopolamine-induced memory dysfunction, blocked beta-amyloid-induced reduction of ACH (Figure 41) and choline acetyltransferase (CHAT), and diminished ACHE activity in the mouse hippocampus. Gintonin also blocked amyloid plaque-induced changes in ACH, CHAT, and ACHE in a transgenic AD model. These findings for gintonin are consistent with FDA-approved drugs for the treatment of AD with respect to their hormetic effects at the level of operational mechanisms [130].

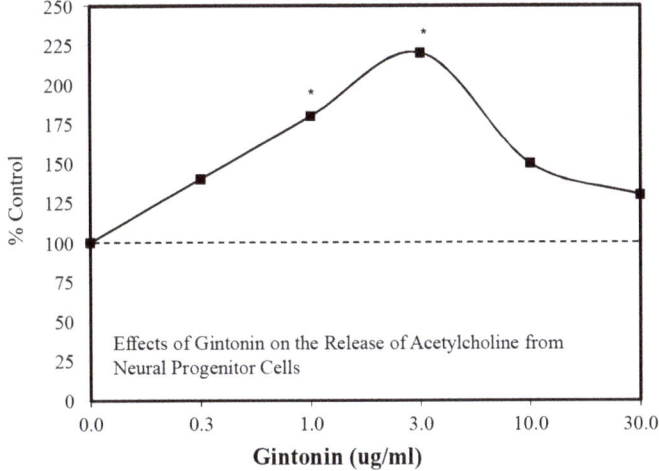

Figure 41. Effects of gintonin on the release of acetylcholine from neural progenitor cells (source: [129,131]). Each * represent statistical significance for a data point.

6.8. Astrocyte Glycogenolysis and Preconditioning

Astrocytes are brain cells that store glycogen. These cells also express lysophosphatidic acid (LPA) receptors. Astrocytes provide energy for neurons via astrocytic glycogenolysis under both physiological and pathological frameworks. Ginseng has been linked to this astrocyte–neuron interaction, since gintonin is an exogenous protein-coupled LPA receptor ligand. As a result of this biological framework, Choi et al. [128] assessed the capacity of gintonin to affect astrocyte glycogenolysis, ATP production, glutamate uptake, and cell viability under a range of biological conditions, including hypoxia and re-oxygenation stress states. The gintonin treatment increased astrocyte glycogenolysis via LPA receptors under both stress and non-stress-related conditions in an hormetic dose–response fashion. Thus, gintonin can mediate astrocyte energy release as well as protect and enhance the adaptive capacity of astrocytes under stress following hormetic dose response processes. These findings have potentially significant neuroprotective implications for public health and clinical application. Gintonin has also been shown to hormetically enhance the blood–brain barrier permeability and brain delivery via the use of LPA receptors, which is a process that may be of utility with respect to new formulations of ginseng mixtures but also combined with other potentially beneficial agents that have poor capacity to cross the blood–brain barrier [126].

6.9. Wound Healing

Several research initiatives have shown that gentonin has the potential to enhance wound healing endogenously as well as with skin (Figure 42) [118,123]. Both studies reflect the capacity of gintonin to mediate these processes via hormetic dose responses, which are linked to LPA receptors. These findings have the potential to provide insight for how ginseng mixtures have been able to successfully treat various types of skin wounds within animal model studies and humans.

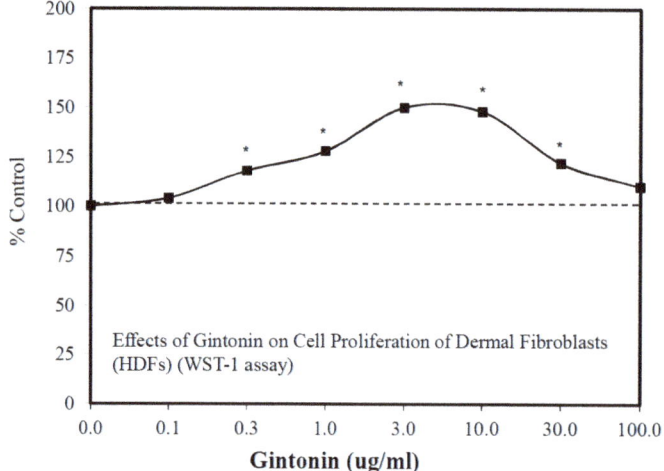

Figure 42. Effects of gintonin on cell proliferation of dermal fibroblasts (HDFs) (WST-1 assay) (source: [123]). Each * represent statistical significance for a data point.

7. Ginseng Mixtures

7.1. Introduction

Ginseng has been a studied in a dose–response fashion via the use of various types of mixtures and individual constituent agents, such Rg1, Rb1, Rb2, Rd, Re, and others. In this section, the occurrence of hormetic dose responses as induced by several types of ginseng mixtures is addressed. Such mixtures include extracts from Korean Red Ginseng (KRG), Ginseng Total Saponins (GTS), and other ginseng mixture extracts [132]. In general, ginseng saponins may be placed into one of three major groups based on chemical structures: protopanaxadiols, protopanaxatriols, and oleanolic acid saponins. Protopanaxadiols (e.g., Rb1, Rb2, Rc, Rd, Rg3) have sugar moieties attached to the 3-position of the dammarene-type triterpine. In contrast, protopanaxatriols (Re, Rf, Rg1, R2, Rh1) have the sugar moieties attached to the 6-position. The roots of ginseng also contain other compounds such as polysaccharides, peptides, polyacetylene alcohols (e.g., panaydol), fatty acids, and minerals.

A comparison of KRG with GTS and various other ginseng extracts reveals that the ginsenoside constituent content of KRG is consistent across studies, with the following approximate common constituent ratios: with Rb1 (33%), Rc (13%), Rb2 (11%), Re (8%), and Rg1 (8%). The remaining constituents (e.g., Rd, Rf, Rh, Rg2) are typically in the 4–5% range. In the total saponin mixture papers of Xia et al. [23] and Hu et al. [22] from the same laboratory, the values were far different than those seen for KRG: Re (27%), Rg 2 (19%), Rg1 (9%), and Rb2 (7%). The remaining ginsenosides ranged from 1.5% to 5.5%. Another ginseng mixture (e.g., Panax notoginseng) provides markedly different proportions of chemical constituents [21]. Some authors purchase the extracts from the same company with the same ginseng extract (G115) with 4% total ginsenosides [13] but did not present the specific constituent values. In general, the marked diversity of ginseng constituent mixtures makes such studies unique experimental systems and difficult to directly compare with other ginseng products.

From an overall perspective, the ginseng mixture studies showing hormetic dose responses used 16 different biological models (Table 1) with eight being neuronal-behavorially related models. These mixture studies also included several pre- and post-conditioning experiments [22–26,133]. The quantitative features of the ginseng mixture hormetic dose response studies had a median maximum stimulation of 155.5% with the stimulatory dose range being 7-fold (Table 4).

Table 4. Hormesis dose responses (median values -% stimulation).

	Mixtures	Rb1	Rd	Rg1	Gintonin	Re
Max Stim	155.5	169.6	146/59.5 (J)	180	172.5	133
Stim Range	7	53.3	10	10	20	25
Sample Size	29	26	6	50	8	7

It is not common for a total ginseng saponin mixture to be compared directly with the effects of specific constituents in the same study. However, in the report of Liao et al. [24], Rb1, Rg1 and GTS mixture (Figure 43) showed hormetic dose responses for spinal cord survival with embryonic Sprague–Dawley rats with both a direct stimulation and preconditioning protocols.

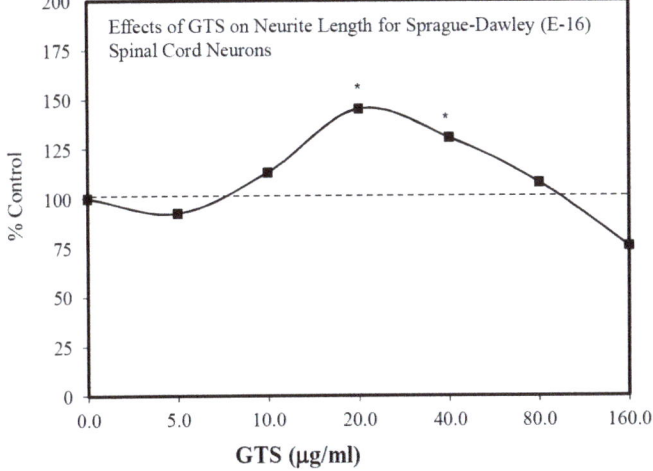

Figure 43. Effects of GTS on neurite length for Sprague–Dawley (E-16) spinal cord neurons (source: [24]). Each * represent statistical significance for a data point.

7.2. Kidney Toxicity

In the case of the KRG studies, hormetic dose responses were reported using five biology models (i.e., Dermal papilla cells, Park et al. [95]; A549 cell-human pulmonary epithelium cells, Song et al. [16,134]; HUVEC [15]; Murine osteoblastic MC3T3 cells [129,131]; LLC-PKI cells [133]) with a focus on possible clinical translation for preventing kidney toxicity during organ transplant procedures [133] and preventing osteoporosis as a result of long-term glucocorticoid treatment [131]. In the case of kidney toxicity, it is well known that the drug FK506 plays a critical role in assuring that a patient will not reject a transplanted organ. However, about 60% of patients report kidney toxicity in this process due to the FK506. The clinical importance of the adverse response to FK506 stimulated consideration to whether various chemopreventive agents might mitigate such adverse effects. While the first efforts in this general area were published by Hisamura et al. [135,136] using green tea extracts and tea polyphenols, it was inspired by a series of papers a decade earlier by Yokozawa et al. [137–140] showing that green tea tannins reduced the progression and severity of renal failure in nephrectomized rats. Subsequently, Hisamura et al. [135] showed green tea extracts/tea polyphenols to protect against FK506-induced toxicity to LLC-PK1 cells that were derived from pig renal tubular epithelium.

These developments led to research showing that KRG could also be effective in preventing nephrotoxicity induced by gentamicin in rat renal tubular cells [141,142] and by chronic exposure to cyclosporine [143]. These findings led Lee et al. [133] to assess whether KRG would prevent the toxicity of FK506 when both were administered at the same time. Using the LLC-PKI-pig kidney epithelial cells as their model, a toxic dose of FK506 was selected to challenge cell survival, reducing it to 60%. However, the KRG reduced significantly the FK506 toxicity in a manner that followed a hormetic dose response (Figure 44), with the optimal response occurring at 50 µM. Mechanistic follow-up studies revealed that the KRG treatment prevented an FK506-induced increase in p-p38, KIM-1, cleaved caspase 3, and increases in TLR-4 mRNA, all of which comprised key components of the toxicity pathways. A subsequent supportive study by Zhang et al. [144] reported that Panax notoginseng saponin (PNS) protected against polymyxin E-induced nephrotoxicity in an in vivo mouse (IM administration) study (Figure 45). Follow-up experiments with mouse renal tubular cells showed that PNS enhanced cell viability and the expression of BCL-2 while restoring mitochondrial function.

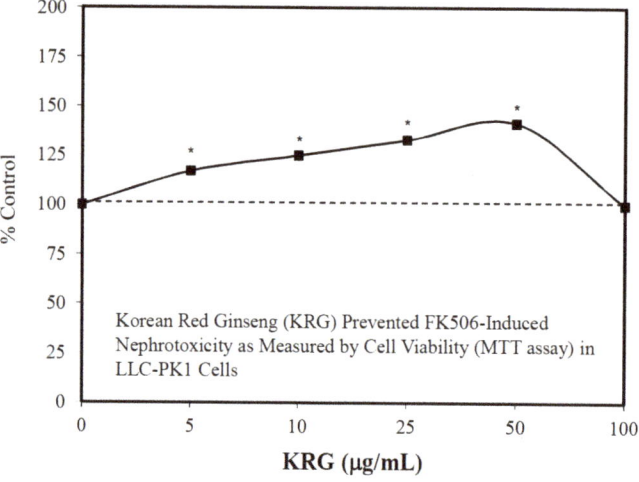

Figure 44. Korean Red Ginseng (KRG) prevented FK506-induced nephrotoxicity as measured by cell viability (MTT assay) in LLC-PK1 cells (source: [133]). Each * represent statistical significance for a data point.

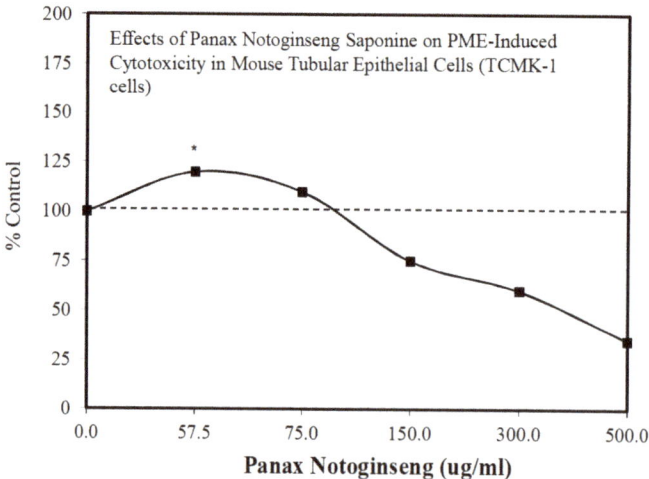

Figure 45. Effects of Panax notoginseng saponine on PME-induced cytotoxicity in mouse tubular epithelial cells (TCMK-1 cells) (source: [144]). Each * represent statistical significance for a data point.

7.3. Bone Toxicity

KRG reversed the toxic effect of dexamethasone on osteobastic MC3T3-E1 cells as measured by multiple toxicity endpoints [131]. Of particular interest was that the KRG prevented the capacity of dexamethasone to decrease the expression of osteogenic gene markers (e.g., ALP) in MC3T3-E1 cells in a hormetic fashion (Figure 46). These findings provide a foundation to further explore whether ginseng may be able to reduce glucocorticoid induced osteoporosis in an in vivo rodent model.

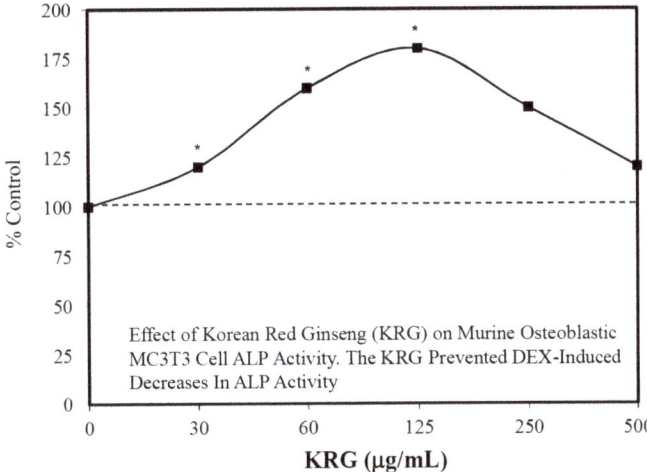

Figure 46. Effect of Korean Red Ginseng (KRG) on murine osteoblastic MC3T3 Cell ALP activity. The KRG prevented DEX-induced decreases in ALP activity (source: [131]). Each * represent statistical significance for a data point.

7.4. Learning and Memory

Considerable research was undertaken on the effects of ginseng extracts on a range of behavioral parameters in animal models and humans by VD Petkov in Bulgaria during the mid 1950s to mid 1980s. Some of these investigations suggested a biphasic dose dependency. For example, Petkov [145] reported that orally administered ginseng extract at 20 mg/kg for three days enhanced learning and memory in rats undergoing punishment-reinforced maze training. However, this improved learning response was not only absent at the dose of 100 mg/kg but decreased relative to the control group. This biphasic dose dependency was subsequently explored in male Wistar rats in a series of different endpoint specific behavior/learning experiments using six doses with a dose range from 3 to 300 mg/kg with these treatments administered over 10 consecutive days. Training began on the 10th day, one hour following the last ginseng treatment. Learning retention testing was administered from 24 h out to 14 days following the cessation of the training sessions. The authors reported the occurrence of biphasic dose responses for multiple endpoint tests (e.g., multiple learning/memory Shuttle box tests, two-way avoidance and punishment reinforcement testing, step-down passive avoidance tests, staircase maze testing). In each case, the dose response was biphasic, with the optimal dose ranging from 10 to 30 mg/kg, depending on the endpoint and experiment. These findings confirmed earlier reports emphasizing the biphasic nature of the ginseng extract effects. Petkov and Mosharrof [146] noted that multiple researchers assessing others drugs with cognition activating effects reported similar biphasic dose responses, creating a type of hormetic "therapeutic window".

7.5. Brain Traumatic Injury

The IP administration of GTS has also been shown to reduce traumatic brain injury in male rats (Figure 47) [22,23] in a hormetic manner. These findings were consistent with the report that Panex ginseng extracts protect astrocytes from hydrogen peroxide-induced toxicity during preconditioning experiments [26].

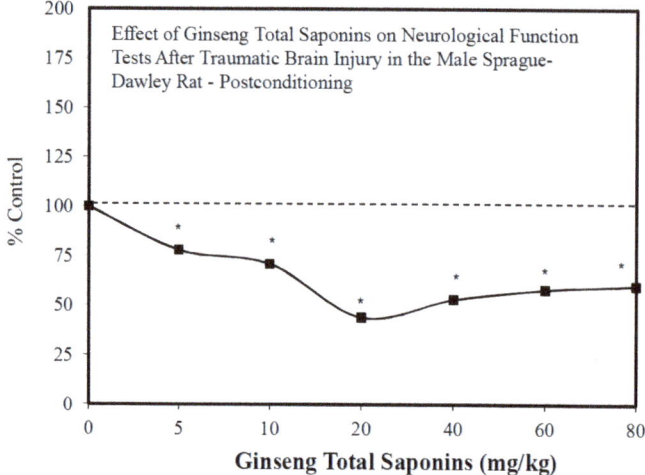

Figure 47. Effect of ginseng total saponins on neurological function tests after traumatic brain injury in the male Sprague–Dawley rat post-conditioning (source: [23]).

7.6. Muscle Injury

Orally administered ginseng extract (G115 extract) (4% ginsenosides) was also protective of muscle from exercise-induced stress regardless of which type of muscle fiber was studied with Wistar rats [12,13]. The protection started at the lowest dose tested (3 mg/kg), continuing to 100 mg/kg. The ginseng was administered daily for a three-month period. At the end of the three-month period, the animals were given an acute exercise stress experience using a treadmill [i.e., 20 m/min (0% gradient) for 80 min/day]. One week prior to the intense exercise, the rats were acclimated on the treadmill at 15 min/day with the speed increasing from 10 to 20 m/min. In traditional oriental medicine, the prescription for ginseng has been reported to be between 10 and 100 mg/kg, thereby excluding the low (3 mg/kg) and high (500 mg/kg) doses used in the Voces et al. [13] studies. Therefore, the protection is seen at about one-third of the lowest recommended dose. Of further interest is that Yu et al. [147] showed that oral Rg1 supplementation at 0.1 mg/kg significantly protected against exercise-induced oxidative stress in skeletal muscle.

7.7. Liver Injury and Repair

In Traditional Chinese Medicine (TCM), Panax has been employed to treat patients for a spectrum of liver diseases. According to Hui et al. [148], Panax nontoginseng saponins (PNS) have been effective in the treatment of liver fibrosis. Likewise, PNS has been protective against triptolide [149] and ethanol [150]-induced liver damage. These findings lead Zhong et al. [151] to hypothesize that PNS may have protective effects against damage resulting from partial hepatectomy (PH). In their follow-up investigations, the effect of PNS on liver regeneration following PH was assessed in a mouse model. This in vivo experiment was preceded by an in vitro primary hepatocyte cell culture study that assessed the effects of a broad range of PNS concentrations (0.01–0.50 µg/mL) on cell viability/cell proliferation assays. In the in vitro experiments, the PNS induced an hormetic–biphasic concentration response over the 50-fold concentration range with the maximum stimulation being 122% compared to a control value of 100% (Figure 48). A follow-up experiment using a marker for cell proliferation also showed a biphasic concentration response with the same optimized concentration between the two experiments. Then, this optimized concentration was selected for a follow up in vivo experiment to test the capacity of PNS to enhance liver regeneration in the PH study protocol. The PNS treatment in the in vivo study resulted in an increase in the liver to body weight ratio, lower levels of AST/ALS and other biomarkers of less injury, and enhanced regeneration. Mechanistic evaluation linked these enhanced recovery activities with the upregulation of P13/AKT/mTOR and the AKT/Bad cell pathways. According to the authors, this study provides support for the use of PNS in clinical settings for patients experiencing PH and perhaps other types of liver damage.

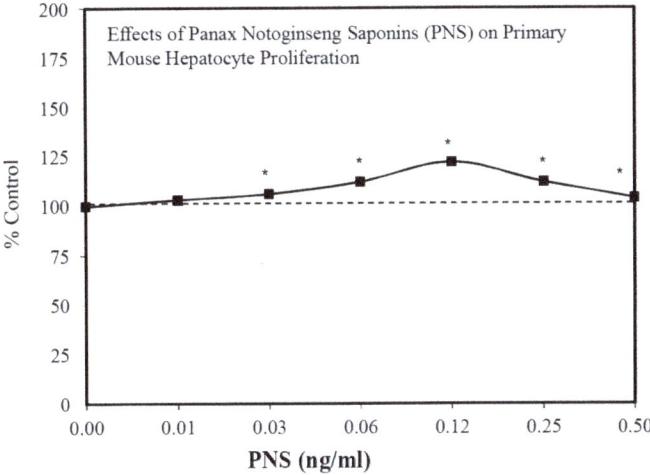

Figure 48. Effects of Panax Notoginseng Saponins (PNS) on primary mouse hepatocyte proliferation (source: [151]).

8. Discussion

The present assessment reveals that hormetic dose responses have been commonly reported in the biomedical literature for ginseng constituents and mixtures. While this assessment addresses the principal ginseng mixtures and constituents hormetic effects have also been reported in less well-studied constituents (e.g., RH2 [52], Rc [110] and Rg 3 [106]). The range of endpoints assessed has been broad but dominated by the area of neuroprotection. The areas of greatest interest have been those dealing with cellular/animal models for AD [48] and PD [41,42] disease, followed by stroke [51,52,152,153], neuronal health/regeneration based on studies with spinal cord [24,107]/sciatic nerve [62] injuries, and pain [113]. It is remarkable that this broad range of endpoints from a similarly wide variety of biological models and experimental approaches (e.g., pre-post-conditioning, non-conditioning, different mediators of damage) display hormetic dose responses. These results have also been reported by numerous independent research groups. In most studies, there has been substantial mechanism-receptor/pathway findings to account for the protective effects.

There have been other targeted research areas for the chemoprotective properties of ginseng. For example, there has been substantial research concerning the capacity of Rb1 to prevent symptoms of diabetes within an hormetic dose–response context [82,83]. Given the widespread occurrence of diabetes within the human population, there has been interest in using ginseng products in the treatment of type 2 diabetes. However, the biphasic nature of the hormetic dose response poses important challenges to identify endpoint specific optimal doses, as well as how close the optimal dose may be to potentially harmful higher doses along with the issue of human inter-individual variability.

The ginseng hormetic findings have also shown potential application for the treatment of corneal lesions with chemoprotection findings for both in vitro and in vivo studies [125]. In a similar fashion, ginseng extract treatment reduced the occurrence of FK506-induced kidney toxicity in a spectrum of model experimental systems [133]. These findings have potential practical relevance, since a very high proportion of organ transplant patients that receive FK506 to prevent organ rejection develop kidney toxicity.

Regardless of the biological model, endpoint measured, constituent studied, or mixture type employed, the quantitative features of the dose responses have been similar and consistent with the vast literature for hometic dose responses in plants and animals in vitro and in vivo settings [4,153,154]. The maximum stimulations with ginseng have been generally within the 130–180% range, while the width of the stimulation for the above respective comparison groups is less than 50-fold (Table 4). While the principal focus has been has been on assessing the low-dose stimulation, the high dose inhibitory aspect of the hormetic dose response is often more limited, as some studies do not evaluate responses greater than the threshold or even achieve a threshold. Further, the assessment of mechanism for the low-dose stimulation was also more extensively pursued than for the higher dose responses. An extensive mechanistic assessment of hormetic dose responses [13] includes mechanisms for some hormetic dose responses in both the low and high dose zones for those interested.

While efforts have been made to assess the pharmacokinetic characteristics of ginsenosides, there is a general lack of comprehensive studies in the area. The ginsenosides have chemically complex structures and a diverse range of biotransformation pathways, making generalizations difficult. However, most of the ginsenosides have low gastrointestinal absorption, being less than 5–10% [155–157]. The half-life in humans for several of the ginsenosides falls within the 18–24 h. duration [53]. Furthermore, the concentrations of ginsenosides are typically about 10-fold higher in the plasma than in the brain, suggesting that there is limited permeability through the blood–brain barrier. These observations indicate that there is likely to be a considerable range of cellular concentrations of various ginsenoside constituents.

A review of the ginseng hormesis literature reveals that a strong majority have utilized in vitro methods with cell cultures. However, nearly 20 studies utilized in vivo animal model studies assessing responses in a diverse set of organs, including the brain (TBI, stroke, AD pathology, behavior), skeletal muscle, heart, peripheral nerves, pain, and various diabetic disease endpoints. While most of the in vivo studies employed an IP administration, several papers administered the ginsenoside via the oral route. Of interest is that three of these oral studies dealt with brain endpoints such as AD pathology [129], depression behavior and BNDF [28], and learning behavior [146]. This suggests that some ginsenoside constituents and their mixtures can have biological effects on neuronal endpoints at relatively low concentrations. The optimal exposure in the Petkov and Mosharrof [146] study was 10 mg/kg, which is a dose that is commonly used by humans.

It has been widely emphasized that ginsenosides and their metabolites have poor bioavailability and cannot reach the intended biological targets when administered orally [158]. However, there are a large number of studies demonstrating that orally administered ginseng mixtures/constituents have biologically significant responses at doses that are in the low to moderate range, affecting a broad range of organs and endpoints. These responses are seen for multiple organs such as the liver [100,159], kidney [133], brain/behavior [53,160], skeletal muscle [12,13,161,162], and others in experimental systems. Furthermore, a long-term (90 day) oral consumption of ginseng extract markedly reduced the susceptibility of both young (6-month-old) and intermediate-aged (18-month-old) rats to acute ischemia reperfusion injury following a preconditioning exposure [163]. Therefore, these examples indicate that there is convincing evidence that the statement by Yu et al. [158] relating to oral ginseng not reaching biological targets to have many exceptions and can not therefore be seen as reflecting a reliable generalization.

Despite the rather extensive number of reports in the biomedical literature that demonstrate that hormetic dose responses are common for ginseng effects, this is the first paper to provide an integrated synthesis of this topic. The implications of the present findings have the potential to be significant, since a very broad array of cell types and endpoints have been reported to display hormetic dose responses, often with variable optimal dose ranges. Humans ingesting ginseng mixtures in the 500 to several thousand mg/day range are likely to be common. Such exposures are expected to have the potential to induce a spectrum of biological effects, with some likely in hormetic optimal dose zone. However, despite the substantial recognition that ginseng dose responses are very commonly hormetic, the clarification of what the effects will be on human populations remain to be resolved. Furthermore, the large number of hormetic dose response observations in the experimental studies reported here should also encourage researchers to carefully consider their study design strategies with respect to the number and spacing of doses.

Funding: EJC acknowledges longtime support from the US Air Force (AFOSR FA9550-19-1-0413) and ExxonMobil Foundation (S18200000000256). The U.S. Government is authorized to reproduce and distribute for governmental purposes notwithstanding any copyright notation thereon. The views and conclusions contained herein are those of the author and should not be interpreted as necessarily representing policies or endorsement, either expressed or implied. Sponsors had no involvement in study design, collection, analysis, interpretation, writing and decision to and where to submit for publication consideration.

Conflicts of Interest: The author declares no conflict of interest.

References

1. Fujitani, I. Essay on the chemistry and pharmacology of ginseng root. *Arch. Int. Pharmacodyn. Ther.* **1905**, *14*, 355.
2. Calabrese, E.J.; Baldwin, L.A. Defining hormesis. *Hum. Exp. Toxicol.* **2002**, *21*, 91–97. [CrossRef] [PubMed]
3. Calabrese, E.J.; Mattson, M.P. How does hormesis impact biology, toxicology, and medicine? *Aging Mech. Dis.* **2017**, *3*, 13. [CrossRef] [PubMed]
4. Calabrese, E.J.; Blain, R.B. The hormesis database: The occurrence of hormesis dose responses in the toxicological literature. *Regul. Toxicol. Pharmacol.* **2011**, *61*, 73–81. [CrossRef]
5. Calabrese, E.J. Biphasic dose responses in biology, toxicology and medicine: Accounting for their generality and quantitative feature. *Environ. Pollut.* **2013**, *182*, 452–460. [CrossRef]
6. Calabrese, E.J. Preconditioning is hormesis. Part 1: Documentation, dose-response features and mechanistic foundations. *Pharmacol. Res.* **2016**, *110*, 242–264. [CrossRef]
7. Calabrese, E.J. Hormesis: Why it is important to toxicology and toxicologists. *Environ. Chem. Toxicol.* **2008**, *27*, 1451–1474. [CrossRef]
8. Calabrese, E.J. Hormetic mechanisms. *Crit. Rev. Toxicol.* **2013**, *43*, 580–606. [CrossRef]
9. Calabrese, E.J.; Dhawan, G.; Kapoor, R.; Mattson, M.P.; Rattan, S.I. Curcumin and hormesis with particular emphasis on neural cells. *Food Chem. Toxicol.* **2019**, *129*, 399–404. [CrossRef]
10. Calabrese, E.J.; Calabrese, V.; Tsatsakis, A.; Giordano, J.J. Hormesis and Ginkgo biloba (GB): Numerous biological effects of GB are mediated via hormesis. *Aging Res. Rev.* **2020**, in press. [CrossRef]
11. Calabrese, E.J.; Tsatsakis, A.M.; Agathokleous, E.; Giordano, J.; Calabrese, V. Hormesis and Green Tea. *Dose-Response* **2020**, in press.
12. Voces, J.; Alvarez, A.I.; Vila, L.; Ferrando, A.; Cabral de Oliverira, C.; Prieto, H.G. Effects of administration of the standardized Panax ginseng extract G115 on hepatic antioxidant function after exhaustive exercise. *Comp. Biochem. Physiol. Part C* **1999**, *123*, 175–184. [CrossRef]
13. Voces, J.; Cabral de Oliveira, A.C.; Prieto, J.G.; Vila, L.; Perez, A.C.; Duarte, E.D.G.; Alvarez, A.I. Ginseng administration protects skeletal muscle from oxidative stress induced acute exercise in rats. *Braz. J. Med. Biol. Res.* **2004**, *37*, 1863–1871. [CrossRef] [PubMed]
14. Li, Y.; Xiao, Z.; Li, B.; Wang, H.; Qi, J.; Wang, Y. Ginsenoside exhibits concentration-dependent dual effects on HepG2 cell proliferation via regulation of c-Myc and HNF-4a. *Eur. J. Pharm.* **2016**, *792*, 26–32. [CrossRef]
15. Sung, W.N.; Kwok, H.H.; Rhee, M.H.; Yue, R.Y.K.; Wong, R.N.S. Korean Red Ginseng extract induces angiogenesis through activation of glucocorticoid receptor. *J. Ginseng Res.* **2017**, *41*, 477–486. [CrossRef]

16. Song, H.; Lee, Y.J. Inhibition of hypoxia-induced cyclooxygenase-2 by Korean Red Ginseng is dependent on peroxisome proliferator-activated receptor gamma. *J. Ginseng Res.* **2017**, *41*, 240–246. [CrossRef]
17. Seghinsara, A.M.; Shoorei, H.; Taheri, A.A.H.; Khaki, A.; Shokoohi, M.; Tahmasebi, M.; Khaki, A.A.; Eyni, H.; Ghorbani, S.; Rad, H.R.; et al. Panax ginseng extract improves follicular development after mouse preantral follicle 3D culture. *Cell J.* **2019**, *21*, 210–219.
18. Lim, B.V.; Shin, M.C.; Jang, M.J.; Lee, T.H.; Kim, Y.P.; Kim, H.B.; Lee, K.S.; Kim, H.; Kim, E.H.; Kim, C.J. Ginseng radix increases cell proliferation in dentate gyrus of rats with streptozotocin-induced diabetes. *Biol. Pharm. Bull.* **2002**, *25*, 1550–1554. [CrossRef]
19. Kanzaki, T.; Morisaki, N.; Shiina, R.; Saito, Y. Role of transforming growth factor-beta pathway in the mechanism of wound healing by saponin from Ginseng Radix rubra. *Br. J. Pharmacol.* **1998**, *125*, 255–262. [CrossRef]
20. Morisaki, N.; Watanebe, S.; Tezuka, M.; Zenibayashi, M.; Shiina, R.; Koyama, N.; Kanzaki, T.; Saito, Y. Mechanism of angiogenic effects of saponin from ginseng Radix rubra in human umbilical vein endothelial cells. *Br. J. Pharmacol.* **1995**, *115*, 1188–1193. [CrossRef]
21. Shi, X.; Yu, W.; Yang, T.; Liu, W.; Zao, Y.; Sun, Y.; Cahi, L.; Gao, Y.; Dong, B.; Zhu, L. *Panax notoginseng* saponins provide neuroprotection by regulating NgR1/RhoA/ROCK2 pathway expression, in vitro and in vivo. *J. Ethnopharmacol.* **2016**, *190*, 301–312. [CrossRef] [PubMed]
22. Hu, B.Y.; Liu, X.J.; Qiang, R.; Jiang, Z.L.; Xu, L.H.; Wang, G.H.; Li, X.; Peng, B. Treatment with ginseng total saponins improves the neurorestoration of rat after traumatic brain injury. *J. Ethnopharmacol.* **2014**, *155*, 1243–1255. [CrossRef] [PubMed]
23. Xia, L.; Jiang, Z.-J.; Wang, G.-H.; Hu, B.-Y.; Ke, K.-F. Treatment with ginseng total saponins reduces the secondary brain injury in rat after cortical impact. *J. Neurosci. Res.* **2012**, *90*, 1424–1436. [CrossRef] [PubMed]
24. Liao, B.; Newmark, H.; Zhou, R. Neuroprotective effects of ginseng total saponin and ginsenosides Rb1 and Rg1 on spinal cord neurons in vitro. *Exp. Neurol.* **2002**, *173*, 224–234. [CrossRef]
25. Zhang, C.; Li, C.; Chen, S.; Li, Z.; Ma, L.; Ji, X.; Wang, K.; Bao, J.; Liang, Y.; Chem, M.; et al. Hormetic effect of panaxatriol saponins confers neuroprotection in PC12 cells and zebrafish through P13K/AKT/mTOR and AMPK/SIRT1FOX03 pathways. *Sci. Rep.* **2017**, *7*, 41082. [CrossRef]
26. Naval, M.V.; Gomez-Serranillo, A.P.; Carretero, M.E.; Villar, A.M. Neuroprotective effect of a ginseng (Panax ginseng) root extract on astrocytes primary culture. *J. Ethnopharmacol.* **2007**, *112*, 262–270. [CrossRef]
27. Gao, Y.; Li, J.; Chu, S.; Zhang, Z.; Chen, N.; Li, L.; Zhang, L. Ginsenoside Rg1 protects mice against streptozotocin–induced type 1 diabetic by modulating the NLRP3 and Keap1/Nrf2/HO-1 pathways. *Eur. J. Pharm.* **2020**, *866*, 172801. [CrossRef]
28. Boonlert, W.; Benya-Aphikul, H.; Welbat, J.M.; Rodsiri, R. Ginseng extract G115 attenuates ethanol-induced depression in mice b increasing brain BDNF levels. *Nutrients* **2017**, *9*, 931. [CrossRef] [PubMed]
29. Shen, L.; Zhang, J. NMDA receptor and iNOs are involved in the effects of ginsenoside Rg1 on hippocampal neurogenesis in ischemic gerbils. *Neurol. Res.* **2007**, *29*, 270–273. [CrossRef] [PubMed]
30. Shi, A.W.; Wang, X.B.; Lu, F.X.; Zhu, M.M.; Kong, X.Q.; Cao, K.J. Ginsenoside Rg1 promotes endothelial progenitor cell migration and proliferation. *Acta Pharmacol. Sin.* **2009**, *30*, 299–306. [CrossRef] [PubMed]
31. Xu, F.T.; Li, H.M.; Yin, Q.S.; Cui, S.E.; Liu, D.L.; Nan, H.; Han, Z.A.; Xu, K.M. Effect of ginsenoside Rg1 on proliferation and neural phenotype differentiation of human adipose-derived stem cells in vitro. *Can. J. Physiol. Pharmacol.* **2014**, *92*, 467–475. [CrossRef]
32. Dong, J.; Zhu, G.; Wang, T.C.; Shi, F.S. Ginsenoside Rg1 promotes neural differentiation of mouse adipose-derived stem cells via the miRNA-124 signaling pathway. *J. Zhejiang Univ. Sci. B* **2017**, *18*, 445–448. [CrossRef]
33. Liu, J.W.; Tian, S.J.; Barry, D.; Luu, B. Panaxadiol glycosides that induce neuronal differentiation in neurosphere stem cells. *J. Nat. Prod.* **2007**, *70*, 1329–1334. [CrossRef] [PubMed]
34. Liang, Z.J.; Lu, Z.; Zhu, D.D.; Yi, X.L.; Wu, F.X.; He, N.; Tang, C.; Wei, C.Y.; Li, I.; Li, H.M. Ginsenoside Rg1 accelerates paracrine activity and adipogenic differentiation of human breast adipose-derived stem cells in a dose-dependent manner in vitro. *Cell Transplant.* **2019**, *28*, 286–295. [CrossRef] [PubMed]
35. Gao, J.; Wan, F.; Tian, M.; Li, Y.; Li, Y.; Zhang, J.; Wang, Y.; Huang, X.; Zhang, L.; Si, Y.C. Effects of ginsenoside-Rg1 on the proliferation and glial-like directed differentiation of embryonic rat cortical neural stem cells in vitro. *Mol. Med. Rep.* **2017**, *16*, 8875–8881. [CrossRef] [PubMed]

36. Wang, P.; Wei, X.; Zhou, Y.; Wang, Y.P.; Yang, K.; Zhang, F.J.; Jiang, R. Effect of ginsenoside Rg1 on proliferation and differentiation of human dental pulp cells in vitro. *Aust. Dent. J.* **2012**, *57*, 157–165. [CrossRef]
37. Yin, L.-H.; Cheng, W.-X.; Qin, A.-S.; Sun, K.M.; Zhong, M.; Wang, J.K.; Gao, W.Y.; Yu, Z.H. Effects of ginsenoside (Rg1) on the proliferation and osteogenic differentiation of human periodontal ligament stem cells. *Chin. J. Integr. Med.* **2015**, *21*, 676–681. [CrossRef]
38. Kim, S.H.; Choi, K.H.; Lee, D.K.; Oh, J.M.; Hwang, J.Y.; Park, C.H.; Lee, C.K. Ginsenoside Rg1 improves in vitro-produced embryo quality by increasing glucose uptake in procine blastocytes. *Asian-Australas. J. Anim. Sci.* **2016**, *29*, 1095–1101. [CrossRef]
39. Li, Y.B.; Wang, Y.; Tang, J.P.; Chen, D.; Wang, S.L. Neuroprotective effects of ginsenoside Rg1-induced neural stem cell transplantation on hypoxic-ischemic encephalopathy. *Neural Regen. Res.* **2015**, *5*, 753–759.
40. Chen, C.; Ahou, Y.C.; Chen, Y.; Zhu, Y.G.; Fang, F.; Chen, L.M. Ginsenoside Rg1 reduces MPTP-induced substantia nigra neuron loss by suppressing oxidative stress. *Acta Pharmacol. Sin.* **2005**, *26*, 56–62. [CrossRef]
41. Gao, Q.G.; Chen, W.F.; Xie, J.X.; Wong, M.S. Ginsenoside Rg1 protect against 6-OHDA–induced neurotoxicity in neuroblastoma SK-N-SH cells via IGF-1 receptor and estrogen receptor pathways. *J. Neurochem.* **2009**, *109*, 1338–1347. [CrossRef] [PubMed]
42. Ge, K.L.; Chen, W.F.; Xie, J.X.; Wong, M.S. Ginsenoside Rg1 protects against 6-OHDA-induced toxicity in MES23.5 cells via Akt and ERK signaling pathways. *J. Ethnopharmacol.* **2010**, *127*, 118–123. [CrossRef] [PubMed]
43. Fernandez-Moriano, C.; Gonzalez-Burgos, E.; Iglesian, I.; Lozano, R.; Gomez-Serranillos, M.P. Evaluation of the adaptogenic potential exerted by ginsenosides Rb1 and Rg1 against oxidative stress-mediated neurotoxicity in an in vitro neuronal model. *PLoS ONE* **2017**, *12*, e0182933. [CrossRef]
44. Chan, R.Y.; Chen, W.F.; Dong, A.; Guo, D.A.; Wong, M.S. Estrogen-like activity of ginsenoside Rg1 derived from *Panax notoginseng*. *J. Clin. Endocrinol. Metab.* **2002**, *87*, 3691–3695. [CrossRef] [PubMed]
45. Green, P.S.; Gridley, K.E.; Simpkins, J.W. Estradiol protects against beta-amyloid (25-3)5-induced toxicity in SK-N-SH human neuroblastoma cells. *Neurosci. Lett.* **1996**, *218*, 165–168. [CrossRef]
46. Xu, H.; Gouras, G.K.; Greefield, J.P.; Vincent, B.; Naslund, J.; Mazzarelli, L.; Fried, G.; Jovanoic, J.N.; Seeger, M.; Relkin, N.R.; et al. Estrogen reduces neuronal generation of Alzheimer beta-amyloid peptides. *Nat. Med.* **1998**, *4*, 447–451. [CrossRef]
47. Goodenough, S.; Schafer, M.; Behl, C. Estrogen-induced cell signaling in a cellular model of Alzheimer's disease. *J. Steroid Biochem. Mol. Biol.* **2003**, *84*, 301–305. [CrossRef]
48. Gong, L.; Li, S.L.; Li, H.; Zhang, L. Ginsenoside Rg1 protects primary cultured rat hippocampal neurons from cell apoptosis induced by B-amyloid protein. *Pharm. Biol.* **2011**, *49*, 501–507. [CrossRef]
49. Nie, L.; Xia, J.; Li, H.; Zhang, Z.; Yang, Y.; Huang, X.; He, Z.; Liu, J.; Yang, X. Ginsenoside Rg1 ameliorates behavioral abnormalities and modulates the hippocampal proteomic change in triple transgenic mice of Alzheimer's Disease. *Oxid. Med. Cell. Longev.* **2017**, *2017*, 6473506. [CrossRef]
50. Zhang, X.; Wang, J.; Xing, Y.; Gong, L.; Li, H.; Wu, Z.; Li, Y.; Wang, J.; Wang, Y.; Dong, L.; et al. Effects of ginsenoside Rg1 or 17b-estradiol on a cognitively impaired, ovariectomized rat model of Alzheimer's Disease. *Neuroscience* **2012**, *220*, 191–200. [CrossRef]
51. Chu, S.F.; Zhang, Z.; Zhou, X.; He, W.B.; Chen, C.; Luo, P.; Liu, D.D.; Gong, H.F.; Wang, Z.Z.; Sun, H.S.; et al. Ginsenoside Rg1 protects against ischemic/reperfusion-induced neuronal injury through miR-144/Nrf2/ARE pathway. *Acta Pharmacol. Sin.* **2019**, *40*, 13–25. [CrossRef] [PubMed]
52. Cheng, Z.; Zhang, M.; Ling, C.; Zhu, Y.; Ren, H.; Hong, C.; Qin, J.; Lu, T.; Wang, J. Neuroprotective effects of ginsenosides against cerebral ischemia. *Molecules* **2019**, *24*, 1102. [CrossRef] [PubMed]
53. Li, M.; Guam, Y.; Liu, N.; Shao, C.; Liu, Z.; Chen, J.; Wang, Q.; Pan, X.; Sun, H.; Ahang, Y. Brain concentration of ginsenosides and pharmacokinetics after oral administration of mountain-cultivated ginseng. *J. Chin. Chem. Soc.* **2017**, *64*, 395–403. [CrossRef]
54. Li, Y.; Suo, L.; Li, H.; Xue, W. Protective effects of ginsenoside Rg1 against oxygen-glucose-deprivation-induced apoptosis in neural stem cells. *J. Neurol. Sci.* **2017**, *373*, 107–112. [CrossRef] [PubMed]
55. Lu, M.C.; Lai, T.Y.; Hwang, J.M.; Chen, H.T.; Chang, S.H.; Tsai, F.J.; Wang, H.L.; Lin, C.C.; Kuo, W.W.; Huang, C.Y. Proliferation- and migration-enhancing effects of ginseng and ginsenoside Rg1 though IGF-I- and FGF-2-signaling pathways on RSC96 Schwann cells. *Cell Biochem. Funct.* **2009**, *27*, 186–192. [CrossRef]

56. Chan, L.S.; Yue, P.Y.K.; Wong, Y.Y.; Wong, R.N.S. MicroRNA-15b contributes to ginsenoside-Rg1-induced angiogenesis through increased expression of VEGFR-2. *Biochem. Pharmacol.* **2013**, *86*, 392–400. [CrossRef] [PubMed]
57. Wang, W.X.; Wang, W.; Chen, H.J. Study progression in neuroprotective effects of ginsenoside Rg1. *J. Bethune Med. Coll.* **2005**, *10*, 291–293.
58. Wei, C.B.; Jia, J.P.; Wang, F. Effects of ginsenosides Rg1 and Rb1 on metabolism pathway of amyloid protein. *Chin. J. Inf. Tradit. Chin. Med.* **2008**, *9*, 28–30.
59. Zhang, Z.J.; Jiang, W. Effects and its mechanism of ginsenosides on dilating rabbit basal artery. *J. Heart* **2003**, *15*, 313–315.
60. Lu, Z.F.; Shen, Y.X.; Zhang, P. Ginsenoside Rg1 promote proliferation and neurotrophin expression of olfactory ensheating cells. *J. Asian Nat. Res.* **2010**, *12*, 265–272. [CrossRef]
61. Zhou, P.; Dong, L.L.; Yang, Z.J.; Fang, Z. A study of effects of ginsenoside Rg1 on regeneration of rat sciatic nerves. *Inn. Mong. Med. J.* **2011**, *43*, 413–415.
62. Huo, D.-S.; Zhang, M.; Cai, Z.-P.; Dong, C.-X.; Wang, H.; Yang, Z.-J. The role of nerve growth factor in ginsenoside Rg1-induced regeneration of injured rat sciatic nerve. *J. Toxicol. Environ. Health Part A* **2015**, *78*, 1328. [CrossRef] [PubMed]
63. Xu, A.M.; Li, C.B.; Liu, Q.L.; Yang, H.; Li, P. Ginsenoside Rg1 protects H9c2 cells against nutritional stress-induced injury via aldolase/AMPK/PINK1. *J. Cell. Biochem.* **2019**, *120*, 18388–18397. [CrossRef]
64. Tong, L.S.; Chao, C.Y. Effects of ginsenoside Rg1 of Panax ginseng on mitosis in human blood lymphocytes in vitro. *Am. J. Chin. Med.* **1980**, *8*, 254–267. [CrossRef] [PubMed]
65. Liu, J.; Wang, S.; Liu, H.; Yang, L.; Nan, G. Stimulatory effect of saponin from Panax ginseng on immune function of lymphocytes in the elderly. *Mech. Ageing Dev.* **1995**, *83*, 43–53. [CrossRef]
66. Zhang, Y.Z.; Yan, L.; Kang, X.P.; Dou, C.Y.; Zhou, R.G.; Huang, S.Q.; Peng, L.; Wen, L. Ginsenoside Rb1 confers neuroprotection via promotion of glutamate transporters in a mouse model of Parkinson's disease. *Neuropharmacology* **2013**, *131*, 223–237. [CrossRef]
67. Tohda, C.; Matsumoto, N.; Zou, K.; Meselhy, M.R.; Komatsu, K. AB (25-35)-induced memory impairment, axonal atrophy, and synaptic loss are ameliorated by MI, a metabolite of protopanaxadiol-type saponins. *Neuropsycopharmacology* **2004**, *29*, 860–868. [CrossRef]
68. Kim, Y.C.; Kim, S.R.; Markelonis, G.J.; Oh, T.H. GInsenosides RB1 and Rg3 protect cultured rat cortical cells from glutamate-induced neurodegeneration. *J. Neurosci. Res.* **1998**, *53*, 426–432. [CrossRef]
69. Ni, N.; Liu, Q.; Ren, H.; Wu, D.; Luo, C.; Li, P.; Wan, J.B.; Su, H. Ginsenoside Rb1 protects rat neural progenitor cells against oxidative injury. *Molecules* **2014**, *19*, 3012–3024. [CrossRef]
70. Hadlock, T.; Sunback, C.; Hunter, D.; Cheney, M.; Vacanti, J.P. A polymer foam conduit seeded with Schwann cells promotes guided peripheral nerve regeneration. *Tissue Eng.* **2000**, *6*, 119–127. [CrossRef] [PubMed]
71. Chang, C.J. The effect of pulse-released nerve growth factor from genipin-crosslinked gelatin in Schwann cell-seeded polycaprolactone conduits on large-gap peripheral nerve regeneration. *Tissue Eng. Part A* **2009**, *15*, 547–557. [CrossRef] [PubMed]
72. Huang, J.; Ye, Z.; Hu, Z.; Lu, L.; Luo, Z. Electrical stimulation induces calcium-dependent release of NGF from cultured Schwann cells. *Glia* **2010**, *58*, 622–631. [CrossRef] [PubMed]
73. Huang, J.; Hu, X.; Lu, L.; Ye, Z.; Zhang, Q.; Luo, Z. Electrical regulation of Schwann cells using conductive polypyrrole/chitosan polymers. *J. Biomed. Mater. Res.* **2010**, *93A*, 164–174. [CrossRef] [PubMed]
74. He, J.; Ding, W.L.; Li, F.; Li, F.; Wang, W.J.; Zhu, H. Panaxydol treatment enhances the biological properties of Schwann cells in vitro. *Chem.-Biol. Interact.* **2009**, *177*, 34–39. [CrossRef]
75. Liang, W.; Ge, S.; Yang, L.; Yang, M.; Ye, Z.M.; Yan, M.; Du, J.; Luo, Z. Ginsenosides RB1 and Rg1 promote proliferation and expression of neurotrophic factors in primary Schwann cell cultures. *Brain Res.* **2010**, *1357*, 18–25. [CrossRef]
76. Xia, R.; Zhao, B.; Wu, Y.; Hou, J.B.; Zhang, L.; Xu, J.J.; Xia, Z.Y. Ginsenoside Rb1 preconditioning enhances eNOS expression and attenuates myocardial ischemia/reperfusion injury in diabetic rats. *J. Biomed. Biotechnol.* **2011**, *2011*, 767930. [CrossRef]
77. Li, J.; Shao, Z.H.; Xie, J.Z.; Wang, C.Z.; Ramachandran, S.; Yin, J.J.; Aung, H.; Li, C.Q.; Qin, G.; Vanden Hoek, T.; et al. The effects of ginsenoside Rb1 on JNK in oxidative injury in cardiomyocytes. *Arch. Pharmacal Res.* **2012**, *35*, 1259–1267. [CrossRef]

78. Wu, Y.; Xia, Z.Y.; Dou, J.J.; Zhang, L.; Xu, J.J.; Zhao, B.; Lei, S.Q.; Liu, H.M. Rb1 against myocardial ischemia/reperfusion injury in streptozotocin-induced diabetic rats. *Mol. Biol. Rep.* **2011**, *38*, 4327–4335. [CrossRef]
79. Yan, X.; Tian, J.; Wu, H.; Liu, Y.; Ren, J.; Zheng, S.; Zhang, C.; Yang, C.; Li, Y.; Wang, S. Ginsenoside Rb1 protects neonatal rat cardiomyocytes from hypoxia/ischemia induced apoptosis and inhibits activation of the mitochondrial apoptotic pathway. *Evid.-Based Complement. Altern. Med.* **2014**, *2014*, 149195. [CrossRef]
80. Yan, X.; Xue, J.; Wang, S.; Liu, Y.; Zheng, S.; Zhang, C.; Yang, C. Ginsenodie-Rb1 protests hypoxic-and ischemic-damaged cardiomyocyte by regulating expression of miRNAs. *Evid.-Based Complement. Altern. Med.* **2015**, *2015*, 171306. [CrossRef]
81. Yang, C.; Li, B.; Liu, Y.; Xing, Y. Ginsenoside Rb1 protects cardiomyocyres from oxygen-glucose deprivation injuries by targeting microRNA-21. *Exp. Ther. Med.* **2019**, *17*, 3709–3716. [PubMed]
82. Shang, W.; Yang, Y.; Jiang, B.; Jin, H.; Zhou, L.; Liu, S.; Chen, M. Ginsenoside Rb1 promotes adipogenesis in 3T3-L1 cells by enhancing PPARy2 and C/EBPa gene expression. *Life Sci.* **2007**, *80*, 618–625. [CrossRef] [PubMed]
83. Shang, W.; Yang, Y.; Zhou, L.; Jiang, B.; Jin, H.; Cjen, M. Ginsenoside Rb1 stimulates glucose uptake through insulin-like signaling pathway in 3T3-L1 adipocytes. *J. Endocrinol.* **2008**, *198*, 561–569. [CrossRef] [PubMed]
84. Mu, Q.; Fang, X.; Li, X.; Zhao, D.; Mo, F.; Jiang, G.; Yu, N.; Zhang, Y.; Guo, Y.; Fu, M.; et al. Ginsenoside Rb1 promotes browning through regulation of PPARy in 3T3-L1 adipocytes. *Biochem. Biophys. Res. Commun.* **2015**, *466*, 530–535. [CrossRef] [PubMed]
85. Hosseini, S.S.; Tabandeh, M.R.; Namin, A.S.M. Promoting effect of ginsenoside Rb1 for GLUT-4 gene expression and cellular synthesis in C1C12 cells. *Int. J. Pharm. Res. Allied Sci.* **2016**, *5*, 151–158.
86. Lee, G.Y.; Park, K.G.; Namgoong, S.; Han, S.K.; Jeong, S.H.; Dhong, E.S.; Kim, W.K. Effects of Panax ginseng extract on human dermal fibroblast proliferation and collagen synthesis. *Int. Wound J.* **2015**, *13* (Suppl. S1), 42–46.
87. Kim, Y.G.; Sumiyoshi, M.; Kawahira, K.; Sakanaka, M.; Kimura, Y. Effects of Red Ginseng extract on ultraviolet B-irradiated skin change in C57Bl mice. *Phytother. Res.* **2008**, *22*, 1423–1427. [CrossRef]
88. Kim, W.K.; Song, S.Y.; Oh, W.K.; Kaewsuwan, S.; Tran, T.L.; Kim, W.S.; Sung, J.H. Wound-healing effect of ginsenosdide Rd from leaves of Panax ginseng via cyclic AMP-dependent protein kinase patway. *Eur. J. Pharm.* **2013**, *702*, 285–293. [CrossRef]
89. Kimura, Y.; Sumiyoshi, M.; Kawahira, K.; Sakanaka, M. Effects of ginseng saponins isolated from Red Ginseng roots on burn wound healing in mice. *Br. J. Pharmacol.* **2006**, *148*, 860–870. [CrossRef]
90. Shedoeva, A.; Leavesley, D.; Upton, Z.; Fan, C. Wound healing and the use of medicinal plants. *Evid.-Based Complement. Altern. Med.* **2019**, *2019*, 2684108. [CrossRef]
91. Calabrese, E.J. Stimulating hair growth via hormesis: Experimental foundations and clinical implications. *Pharmacol. Res.* **2020**, *152*, 104599. [CrossRef]
92. Kubo, M.; Matsuda, H.; Fukui, M.; Nakai, Y. Development studies of cuticle drugs from natural resources. 1. Effects of crude drug extracts on hair growth in mice. *Yakugaku Zasshi J. Pharm. Soc. Jpn.* **1988**, *108*, 971–978. [CrossRef]
93. Shin, H.S.; Park, S.Y.; Hwang, E.S.; Lee, D.G.; Song, G.T.; Mavlonov, T.H. The inductive effect of ginsenosdie F2 on hair growth by altering the ENT signal pathway in telogen mouse cells. *Eur. J. Pharm.* **2014**, *730*, 82–89. [CrossRef] [PubMed]
94. Shin, H.S.; Park, S.Y.; Hwang, E.S.; Lee, D.G.; Mavlonov, T.H. Ginsenoside F2 reduces hair loss by controlling apoptosis through the sterol regulatory element-binding protein cleavage activating protein and transforming growth factor-b pathways in a dihydrotestosterone-induced mouse model. *Biol. Pharm. Bull.* **2014**, *37*, 755–763. [CrossRef] [PubMed]
95. Park, G.H.; Park, K.Y.; Cho, H.I.; Lee, S.M.; Han, J.S.; Won, C.H.; Chang, S.E.; Lee, M.W.; Choi, J.H.; Moon, K.C.; et al. Red ginseng extract promotes the hair growth in cultured human hair follicles. *J. Med. Food* **2015**, *18*, 354–362. [CrossRef]
96. Zhang, H.; Su, Y.; Wang, J.; Gao, F.; Yang, F.; Li, G. Ginsenoside Rb1 promotes the growth of mink hair follicle via P13K/AKT/GSK-3B signaling pathway. *Life Sci.* **2019**, *229*, 210–218. [CrossRef] [PubMed]
97. Kim, J.H.; Yi, S.M.; Choi, J.E.; Son, S.E. Study of the efficacy of Korean red Ginseng in the treatment of androgenic alopecia. *J. Ginseng Res.* **2009**, *33*, 223–228.

98. Yokozawa, T.; Kiu, Z.W.; Dong, E.B. A study of ginsenoside-Rd in a renal ischemia-reperfusion model. *Nephron* **1998**, *78*, 201–206. [CrossRef]
99. Yokozawa, T.; Owada, S. Effect of ginsenoside-Rd in cephaloridine-induced renal disorder. *Nephron* **1999**, *81*, 200–207. [CrossRef]
100. Yokozawa, T.; Satoh, A.; Cho, E.J. Ginsenoside-rd attenuates oxidative damage related to aging in senescence-accelerated mice. *J. Pharm. Pharmacol.* **2004**, *56*, 107–113. [CrossRef]
101. Lopez, M.V.N.; Gomez-Serranillo Cuadrado, M.P.G.S.; Ruiz-Poveda, O.M.P.; Del Fresno, A.M.V.; Accame, M.E.C. Neuroprotective effect of individual ginsenosides on astrocytes primary culture. *Biochem. Biophys Acta* **2007**, *1770*, 1308–1316. [CrossRef] [PubMed]
102. Ye, R.; Han, J.; Zhao, L.; Cao, R.; Rao, Z.; Zhao, G. Protection effects of ginsenoside Rd on PC 12 cells against hydrogen peroxide. *Biol. Pharm. Bull.* **2008**, *31*, 1923–1927. [CrossRef] [PubMed]
103. Ye, R.; Kong, X.; Yang, Q.; Zhang, Y.; Zhao, G. Ginsenoside RD attenuates redox imbalance and improves stroke outcome after focal cerebral ischemia in aged mice. *Neuropharmacology* **2011**, *61*, 815–824. [CrossRef] [PubMed]
104. Lin, T.; Liu, Y.; Shi, M.; Li, L.; Liu, Y.; Zhao, G. Promotive effect of ginsenoside Rd on proliferation of neural stem cells in vivo and in vitro. *J. Ethnopharmacol.* **2012**, *142*, 754–761. [CrossRef]
105. Liu, Y.; Zhang, R.-Y.; Zhao, J.; Dong, Z.; Feng, D.-Y.; Wu, R.; Shi, M.; Zhao, G. Ginsenoside Rd protects SH-SY5Y cells against 1-methyl-4-phenylpyridinium induced injury. *Int. J. Mol. Sci.* **2015**, *16*, 14395–14408. [CrossRef]
106. Kim, D.H.; Kim, D.W.; Jung, B.H.; Lee, J.H.; Lee, H.; Hwang, G.S.; Kang, K.S.; Lee, J.W. Ginsenoide Rb2 suppresses the glutamate-mediated oxidative stress and neuronal cell death in HT22 cells. *J. Ginseng Res.* **2019**, *41*, 326–334. [CrossRef]
107. Wang, B.; Zhu, Q.; Man, X.; Guo, L.; Hao, L. Ginsenoside Rd inhibits apoptosis following spinal cord ischemia/reperfusion injury. *Neural Regen. Res.* **2014**, *9*, 1678–1687.
108. Yang, I.; Deng, Y.; Xu, S.; Zeng, X. In vivo pharmacokinetic and metabolism studies of ginsenoside Rd. *J. Chromatogr. B Analyt. Technol. Biomed. Life Sci.* **2007**, *854*, 77–84. [CrossRef]
109. Wang, Y.; Li, X.; Wang, X.; Lau, W.; Wang, Y.; Xing, Y.; Zhang, X.; Ma, X.; Gao, F. Ginsenoside Rd attenuates myocardial ischemia/reperfusion injury via AKT, GSK-3B signaling and inhibition of the mitochondria-dependent apoptotic pathway. *PLoS ONE* **2013**, *8*, e70956.
110. Lee, D.; Lee, D.S.; Jung, K.; Hwang, G.S.; Lee, H.L.; Yamabe, N.; Lee, H.J.; Eom, W.; Kim, K.H.; Kang, K.S. Protective effect of ginsenoside Rb1 against tacrolimus-induced apoptosis in renal proximal tubular LLC-PK1 cells. *J. Ginseng Res.* **2018**, *42*, 75–80. [CrossRef]
111. Purup, S.; Larsen, E.; Christensen, L.P. Differential effects of falcarinol and related aliphatic C17-polyacetylene on intestinal cell proliferation. *J. Agric. Food Chem.* **2009**, *57*, 8290–8296. [CrossRef] [PubMed]
112. Nie, B.M.; Jiang, X.Y.; Cai, J.X.; Fum, S.L.; Yang, L.M.; Lin, L.; Hang, Q.; Lu, P.L.; Lu, Y. Panaxydol and panaxynol protect cultured cortical neurons against AB25-35-induced toxicity. *Neuropharmacology* **2008**, *54*, 845–853. [CrossRef] [PubMed]
113. Ahn, E.J.; Choi, G.J.; Kang, H.; Baek, C.W.; Jung, Y.H.; Woo, Y.C.; Bang, S.R. Antinociceptive effects of ginsenoside Rg3 in a rat model of incisional pain. *Eur. Surg. Res.* **2016**, *57*, 211–223. [CrossRef] [PubMed]
114. Wang, M.; Chen, X.; Jin, W.; Xu, X.; Li, X.; Sun, L. Ginsenoside Rb3 exerts protective properties against cigarette smoke extract-induced cell injury by inhibiting the p38 MAPK/NF-κB and TGF-β1/VEGF pathways in fibroblasts and epithelial cells. *Biomed. Pharmacother.* **2018**, *108*, 1751–1758. [CrossRef] [PubMed]
115. Park, M.W.; Ha, J.; Chung, S.H. 20(S)-ginsenoside Rg3 enhances glucose-stimulated insulin secretion and activates AMPK. *Biol. Pharm. Bull.* **2008**, *31*, 748–751. [CrossRef]
116. Wright, S.M.; Allman, E. Inhibition of Herbes Simplex virues, Types 1 and 2, by ginsenoside 20(s)-Rg3. *J. Microbiol. Biotechnol.* **2020**, *30*, 101–108. [CrossRef]
117. Song, J.H.; Choi, H.J.; Song, H.H.; Hong, E.H.; Lee, B.R.; Oh, S.R.; Choi, K.; Yeo, S.G.; Lee, Y.P.; Cho, S.; et al. Antiviral activity of ginsenosides against coxsackievirus B, enterovirus 71, and human rhinovirus 3. *J. Ginseng Res.* **2014**, *38*, 173–179. [CrossRef]
118. Huang, G.D.; Zhong, X.F.; Deng, A.Y.; Zeng, R. Proteomic analysis of ginsenoside Re attenuates hydrogen peroxide-induced oxidative stress in human umbilical vein endothelial cells. *Food Funct.* **2016**, *7*, 2451–2461. [CrossRef]

119. Yang, K.; Luo, Y.; Lu, S.; Hu, R.; Du, R.; Liao, P.; Sun, G.; Sun, X. Salvianolic acid B and ginsenoside Re synergistically protect against Ox-LDL-induced endothelial apoptosis through the antioxidative and anti-inflammatory mechanisms. *Front. Pharmacol.* **2018**, *9*, 662. [CrossRef]
120. Wang, L.; Yuan, D.; Zhang, D.; Zhang, W.; Liu, C.; Cheng, H.; Song, Y.; Tan, Q. Ginsenoside Re promotes nerve regeneration by facilitating the proliferation, differentiation and migration of Schwann Cells via the ERK- and JNK-dependent pathway in rat model of sciatic nerve crush injury. *Cell. Mol. Neurobiol.* **2015**, *35*, 827–840. [CrossRef]
121. Liu, M.; Bai, X.; Yu, S.; Zhao, W.; Qiao, J.; Liu, Y.; Zhao, D.; Wang, J.; Wang, S. Ginenoside Re inhibits ROS/ASK-1dependent mitochondrial apoptosis pathway and activation of Nrf2-antioxidant response in beta-amyloid challenged SH-SY5Y cells. *Molecules* **2019**, *24*, 2687. [CrossRef] [PubMed]
122. Lee, S.; Kim, M.G.; Ko, S.K.; Kim, H.K.; Leem, K.H.; Kim, Y.J. Protective effect of ginsenoside Re on acute gastric mucosal lesion induced b compound 48/80. *J. Ginseng Res.* **2014**, *38*, 8–96. [CrossRef] [PubMed]
123. Lee, R.; Lee, N.-E.; Hwang, H.; Rhim, H.; Cho, I.-H.; Nah, S.-Y. Ginseng gintonin enhances hyaluronic acid and collagen release from human dermal fibroblasts through lysophosphatidic acid receptor interaction. *Molecules* **2019**, *24*, 4438. [CrossRef] [PubMed]
124. Lee, A.E.; Park, S.D.; Hwang, H.; Choi, S.H.; Lee, R.M.; Nam, S.M.; Choi, J.H.; Rhim, H.; Cho, I.H.; Kim, H.C.; et al. Effects of a gintonin-enriched fraction on hair growth: An in vitro and in vivo study. *J. Ginseng Res.* **2020**, *44*, 168–177. [CrossRef]
125. Kim, H.J.; Kim, J.Y.; Lee, B.H.; Choi, S.H.; Rhim, H.; Kim, H.C.; Ahn, S.Y.; Jeong, S.W.; Jang, M.; Cho, I.H.; et al. Gintonin, an exogenous ginseng-derived LPA receptor ligand, promotes corneal wound healing. *J. Vet. Sci.* **2017**, *18*, 387–397. [CrossRef]
126. Kim, D.G.; Jang, M.; Choi, S.H.; Kim, H.J.; Jhun, H.; Kim, H.C.; Rhim, H.; Cho, I.H.; Nah, S.Y. Gintonin, a ginseng-derived exogenous lysophosphatidic acid receptor ligand, enhances blood-brain barrier permeability and brain delivery. *Int. J. Biol. Macromol.* **2018**, *114*, 1325–1337. [CrossRef]
127. Hwang, S.H.; Lee, B.H.; Choi, S.H.; Kim, H.J.; Won, K.J.; Lee, H.M.; Rhim, H.; Kim, H.C.; Nah, S.Y. Effects of gintonin on the proliferation, migration, and tube formation of human umbilical-vein endothelial cells: Involvement of lysophosphatidic acid receptors and vascular endothelial growth factor signaling. *J. Ginseng Res.* **2016**, *40*, 325–333. [CrossRef]
128. Choi, S.H.; Kim, H.J.; Cho, H.J.; Park, S.D.; Lee, N.E.; Hwang, S.H.; Cho, I.H.; Hwang, H.; Rhim, H.; Kim, H.C.; et al. Gintonin, a ginseng-derived exogenous lysophophatidic acid receptor ligand, protects astrocytes from hypoxic and re-oxygenation stresses through stimulation of astrocytic glycogenolysis. *Mol. Neurobiol.* **2019**, *56*, 3280–3294. [CrossRef]
129. Kim, H.J.; Shin, E.J.; Lee, B.H.; Choi, S.H.; Jung, S.W.; Cho, I.K.; Hwang, S.H.; Kim, J.Y.; Han, J.S.; Chung, C.H.; et al. Oral administration of gintonin attenuates cholinergic impairments by scopolamine, amyloid-B protein, and mouse model of Alzheimer's Disease. *Mol. Cells* **2015**, *38*, 796–805. [CrossRef]
130. Calabrese, E.J. Alzheimer's Disease drugs: An application of the hormetic dose-response model. *Crit. Rev. Toxicol.* **2008**, *38*, 419–452. [CrossRef]
131. Kim, J.; Lee, H.; Kang, K.S.; Chun, K.H.; Hwang, G.S. Protective effect of Korean Red Ginseng against glucocorticoid-induced osteoporosis in vitro and in in vivo. *J. Ginseng Res.* **2015**, *39*, 46–53. [CrossRef] [PubMed]
132. Attele, A.S.; Wua, J.A.; Yuan, C.S. Ginseng pharmacology, multiple constituents and multiple actions. *Biochem. Pharmacol.* **1999**, *58*, 1685–1693. [CrossRef]
133. Lee, D.; Kang, K.S.; Yu, J.S.; Woo, J.Y.; Hwang, G.S.; Eom, D.W.; Baek, S.H.; Lee, H.L.; Kim, K.H.; Yamabe, N. Protective effect of Korean Red Ginseng against FK506-induced damage in LLC-PKI cells. *J. Ginseng Res.* **2017**, *41*, 284–289. [CrossRef] [PubMed]
134. Song, H.; Park, J.; Choi, K.O.; Lee, J.; Chen, J.; Park, H.J.; Yu, B.I.; Iida, M.; Rhyu, M.R.; Lee, Y.J. Ginsenoside Rf inhibits cyclooxygenase-2 induction via peroxisome proliferator-activated receptor gamma in A549 cells. *J. Ginseng Res.* **2019**, *43*, 319–325. [CrossRef]
135. Hisamura, F.; Kojima-Yuasa, A.; Kennedy, D.O.; Matsui-Yuasa, I. Protective effect of green tea extract and tea polyphenols against FK506-induced cytotoxicity in renal cells. *Pharmacol. Toxicol.* **2006**, *98*, 192–196. [CrossRef]

136. Hisamura, F.; Kojima-Yuasa, A.; Huang, X.D.; Kennedy, D.O.; Opare, D.; Matsui-Yuasa, I. Synergistic effect of green tea polyphenols on their protection against FK506-induced cytotoxicity in renal cells. *Am. J. Chin. Med.* **2008**, *36*, 615–624. [CrossRef]
137. Yokozawa, T.; Oura, H.; Sakanaka, S.; Ishigaki, S.; Kim, M. Depressor effect of tannin in green tea on rats with renal hypertension. *Biosci. Biotechnol. Biochem.* **1994**, *58*, 855–858. [CrossRef]
138. Yokozawa, T.; Chung, H.Y.; Lin, A.H.; Oura, H. Effectiveness of green tea tannin on rats with chronic renal failure. *Biosci. Biotechnol. Biochem.* **1996**, *60*, 1000–1005. [CrossRef]
139. Yokozawa, T.; Dong, E.; Oura, H.; Nonoka, G.; Nishioka, I. Magnesium lithospermate B ameliorates cisplatin-induced injury in cultured renal epithelial cells. *Exp. Toxicol. Pathol* **1997**, *49*, 343–346. [CrossRef]
140. Yokozawa, T.; Cho, E.J.; Nakagawa, T. Influence of green tea polyphenols tea tannin on rats with chronic renal failure. *J. Agric. Food Chem.* **2003**, *51*, 2424–2425. [CrossRef]
141. Lee, Y.K.; Chin, Y.W.; Choi, Y.H. Effects of Korean red ginseng extract on acute renal failure induced by gentamicin and pharmacokinetic changes by metformin in rats. *Food Chem. Toxicol.* **2013**, *59*, 153–159. [CrossRef] [PubMed]
142. Shin, H.S.; Yu, M.; Kim, M.; Choi, H.S.; Kang, D.H. Renoprotective effect of red ginseng in gentamicin-induced acute kidney injury. *Lab. Investig.* **2014**, *94*, 1147–1160. [CrossRef] [PubMed]
143. Doh, K.C.; Lim, S.W.; Piao, S.G.; Jin, L.; Heo, S.B.; Zheng, Y.F.; Bae, S.K.; Hwang, C.H.; Min, K.I.; Chung, B.H.; et al. Ginseng treatment attenuates chronic cyclosporine nephropathy via reducing oxidative stress in an experimental mouse model. *Am. J. Nephrol.* **2013**, *37*, 421–433. [CrossRef]
144. Zhang, Y.; Chi, X.; Wang, Z.; Bi, S.; Wang, Y.; Shi, F.; Hu, S.; Wang, H. Protective effects of *Panax notoginseng* saponins on PME-induced nephrotoxicity in mice. *Biomed. Pharmacother.* **2019**, *116*, 108970. [CrossRef] [PubMed]
145. Petkov, V. Effect of ginseng on the brain biogenic monoamines and 3',5'-AMP system. *Arzneim. Forsch./Drug Res.* **1978**, *28*, 388–393.
146. Petkov, V.D.; Mosharrof, A.H. Effects of standardized ginseng extract on learning, memory and physical capabilities. *Am. J. Chin. Med.* **1987**, *15*, 19–29. [CrossRef]
147. Yu, S.H.; Huang, H.Y.; Korivi, M.; Hsu, M.F.; Huang, C.Y.; Hou, C.W.; Chen, C.Y.; Kao, C.L.; Lee, R.P.; Lee, S.D.; et al. Oral Rg1 supplementation strengthens antioxidant defense system against exercise-induced oxidative stress in rat skeletal muscles. *J. Int. Soc. Sports Nutr.* **2012**, *9*, 23. [CrossRef]
148. Hui, J.; Gao, J.; Wang, Y., Zhang, J.; Han, Y.M.; Wei, L.; Wu, J. *Panax notoginseng* saponins ameliorates experimental hepatic fibrosis and hepatic stellae cell proliferation by inhibiting the Jak2.State3 pathways. *J. Tradit. Chin. Med.* **2016**, *36*, 217–224. [CrossRef]
149. Zhou, L.; Zhou, C.; Feng, Z.; Liu, Z.; Ahu, H.; Zhou, X. Triptolide-induced hepatotoxicity can be alleviated when combined with *Panax notoginseng* saponins and Catapol. *J. Ethnopharmacol.* **2018**, *214*, 232–329. [CrossRef]
150. Ding, R.B.; Tian, K.; Cao, Y.W.; Bao, J.L.; Wang, M.; He, C.; Hu, Y.; Su, H.; Wan, J.B. Protective effect of *Panax notoginseng* saponins on acute ethanol-induced liver injury is associated with ameliorating hepatic lipid accumulation and reducing ethanol-mediated oxidative stress. *J. Agric. Food Chem.* **2015**, *63*, 2413–2422. [CrossRef]
151. Zhong, H.; Wu, H.; Bai, H.; Wang, M.; Wen, J.; Gong, J.; Miao, M.; Yuan, F. *Panax notoginseng* saponins promote liver regeneration through activation of the P13/AKTmTOR cell proliferation pathway and upregulation of the AKT/BAD cell survival pathway in mice. *BMC Complement. Altern. Med.* **2019**, *19*, 22. [CrossRef] [PubMed]
152. Calabrese, E.J.; Blain, R.B. The occurrence of hormestic dose responses in the toxicological literature. The hormesis database: An overview. *Toxicol. Appl. Pharmacol.* **2005**, *202*, 289–301. [CrossRef] [PubMed]
153. Xie, W.; Zhou, P.; Sun, Y.; Meng, X.; Dai, Z.; Sun, G.; Sun, X. Protective effects and target network analysis of Ginsenoside Rg1 in cerebral ischemia and reperfusion injury: A comprehensive overview of experimental studies. *Cells* **2018**, *7*, 270. [CrossRef] [PubMed]
154. Calabrese, E.J.; Blain, R.B. Hormesis and plant biology. *Environ. Pollut.* **2009**, *157*, 42–48. [CrossRef] [PubMed]
155. Qi, L.W.; Wang, C.Z.; Yuan, C.S. Isolation and analysis of ginseng: Advances and challenges. *Nat. Prod. Rep.* **2011**, *28*, 467–495. [CrossRef] [PubMed]
156. Peng, D.; Wang, H.; Qu, C.; Xie, L.; Wicks, S.M.; Xie, J. Ginsenoside Re: Its chemistry, metabolism and pharmacokinetics. *Chin. Med.* **2012**, *7*. [CrossRef] [PubMed]

157. Li, J.; Dai, Y.-L.; Zheng, F.; Xu, C.-E.; Feng, L.; Wang, X.-Y.; Zheng, B.-S.; Yu, S.-S. Oral absorption and in vivo biotransformation of ginsenosides. *Chin. J. Biol.* **2014**, *27*, 1633–1636.
158. Yu, S.E.; Mwesige, B.; Yi, Y.S.; Yoo, B.C. Ginsenosides: The need to move forward from bench to clinical trials. *J. Ginseng Res.* **2019**, *43*, 361–367.
159. Ki, S.H.; Yang, J.H.; Ku, S.K.; Kim, S.C.; Kim, S.C.; Kim, Y.W.; Cho, I.J. Red ginseng extract protects against carbon tetrachloride-induced liver fibrosis. *J. Ginseng Res.* **2013**, *37*, 45–53. [CrossRef]
160. Hou, J.; Xue, J.; Lee, M.; Yu, J.; Sung, C. Long-term administration of ginsenoside Rh1 enhances learning and memory b promoting cell survival in the mouse hippocampus. *Int. J. Mol. Med.* **2014**, *33*, 234–240. [CrossRef]
161. Fu, Y.; Ji, L.L. Chronic ginseng consumption attenuates age-associated oxidative stress in rats. *J. Nutr.* **2003**, *133*, 3603–3609. [CrossRef] [PubMed]
162. Jeong, H.J.; So, H.K.; Jo, A.; Kim, H.B.; Lee, S.J.; Bae, G.U.; Kang, J.S. Ginsenoside Rg1 augments oxidative metabolism and anabolic response to skeletal muscle in mice. *J. Ginseng Res.* **2019**, *43*, 475–481. [CrossRef] [PubMed]
163. Luo, P.; Dong, G.; Liu, L.; Zhou, H. The long-term consumption of ginseng extract reduces the susceptibility of intermediate-aged heart to acute ischemia reperfusion injury. *PLoS ONE* **2015**, *10*, e0144733. [CrossRef] [PubMed]

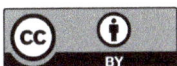

© 2020 by the author. Licensee MDPI, Basel, Switzerland. This article is an open access article distributed under the terms and conditions of the Creative Commons Attribution (CC BY) license (http://creativecommons.org/licenses/by/4.0/).

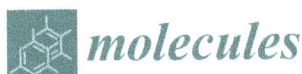

Review

Therapeutic Emergence of Rhein as a Potential Anticancer Drug: A Review of Its Molecular Targets and Anticancer Properties

Sahu Henamayee [1], Kishore Banik [1], Bethsebie Lalduhsaki Sailo [1], Bano Shabnam [1], Choudhary Harsha [1], Satti Srilakshmi [2], Naidu VGM [2], Seung Ho Baek [3], Kwang Seok Ahn [4,*] and Ajaikumar B Kunnumakkara [1,*]

1. Cancer Biology Laboratory and DBT-AIST International Laboratory for Advanced Biomedicine (DAILAB), Department of Biosciences and Bioengineering, Indian Institute of Technology (IIT) Guwahati, Assam 781039, India; henamayeesahu@yahoo.com (S.H.); kishore.banik@iitg.ac.in (K.B.); b.sailo@iitg.ac.in (B.L.S.); bano176106104@iitg.ac.in (B.S.); harsha.choudhary@iitg.ac.in (C.H.)
2. Department of Pharmacology & Toxicology, National Institute of Pharmaceutical Education and Research (NIPER, Guwahati), Assam 781125, India; srilakshmisatthi@gmail.com (S.S.); vgmnaidu@gmail.com (N.V.)
3. College of Korean Medicine, Dongguk University, 32 Dongguk-ro, Ilsandong-gu, Goyang-si, Gyeonggi-do 10326, Korea; baekone99@gmail.com
4. Department of Science in Korean Medicine, Kyung Hee University, 24 Kyungheedae-ro, Dongdaemun-gu, Seoul 02447, Korea
* Correspondence: ksahn@khu.ac.kr (K.S.A.); kunnumakkara@iitg.ac.in or ajai78@gmail.com (A.B.K.); Tel.: +82-2-961-2316 (K.S.A.)

Academic Editors: Sokcheon Pak and Soo Liang Ooi
Received: 7 April 2020; Accepted: 7 May 2020; Published: 12 May 2020

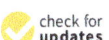

Abstract: According to the World Health Organization (WHO), cancer is the second-highest cause of mortality in the world, and it kills nearly 9.6 million people annually. Besides the fatality of the disease, poor prognosis, cost of conventional therapies, and associated side-effects add more burden to patients, post-diagnosis. Therefore, the search for alternatives for the treatment of cancer that are safe, multi-targeted, effective, and cost-effective has compelled us to go back to ancient systems of medicine. Natural herbs and plant formulations are laden with a variety of phytochemicals. One such compound is rhein, which is an anthraquinone derived from the roots of *Rheum* spp. and *Polygonum multiflorum*. In ethnomedicine, these plants are used for the treatment of inflammation, osteoarthritis, diabetes, and bacterial and helminthic infections. Increasing evidence suggests that this compound can suppress breast cancer, cervical cancer, colon cancer, lung cancer, ovarian cancer, etc. in both in vitro and in vivo settings. Recent studies have reported that this compound modulates different signaling cascades in cancer cells and can prevent angiogenesis and progression of different types of cancers. The present review highlights the cancer-preventing and therapeutic properties of rhein based on the available literature, which will help to extend further research to establish the chemoprotective and therapeutic roles of rhein compared to other conventional drugs. Future pharmacokinetic and toxicological studies could support this compound as an effective anticancer agent.

Keywords: rhein; cancer; phytochemical; molecular targets; chemoprevention; chemotherapy

1. Introduction

Cancer is the second leading cause of death globally, killing around 9.6 million people annually [1]. Despite the significant advances in the field of cancer therapy, major limitations such as drug inefficacy, drug resistance, distant metastasis, associated side-effects, and toxicity hinder the use of chemotherapeutic approaches [2–9]. Therefore, there is an urgent need to discover novel therapeutic agents, as the number of cancer-related deaths will increase dramatically in the coming years [1]. It is now evident that naturally derived bioactives have been a boon to human civilization since time immemorial. The Ayurveda, the Chinese Pharmacopoeia (2005), Unani and other Indian systems of medicine demonstrate the importance of these multi-targeted phytochemicals for the prevention and treatment of different diseases in humans [10,11]. Besides, there is also evidence that our daily diet has a significant protective role, guarding us against oxidative stress and various disorders [12–22]. It is well established that natural compounds rich in antioxidants can activate different survival pathways and protect normal cells from the adverse effects of anticancer therapies [23,24]. Additionally, many of these dietary ingredients are known to directly or indirectly increase the actions of many chemotherapeutic drugs, which in turn enhances their therapeutic potential, as evident from many preclinical and clinical studies [25–32]. Again, the chemoprotective and chemosensitizing effects of natural products have widened the research arena to include compounds beyond conventional anticancer drugs [33–38]. One such compound is rhein, a naturally derived aglycone from rhubarb leaves. Traditional practices show that the rhubarb plant (*Rheum officinale*) was widely prescribed due to its anticathartic and antistomachic properties. Its therapeutic potential also includes antibacterial, antidiabetic, antiinflammatory and anticancer activities [39–44]. Additionally, one of the metabolic precursors of rhein, diacerein, has shown significant results in easing pain and improving matrix synthesis in the treatment of osteoarthritis [45]. A large number of preclinical studies have demonstrated the anticancer activities of rhein against breast cancer, cervical cancer, nasopharyngeal cancer, tongue cancer, pancreatic cancer, ovarian cancer, and hepatocellular carcinoma, in addition to its pro-apoptotic, antiproliferative, and antiangiogenic properties [46–57]. In addition, preclinical studies have shown that as an antineoplastic compound, rhein potentiated the cytotoxic effect of chemotherapeutic drugs, minimized side-effects, enhanced tolerability, and reduced multidrug resistance [57]. Although this anthraquinone glycoside has a broad spectrum of therapeutic potential, it shows poor systemic ability and remains unexplored due to its highly hydrophobic structure [58]. However, there are formulations that can overcome these issues [59–61]. The broad aim of this article was to provide an overall framework describing the nature, chemistry, ethnopharmacological uses, biological activities, molecular targets, and the chemoprotective, chemopreventive and therapeutic potential of rhein in different cancers.

2. Rhein in Nature

Nature offers many safe, effective, and affordable curatives for many chronic ailments, which are mainly obtained from plants. These phytochemicals are extracted from different parts of plants and many act as dietary supplements and have significant health benefits [62–64]. The compound rhein which has shown many medicinal properties, is one of the major phytochemical components of plants like *Aloe barbadensis* (Family Asphodelaceae), *Rheum* spp., *Polygonum multiflorum*, *P. cuspidatum* (Family Polygonaceae), *Cassia occidentalis* (Family Fabaceae), etc., as described later [65,66]. Various sources of rhein are depicted in Figure 1. Studies have shown that the Chinese medicine Da Huang or Chinese rhubarb, used for treating inflammation in humans, is composed of three different *Rheum* species, i.e., *R. palmatum* L., *R. tanguticum*, and *R. officinale*, all of which contain rhein [67].

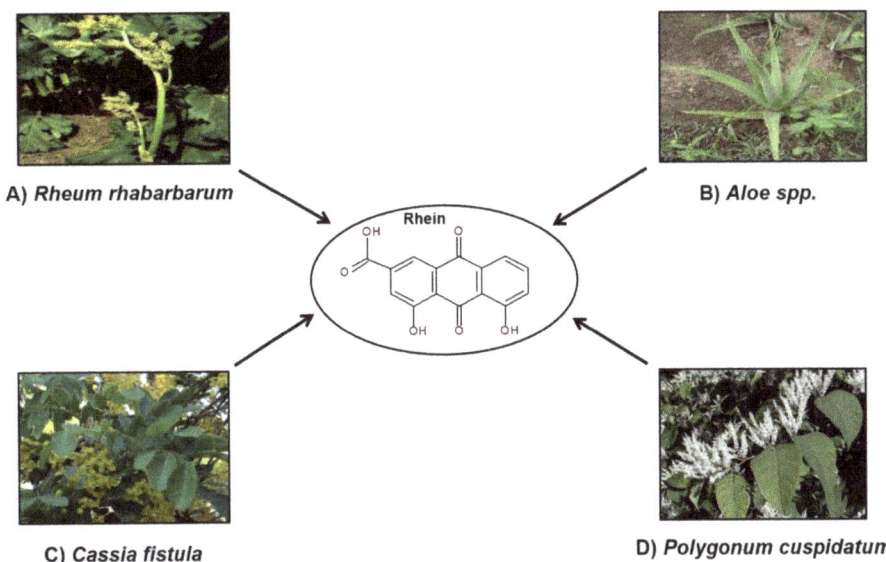

Figure 1. Sources of rhein: (**A**) *Rheum rhabarbarum* (Kay Yatskievych/ www.discoverlife.org); (**B**) *Aloe spp.* (Pankaj Oudhia/ www.discoverlife.org); (**C**) *Cassia fistula* (John Pickering/ www.discoverlife.org); (**D**) *Polygonum cuspidatum* (Les Mehrhoff/ www.discoverlife.org).

The foliar parts of cultivated species of *Rheum* are usually edible [68]. Potential larvicidal and anticancerous activities were observed in isolates of rhein from extracts of yellow *Cassia fistula* flowers [69,70].

3. Ethnopharmacological Uses of Plants Containing Rhein

Plants containing rhein have been used in different systems of traditional medicine for the prevention and treatment of different diseases. The 1000-year-old Chinese Pharmacopoeia suggests the use of the Rhei Rhizoma or rhubarb components as a laxative because they stimulate the secretion of bile into the intestines and support the expulsion of toxic waste matter. In addition, the components of rhubarb are also involved in hepatoprotection and antibacterial activity [71,72]. The Chinese Pharmacopoeia (1997) suggests a potential use of the herb *P. multiflorum* for blood cleansing and improving blood circulation [73]. The root extracts of this plant, popularly known as Heshouwu in China, are used for their antiobesity properties [74]. The use of the herb *P. multiflorum* was cited in the literature of the Tang dynasty and the Song dynasty and the 2010 edition of the Chinese Pharmacopoeia. Its formulation with other herbs reduces its toxicity and acts over several human health disorders. There have been 242 patented formulations of the plant *P. multiflorum* with other herbs such as *Radix rehmanniae*, *R. astragalus*, *R. ophiopogonis*, *Salviae miltiorrhizae*, and *Angelica sinensis*, all with different pharmacological properties. The associated studies demonstrated that combining *P. multiflorum* with other herbs enhanced its beneficial effects on human health, such as longer serum retention of its bioactive compounds and decreased toxicity [75]. In a clinical study on 312 patients, the alcoholic extracts of rhubarb showed a significant effect in the treatment of gastric and duodenal ulcer bleeding [76]. Another traditional Chinese medicine, San-Huang-Xie-Xin-Tang (SHXXT), composed of three herbs, Radix et Rhizoma Rhei (*Rheum palmatum* L.), Radix scutellaria (*Scutellaria baicalensis* Georgi), and Rhizoma coptidis (*Coptis chinensis* Franch), was shown to be involved in attenuating inflammation of the airways, colon, and blood vessels [77]. The Banxia Xiexin Decoction (BXD), one of its active components being rhein, is prescribed to ease various inflammatory disorders like gastritis and upper airway inflammation [78]. The BXD was also effective in curing colon cancer in animals [79].

Additionally, studies demonstrated that the combination of cisplatin and the BXD decoction induced apoptosis in A549 human lung cancer cells [80]. A decoction of the herbs *Rheum palmatum* L., *Artemisia annua* L., and *Gardenia jasminoides* Ellis, popularly known as Yin-Chen-Hao-Tang (YCHT), is primarily used to treat several liver disorders. Pharmacokinetic studies have shown that the compounds rhein, geniposide and 6,7-dimethylesculetin, isolated from YCHT, enhanced the synergistic and therapeutic benefits, as demonstrated in animal models [81].

The Indian system of medicine Ayurveda suggests the use of *R. australe* (one of the sources of rhein), commonly found in the Himalayas, for curing multiple chronic diseases, including cancers of liver, breast and prostate [65]. The rhizomes of another species of *Rheum*, *R. emodi* showed antihelminthic, antiulcerative and anticancerous activities [82]. Its extract was also reported to be effective in curing *Helicobacter-pylori*-induced ulcers in animals [72]. Recent reports have demonstrated the antiinflammatory activity of anthraquinones found in *Cassia sp.* in the treatment of airway-associated allergies [83].

4. Chemistry of Rhein

The rhein molecule, or 4,5-dihydroxy-9,10-dioxoanthracene-2-carboxylic acid, is a planar compound with three fused benzene rings, has a molecular mass of 283.22 g/mol and the molecular formula $C_{15}H_8O_6$ [84]. It is also popularly known as Rhubarb Yellow. Rhein is found in its free form or as glucosides in the Fabaceae and Polygonaceae family of plants [85]. This compound is water-insoluble, meaning it has low systemic bioavailability. However, the lipophilic nature of this compound permits it to easily get into cells [86]. As this compound has a highly stable structure, various hydrophilic and lipophilic nano-formulations have been developed to improve its oral absorption, bioavailability, and sustained targeted release [59]. A conjugate of rhein, rhein–DOTA (1,4,7,10-tetraazacyclododecane-1,4,7,10-tetraacetic acid) has been used to treat sarcoma and owing to its remarkable necrosis avidity; studies suggest that it could be used as a significant probe for PET/CT-imaging-mediated early detection of response to antitumor therapy [87].

The plasma concentration of rhein has also been compared with other anthraquinones found in traditional Chinese medicine, such as Rhei Rhizoma (used for treating various neuroinflammatory disorders and osteoarthritis) [88,89]. It was observed that there was a significant increase in serum concentrations of rhein, 12 hours after oral administration of Rhei Rhizoma, where the peak serum concentration was reported to be 126.50 ng/mL, which is comparably higher than rhein alone [90].

5. Biological Activities of Rhein

Rhein has been actively explored for its pharmacological benefits to human health. Many biological properties of rhein have been studied, such as curing inflammatory disorders like upper airway inflammation, asthma, gastritis, and fatty liver and protecting against cerebral ischemic injury, diabetic nephropathy, etc. [42,78,79,91,92]. Several studies have shown that rhein is an effective antidiabetic, antiosteoarthritic and anticathartic agent [39,40,44,45,60]. The antibacterial properties of rhein have been observed in the rhizomes of rhubarb (*R. officinale*) [93]. Some other studies have demonstrated that rhein has a higher antioxidative potential than another anthroquinone component of *P. multiflorum*, aloe-emodin. In addition, the chemiluminescent data for the free-radical-scavenging activity of rhein suggested that it is more effective than antioxidants like α-tocopherol and Vitamin C [94]. Rhein, and its derivatives and analogs, are known to show the anticancer activity against various cancers, as shown in Figure 2 and Table 1, which is of paramount interest.

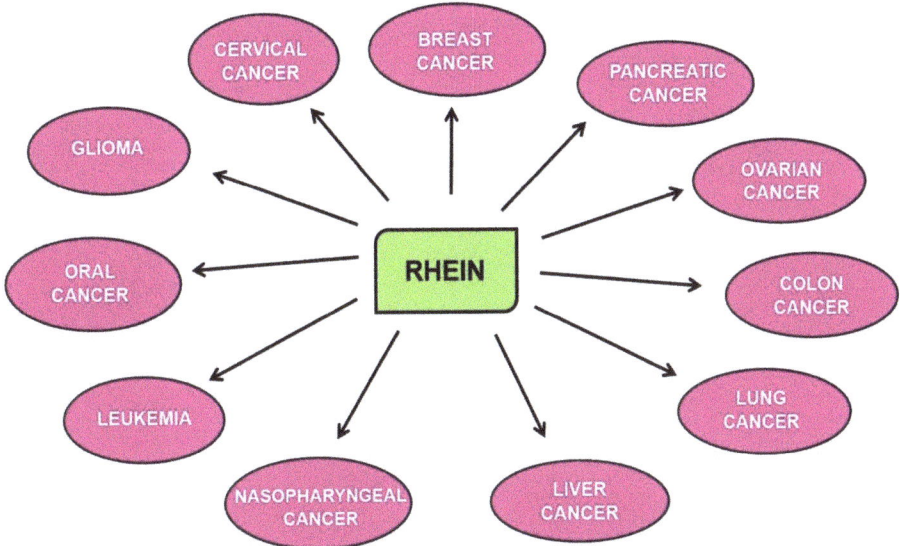

Figure 2. Anticancer activity of rhein in different cancers.

6. Molecular Targets of Rhein

Increasing lines of evidence suggest the anticancer activity of rhein against different cancers, as depicted in Figure 2 [43,46,54]. Rhein has been shown to inhibit the distinct hallmarks of cancer, including cell proliferation, angiogenesis, migration, epithelial to mesenchymal transition (EMT), etc. These cellular processes are regulated via the modulation of several cellular molecules such as enzymes, transcription factors, kinases, cell-cycle proteins, growth factors, oncoproteins, tumor suppressor proteins, apoptotic proteins, etc., as shown in Figure 3 [52–56]. Many important molecular pathways or proteins regulating the survival of cancerous cells are targets of rhein, including the sonic hedgehog pathway, serine-threonine kinases like Akt kinase, etc. [46]. Rhein is also known to exert its anti-inflammatory effect by modulation of nuclear factor—kappa light chain enhancer of activated B cells (NF-κB), which subsequently regulates the downstream nitric oxide synthase pathway [95]. The other important nuclear targets of this phytochemical include p53 and p21/WAF proteins, which aid in the induction of apoptosis [96]. The rhein-induced mitochondrial apoptotic pathway is activated by increased levels of Fas, cleaved caspases-3, -8, -9, poly(ADP-ribose) polymerase (PARP), etc. and decreased expression of B cell lymphoma 2 (Bcl-2), cyclin A and cyclin-dependant kinases (CDK) [97]. The antitumorigenic effects of this compound in ovarian cancer cells is exerted through inhibition of the phosphorylation of mitogen-activated protein kinase (MAPK) pathway elements like mitogen-activated protein kinase kinase (MEK) and extracellular-signal-regulated kinase (ERK) [47]. Under hypoxic conditions, rhein has also been shown to enhance cytotoxicity in colorectal cancer cells (CRC) by modulating the expression of hypoxia-inducible factor-1 alpha (HIF-1α) expression, which acts on immunosuppressive molecules such as the downstream elements programmed cell death ligand-1 (PD-L1), vascular endothelial growth factor (VEGF), cyclooxygenase 2 (COX-2) and galectin-1 [98]. The different pathways modulated by rhein are discussed below.

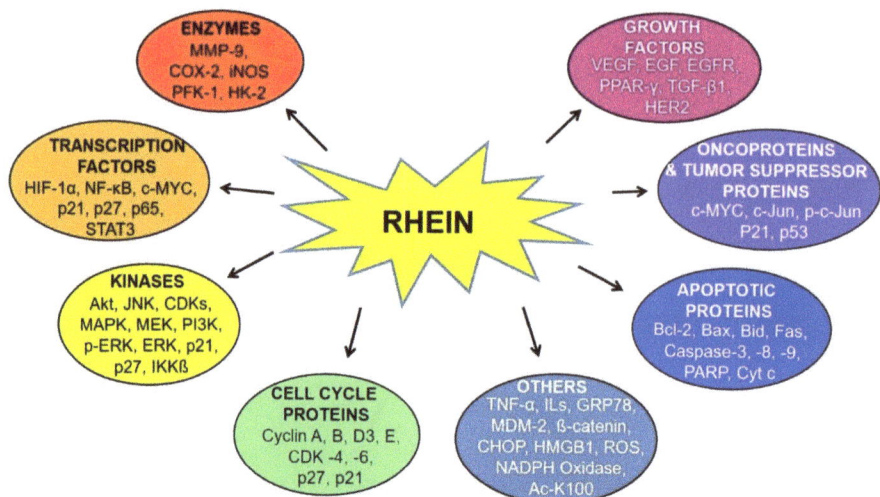

Figure 3. Molecular targets of rhein. Abbreviations: Ac-K100: acetylated lysine; Bax: Bcl-2-associated X protein; Bcl-2: B cell lymphoma 2; Bid: BH3 interacting domain death agonist; CDK: cyclin-dependent kinase; CHOP: CCAAT/enhancer-binding protein homologous protein; COX-2: cyclooxygenase 2; Cyt c: cytochrome c; EGF: extracellular growth factor; Fas: FS-7-associated surface antigen; GRP78: 78 kDa glucose regulated protein; HER-2: human epidermal growth factor receptor 2; HIF-1α: hypoxia-inducible factor 1 alpha; HK-2: hexokinase 2; HMGB1: high-mobility-group-box-1; IKKβ: inhibitor of nuclear factor kappa-B kinase subunit beta; IL: interleukin; iNOS: inducible nitric oxide synthase; JNK: c-Jun N-terminal kinase; MAPK: mitogen-activated protein kinase; MDM2: murine double minute-2; MEK: mitogen-activated protein kinase kinase; MMP-9: Matrix metalloproteinase-9; NADPH: nicotinamide adenine dinucleotide phosphate; NF-κB: nuclear factor kappa light chain enhancer of activated B cells; PARP: poly ADP ribose polymerase; p-c-Jun: phosphorylated c-Jun; pERK: phosphorylated extracellular signal-regulated kinase; PFK-1: phosphofructokinase-1; PI3K: phosphoinositide 3-kinase; PPAR-γ: peroxisome proliferator-activated receptor gamma; ROS: reactive oxygen species; STAT3: signal transducer and activator of transcription 3; TGF-β1: transforming growth factor beta 1; TNF-α: tumor necrosis factor alpha and VEGF: vascular endothelial growth factor.

6.1. MAPK Signaling Pathway

The MAPK signaling pathway plays a vital role in cell proliferation and survival. These molecules influence the group of responsive enzymes recruited to deal with cellular stress caused by heat, osmosis, cytokines and ultraviolet (UV) irradiation [99]. The MAPK family of proteins are also involved in the generation of mitogenic responses and the production of stress response proteins in different cells of the body. The three major MAPK families are ERKs, Jun amino-terminal kinases (JNKs) and stress-activated protein kinases (p38/SAPKs) [100–104]. A recent study showed that HeLa cervical cancer cells underwent apoptosis upon modulation of the MAPK pathway by rhein. It was demonstrated that due to the binding of rhein lysinate (RHL or a salt of rhein and lysine), the phosphorylation of ERK1/2, JNK and p38 MAPK was enhanced, which activated growth-inhibitory pathways including the regulation of apoptotic proteins like increased levels of cleaved caspase-3/7 and PARP [48].

6.2. Wnt Signaling Pathway

As discussed earlier, rhein can inhibit cell proliferation in various cancer cells by targeting β-catenin, PI3K/Akt, ERK, p38 MAPK, JNK and fat mass and obesity-associated genes (FTO). Cyclin D1, one of the major cell-cycle mediator proteins, is overexpressed in the cancer cells due to the increased β-catenin levels. Thus, there is a crucial role of β-catenin, a component of the Wnt signaling pathway, in activating the genes for growth regulation involving cellular survival, proliferation and metastasis [105–109]. It was shown that rhein induced cell-cycle arrest at the G0/G1 and S phases in A549 lung cancer cells and BEL-7402 hepatocellular cancer cells, respectively [54,110]. It was demonstrated that rhein induced apoptosis in A549 cells due to the enhanced levels of GRP78 and reduced CDK-4, -6 and cyclin E (some of the molecular components of the Wnt pathway) [110]. Studies also showed that rhein suppressed the active levels of β-catenin in HepG2 human liver cancer cells and HeLa cervical cancer cells, which resulted in a cell-cycle arrest at the S phase [111]. Similarly, rhein induced cell-cycle arrest at the S-phase in BEL-7402 cells. The suppression of c-Myc, a target of the Wnt/β-catenin pathway, and the induction of caspase-3 by rhein suppressed the proliferation and survival of these cells [54].

6.3. NF-κB Signaling Pathway

One of the most rapid-acting transcription factors mediating inflammatory processes is nuclear factor-kappa B (NF-κB) [112–117]. It is kept inactive in the cell by the binding of IκB. Harmful stimuli like stress, UV, bacterial or viral antigens, cytokines, or free radicals, reactive oxygen species (ROS) cause IκB kinases to phosphorylate the IκB protein that translocates NF-κB to the nucleus for the transcription of different genes involved in inflammation and cancer. Therefore, active NF-κB leads to stimulation of an inflammatory response or immune response and promotes cell survival and cell proliferation [118–124]. Thus, putting a check on the activation of NF-κB and its accessory pathways can lead to the suppression of inflammation, angiogenesis, and carcinogenesis [62,125–133]. Studies have defined the role of many natural inhibitors of NF-κB that are obtained from the diet, which reduce inflammation and restore energy balance in humans [29,134]. This safe, well-tolerated natural compound was shown to inhibit LPS-induced NF-κB activation and regulatory pathways in RAW 264.7 macrophages by inhibiting the protein, inhibitor of nuclear factor kappa-B kinase subunit beta (IKKβ). It was also observed that rhein induced an antiinflammatory effect by modulating the expression of NF-κB and its downstream elements such as intracellular ROS, inducible nitric oxide synthase (iNOS), interleukin (IL)-6, and pro-inflammatory factors like IL-1β and high-mobility-group-box-1 (HMGB1) [135].

6.4. HIF-1 Signaling Pathway

Studies on the exposure of tumor cells to hypoxic conditions have shown enhanced levels of COX-2, PD-L1, IL-10, VEGF, galectin-1, and transforming growth factor-β1 (TGF-β1) [136]. These immunosuppressing molecules stop immune cell differentiation, drive apoptosis of T cells, and inhibit the development of dendritic cells. The transcription of these immunosuppressive molecules is driven by HIF-1α, which is produced due to hypoxia in tumor cells [137]. In a recent study involving breast cancer cells MCF-7 and MDA-MB-435, rhein was reported to play an important role in reducing tumor growth and vasculogenesis by inhibiting the expression of HIF-1α. The effect of rhein was also observed in hypoxia-induced angiogenesis in these cells, where HIF-1α and VEGF levels were reduced [138].

6.5. Other Signaling Pathways Regulated by Rhein

Matrix metalloproteinases (MMPs), a family of zinc proteases, help cancer cells to invade by degrading the extracellular matrix and the basal membrane [139]. They disrupt the structure of healthy tissues and thereby enhance disease progression. The MAPK family of proteins are modulated by ROS-mediated MMP activation to help in the invasion of tumors [2]. Gastric cancer cells have increased expression of upstream regulators NF-κB and activator protein (AP)-1 that direct the MMP gene activity. Studies have shown that rhein may act by suppressing JNK1/2 or p38 to modulate MMP through AP-1 expression [53]. Ser/Thr–Pro regulated protein phosphorylation is involved in epithelial cell proliferation and transformation [140]. The Pin1-driven Ser/Thr–Pro can activate oncoproteins like NF-κB and AP-1 and also destabilize tumor-suppressor genes like p53 by phosphorylation of Ser/Thr–Pro. Thus, the regulation of these proteins by rhein can provide a therapeutic target to kill cancer cells. It has been shown that the suppression of Pin1 in cancer cells leads to apoptosis or suppression of expression of the onco-proteins [141]. Studies have shown that rhein also targets the formation of the Pin1/c-Jun complex, which is an essential regulator of the cyclin D1 gene in the G2/M phase of cell-cycle progression. The disruption of pc-Jun (Ser73) and Pin1 bond was induced by rhein, which ultimately led to the cell cycle arrest in G2/M phase [142].

The pathways that induce cell death by apoptosis include two regulatory pathways. One pathway involves death-receptor-mediated caspase-8 activation, which can stimulate downstream caspase-3. Another pathway that induces apoptosis is mitochondria-mediated. The release of cytochrome c (Cyt c) from mitochondria leads to the activation of procaspase-9, which initiates an apoptosis-symbolic apoptosome formation composed of dATP (deoxyadenosine triphosphate), Apaf-1, procaspase-9 and Cyt c [143]. Apoptosome formation causes the activation of caspase-3, -6 and -7. Several studies have shown that rhein increases intracellular levels of nitric oxide, ROS, and Ca^{2+}, stimulates apoptosis, and inhibits cell proliferation and angiogenesis both in vitro and in vivo [143]. Bim, a pro-apoptotic Bcl-2-family protein, is a critical mediator of rhein-induced apoptosis. Rhein activated forkhead box O3a (FOXO3a), an inducer of Bim expression, in MCF-7 and HepG2 cells, which in turn enhanced the Bim protein levels [144]. Elevated levels of ROS modulated apoptosis by affecting the mitochondrial membrane permeability (MMPE) and causing subsequent loss of membrane potential ($\Delta\Psi m$) [43]. Some other studies have shown the role of MMPE in apoptosis induction, triggering the release of Cyt c [145]. Therefore, studies have demonstrated the apoptotic effect of rhein via modulation of ROS, MMPE, and caspases-3, -8, and -9, in SCC-4, A549 and HL-60 cancer cells [43,110,145].

Rhein, being a planar molecule, has a significant structural advantage of being easily intercalated into the DNA molecule. Thus, an increase in DNA length consequently disrupts gene function. Rhein induced the DNA damage in targeted cancerous cells by inducing the apoptotic pathways that led to cell-cycle arrest [43]. Thus, rhein is a multitargeted compound, and its plausible mechanism of action, as evidenced by several studies, is shown in Figure 4.

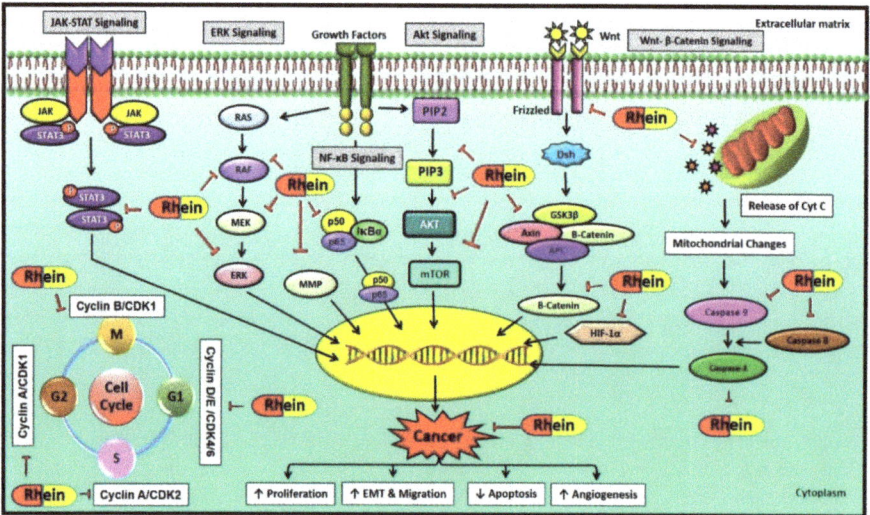

Figure 4. Mechanism of action of rhein. Abbreviations: APC: adenomatous polyposis coli; CDK: cyclin-dependent kinase; Dsh: dishevelled; EMT: epithelial to mesenchymal transition; ERK: extracellular signal-regulated kinase; GSK3β: glycogen synthase kinase 3β; HIF-1α: hypoxia-inducible factor 1 alpha; JAK: Janus kinase; MEK: mitogen-activated protein kinase kinase; MMP: matrix metalloproteinase; mTOR: mammalian target of rapamycin; NF-κB: nuclear factor kappa light chain enhancer of activated B cells; PIP2: phosphatidylinositol 4,5-bisphosphate; PIP3: phosphatidylinositol (3,4,5)-trisphosphate; and STAT: signal transducer and activator of transcription.

Table 1. Chemopreventive activity of rhein in different cancers.

Cancer	In Vitro/In Vivo /Ex Vivo	Model	Mechanism of Action	References
Breast cancer	In vivo	4T1 xenograft mice	Caspase-3, -8, -9↑, TNF-α↑, IL-6↑	[146]
	In vitro and in vivo	MCF-7, SK-Br-3, and MDA-MB-231 cells	p-EGFR↓, p-MEK↓, p-ERK↓	[46]
		MCF-7 injected BALB/c athymic mice		
	In vitro	SK-Br-3	p-HER-2↓, NF-κB↓, p53↑, p21↑	[147]
	In vitro	MCF-7	Cleaved caspase↑, p-Akt↓, FOXO3a↑, Bim↑	[144]
	In vitro	MCF-7, MDA-MB-435s	PI3K↓, p-Akt↓, p-ERK↓, NF-κB↓, HIF-1α↓, EGF↓	[138]
			Hsp90α↓, COX-2↓, HER-2↓, VEGF(165)↓, p-I-κB↓	
	In vitro	MDA-MB-231	Beclin-1↑, LC3-II/LC3-I↑, p62↓	[148]
Cervical cancer	In vitro	HeLa	MAPK↑, JNK↑, p-ERK↑,	[48]
			cleaved PARP↑, Caspase-3, -7↑	
	In vitro	HeLa	β-catenin↓, S phase arrest↑	[111]
	In vitro	CaSki	Cyt c↑, Caspase-3, -8, -9↑, Fas↑, p53↑, p21↑, Bcl-2↓,	[149]
			ΔΨm↓, cleaved Bid↑, cleaved PARP↑	
Colon cancer	In vitro	Caco-2	p-ERK1/2↑ (at higher concentrations of rhein)	[150]
	In vitro	HT29, HCT116, Colo205, SW620	HIF-1α↓, PD-L1↓, VEGF↓, COX-2↓, galectin-1↓	[98]
	In vitro	HCT116, SW620	p-STAT3↓	[151]
Glioma	In vitro	F98	ERK1/2↓	[152]
	In vitro	T98G, U87, U251	Ac-K100↑, NDRG1↑	[153]
Leukemia	In vivo	EU-1 injected SCID mice	MDM2↓, p53↑	[154]
	In vitro	HL-60	Cleaved caspase↑, cleaved PARP↑, cleaved Bid↑, ΔΨm↓	[145]
	In vitro	NB4	p-ERK↑, Caspase-3↑	[155]
Liver cancer	In vitro and in vivo	HepG2, HepG2 injected BALB/c-nu mice	β-catenin↓, S phase arrest	[111]
	In vitro	HepG2	CD95↑, p53↑, p21/WAF↑, mCD95L↑, sCD95L↑	[96]
	In vitro	BEL-7402	c-Myc↓, Caspase-3↑, S phase arrest	[54]

Table 1. Cont.

Cancer	In Vitro/In Vivo /Ex Vivo	Model	Mechanism of Action	References
	In vitro	HepG2	p-Akt↓, FOXO↑, Bim↑, CHOP↑, p-eIF2α↑, p-ERK↓, Caspase-3, -8, -9↑	[144]
	In vitro	HepaRG	ROS↑, ΔΨm↓, Bcl-2↓, Cyclin A↓, S-phase arrest↑	[97]
	In vitro	SMMC-7721, SMMC-7721/DOX	ATP synthesis↓, inner ΔΨm↓	[156]
	In vitro	HepG2, Huh7	ROS↑, p-c-Jun↑, Caspase-3↑	[55]
Lung cancer	In vitro and in vivo	PC-9, H460, A549, H460 xenograft mice	STAT3↓, Bax↑, Bcl-2↓, G2/M phase arrest↑	[157]
	In vitro	A549	p-PI3K↓, Akt↓, mTOR↓, Bcl-2↓	[158]
	In vitro	A549	G0/G1 phase arrest↑, GADD153↑, GRP78↑, Cyt c↑, Caspase-8↑, Bax↑,Bcl-2↓, Cleaved Bid↑, Cyclin D3↓, Cyclin E↓, CDK-4↓, CDK-6↓, ROS↑, p53↑, p21↑, ΔΨm↓	[110]
Nasopharyngeal cancer	In vitro	NPC	GRP78↑, ATF6↑, CHOP↑, ROS↑, Caspase-3, -8, -9↑	[49]
Ovarian cancer	In vitro	SKOV3-PM4	Rac1↓, ROS↓, MAPK↓, TIMP-1↑, TIMP-2↑,AP-1↓	[53]
	In vitro	A2780, OV2008	MMP↓	[159]
Pancreatic cancer	In vitro and in vivo	AsPC-1, Patu8988T, BxPC-3,PANC-1 injected BALB/c athymic mice	p-STAT3↓	[52]
	In vitro and in vivo	AsPC-1, BxPC-3, HPAF-2, MiaPaCa2, Panc-1, MiaPaCa2 injected athymic Balb/c mice	HIF-1α↓, PFK-1↓, HK-II↓, Glut-1↓	[160]
Oral cancer	In vivo	SCC-4	p53↓, cyclin A & E↓, ER Ca^{2+}↑, ROS↑, Caspase-3, -8, -9↑, Bcl-2↓, Cyt c↑	[43]
	In vitro	SCC-4	MMP-9↓	[50]

↑: Upregulated; ↓: Downregulated.

7. Chemopreventive and Therapeutic Properties of Rhein for Different Cancers

Mounting evidence shows that the multitargeted compound rhein is minimally toxic, affordable and effective for the prevention and treatment of different types of cancers, as listed in Table 1. The following part of the review enumerates the anticancer potential of rhein for different cancers.

7.1. Breast Cancer

Breast cancer is the most commonly occurring cancer and leading cause of mortality in females worldwide [1,107,161–165]. A number of studies have been carried out to investigate the role of rhein in the prevention and treatment of breast cancer both in in vitro and in vivo. This compound suppressed proliferation and inhibited breast cancer in mice. For instance, the administration of rhein has been shown to suppress tumor growth in 4T1-cell-induced mouse xenografts [146]. This study also showed that rhein in combination with atezolizumab synergistically elevated the expression of apoptotic protein such as Bax and caspases-3, -8, and -9, and decreased that of Bcl-2 [146]. In another study, it was reported that rhein inhibited the phosphorylation of Akt and activated FOXO3a and further stimulated the activity of the pro-apoptotic protein Bim, which led to the cleavage of caspase proteins and subsequent induction of apoptosis in MCF-7 cells [144]. Rhein was also shown to inhibit NF-κB activation and its downstream targets HIF-1α and VEGF165 in breast cancer cells, MCF-7 and MDA-MB-435 [138]. In addition, rhein was shown to inhibit phosphorylation of HER-2 protein in SK-Br-3 cells in vitro, thus showing its potential in the development of therapies for HER-2-positive breast cancer [147]. Not only rhein, but also its derivatives showed promising effects in breast cancer. For example, a novel rhein-derived compound, 4F, was found to induce autophagy in MDA-MB-231 cells by upregulating the expression of beclin-1 and causing the degradation of p62 [148]. Furthermore, it was observed that an analog of rhein, rhein lysinate (RHL), inhibited phosphorylation of EGFR, MEK, c-Raf, and ERK and induced apoptosis in MCF-7, SK-Br-3, and MDA-MB-231 cells [46]. This study also demonstrated that rhein has the potential to sensitize breast cancer cells to taxol by decreasing the levels of phospho-epidermal growth factor receptor (p-EGFR), thus unravelling the potential of this anthraquinone for the management of drug resistance in breast cancer cells [46].

7.2. Cervical Cancer

Globally, cervical cancer is one of the leading causes of cancer-related deaths among women, with annual incidence rates of 500,000 patients [1,166]. Several studies have showcased the anticancer potential of rhein in cervical cancer. For instance, rhein was shown to inhibit β-catenin and c-Myc, which are highly overexpressed in cervical cancer cells, by suppressing the phosphorylation of GSK3β and inducing S-phase cell-cycle arrest in HeLa cells [111]. In another study, Ip et al. (2007) showed that in Ca Ski cervical cancer cells, rhein induced apoptosis via the mitochondrial pathway. It was observed that treatment with rhein induced Ca^{2+} release from the endoplasmic reticulum, which was followed by disruption of the mitochondrial membrane potential due to the release of Cyt c, activated caspase-3 and PARP cleavage, leading to apoptosis in these cells [149]. The rhein derivative RHL was also found to inhibit the proliferation of HeLa cells in a dose- and time-dependent manner through the phosphorylation and activation of the downstream regulators of MAPKs such as JNK, p38 MAPK and ERK1/2, thereby inducing the activation of apoptotic proteins like cleaved caspase-3/7 and PARP [48].

7.3. Colon Cancer

Colon cancer is the third leading cause of cancer-related deaths worldwide. The anticancer potential of rhein against colon cancer has been reported by both in vitro and in vivo studies. For example, rhein has been shown to inhibit the proliferation of Caco-2 cells by modulating the MAPK pathway [150]. It was also observed that rhein induced apoptosis in HCT-116 and SW620 cells by suppressing phospho-signal transducer and activator of transcription 3 (p-STAT3), Bcl-2, cyclin D1, and cyclin B1 [151]. Moreover, in HT29 cells, rhein showed a suppressive activity over the elevated expression of

HIF-1α and several immunosuppressive molecules like PD-L1, VEGF, COX-2, IL-10, etc., that were found to be involved in the survival of these cancer cells. [98]. Although rhein showed significant cytotoxicity in colon cancer cell line COLO 320 DM, it was found to be safe and did not cause DNA damage to normal colon cells, thus exhibiting selective toxicity [69]. In addition, recent studies on animal models of colon cancer have shown possible involvement of rhein in alleviating tumor proliferation via the activation of MAPK/NF-κB pathways [79].

7.4. Glioma

Glioma and glioblastoma are some of the severe forms of rapidly developing brain tumors [7,153]. Rhein and its derivatives have shown significant effect in suppressing the proliferation and survival of these cancer cells. For example, the treatment of rhein suppressed the activation of ERK1/2 by and elevated Bcl-2 and caspase-3 levels, induced apoptosis and cell-cycle arrest in rat F98 (sub-S phase arrest) and human Hs683 (G2/M phase arrest) glioma cell lines [152]. In another study, a novel rhein-derived compound, hydroxyethyl hydroxamic acid (SYSUP007), was found to suppress the proliferation, invasion, and migration of glioblastoma cells T98G and U251. Additionally, the treatment of glioblastoma cells with this formulation was shown to inhibit MMP-9 and SGK-1, which are involved in drug resistance and tumor development, and also this formulation induced the expression of Ac-K100 (acetylated lysine) in these cells [153].

7.5. Leukemia

Mutation in immature lymphocytes leads to uncontrolled or non-functional development of the derived blood cells. These cancerous cells in lymphoblasts or acute lymphoblastic leukemia (ALL) are the cause of 25% of all childhood cancers [167]. The antileukemic effect of rhein was studied on the acute promyelocytic leukemia cell lines NB4 and HL-60 [146,163]. Rhein was shown to target the Bid protein, which caused the loss of mitochondrial potential due to Cyt c efflux and induced the cleavage of an apoptotic executioner caspase, caspase-3, in HL-60 cells [145]. Besides the involvement of mitochondrial and caspase pathway, studies have shown that rhein also targets the signalling complexes p-ERK, PI3K, and p-Akt, which leads to the apoptosis of human NB4 cells [155]. In another study, the rhein-derived compound AQ-101 was shown to disrupt MDM2 protein interaction and controlled the proliferation of ALL cells in vitro and in vivo by modulating the expression of p53 [154].

7.6. Liver Cancer

Liver cancer is the second leading cause of cancer-related deaths and the sixth-most common form of cancer in the world [168–176]. The anticancerous activities of rhein have been well studied in liver cancer. An in vitro study on the effect of rhein against HepaRG cells showed that it induced cell cycle arrest at S phase by modulating the expression of cyclin E, p53, p21, cyclin A, and CDK-2 [97]. Another study on the effect of rhein against arrested Hep G2 cells revealed that rhein arrested cell growth in the G1 phase of the cell cycle by inducing p53 and p21/WAF1 proteins [96]. Recent studies have shown that this compound induces apoptosis and G0/G1 cell-cycle arrest via regulation of ROS in both HepG2 and Huh7 cells [55].

As an essential apoptotic inducer, the Bim protein plays a vital role in inducing angiogenesis and tumorigenesis in cancer cells. Rhein-mediated modulation of phosphorylation of Akt and FOXO3a induced Bim secretion and caused apoptosis in HepG2 cells [144]. It was shown that rhein also incited the release of mitochondrial Cyt c and hindered the synthesis of ATP, which induced apoptosis due to the loss of mitochondrial membrane potential in HepaRG cells and SMMC-7721/DOX cells, respectively [97,156]. In another study, it was reported that the proliferation of hepatocellular cells, BEL-7402 was significantly decreased by rhein via regulation of caspase-3 and oncogene c-Myc [54]. The anticancer effect of rhein was also studied in in vivo models of liver cancer. For example, rhein was shown to inhibit HepG2-induced xenograft tumorigenesis in animals, by suppressing β-catenin expression and GSK3β levels to reduce the tumor growth. This antiproliferative activity of rhein on cell proliferation of HepG2 liver cancer cells was also due to the decrease of β-catenin, induced by modulation of p53 and K-ras proteins [111].

7.7. Lung Cancer

Lung cancer is the most diagnosed cancer in the world [1,177–184]. Many reports have also highlighted the potential therapeutic effects of rhein against lung cancer. Bu et al. (2020) demonstrated that rhein induced apoptosis in A549 cells by modulating the expression of p-AMPK, mTOR, and Bcl-2 proteins [158]. The reduced Bcl-2 expression, Cyt c efflux, the rapid loss of ΔΨm and enhanced caspase-3 activity led to apoptosis in these cells. Moreover, treatment with rhein also resulted in increased expression levels of p53 and p21 and decreased levels of CDK-4 and -6 and cyclin E, which led to G0/G1 cell-cycle arrest [110]. Some preclinical studies also showed the regulation of STAT3, Bax, and Bcl-2 expression pathway by rhein in A549 cells. It was shown that the treatment of rhein halted the cell cycle at G2/M phase via downregulation of cyclin B1, MDM2, and p-53 expression levels in H460 and PC-9 cells [157].

7.8. Nasopharyngeal Cancer (NPC)

The anticancer activity of rhein has also been reported in NPC, a rare form of head and neck cancer. It was shown that treatment with rhein modulated the activating transcription factor (ATF)6 and p-ERK-regulated induction of endoplasmic reticulum (ER) stress-associated apoptosis factor and CCAAT/enhancer-binding protein homologous protein (CHOP) in a dose- and time-dependent manner. The observed changes in the levels of cytosolic Ca^{2+}, ROS, and MMP had an antiproliferative impact in these cells. It was also shown that rhein modulated the activities of caspase-8 and -9 via the activation of CHOP and caspase-3 [49].

7.9. Ovarian Cancer

Ovarian cancer is a cancer that develops in the ovaries. Rac1, a small G protein family member, influences cell migration and invasion by generating ROS in these cancer cells. Rhein was shown to reduce the activity of Rac1 and AP-1, thereby regulating its downstream ROS-dependent signaling axis p38/JNK MAPK in SKOV3-PM4 cells, and attenuating cellular proliferation, migration, and invasion [53]. Rhein also inhibited matrix metalloproteinases in A2780 and OV2008 cell lines [159].

7.10. Pancreatic Cancer (PC)

Cancers of the pancreas are some of the most lethal forms of cancer [64]. Rhein, along with EGFR inhibitors, was shown to inhibit STAT3 in PC. The combination of rhein along with the EGFR inhibitor erlotinib against PANC-1 and BxPC-3 xenograft mouse models displayed a synergistic effect by diminishing the expression of p-STAT3 and p-EGFR. Additionally, it also inhibited Bcl-2 levels and enhanced Bax levels in the in vivo models [52]. Rhein was also shown to counter the Warburg effect in MiaPaCa2 cells. The preclinical studies suggested that there was a decrease in levels of HIF-α and associated proteins and PFK (phosphofructokinase)-1 after the treatment with rhein. Thus, rhein helped to improve the glucose homeostasis in these cancer cells [160].

7.11. Oral Cancer

Cancers of the oral cavity is a major health concern worldwide [1]. Few studies have shown the efficacy of rhein against oral cancer. Rhein was reported to have an essential role in preventing the migration and invasion of SCC-4 cells by suppressing the activity of the MMP-9 gene [50]. It led to DNA damage in these cells via inhibition of mRNA expression of DNA-repair-associated genes like O(6)-methylguanine-DNA methyltransferase (MGMT) [51]. Moreover, the compound also induced S-phase arrest in SCC-4 cells by inhibiting cyclin B1 and cyclin A in vitro. In addition, there was an induction of caspase-3 proteases and reduction in Bcl-2 levels in the cells treated with rhein. It was also seen that ROS and Ca^{+2} levels could be involved in rhein-induced apoptosis [43].

8. Toxicity of Rhein

Toxicity is often associated with the use of drugs and medicines, and remains a major challenge related to drug safety and clinical applications. The toxicity of rhein has been reported in a few studies. For example, Xianghong et al. (2010) showed the acute hepatotoxicity associated with the plant extracts of *P. multiforum* in mice, which was due to one of its anthraquinone components, rhein [185]. Rhein also induced toxicity at the dosage of 6.25–50 µM in hepatocytes in vitro [185]. In another investigation, it was observed that rhein induced apoptosis in renal epithelial HK-2 cells through the uncoupling protein (UCP)-2-related mitochondrial pathway [186]. In addition, the dose-dependent effects of rhein exerted a toxic effect in hepatic HL-7702 cells via the oxidative stress-involved mitochondria-mediated apoptotic pathway. After 12 hours of treatment, a significant apoptotic effect was observed at 50 µM and 100 µM concentrations of rhein [187]. However, in most of the studies, it was observed that very high concentrations of rhein induced toxicity in normal cells.

9. Conclusions

Rhein, isolated from rhubarb herbs, an ancient Chinese medicine, has been in use for thousands of years. In developing parts of world like India and Africa, around 65% and 80% of the population, respectively, make use of phytomedicines. To obtain the maximum benefit from these multitargeted phytochemicals in the prevention and treatment of chronic diseases, they have been used in conjunction with monotargeted modern medicines [188–192]. Rhein was shown to induce the anticancerous effect through multiple mechanisms. This compound rhein has the potential to modulate various key regulatory pathways like NF-κB, PI3K/Akt, MAPKs, etc., which are important for the regulation of several chronic diseases like arthritis, renal dysfunction, neuronal dysfunction, etc. There are many more unidentified cellular molecules that interact with rhein, which are involved in inducing cytotoxicity in the cancer cells. The research into its potential effects with other established anticancer drugs and nanomatrix formulation is still in its infancy. This novel compound lacks momentum in research due to its high hydrophobicity which leads to its low bioavailability. Thus, with improvement in its physicochemical dynamics, this multimodal molecule could be of more value to human health.

With the discovery of induction routes of cancer, the race to identify a cure has accelerated [90]. To translate phytochemicals into clinical setting, the efficiency of the drugs needs to be improved through enhancing the drug interactions, drug dynamics, and other pharmacokinetic parameters [193]. Although the biological effect of *Rheum* rhizomes in several polyherbal extracts are of high ethnopharmacological importance, there are fewer data available from pharmacokinetic studies of rhein alone. As the source of rhein is botanical, it could significantly decrease the expenses involved in treating cancer. Apart from the need to conduct more in vitro and in vivo studies, clinical trials have to be performed with rhein to validate its anticancerous therapeutic potential. Prior to clinical trials with this compound, it will be necessary to identify the safe levels of this compound with regard to active blood levels, retention ability, and disposed metabolites [90]. Thus, this novel compound could be of high value to human health when used at appropriate concentrations and in the form of formulations with enriched bioavailability and upgraded pharmacodynamics.

Funding: This work was supported by the project BT/556/NE/U-EXCEL/2016 awarded to Ajaikumar B Kunnumakkara by Department of Biotechnology (DBT), Government of India on 31.03.2017. The author Henamayee Sahu acknowledges ICMR, New Delhi, India, the author Kishore Banik acknowledges UGC, New Delhi, India and the author Bethsebie Lalduhsaki Sailo acknowledges DST-INSPIRE for providing respective fellowships. This work was also supported by a National Research Foundation of Korea (NRF) grant funded by the Korean government (MSIP) (NRF-2018R1D1A1B07042969).

Conflicts of Interest: The authors declare no competing interests.

Abbreviations

Ac-K100	Acetylated lysine
ATF6	Activating transcription factor 6
ATP	Adenosine triphosphate
Bax	Bcl-2-associated X protein
Bcl-2	B cell lymphoma 2
Bid	BH3 interacting domain death agonist
CD	Cluster of differentiation
c-PARP	cleaved- Poly ADP ribose polymerase
CHOP	CCAAT/enhancer-binding protein homologous protein
COX-2	Cyclooxygenase 2
EGFR	Epidermal growth factor receptor
ER	Endoplasmic reticulum
ERK	Extracellular signal-regulated kinase
FOXO	Class O of Forkhead box transcription factors
FOXO3a	Forkhead box O3a
Fas	FS-7-associated surface antigen
GADD153	Growth arrest and DNA damage153
Glut-1	Glucose transporter1
GRP78	78 kDa Glucose-regulated protein
HER-2	Human epidermal growth factor receptor 2
HIF-1α	Hypoxia-inducible factor 1 alpha
HK-II	Hexokinase2
HMGB1	High-mobility-group-box-1
IL-6	Interleukin-6
IL-1β	Interleukin-1 beta
IKKβ	Inhibitor of nuclear factor kappa –B kinase subunit beta
JNK	c-Jun N-terminal kinase
mTOR	Mammalian target of rapamycin
MAPK	Mitogen-activated protein kinase
mCD95L	Membrane-bound CD95 ligand
MDM2	Murine double minute 2
MEK	Mitogen-activated protein kinase kinase
MMP	Matrix metalloproteinase
NO	Nitric oxide
NADPH oxidase	Nicotinamide adenine dinucleotide phosphate oxidase
NDRG1	N-myc downstream regulated 1
NF-κB	Nuclear factor- kappa light chain enhancer of activated B cells
p-Akt	Phosphorylated Akt
PARP	Poly ADP ribose polymerase
PFK-1	Phosphofructokinase-1
p-HER-2	Phosphorylated human epidermal growth factor receptor 2
p-EGFR	Phosphorylated epidermal growth factor receptor
p-c-Jun	Phosphorylated c-Jun
p-eIF2α	Phosphorylated eukaryotic initiation factor 2 alpha
RAC1	Ras-related C3 botulinum toxin substrate 1
ROS	Reactive oxygen species
sCD95L	Soluble CD95 ligand
STAT3	Signal transducer and activator of transcription 3
TIMP	Tissue inhibitor of metalloproteinase
TNF-α	Tumor necrosis factor- alpha
UPR	Unfolded protein response
VEGF	Vascular endothelial growth factor

References

1. Bray, F.; Ferlay, J.; Soerjomataram, I.; Siegel, R.L.; Torre, L.A.; Jemal, A. Global cancer statistics 2018: GLOBOCAN estimates of incidence and mortality worldwide for 36 cancers in 185 countries. *CA A Cancer J. Clin.* **2018**, *68*, 394–424. [CrossRef] [PubMed]
2. Devi Khwairakpam, A.; Monisha, J.; Roy, N.K.; Bordoloi, D.; Padmavathi, G.; Banik, K.; Khatoon, E.; Kunnumakkara, A.B. Vietnamese coriander inhibits cell proliferation, survival and migration via suppression of Akt/mTOR pathway in oral squamous cell carcinoma. *J. Basic Clin. Physiol. Pharmacol.* **2019**. [CrossRef] [PubMed]
3. Banik, K.; Harsha, C.; Bordoloi, D.; Lalduhsaki Sailo, B.; Sethi, G.; Leong, H.C.; Arfuso, F.; Mishra, S.; Wang, L.; Kumar, A.P.; et al. Therapeutic potential of gambogic acid, a caged xanthone, to target cancer. *Cancer Lett.* **2018**, *416*, 75–86. [CrossRef] [PubMed]
4. Padmavathi, G.; Roy, N.K.; Bordoloi, D.; Arfuso, F.; Mishra, S.; Sethi, G.; Bishayee, A.; Kunnumakkara, A.B. Butein in health and disease: A comprehensive review. *Phytomed. Int. J. Phytother. Phytopharm.* **2017**, *25*, 118–127. [CrossRef] [PubMed]
5. Roy, N.K.; Deka, A.; Bordoloi, D.; Mishra, S.; Kumar, A.P.; Sethi, G.; Kunnumakkara, A.B. The potential role of boswellic acids in cancer prevention and treatment. *Cancer Lett.* **2016**, *377*, 74–86. [CrossRef]
6. Monisha, J.; Jaiswal, A.; Banik, K.; Choudhary, H.; Singh, A.K.; Bordoloi, D.; Kunnumakkara, A.B. Cancer Cell Chemoresistance: A Prime Obstacle in Cancer Therapy. In *Cancer Cell Chemoresistance and Chemosensitization*; World Scientific: Singapore, 2018; pp. 15–49.
7. Khwairakpam, A.D.; Monisha, J.; Banik, K.; Choudhary, H.; Sharma, A.; Bordoloi, D.; Kunnumakkara, A.B. Chemoresistance in Brain Cancer and Different Chemosensitization Approaches. In *Cancer Cell Chemoresistance and Chemosensitization*; World Scientific: Singapore, 2018; pp. 107–127.
8. Padmavathi, G.; Monisha, J.; Banik, K.; Thakur, K.K.; Choudhary, H.; Bordoloi, D.; Kunnumakkara, A.B. Different chemosensitization approaches to overcome chemoresistance in prostate cancer. In *Cancer Cell Chemoresistance and Chemosensitization*; World Scientific: Singapore, 2018; pp. 583–613.
9. Javadi, M.; Roy, N.K.; Sharma, A.; Banik, K.; Ganesan, P.; Bordoloi, D.; Kunnumakkara, A.B. Chemoresistance and chemosensitization in Melanoma. In *Cancer Cell Chemoresistance and Chemosensitization*; World Scientific: Singapore, 2018; pp. 479–527.
10. Chinese Pharmacopoeia Commission. *Pharmacopoeia of the People's Republic of China*; Chemical Industry Press: Beijing, China, 2005; p. 17.
11. Kunnumakkara, A.B.; Banik, K.; Bordoloi, D.; Harsha, C.; Sailo, B.L.; Padmavathi, G.; Roy, N.K.; Gupta, S.C.; Aggarwal, B.B. Googling the Guggul (Commiphora and Boswellia) for Prevention of Chronic Diseases. *Front. Pharmacol.* **2018**, *9*, 686. [CrossRef]
12. Khwairakpam, A.D.; Bordoloi, D.; Thakur, K.K.; Monisha, J.; Arfuso, F.; Sethi, G.; Mishra, S.; Kumar, A.P.; Kunnumakkara, A.B. Possible use of Punica granatum (Pomegranate) in cancer therapy. *Pharmacol. Res.* **2018**, *133*, 53–64. [CrossRef]
13. Lu, K.; Zhang, C.; Wu, W.; Zhou, M.; Tang, Y.; Peng, Y. Rhubarb extract has a protective role against radiation-induced brain injury and neuronal cell apoptosis. *Mol. Med. Rep.* **2015**, *12*, 2689–2694. [CrossRef]
14. Kashyap, D.; Tuli, H.S.; Yerer, M.B.; Sharma, A.; Sak, K.; Srivastava, S.; Pandey, A.; Garg, V.K.; Sethi, G.; Bishayee, A. Natural product-based nanoformulations for cancer therapy: Opportunities and challenges. *Semin. Cancer Biol.* **2019**. [CrossRef]
15. Merarchi, M.; Sethi, G.; Shanmugam, M.K.; Fan, L.; Arfuso, F.; Ahn, K.S. Role of Natural Products in Modulating Histone Deacetylases in Cancer. *Molecules* **2019**, *24*. [CrossRef]
16. Shanmugam, M.K.; Warrier, S.; Kumar, A.P.; Sethi, G.; Arfuso, F. Potential Role of Natural Compounds as Anti-Angiogenic Agents in Cancer. *Curr. Vasc. Pharmacol.* **2017**, *15*, 503–519. [CrossRef] [PubMed]
17. Tewari, D.; Nabavi, S.F.; Nabavi, S.M.; Sureda, A.; Farooqi, A.A.; Atanasov, A.G.; Vacca, R.A.; Sethi, G.; Bishayee, A. Targeting activator protein 1 signaling pathway by bioactive natural agents: Possible therapeutic strategy for cancer prevention and intervention. *Pharmacol. Res.* **2018**, *128*, 366–375. [CrossRef] [PubMed]
18. Hsieh, Y.S.; Yang, S.F.; Sethi, G.; Hu, D.N. Natural bioactives in cancer treatment and prevention. *BioMed Res. Int.* **2015**, *2015*, 182835. [CrossRef] [PubMed]
19. Yang, S.F.; Weng, C.J.; Sethi, G.; Hu, D.N. Natural bioactives and phytochemicals serve in cancer treatment and prevention. *Evid. Based Complementary Altern. Med. Ecam* **2013**, *2013*, 698190. [CrossRef]

20. Prasannan, R.; Kalesh, K.A.; Shanmugam, M.K.; Nachiyappan, A.; Ramachandran, L.; Nguyen, A.H.; Kumar, A.P.; Lakshmanan, M.; Ahn, K.S.; Sethi, G. Key cell signaling pathways modulated by zerumbone: Role in the prevention and treatment of cancer. *Biochem. Pharmacol.* **2012**, *84*, 1268–1276. [CrossRef]
21. Ramachandran, L.; Manu, K.A.; Shanmugam, M.K.; Li, F.; Siveen, K.S.; Vali, S.; Kapoor, S.; Abbasi, T.; Surana, R.; Smoot, D.T.; et al. Isorhamnetin inhibits proliferation and invasion and induces apoptosis through the modulation of peroxisome proliferator-activated receptor gamma activation pathway in gastric cancer. *J. Biol. Chem.* **2012**, *287*, 38028–38040. [CrossRef]
22. Yarla, N.S.; Bishayee, A.; Sethi, G.; Reddanna, P.; Kalle, A.M.; Dhananjaya, B.L.; Dowluru, K.S.; Chintala, R.; Duddukuri, G.R. Targeting arachidonic acid pathway by natural products for cancer prevention and therapy. *Semin. Cancer Biol.* **2016**, *40–41*, 48–81. [CrossRef]
23. Thakur, K.K.; Bordoloi, D.; Prakash, J.; Javadi, M.; Roy, N.K.; Kunnumakkara, A.B. Different Chemosensitization Approaches for the Effective Management of HNSCC. In *Cancer Cell Chemoresistance and Chemosensitization*; World Scientific: Singapore, 2018; pp. 399–423.
24. Padmavathi, G.; Bordoloi, D.; Banik, K.; Javadi, M.; Singh, A.K.; Kunnumakkara, A.B. Mechanism of Chemoresistance in Bone Cancer and Different Chemosensitization Approaches. In *Cancer Cell Chemoresistance and Chemosensitization*; World Scientific: Singapore, 2018; pp. 81–106.
25. Bordoloi, D.; Monisha, J.; Roy, N.K.; Padmavathi, G.; Banik, K.; Harsha, C.; Wang, H.; Kumar, A.P.; Arfuso, F.; Kunnumakkara, A.B. An Investigation on the Therapeutic Potential of Butein, A Tretrahydroxychalcone Against Human Oral Squamous Cell Carcinoma. *Asian Pac. J. Cancer Prev. APJCP* **2019**, *20*, 3437–3446. [CrossRef]
26. Girisa, S.; Shabnam, B.; Monisha, J.; Fan, L.; Halim, C.E.; Arfuso, F.; Ahn, K.S.; Sethi, G.; Kunnumakkara, A.B. Potential of Zerumbone as an Anti-Cancer Agent. *Molecules* **2019**, *24*. [CrossRef]
27. Sailo, B.L.; Banik, K.; Padmavathi, G.; Javadi, M.; Bordoloi, D.; Kunnumakkara, A.B. Tocotrienols: The promising analogues of vitamin E for cancer therapeutics. *Pharmacol. Res.* **2018**, *130*, 259–272. [CrossRef]
28. Ranaware, A.M.; Banik, K.; Deshpande, V.; Padmavathi, G.; Roy, N.K.; Sethi, G.; Fan, L.; Kumar, A.P.; Kunnumakkara, A.B. Magnolol: A Neolignan from the Magnolia Family for the Prevention and Treatment of Cancer. *Int. J. Mol. Sci.* **2018**, *19*. [CrossRef] [PubMed]
29. Monisha, J.; Padmavathi, G.; Roy, N.K.; Deka, A.; Bordoloi, D.; Anip, A.; Kunnumakkara, A.B. NF-kappaB Blockers Gifted by Mother Nature: Prospectives in Cancer Cell Chemosensitization. *Curr. Pharm. Des.* **2016**, *22*, 4173–4200. [CrossRef] [PubMed]
30. Padmavathi, G.; Rathnakaram, S.R.; Monisha, J.; Bordoloi, D.; Roy, N.K.; Kunnumakkara, A.B. Potential of butein, a tetrahydroxychalcone to obliterate cancer. *Phytomed. Int. J. Phytother. Phytopharm.* **2015**, *22*, 1163–1171. [CrossRef] [PubMed]
31. Liskova, A.; Stefanicka, P.; Samec, M.; Smejkal, K.; Zubor, P.; Bielik, T.; Biskupska-Bodova, K.; Kwon, T.K.; Danko, J.; Büsselberg, D.; et al. Dietary phytochemicals as the potential protectors against carcinogenesis and their role in cancer chemoprevention. *Clin. Exp. Med.* **2020**, *20*, 173–190. [CrossRef] [PubMed]
32. Kunnumakkara, A.B.; Sung, B.; Ravindran, J.; Diagaradjane, P.; Deorukhkar, A.; Dey, S.; Koca, C.; Yadav, V.R.; Tong, Z.; Gelovani, J.G.; et al. γ-Tocotrienol inhibits pancreatic tumors and sensitizes them to gemcitabine treatment by modulating the inflammatory microenvironment. *Cancer Res.* **2010**, *70*, 8695–8705. [CrossRef]
33. Bordoloi, D.; Roy, N.K.; Monisha, J.; Padmavathi, G.; Kunnumakkara, A.B. Multi-Targeted Agents in Cancer Cell Chemosensitization: What We Learnt from Curcumin Thus Far. *Recent Pat. Anti-Cancer Drug Discov.* **2016**, *11*, 67–97. [CrossRef]
34. Banik, K.; Ranaware, A.M.; Harsha, C.; Nitesh, T.; Girisa, S.; Deshpande, V.; Fan, L.; Nalawade, S.P.; Sethi, G.; Kunnumakkara, A.B. Piceatannol: A natural stilbene for the prevention and treatment of cancer. *Pharmacol. Res.* **2020**, *153*, 104635. [CrossRef]
35. Banik, K.; Sailo, B.L.; Thakur, K.K.; Jaiswal, A.; Monisha, J.; Bordoloi, D.; Kunnumakkara, A.B. Potential of different chemosensitizers to overcome chemoresistance in cervical cancer. In *Cancer Cell Chemoresistance and Chemosensitization*; World Scientific: Singapore, 2018; pp. 163–179.
36. Sailo, B.L.; Bordoloi, D.; Banik, K.; Khwairakpam, A.D.; Roy, N.K.; Prakash, J.; Kunnumakkara, A.B. Therapeutic strategies for chemosensitization of renal cancer. In *Cancer Cell Chemoresistance and Chemosensitization*; World Scientific: Singapore, 2018; pp. 615–639.
37. Sailo, B.L.; Javadi, M.; Jaiswal, A.; Prakash, J.; Roy, N.K.; Thakur, K.K.; Banik, K.; Bordoloi, D.; Kunnumakkara, A.B. Molecular Alterations Involved in Pancreatic Cancer Chemoresistance and Chemosensitization Strategies. In *Cancer Cell Chemoresistance and Chemosensitization*; World Scientific: Singapore, 2018; pp. 557–581.

38. Choudhary, H.; Thakur, K.K.; Sharma, A.; Roy, N.K.; Khwairakpam, A.D.; Bordoloi, D.; Kunnumakkara, A.B. Strategies to Overcome Chemoresistance in Ovarian Cancer. In *Cancer Cell Chemoresistance and Chemosensitization*; World Scientific: Singapore, 2018; pp. 529–555.
39. Mohammed, A.; Ibrahim, M.A.; Tajuddeen, N.; Aliyu, A.B.; Isah, M.B. Antidiabetic potential of anthraquinones: A review. *Phytother. Res.* **2020**, *34*, 486–504. [CrossRef]
40. Zhou, Y.X.; Xia, W.; Yue, W.; Peng, C.; Rahman, K.; Zhang, H. Rhein: A Review of Pharmacological Activities. *Evid. Based Complementary Altern. Med.* **2015**, *2015*, 578107. [CrossRef]
41. Zhang, Y.; Fan, S.; Hu, N.; Gu, M.; Chu, C.; Li, Y.; Lu, X.; Huang, C. Rhein Reduces Fat Weight in db/db Mouse and Prevents Diet-Induced Obesity in C57Bl/6 Mouse through the Inhibition of PPARgamma Signaling. *PPAR Res.* **2012**, *2012*, 374936. [CrossRef]
42. Sheng, X.; Wang, M.; Lu, M.; Xi, B.; Sheng, H.; Zang, Y.Q. Rhein ameliorates fatty liver disease through negative energy balance, hepatic lipogenic regulation, and immunomodulation in diet-induced obese mice. *Am. J. Physiol. Endocrinol. Metab.* **2011**, *300*, e886–e893. [CrossRef] [PubMed]
43. Lai, W.W.; Yang, J.S.; Lai, K.C.; Kuo, C.L.; Hsu, C.K.; Wang, C.K.; Chang, C.Y.; Lin, J.J.; Tang, N.Y.; Chen, P.Y.; et al. Rhein induced apoptosis through the endoplasmic reticulum stress, caspase- and mitochondria-dependent pathways in SCC-4 human tongue squamous cancer cells. *In Vivo* **2009**, *23*, 309–316.
44. Zheng, J.M.; Zhu, J.M.; Li, L.S.; Liu, Z.H. Rhein reverses the diabetic phenotype of mesangial cells over-expressing the glucose transporter (GLUT1) by inhibiting the hexosamine pathway. *Br. J. Pharmacol.* **2008**, *153*, 1456–1464. [CrossRef] [PubMed]
45. Li, H.; Liang, C.; Chen, Q.; Yang, Z. Rhein: A potential biological therapeutic drug for intervertebral disc degeneration. *Med. Hypotheses* **2011**, *77*, 1105–1107. [CrossRef] [PubMed]
46. Lin, Y.J.; Zhen, Y.S. Rhein lysinate suppresses the growth of breast cancer cells and potentiates the inhibitory effect of Taxol in athymic mice. *Anti-Cancer Drugs* **2009**, *20*, 65–72. [CrossRef]
47. Lin, Y.J.; Zhen, Y.Z.; Shang, B.Y.; Zhen, Y.S. Rhein lysinate suppresses the growth of tumor cells and increases the anti-tumor activity of Taxol in mice. *Am. J. Chin. Med.* **2009**, *37*, 923–931. [CrossRef]
48. Zhen, Y.Z.; Lin, Y.J.; Gao, J.L.; Zhao, Y.F.; Xu, A.J. Rhein lysinate inhibits cell growth by modulating various mitogen-activated protein kinases in cervical cancer cells. *Oncol. Lett.* **2011**, *2*, 129–133. [CrossRef]
49. Lin, M.L.; Chen, S.S.; Lu, Y.C.; Liang, R.Y.; Ho, Y.T.; Yang, C.Y.; Chung, J.G. Rhein induces apoptosis through induction of endoplasmic reticulum stress and Ca^{2+}-dependent mitochondrial death pathway in human nasopharyngeal carcinoma cells. *Anticancer Res.* **2007**, *27*, 3313–3322.
50. Chen, Y.Y.; Chiang, S.Y.; Lin, J.G.; Ma, Y.S.; Liao, C.L.; Weng, S.W.; Lai, T.Y.; Chung, J.G. Emodin, aloe-emodin and rhein inhibit migration and invasion in human tongue cancer SCC-4 cells through the inhibition of gene expression of matrix metalloproteinase-9. *Int. J. Oncol.* **2010**, *36*, 1113–1120. [CrossRef]
51. Chen, Y.Y.; Chiang, S.Y.; Lin, J.G.; Yang, J.S.; Ma, Y.S.; Liao, C.L.; Lai, T.Y.; Tang, N.Y.; Chung, J.G. Emodin, aloe-emodin and rhein induced DNA damage and inhibited DNA repair gene expression in SCC-4 human tongue cancer cells. *Anticancer Res.* **2010**, *30*, 945–951.
52. Yang, L.; Lin, S.; Kang, Y.; Xiang, Y.; Xu, L.; Li, J.; Dai, X.; Liang, G.; Huang, X.; Zhao, C. Rhein sensitizes human pancreatic cancer cells to EGFR inhibitors by inhibiting STAT3 pathway. *J. Exp. Clin. Cancer Res.* **2019**, *38*, 31. [CrossRef] [PubMed]
53. Zhou, G.; Peng, F.; Zhong, Y.; Chen, Y.; Tang, M.; Li, D. Rhein suppresses matrix metalloproteinase production by regulating the Rac1/ROS/MAPK/AP-1 pathway in human ovarian carcinoma cells. *Int. J. Oncol.* **2017**, *50*, 933–941. [CrossRef]
54. Shi, P.; Huang, Z.; Chen, G. Rhein induces apoptosis and cell cycle arrest in human hepatocellular carcinoma BEL-7402 cells. *Am. J. Chin. Med.* **2008**, *36*, 805–813. [CrossRef] [PubMed]
55. Wang, A.; Jiang, H.; Liu, Y.; Chen, J.; Zhou, X.; Zhao, C.; Chen, X.; Lin, M. Rhein induces liver cancer cells apoptosis via activating ROS-dependent JNK/Jun/caspase-3 signaling pathway. *J. Cancer* **2020**, *11*, 500–507. [CrossRef]
56. He, Z.H.; He, M.F.; Ma, S.C.; But, P.P. Anti-angiogenic effects of rhubarb and its anthraquinone derivatives. *J. Ethnopharmacol.* **2009**, *121*, 313–317. [CrossRef] [PubMed]
57. Chai, S.; To, K.K.; Lin, G. Circumvention of multi-drug resistance of cancer cells by Chinese herbal medicines. *Chin. Med.* **2010**, *5*, 26. [CrossRef] [PubMed]
58. Xu, H.; Lu, Y.; Zhang, T.; Liu, K.; Liu, L.; He, Z.; Xu, B.; Wu, X. Characterization of binding interactions of anthraquinones and bovine beta-lactoglobulin. *Food Chem.* **2019**, *281*, 28–35. [CrossRef]

59. Feng, H.; Zhu, Y.; Fu, Z.; Li, D. Preparation, characterization, and in vivo study of rhein solid lipid nanoparticles for oral delivery. *Chem. Biol. Drug Des.* **2017**, *90*, 867–872. [CrossRef]
60. Gómez-Gaete, C.; Retamal, M.; Chávez, C.; Bustos, P.; Godoy, R.; Torres-Vergara, P. Development, characterization and in vitro evaluation of biodegradable rhein-loaded microparticles for treatment of osteoarthritis. *Eur. J. Pharm. Sci.* **2017**, *96*, 390–397. [CrossRef]
61. Yuan, Z.; Gu, X. Preparation, characterization, and in vivo study of rhein-loaded poly (lactic-co-glycolic acid) nanoparticles for oral delivery. *Drug Des. Dev.* **2015**, *9*, 2301. [CrossRef]
62. Kunnumakkara, A.B.; Sailo, B.L.; Banik, K.; Harsha, C.; Prasad, S.; Gupta, S.C.; Bharti, A.C.; Aggarwal, B.B. Chronic diseases, inflammation, and spices: How are they linked? *J. Transl. Med.* **2018**, *16*, 14. [CrossRef] [PubMed]
63. Khwairakpam, A.D.; Damayenti, Y.D.; Deka, A.; Monisha, J.; Roy, N.K.; Padmavathi, G.; Kunnumakkara, A.B. Acorus calamus: A bio-reserve of medicinal values. *J. Basic Clin. Physiol. Pharmacol.* **2018**, *29*, 107–122. [CrossRef] [PubMed]
64. Kunnumakkara, A.B.; Sung, B.; Ravindran, J.; Diagaradjane, P.; Deorukhkar, A.; Dey, S.; Koca, C.; Tong, Z.; Gelovani, J.G.; Guha, S.; et al. Zyflamend suppresses growth and sensitizes human pancreatic tumors to gemcitabine in an orthotopic mouse model through modulation of multiple targets. *Int. J. Cancer* **2012**, *131*, E292–E303. [CrossRef] [PubMed]
65. Rokaya, M.B.; Munzbergova, Z.; Timsina, B.; Bhattarai, K.R. *Rheum* australe D. Don: A review of its botany, ethnobotany, phytochemistry and pharmacology. *J. Ethnopharmacol.* **2012**, *141*, 761–774. [CrossRef] [PubMed]
66. Yang, F.; Zhang, T.; Xu, G.; Chou, F.E.; Ito, Y. pH-MODULATED STEPWISE ELUTION CCC AND ITS APPLICATION TO THE PREPARATIVE SEPARATION OF HYDROXYANTHRAQUINONE COMPOUNDS FROM TRADITIONAL CHINESE MEDICINAL HERBS. *J. Liq. Chromatogr. Relat. Technol.* **2001**, *24*, 1617–1628. [CrossRef]
67. Yang, D.Y.; Fushimi, H.; Cai, S.Q.; Komatsu, K. Molecular analysis of *Rheum* species used as Rhei Rhizoma based on the chloroplast matK gene sequence and its application for identification. *Biol. Pharm. Bull.* **2004**, *27*, 375–383. [CrossRef] [PubMed]
68. Cojocaru, A.; Vlase, L.; Munteanu, N.; Stan, T.; Teliban, G.C.; Burducea, M.; Stoleru, V. Dynamic of phenolic compounds, antioxidant activity, and yield of rhubarb under chemical, organic and biological fertilization. *Plants* **2020**, *9*, 355. [CrossRef]
69. Duraipandiyan, V.; Baskar, A.A.; Ignacimuthu, S.; Muthukumar, C.; Al-Harbi, N.A. Anticancer activity of Rhein isolated from Cassia fistula L. flower. *Asian Pac. J. Trop. Dis.* **2012**, *2*, S517–S523. [CrossRef]
70. Duraipandiyan, V.; Ignacimuthu, S.; Gabriel Paulraj, M. Antifeedant and larvicidal activities of Rhein isolated from the flowers of *Cassia fistula* L. *Saudi J. Biol. Sci.* **2011**, *18*, 129–133. [CrossRef]
71. Yang, F.; Xu, Y.; Xiong, A.; He, Y.; Yang, L.; Wan, Y.J.; Wang, Z. Evaluation of the protective effect of Rhei Radix et Rhizoma against alpha-naphthylisothiocyanate induced liver injury based on metabolic profile of bile acids. *J. Ethnopharmacol.* **2012**, *144*, 599–604. [CrossRef]
72. Harsha, C.; Banik, K.; Bordoloi, D.; Kunnumakkara, A.B. Antiulcer properties of fruits and vegetables: A mechanism based perspective. *Food Chem. Toxicol. Int. J. Publ. Br. Ind. Biol. Res. Assoc.* **2017**, *108*, 104–119. [CrossRef]
73. Chinese Pharmacopoeia Commission. *Pharmacopoeia of the People's Republic of China*; Chemical Industry Press: Beijing, China, 1997; pp. 149–150.
74. Choi, R.Y.; Lee, H.I.; Ham, J.R.; Yee, S.T.; Kang, K.Y.; Lee, M.K. Heshouwu (*Polygonum multiflorum* Thunb.) ethanol extract suppresses pre-adipocytes differentiation in 3T3-L1 cells and adiposity in obese mice. *Biomed. Pharmacother.* **2018**, *106*, 355–362. [CrossRef]
75. Lin, L.; Ni, B.; Lin, H.; Zhang, M.; Li, X.; Yin, X.; Qu, C.; Ni, J. Traditional usages, botany, phytochemistry, pharmacology and toxicology of *Polygonum multiflorum* Thunb.: A review. *J. Ethnopharmacol.* **2015**, *159*, 158–183. [CrossRef]
76. Zhou, H.; Jiao, D. 312 cases of gastric and duodenal ulcer bleeding treated with 3 kinds of alcoholic extract rhubarb tablets. *Zhong Xi Yi Jie He Za Zhi = Chin. J. Mod. Dev. Tradit. Med.* **1990**, *10*, 150-1–131-2.
77. Wu, J.; Hu, Y.; Xiang, L.; Li, S.; Yuan, Y.; Chen, X.; Zhang, Y.; Huang, W.; Meng, X.; Wang, P. San-Huang-Xie-Xin-Tang constituents exert drug-drug interaction of mutual reinforcement at both pharmacodynamics and pharmacokinetic level: A review. *Front. Pharmacol.* **2016**, *7*, 448. [CrossRef] [PubMed]

78. Ma, B.L.; Ma, Y.M.; Yan, D.M.; Zhou, H.; Shi, R.; Wang, T.M.; Yang, Y.; Wang, C.H.; Zhang, N. Effective constituents in Xiexin Decoction for anti-inflammation. *J. Ethnopharmacol.* **2009**, *125*, 151–156. [CrossRef]
79. Yan, S.; Yue, Y.; Wang, J.; Li, W.; Sun, M.; Zeng, L.; Wang, X. Banxia Xiexin decoction, a traditional Chinese medicine, alleviates colon cancer in nude mice. *Ann. Transl. Med.* **2019**, *7*. [CrossRef] [PubMed]
80. Kim, H.R.; Lee, G.S.; Kim, M.S.; Ryu, D.G.; So, H.S.; Moon, H.C.; Lee, Y.R.; Yang, S.H.; Kwon, K.B. Effects of Banxia Xiexin Decoction (半夏泻心汤) on Cisplatin-Induced Apoptosis of Human A549 Lung Cancer Cells. *Chin. J. Integr. Med.* **2018**, *24*, 436–441. [CrossRef]
81. Zhang, A.; Sun, H.; Yuan, Y.; Sun, W.; Jiao, G.; Wang, X. An in vivo analysis of the therapeutic and synergistic properties of Chinese medicinal formula Yin-Chen-Hao-Tang based on its active constituents. *Fitoterapia* **2011**, *82*, 1160–1168. [CrossRef]
82. Ibrahim, M.; Khan, A.A.; Tiwari, S.K.; Habeeb, M.A.; Khaja, M.N.; Habibullah, C.M. Antimicrobial activity of Sapindus mukorossi and *Rheum* emodi extracts against H pylori: In vitro and in vivo studies. *World J. Gastroenterol.* **2006**, *12*, 7136–7142. [CrossRef]
83. Xu, W.; Hu, M.; Zhang, Q.; Yu, J.; Su, W. Effects of anthraquinones from *Cassia occidentalis* L. on ovalbumin-induced airways inflammation in a mouse model of allergic asthma. *J. Ethnopharmacol.* **2018**, *221*, 1–9. [CrossRef] [PubMed]
84. Wei, Y.; Zhang, T.; Ito, Y. Preparative separation of rhein from Chinese traditional herb by repeated high-speed counter-current chromatography. *J. Chromatogr. A* **2003**, *1017*, 125–130. [CrossRef] [PubMed]
85. Petralito, S.; Zanardi, I.; Memoli, A.; Annesini, M.C.; Travagli, V. Solubility, spectroscopic properties and photostability of Rhein/cyclodextrin inclusion complex. *Spectrochim. Acta. Part Amol. Biomol. Spectrosc.* **2009**, *74*, 1254–1259. [CrossRef] [PubMed]
86. Jin, Q.; Jiang, C.; Gao, M.; Zhang, D.; Yao, N.; Feng, Y.; Wu, T.; Zhang, J. Target exploration of rhein as a small-molecule necrosis avid agent by post-treatment click modification. *New J. Chem.* **2019**, *43*, 6121–6125. [CrossRef]
87. Zhang, A.; Wu, T.; Bian, L.; Li, P.; Liu, Q.; Zhang, D.; Jin, Q.; Zhang, J.; Huang, G.; Song, S. Synthesis and Evaluation of Ga-68-Labeled Rhein for Early Assessment of Treatment-Induced Tumor Necrosis. *Mol. Imaging Biol.* **2019**. [CrossRef]
88. Hwang, D.S.; Gu, P.S.; Kim, N.; Jang, Y.P.; Oh, M.S. Effects of Rhei Undulati Rhizoma on lipopolysaccharide-induced neuroinflammation in vitro and *in vivo*. *Environ. Toxicol.* **2018**, *33*, 23–31. [CrossRef]
89. Liu, Z.; Lang, Y.; Li, L.; Liang, Z.; Deng, Y.; Fang, R.; Meng, Q. Effect of emodin on chondrocyte viability in an in vitro model of osteoarthritis. *Exp. Ther. Med.* **2018**, *16*, 5384–5389. [CrossRef]
90. Qin, F.; Huang, J.; Huang, X.; Ren, P. Simultaneous determination and pharmacokinetic comparisons of aloe-emodin, rhein, emodin, and chrysophanol after oral administration of these monomers, rhei rhizoma and chaiqin-chengqi-tang, to rats. *J. Liq. Chromatogr. Relat. Technol.* **2011**, *34*, 1381–1390. [CrossRef]
91. Zhao, Q.; Wang, X.; Chen, A.; Cheng, X.; Zhang, G.; Sun, J.; Zhao, Y.; Huang, Y.; Zhu, Y. Rhein protects against cerebral ischemic-/reperfusion-induced oxidative stress and apoptosis in rats. *Int. J. Mol. Med.* **2018**, *41*, 2802–2812. [CrossRef]
92. Zhang, Q.; Liu, L.; Lin, W.; Yin, S.; Duan, A.; Liu, Z.; Cao, W. Rhein reverses Klotho repression via promoter demethylation and protects against kidney and bone injuries in mice with chronic kidney disease. *Kidney Int.* **2017**, *91*, 144–156. [CrossRef]
93. Cyong, J.; Matsumoto, T.; Arakawa, K.; Kiyohara, H.; Yamada, H.; Otsuka, Y. Anti-Bacteroides fragilis substance from rhubarb. *J. Ethnopharmacol.* **1987**, *19*, 279–283. [CrossRef] [PubMed]
94. Vargas, F.; Díaz, Y.; Carbonell, K. Antioxidant and Scavenging Activity of Emodin, Aloe-Emodin, and Rhein on Free-Radical and Reactive Oxygen Species. *Pharm. Biol.* **2004**, *42*, 342–348. [CrossRef]
95. Mendes, A.F.; Caramona, M.M.; De Carvalho, A.P.; Lopes, M.C. Diacerhein and rhein prevent interleukin-1beta-induced nuclear factor-kappaB activation by inhibiting the degradation of inhibitor kappaB-alpha. *Pharmacol. Toxicol.* **2002**, *91*, 22–28. [CrossRef] [PubMed]
96. Kuo, P.L.; Hsu, Y.L.; Ng, L.T.; Lin, C.C. Rhein inhibits the growth and induces the apoptosis of Hep G2 cells. *Planta Med.* **2004**, *70*, 12–16. [CrossRef] [PubMed]
97. You, L.; Dong, X.; Yin, X.; Yang, C.; Leng, X.; Wang, W.; Ni, J. Rhein Induces Cell Death in HepaRG Cells through Cell Cycle Arrest and Apoptotic Pathway. *Int. J. Mol. Sci.* **2018**, *19*. [CrossRef]

98. Yuan, X.; Tian, W.; Hua, Y.; Hu, L.; Yang, J.; Xie, J.; Hu, J.; Wang, F. Rhein enhances the cytotoxicity of effector lymphocytes in colon cancer under hypoxic conditions. *Exp. Ther. Med.* **2018**, *16*, 5350–5358. [CrossRef]
99. Pearson, G.; Robinson, F.; Beers Gibson, T.; Xu, B.E.; Karandikar, M.; Berman, K.; Cobb, M.H. Mitogen-activated protein (MAP) kinase pathways: Regulation and physiological functions. *Endocr. Rev.* **2001**, *22*, 153–183. [CrossRef]
100. Morrison, D.K. MAP kinase pathways. *Cold Spring Harb. Perspect. Biol.* **2012**, *4*. [CrossRef]
101. Dai, X.; Wang, L.; Deivasigamni, A.; Looi, C.Y.; Karthikeyan, C.; Trivedi, P.; Chinnathambi, A.; Alharbi, S.A.; Arfuso, F.; Dharmarajan, A.; et al. A novel benzimidazole derivative, MBIC inhibits tumor growth and promotes apoptosis via activation of ROS-dependent JNK signaling pathway in hepatocellular carcinoma. *Oncotarget* **2017**, *8*, 12831–12842. [CrossRef]
102. Kim, S.M.; Kim, C.; Bae, H.; Lee, J.H.; Baek, S.H.; Nam, D.; Chung, W.S.; Shim, B.S.; Lee, S.G.; Kim, S.H.; et al. 6-Shogaol exerts anti-proliferative and pro-apoptotic effects through the modulation of STAT3 and MAPKs signaling pathways. *Mol. Carcinog.* **2015**, *54*, 1132–1146. [CrossRef]
103. Kannaiyan, R.; Manu, K.A.; Chen, L.; Li, F.; Rajendran, P.; Subramaniam, A.; Lam, P.; Kumar, A.P.; Sethi, G. Celastrol inhibits tumor cell proliferation and promotes apoptosis through the activation of c-Jun N-terminal kinase and suppression of PI3 K/Akt signaling pathways. *Apoptosis Int. J. Program. Cell Death* **2011**, *16*, 1028–1041. [CrossRef] [PubMed]
104. Woo, C.C.; Hsu, A.; Kumar, A.P.; Sethi, G.; Tan, K.H. Thymoquinone inhibits tumor growth and induces apoptosis in a breast cancer xenograft mouse model: The role of p38 MAPK and ROS. *PLoS ONE* **2013**, *8*, e75356. [CrossRef]
105. Fu, M.; Wang, C.; Li, Z.; Sakamaki, T.; Pestell, R.G. Minireview: Cyclin D1: Normal and abnormal functions. *Endocrinology* **2004**, *145*, 5439–5447. [CrossRef] [PubMed]
106. Bhuvanalakshmi, G.; Gamit, N.; Patil, M.; Arfuso, F.; Sethi, G.; Dharmarajan, A.; Kumar, A.P.; Warrier, S. Stemness, Pluripotentiality, and Wnt Antagonism: sFRP4, a Wnt antagonist Mediates Pluripotency and Stemness in Glioblastoma. *Cancers* **2018**, *11*. [CrossRef] [PubMed]
107. Bhuvanalakshmi, G.; Basappa; Rangappa, K.S.; Dharmarajan, A.; Sethi, G.; Kumar, A.P.; Warrier, S. Breast Cancer Stem-Like Cells Are Inhibited by Diosgenin, a Steroidal Saponin, by the Attenuation of the Wnt beta-Catenin Signaling via the Wnt Antagonist Secreted Frizzled Related Protein-4. *Front. Pharmacol.* **2017**, *8*, 124. [CrossRef]
108. Panda, P.K.; Naik, P.P.; Praharaj, P.P.; Meher, B.R.; Gupta, P.K.; Verma, R.S.; Maiti, T.K.; Shanmugam, M.K.; Chinnathambi, A.; Alharbi, S.A.; et al. Abrus agglutinin stimulates BMP-2-dependent differentiation through autophagic degradation of beta-catenin in colon cancer stem cells. *Mol. Carcinog.* **2018**, *57*, 664–677. [CrossRef]
109. Fang, D.; Hawke, D.; Zheng, Y.; Xia, Y.; Meisenhelder, J.; Nika, H.; Mills, G.B.; Kobayashi, R.; Hunter, T.; Lu, Z. Phosphorylation of beta-catenin by AKT promotes beta-catenin transcriptional activity. *J. Biol. Chem.* **2007**, *282*, 11221–11229. [CrossRef]
110. Hsia, T.C.; Yang, J.S.; Chen, G.W.; Chiu, T.H.; Lu, H.F.; Yang, M.D.; Yu, F.S.; Liu, K.C.; Lai, K.C.; Lin, C.C.; et al. The roles of endoplasmic reticulum stress and Ca^{2+} on rhein-induced apoptosis in A-549 human lung cancer cells. *Anticancer Res.* **2009**, *29*, 309–318.
111. Liu, S.; Wang, J.; Shao, T.; Song, P.; Kong, Q.; Hua, H.; Luo, T.; Jiang, Y. The natural agent rhein induces beta-catenin degradation and tumour growth arrest. *J. Cell. Mol. Med.* **2018**, *22*, 589–599. [CrossRef]
112. Puar, Y.R.; Shanmugam, M.K.; Fan, L.; Arfuso, F.; Sethi, G.; Tergaonkar, V. Evidence for the Involvement of the Master Transcription Factor NF-kappaB in Cancer Initiation and Progression. *Biomedicines* **2018**, *6*. [CrossRef]
113. Shin, E.M.; Hay, H.S.; Lee, M.H.; Goh, J.N.; Tan, T.Z.; Sen, Y.P.; Lim, S.W.; Yousef, E.M.; Ong, H.T.; Thike, A.A.; et al. DEAD-box helicase DP103 defines metastatic potential of human breast cancers. *J. Clin. Investig.* **2014**, *124*, 3807–3824. [CrossRef] [PubMed]
114. Ahn, K.S.; Sethi, G.; Chaturvedi, M.M.; Aggarwal, B.B. Simvastatin, 3-hydroxy-3-methylglutaryl coenzyme A reductase inhibitor, suppresses osteoclastogenesis induced by receptor activator of nuclear factor-kappaB ligand through modulation of NF-kappaB pathway. *Int. J. Cancer* **2008**, *123*, 1733–1740. [CrossRef] [PubMed]
115. Sethi, G.; Ahn, K.S.; Sung, B.; Aggarwal, B.B. Pinitol targets nuclear factor-kappaB activation pathway leading to inhibition of gene products associated with proliferation, apoptosis, invasion, and angiogenesis. *Mol. Cancer Ther.* **2008**, *7*, 1604–1614. [CrossRef]

116. Sawhney, M.; Rohatgi, N.; Kaur, J.; Shishodia, S.; Sethi, G.; Gupta, S.D.; Deo, S.V.; Shukla, N.K.; Aggarwal, B.B.; Ralhan, R. Expression of NF-kappaB parallels COX-2 expression in oral precancer and cancer: Association with smokeless tobacco. *Int. J. Cancer* **2007**, *120*, 2545–2556. [CrossRef] [PubMed]

117. Ahn, K.S.; Sethi, G.; Jain, A.K.; Jaiswal, A.K.; Aggarwal, B.B. Genetic deletion of NAD(P)H:quinone oxidoreductase 1 abrogates activation of nuclear factor-kappaB, IkappaBalpha kinase, c-Jun N-terminal kinase, Akt, p38, and p44/42 mitogen-activated protein kinases and potentiates apoptosis. *J. Biol. Chem.* **2006**, *281*, 19798–19808. [CrossRef] [PubMed]

118. Monisha, J.; Roy, N.K.; Bordoloi, D.; Kumar, A.; Golla, R.; Kotoky, J.; Padmavathi, G.; Kunnumakkara, A.B. Nuclear Factor Kappa B: A Potential Target to Persecute Head and Neck Cancer. *Curr. Drug Targets* **2017**, *18*, 232–253. [CrossRef]

119. Ahn, K.S.; Sethi, G.; Aggarwal, B.B. Reversal of chemoresistance and enhancement of apoptosis by statins through down-regulation of the NF-kappaB pathway. *Biochem. Pharmacol.* **2008**, *75*, 907–913. [CrossRef]

120. Manna, S.K.; Aggarwal, R.S.; Sethi, G.; Aggarwal, B.B.; Ramesh, G.T. Morin (3,5,7,2′,4′-Pentahydroxyflavone) abolishes nuclear factor-kappaB activation induced by various carcinogens and inflammatory stimuli, leading to suppression of nuclear factor-kappaB-regulated gene expression and up-regulation of apoptosis. *Clin. Cancer Res. Off. J. Am. Assoc. Cancer Res.* **2007**, *13*, 2290–2297. [CrossRef]

121. Chua, A.W.; Hay, H.S.; Rajendran, P.; Shanmugam, M.K.; Li, F.; Bist, P.; Koay, E.S.; Lim, L.H.; Kumar, A.P.; Sethi, G. Butein downregulates chemokine receptor CXCR4 expression and function through suppression of NF-kappaB activation in breast and pancreatic tumor cells. *Biochem. Pharmacol.* **2010**, *80*, 1553–1562. [CrossRef]

122. Shanmugam, M.K.; Manu, K.A.; Ong, T.H.; Ramachandran, L.; Surana, R.; Bist, P.; Lim, L.H.; Kumar, A.P.; Hui, K.M.; Sethi, G. Inhibition of CXCR4/CXCL12 signaling axis by ursolic acid leads to suppression of metastasis in transgenic adenocarcinoma of mouse prostate model. *Int. J. Cancer* **2011**, *129*, 1552–1563. [CrossRef]

123. Siveen, K.S.; Mustafa, N.; Li, F.; Kannaiyan, R.; Ahn, K.S.; Kumar, A.P.; Chng, W.J.; Sethi, G. Thymoquinone overcomes chemoresistance and enhances the anticancer effects of bortezomib through abrogation of NF-kappaB regulated gene products in multiple myeloma xenograft mouse model. *Oncotarget* **2014**, *5*, 634–648. [CrossRef] [PubMed]

124. Kunnumakkara, A.B.; Guha, S.; Krishnan, S.; Diagaradjane, P.; Gelovani, J.; Aggarwal, B.B. Curcumin potentiates antitumor activity of gemcitabine in an orthotopic model of pancreatic cancer through suppression of proliferation, angiogenesis, and inhibition of nuclear factor-κB–regulated gene products. *Cancer Res.* **2007**, *67*, 3853–3861. [CrossRef] [PubMed]

125. Kunnumakkara, A.B.; Nair, A.S.; Ahn, K.S.; Pandey, M.K.; Yi, Z.; Liu, M.; Aggarwal, B.B. Gossypin, a pentahydroxy glucosyl flavone, inhibits the transforming growth factor beta-activated kinase-1-mediated NF-kappaB activation pathway, leading to potentiation of apoptosis, suppression of invasion, and abrogation of osteoclastogenesis. *Blood* **2007**, *109*, 5112–5121. [CrossRef] [PubMed]

126. Li, F.; Shanmugam, M.K.; Siveen, K.S.; Wang, F.; Ong, T.H.; Loo, S.Y.; Swamy, M.M.; Mandal, S.; Kumar, A.P.; Goh, B.C.; et al. Garcinol sensitizes human head and neck carcinoma to cisplatin in a xenograft mouse model despite downregulation of proliferative biomarkers. *Oncotarget* **2015**, *6*, 5147–5163. [CrossRef] [PubMed]

127. Li, F.; Shanmugam, M.K.; Chen, L.; Chatterjee, S.; Basha, J.; Kumar, A.P.; Kundu, T.K.; Sethi, G. Garcinol, a polyisoprenylated benzophenone modulates multiple proinflammatory signaling cascades leading to the suppression of growth and survival of head and neck carcinoma. *Cancer Prev. Res.* **2013**, *6*, 843–854. [CrossRef]

128. Manu, K.A.; Shanmugam, M.K.; Ramachandran, L.; Li, F.; Fong, C.W.; Kumar, A.P.; Tan, P.; Sethi, G. First evidence that gamma-tocotrienol inhibits the growth of human gastric cancer and chemosensitizes it to capecitabine in a xenograft mouse model through the modulation of NF-kappaB pathway. *Clin. Cancer Res. Off. J. Am. Assoc. Cancer Res.* **2012**, *18*, 2220–2229. [CrossRef]

129. Manu, K.A.; Shanmugam, M.K.; Li, F.; Chen, L.; Siveen, K.S.; Ahn, K.S.; Kumar, A.P.; Sethi, G. Simvastatin sensitizes human gastric cancer xenograft in nude mice to capecitabine by suppressing nuclear factor-kappa B-regulated gene products. *J. Mol. Med.* **2014**, *92*, 267–276. [CrossRef]

130. Manu, K.A.; Shanmugam, M.K.; Ramachandran, L.; Li, F.; Siveen, K.S.; Chinnathambi, A.; Zayed, M.E.; Alharbi, S.A.; Arfuso, F.; Kumar, A.P.; et al. Isorhamnetin augments the *anti*-tumor effect of capecitabine through the negative regulation of NF-kappaB signaling cascade in gastric cancer. *Cancer Lett.* **2015**, *363*, 28–36. [CrossRef]
131. Ghosh, S.; May, M.J.; Kopp, E.B. NF-kappa B and Rel proteins: Evolutionarily conserved mediators of immune responses. *Annu. Rev. Immunol.* **1998**, *16*, 225–260. [CrossRef]
132. Kunnumakkara, A.B.; Diagaradjane, P.; Guha, S.; Deorukhkar, A.; Shentu, S.; Aggarwal, B.B.; Krishnan, S. Curcumin sensitizes human colorectal Cancer xenografts in nude mice to γ-radiation by targeting nuclear factor-κB–regulated gene products. *Clin. Cancer Res.* **2008**, *14*, 2128–2136. [CrossRef]
133. Lin, Y.G.; Kunnumakkara, A.B.; Nair, A.; Merritt, W.M.; Han, L.Y.; Armaiz-Pena, G.N.; Kamat, A.A.; Spannuth, W.A.; Gershenson, D.M.; Lutgendorf, S.K.; et al. Curcumin inhibits tumor growth and angiogenesis in ovarian carcinoma by targeting the nuclear factor-κB pathway. *Clin. Cancer Res.* **2007**, *13*, 3423–3430. [CrossRef] [PubMed]
134. Heymach, J.V.; Shackleford, T.J.; Tran, H.T.; Yoo, S.Y.; Do, K.A.; Wergin, M.; Saintigny, P.; Vollmer, R.T.; Polascik, T.J.; Snyder, D.C.; et al. Effect of low-fat diets on plasma levels of NF-kappaB-regulated inflammatory cytokines and angiogenic factors in men with prostate cancer. *Cancer Prev. Res.* **2011**, *4*, 1590–1598. [CrossRef] [PubMed]
135. Gao, Y.; Chen, X.; Fang, L.; Liu, F.; Cai, R.; Peng, C.; Qi, Y. Rhein exerts pro- and anti-inflammatory actions by targeting IKKbeta inhibition in LPS-activated macrophages. *Free Radic. Biol. Med.* **2014**, *72*, 104–112. [CrossRef] [PubMed]
136. Zhao, X.Y.; Chen, T.T.; Xia, L.; Guo, M.; Xu, Y.; Yue, F.; Jiang, Y.; Chen, G.Q.; Zhao, K.W. Hypoxia inducible factor-1 mediates expression of galectin-1: The potential role in migration/invasion of colorectal cancer cells. *Carcinogenesis* **2010**, *31*, 1367–1375. [CrossRef]
137. Clambey, E.T.; McNamee, E.N.; Westrich, J.A.; Glover, L.E.; Campbell, E.L.; Jedlicka, P.; De Zoeten, E.F.; Cambier, J.C.; Stenmark, K.R.; Colgan, S.P.; et al. Hypoxia-inducible factor-1 alpha-dependent induction of FoxP3 drives regulatory T-cell abundance and function during inflammatory hypoxia of the mucosa. *Proc. Natl. Acad. Sci. USA* **2012**, *109*, E2784–E2793. [CrossRef]
138. Fernand, V.E.; Losso, J.N.; Truax, R.E.; Villar, E.E.; Bwambok, D.K.; Fakayode, S.O.; Lowry, M.; Warner, I.M. Rhein inhibits angiogenesis and the viability of hormone-dependent and -independent cancer cells under normoxic or hypoxic conditions in vitro. *Chem. Biol. Interact.* **2011**, *192*, 220–232. [CrossRef]
139. Kunnumakkara, A.B.; Diagaradjane, P.; Anand, P.; Kuzhuvelil, H.B.; Deorukhkar, A.; Gelovani, J.; Guha, S.; Krishnan, S.; Aggarwal, B.B. Curcumin sensitizes human colorectal cancer to capecitabine by modulation of cyclin D1, COX-2, MMP-9, VEGF and CXCR4 expression in an orthotopic mouse model. *Int. J. Cancer* **2009**, *125*, 2187–2197. [CrossRef]
140. Roy, N.K.; Bordoloi, D.; Monisha, J.; Padmavathi, G.; Kotoky, J.; Golla, R.; Kunnumakkara, A.B. Specific Targeting of Akt Kinase Isoforms: Taking the Precise Path for Prevention and Treatment of Cancer. *Curr. Drug Targets* **2017**, *18*, 421–435. [CrossRef]
141. Bao, L.; Kimzey, A.; Sauter, G.; Sowadski, J.M.; Lu, K.P.; Wang, D.G. Prevalent overexpression of prolyl isomerase Pin1 in human cancers. *Am. J. Pathol.* **2004**, *164*, 1727–1737. [CrossRef]
142. Cho, J.H.; Chae, J.I.; Shim, J.H. Rhein exhibits antitumorigenic effects by interfering with the interaction between prolyl isomerase Pin1 and c-Jun. *Oncol. Rep.* **2017**, *37*, 1865–1872. [CrossRef]
143. Banik, K.; Ranaware, A.M.; Deshpande, V.; Nalawade, S.P.; Padmavathi, G.; Bordoloi, D.; Sailo, B.L.; Shanmugam, M.K.; Fan, L.; Arfuso, F.; et al. Honokiol for cancer therapeutics: A traditional medicine that can modulate multiple oncogenic targets. *Pharmacol. Res.* **2019**, *144*, 192–209. [CrossRef] [PubMed]
144. Wang, J.; Liu, S.; Yin, Y.; Li, M.; Wang, B.; Yang, L.; Jiang, Y. FOXO3-mediated up-regulation of Bim contributes to rhein-induced cancer cell apoptosis. *Apoptosis Int. J. Program. Cell Death* **2015**, *20*, 399–409. [CrossRef] [PubMed]
145. Lin, S.; Fujii, M.; Hou, D.X. Rhein induces apoptosis in HL-60 cells via reactive oxygen species-independent mitochondrial death pathway. *Arch. Biochem. Biophys.* **2003**, *418*, 99–107. [CrossRef] [PubMed]
146. Shen, Z.; Zhu, B.; Li, J.; Qin, L. Rhein Augments Antiproliferative Effects of Atezolizumab Based on Breast Cancer (4T1) Regression. *Planta Med.* **2019**, *85*, 1143–1149. [CrossRef]
147. Lin, Y.J.; Huang, Y.H.; Zhen, Y.Z.; Liu, X.J.; Zhen, Y.S. Rhein lysinate induces apoptosis in breast cancer SK-Br-3 cells by inhibiting HER-2 signal pathway. *Yao Xue Xue Bao = Acta Pharm. Sin.* **2008**, *43*, 1099–1105.

148. Liu, Y.; Zhong, Y.; Tian, W.; Lan, F.; Kang, J.; Pang, H.; Hou, H.; Li, D. An autophagy-dependent cell death of MDA-MB-231 cells triggered by a novel Rhein derivative 4F. *Anti-Cancer Drugs* **2019**, *30*, 1038–1047. [CrossRef]
149. Ip, S.W.; Weng, Y.S.; Lin, S.Y.; Mei, D.; Tang, N.Y.; Su, C.C.; Chung, J.G. The role of Ca^{+2} on rhein-induced apoptosis in human cervical cancer Ca Ski cells. *Anticancer. Res.* **2007**, *27*, 379–389.
150. Aviello, G.; Rowland, I.; Gill, C.I.; Acquaviva, A.M.; Capasso, F.; McCann, M.; Capasso, R.; Izzo, A.A.; Borrelli, F. Anti-proliferative effect of rhein, an anthraquinone isolated from Cassia species, on Caco-2 human adenocarcinoma cells. *J. Cell. Mol. Med.* **2010**, *14*, 2006–2014. [CrossRef]
151. Zhuang, Y.; Bai, Y.; Hu, Y.; Guo, Y.; Xu, L.; Hu, W.; Yang, L.; Zhao, C.; Li, X.; Zhao, H. Rhein sensitizes human colorectal cancer cells to EGFR inhibitors by inhibiting STAT3 pathway. *Oncotargets Ther.* **2019**, *12*, 5281–5291. [CrossRef]
152. Tang, N.; Chang, J.; Lu, H.C.; Zhuang, Z.; Cheng, H.L.; Shi, J.X.; Rao, J. Rhein induces apoptosis and autophagy in human and rat glioma cells and mediates cell differentiation by ERK inhibition. *Microb. Pathog.* **2017**, *113*, 168–175. [CrossRef]
153. Chen, J.; Luo, B.; Wen, S.; Pi, R. Discovery of a novel rhein-SAHA hybrid as a multi-targeted anti-glioblastoma drug. *Investig. New Drugs* **2019**. [CrossRef] [PubMed]
154. Gu, L.; Zhang, H.; Liu, T.; Draganov, A.; Yi, S.; Wang, B.; Zhou, M. Inhibition of MDM2 by a Rhein-Derived Compound AQ-101 Suppresses Cancer Development in SCID Mice. *Mol. Cancer Ther.* **2018**, *17*, 497–507. [CrossRef] [PubMed]
155. Heo, S.K.; Noh, E.K.; Kim, J.Y.; Jegal, S.; Jeong, Y.; Cheon, J.; Koh, S.; Baek, J.H.; Min, Y.J.; Choi, Y.; et al. Rhein augments ATRA-induced differentiation of acute promyelocytic leukemia cells. *Phytomed. Int. J. Phytother. Phytopharm.* **2018**, *49*, 66–74. [CrossRef] [PubMed]
156. Wu, L.; Cao, K.; Ni, Z.; Wang, S.; Li, W.; Liu, X.; Chen, Z. Rhein reverses doxorubicin resistance in SMMC-7721 liver cancer cells by inhibiting energy metabolism and inducing mitochondrial permeability transition pore opening. *Biofactors* **2019**, *45*, 85–96. [CrossRef] [PubMed]
157. Yang, L.; Li, J.; Xu, L.; Lin, S.; Xiang, Y.; Dai, X.; Liang, G.; Huang, X.; Zhu, J.; Zhao, C. Rhein shows potent efficacy against non-small-cell lung cancer through inhibiting the STAT3 pathway. *Cancer Manag. Res.* **2019**, *11*, 1167–1176. [CrossRef] [PubMed]
158. Bu, T.; Wang, C.; Jin, H.; Meng, Q.; Huo, X.; Sun, H.; Sun, P.; Wu, J.; Ma, X.; Liu, Z.; et al. Organic anion transporters and PI3K-AKT-mTOR pathway mediate the synergistic anticancer effect of pemetrexed and rhein. *J. Cell. Physiol.* **2020**, *235*, 3309–3319. [CrossRef] [PubMed]
159. Ren, B.; Guo, W.; Tang, Y.; Zhang, J.; Xiao, N.; Zhang, L.; Li, W. Rhein Inhibits the Migration of Ovarian Cancer Cells through Down-Regulation of Matrix Metalloproteinases. *Biol. Pharm. Bull.* **2019**, *42*, 568–572. [CrossRef]
160. Hu, L.; Cui, R.; Liu, H.; Wang, F. Emodin and rhein decrease levels of hypoxia-inducible factor-1alpha in human pancreatic cancer cells and attenuate cancer cachexia in athymic mice carrying these cells. *Oncotarget* **2017**, *8*, 88008–88020. [CrossRef]
161. Shanmugam, M.K.; Ahn, K.S.; Hsu, A.; Woo, C.C.; Yuan, Y.; Tan, K.H.B.; Chinnathambi, A.; Alahmadi, T.A.; Alharbi, S.A.; Koh, A.P.F.; et al. Thymoquinone Inhibits Bone Metastasis of Breast Cancer Cells Through Abrogation of the CXCR4 Signaling Axis. *Front. Pharmacol.* **2018**, *9*, 1294. [CrossRef]
162. Liu, L.; Ahn, K.S.; Shanmugam, M.K.; Wang, H.; Shen, H.; Arfuso, F.; Chinnathambi, A.; Alharbi, S.A.; Chang, Y.; Sethi, G.; et al. Oleuropein induces apoptosis via abrogating NF-kappaB activation cascade in estrogen receptor-negative breast cancer cells. *J. Cell. Biochem.* **2019**, *120*, 4504–4513. [CrossRef]
163. Wang, C.; Kar, S.; Lai, X.; Cai, W.; Arfuso, F.; Sethi, G.; Lobie, P.E.; Goh, B.C.; Lim, L.H.K.; Hartman, M.; et al. Triple negative breast cancer in Asia: An insider's view. *Cancer Treat. Rev.* **2018**, *62*, 29–38. [CrossRef] [PubMed]
164. Mohan, C.D.; Srinivasa, V.; Rangappa, S.; Mervin, L.; Mohan, S.; Paricharak, S.; Baday, S.; Li, F.; Shanmugam, M.K.; Chinnathambi, A.; et al. Trisubstituted-Imidazoles Induce Apoptosis in Human Breast Cancer Cells by Targeting the Oncogenic PI3K/Akt/mTOR Signaling Pathway. *PLoS ONE* **2016**, *11*, e0153155. [CrossRef] [PubMed]
165. Jia, L.Y.; Shanmugam, M.K.; Sethi, G.; Bishayee, A. Potential role of targeted therapies in the treatment of triple-negative breast cancer. *Anti-Cancer Drugs* **2016**, *27*, 147–155. [CrossRef] [PubMed]

166. Ningegowda, R.; Shivananju, N.S.; Rajendran, P.; Basappa; Rangappa, K.S.; Chinnathambi, A.; Li, F.; Achar, R.R.; Shanmugam, M.K.; Bist, P.; et al. A novel 4,6-disubstituted-1,2,4-triazolo-1,3,4-thiadiazole derivative inhibits tumor cell invasion and potentiates the apoptotic effect of TNFalpha by abrogating NF-kappaB activation cascade. *Apoptosis Int. J. Program. Cell Death* **2017**, *22*, 145–157. [CrossRef]
167. Bhojwani, D.; Yang, J.J.; Pui, C.H. Biology of childhood acute lymphoblastic leukemia. *Pediatric Clin. N. Am.* **2015**, *62*, 47–60. [CrossRef] [PubMed]
168. Stewart, B.W.; Wild, C. *World Cancer Report 2014*; The International Agency for Research on Cancer-IARC Publications: Lyon, France, 2014.
169. Sethi, G.; Chatterjee, S.; Rajendran, P.; Li, F.; Shanmugam, M.K.; Wong, K.F.; Kumar, A.P.; Senapati, P.; Behera, A.K.; Hui, K.M.; et al. Inhibition of STAT3 dimerization and acetylation by garcinol suppresses the growth of human hepatocellular carcinoma in vitro and in vivo. *Mol. Cancer* **2014**, *13*, 66. [CrossRef]
170. Siveen, K.S.; Ahn, K.S.; Ong, T.H.; Shanmugam, M.K.; Li, F.; Yap, W.N.; Kumar, A.P.; Fong, C.W.; Tergaonkar, V.; Hui, K.M.; et al. Y-tocotrienol inhibits angiogenesis-dependent growth of human hepatocellular carcinoma through abrogation of AKT/mTOR pathway in an orthotopic mouse model. *Oncotarget* **2014**, *5*, 1897–1911. [CrossRef]
171. Mohan, C.D.; Bharathkumar, H.; Bulusu, K.C.; Pandey, V.; Rangappa, S.; Fuchs, J.E.; Shanmugam, M.K.; Dai, X.; Li, F.; Deivasigamani, A.; et al. Development of a novel azaspirane that targets the Janus kinase-signal transducer and activator of transcription (STAT) pathway in hepatocellular carcinoma in vitro and in vivo. *J. Biol. Chem.* **2014**, *289*, 34296–34307. [CrossRef]
172. Dai, X.; Ahn, K.S.; Kim, C.; Siveen, K.S.; Ong, T.H.; Shanmugam, M.K.; Li, F.; Shi, J.; Kumar, A.P.; Wang, L.Z.; et al. Ascochlorin, an isoprenoid antibiotic inhibits growth and invasion of hepatocellular carcinoma by targeting STAT3 signaling cascade through the induction of PIAS3. *Mol. Oncol.* **2015**, *9*, 818–833. [CrossRef]
173. Rajendran, P.; Li, F.; Shanmugam, M.K.; Vali, S.; Abbasi, T.; Kapoor, S.; Ahn, K.S.; Kumar, A.P.; Sethi, G. Honokiol inhibits signal transducer and activator of transcription-3 signaling, proliferation, and survival of hepatocellular carcinoma cells via the protein tyrosine phosphatase SHP-1. *J. Cell. Physiol.* **2012**, *227*, 2184–2195. [CrossRef]
174. Rajendran, P.; Li, F.; Manu, K.A.; Shanmugam, M.K.; Loo, S.Y.; Kumar, A.P.; Sethi, G. gamma-Tocotrienol is a novel inhibitor of constitutive and inducible STAT3 signalling pathway in human hepatocellular carcinoma: Potential role as an antiproliferative, pro-apoptotic and chemosensitizing agent. *Br. J. Pharmacol.* **2011**, *163*, 283–298. [CrossRef] [PubMed]
175. Tan, S.M.; Li, F.; Rajendran, P.; Kumar, A.P.; Hui, K.M.; Sethi, G. Identification of beta-escin as a novel inhibitor of signal transducer and activator of transcription 3/Janus-activated kinase 2 signaling pathway that suppresses proliferation and induces apoptosis in human hepatocellular carcinoma cells. *J. Pharmacol. Exp. Ther.* **2010**, *334*, 285–293. [CrossRef] [PubMed]
176. Singh, A.K.; Roy, N.K.; Anip, A.; Banik, K.; Monisha, J.; Bordoloi, D.; Kunnumakkara, A.B. Different methods to inhibit chemoresistance in Hepatocellular carcinoma. In *Cancer Cell Chemoresistance and Chemosensitization*; World Scientific: Singapore, 2018; pp. 378–398.
177. Wang, L.; Syn, N.L.; Subhash, V.V.; Any, Y.; Thuya, W.L.; Cheow, E.S.H.; Kong, L.; Yu, F.; Peethala, P.C.; Wong, A.L.; et al. Pan-HDAC inhibition by panobinostat mediates chemosensitization to carboplatin in non-small cell lung cancer via attenuation of EGFR signaling. *Cancer Lett.* **2018**, *417*, 152–160. [CrossRef] [PubMed]
178. Jung, Y.Y.; Shanmugam, M.K.; Narula, A.S.; Kim, C.; Lee, J.H.; Namjoshi, O.A.; Blough, B.E.; Sethi, G.; Ahn, K.S. Oxymatrine Attenuates Tumor Growth and Deactivates STAT5 Signaling in a Lung Cancer Xenograft Model. *Cancers* **2019**, *11*. [CrossRef] [PubMed]
179. Lee, J.H.; Mohan, C.D.; Basappa, S.; Rangappa, S.; Chinnathambi, A.; Alahmadi, T.A.; Alharbi, S.A.; Kumar, A.P.; Sethi, G.; Ahn, K.S.; et al. The IkappaB Kinase Inhibitor ACHP Targets the STAT3 Signaling Pathway in Human Non-Small Cell Lung Carcinoma Cells. *Biomolecules* **2019**, *9*. [CrossRef]
180. Lee, J.H.; Chinnathambi, A.; Alharbi, S.A.; Shair, O.H.M.; Sethi, G.; Ahn, K.S. Farnesol abrogates epithelial to mesenchymal transition process through regulating Akt/mTOR pathway. *Pharmacol. Res.* **2019**, *150*, 104504. [CrossRef]
181. Baek, S.H.; Ko, J.H.; Lee, J.H.; Kim, C.; Lee, H.; Nam, D.; Lee, J.; Lee, S.G.; Yang, W.M.; Um, J.Y.; et al. Ginkgolic Acid Inhibits Invasion and Migration and TGF-beta-Induced EMT of Lung Cancer Cells Through PI3K/Akt/mTOR Inactivation. *J. Cell. Physiol.* **2017**, *232*, 346–354. [CrossRef]

182. Ong, P.S.; Wang, L.; Chia, D.M.; Seah, J.Y.; Kong, L.R.; Thuya, W.L.; Chinnathambi, A.; Lau, J.Y.; Wong, A.L.; Yong, W.P.; et al. A novel combinatorial strategy using Seliciclib((R)) and Belinostat((R)) for eradication of non-small cell lung cancer via apoptosis induction and BID activation. *Cancer Lett.* **2016**, *381*, 49–57. [CrossRef]
183. Lee, J.H.; Kim, C.; Sethi, G.; Ahn, K.S. Brassinin inhibits STAT3 signaling pathway through modulation of PIAS-3 and SOCS-3 expression and sensitizes human lung cancer xenograft in nude mice to paclitaxel. *Oncotarget* **2015**, *6*, 6386–6405. [CrossRef]
184. Lee, J.H.; Kim, C.; Lee, S.G.; Sethi, G.; Ahn, K.S. Ophiopogonin D, a Steroidal Glycoside Abrogates STAT3 Signaling Cascade and Exhibits Anti-Cancer Activity by Causing GSH/GSSG Imbalance in Lung Carcinoma. *Cancers* **2018**, *10*. [CrossRef]
185. Xianghong, S.; Yuwei, S.; Hong, L.; Wei, S. Influence of main component of Heshouwu such as emodin, rhein and toluylene glycoside on hepatic cells and hepatoma carcinoma cell. *Mod. J. Integr. Tradit. Chin. West. Med.* **2010**, *19*, 1315–1319.
186. Mao, Y.; Zhang, M.; Yang, J.; Sun, H.; Wang, D.; Zhang, X.; Yu, F.; Li, J. The UCP2-related mitochondrial pathway participates in rhein-induced apoptosis in HK-2 cells. *Toxicol. Res.* **2017**, *6*, 297–304. [CrossRef] [PubMed]
187. Bounda, G.A.; Zhou, W.; Wang, D.D.; Yu, F. Rhein elicits in vitro cytotoxicity in primary human liver HL-7702 cells by inducing apoptosis through mitochondria-mediated pathway. *Evid. Based Complementary Altern. Med.* **2015**. [CrossRef] [PubMed]
188. Roy, N.K.; Parama, D.; Banik, K.; Bordoloi, D.; Devi, A.K.; Thakur, K.K.; Padmavathi, G.; Shakibaei, M.; Fan, L.; Sethi, G.; et al. An Update on Pharmacological Potential of Boswellic Acids against Chronic Diseases. *Int. J. Mol. Sci.* **2019**, *20*. [CrossRef]
189. Abotaleb, M.; Kubatka, P.; Caprnda, M.; Varghese, E.; Zolakova, B.; Zubor, P.; Opatrilova, R.; Kruzliak, P.; Stefanicka, P.; Büsselberg, D. Chemotherapeutic agents for the treatment of metastatic breast cancer: An update. *Biomed. Pharmacother.* **2018**, *101*, 458–477. [CrossRef] [PubMed]
190. Kapinova, A.; Stefanicka, P.; Kubatka, P.; Zubor, P.; Uramova, S.; Kello, M.; Mojzis, J.; Blahutova, D.; Qaradakhi, T.; Zulli, A.; et al. Are plant-based functional foods better choice against cancer than single phytochemicals? A critical review of current breast cancer research. *Biomed. Pharmacother.* **2017**, *96*, 1465–1477. [CrossRef]
191. Harikumar, K.D.; Kunnumakkara, A.B.; Sethi, G.; Diagaradjane, P.; Anand, P.; Pandey, M.K.; Gelovani, J.; Krishnan, S.; Guha, S.; Aggarwal, B.B. Resveratrol, a multitargeted agent, can enhance antitumor activity of gemcitabine in vitro and in orthotopic mouse model of human pancreatic cancer. *Int. J. Cancer* **2010**, *127*, 257–268. [CrossRef]
192. Sung, B.; Kunnumakkara, A.B.; Sethi, G.; Anand, P.; Guha, S.; Aggarwal, B.B. Curcumin circumvents chemoresistance in vitro and potentiates the effect of thalidomide and bortezomib against human multiple myeloma in nude mice model. *Mol. Cancer. Ther.* **2009**, *8*, 959–970, Erratum in 2009, 8, 1398. [CrossRef]
193. Kunnumakkara, A.B.; Bordoloi, D.; Sailo, B.L.; Roy, N.K.; Thakur, K.K.; Banik, K.; Shakibaei, M.; Gupta, S.C.; Aggarwal, B.B. Cancer drug development: The missing links. *Exp. Biol. Med.* **2019**, *244*, 663–689. [CrossRef]

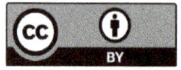 © 2020 by the authors. Licensee MDPI, Basel, Switzerland. This article is an open access article distributed under the terms and conditions of the Creative Commons Attribution (CC BY) license (http://creativecommons.org/licenses/by/4.0/).

MDPI
St. Alban-Anlage 66
4052 Basel
Switzerland
Tel. +41 61 683 77 34
Fax +41 61 302 89 18
www.mdpi.com

Molecules Editorial Office
E-mail: molecules@mdpi.com
www.mdpi.com/journal/molecules

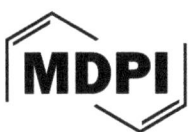

www.ingramcontent.com/pod-product-compliance
Lightning Source LLC
LaVergne TN
LVHW070243100526
838202LV00015B/2171